Drug Utilization Research

Drug Utilization Research

Methods and Applications

EDITORS

Monique Elseviers
University of Antwerp, Belgium

Björn Wettermark
Karolinska Institutet, Sweden

Anna Birna Almarsdóttir
University of Southern Denmark, Denmark

Morten Andersen
Karolinska Institutet, Sweden

Ria Benko
University of Szeged, Hungary

Marion Bennie
University of Strathclyde, Scotland

Irene Eriksson
Karolinska Institutet, Sweden

Brian Godman
Karolinska Institutet, Sweden

Janet Krska
Universities of Greenwich and Kent, United Kingdom

Elisabetta Poluzzi
University of Bologna, Italy

Katja Taxis
University of Groningen, The Netherlands

Vera Vlahović-Palčevski
University of Rijeka, Croatia

Robert Vander Stichele
Ghent University, Belgium

WILEY Blackwell

Registered office: John Wiley & Sons, Ltd, The Atrium, Southern Gate, Chichester, West Sussex, PO19 8SQ, UK

Editorial offices: 9600 Garsington Road, Oxford, OX4 2DQ, UK
The Atrium, Southern Gate, Chichester, West Sussex, PO19 8SQ, UK
111 River Street, Hoboken, NJ 07030-5774, USA

For details of our global editorial offices, for customer services and for information about how to apply for permission to reuse the copyright material in this book please see our website at www.wiley.com/wiley-blackwell

Library of Congress Cataloging-in-Publication Data

Names: Elseviers, Monique, editor.
Title: Drug utilization research : methods and applications / editors, Monique Elseviers [and 12 others].
Description: Chichester, West Sussex : Hoboken, NJ : John Wiley & Sons Inc., 2016. | Includes bibliographical references and index.
Identifiers: LCCN 2015039626 | ISBN 9781118949788 (cloth)
Subjects: | MESH: Drug Utilization. | Biomedical Research. | Drug Evaluation. | Health Policy. | Pharmacoepidemiology--methods. | Pharmacovigilance.
Classification: LCC RM301.25 | NLM WB 330 | DDC 615.1072/4--dc23 LC record available at http://lccn.loc.gov/2015039626

A catalogue record for this book is available from the British Library.

Wiley also publishes its books in a variety of electronic formats. Some content that appears in print may not be available in electronic books.

Set in 8.5/12pt Meridien LT Std by Aptara Inc., New Delhi, India

Printed in Singapore by C.O.S. Printers Pte Ltd

1 2016

Contents

List of contributors

Niels Adriaenssens
Centre for General Practice Department of Primary and Interdisciplinary Care (ELIZA) and
Laboratory of Medical Microbiology
Vaccine & Infectious Disease Institute (VAXINFECTIO)
University of Antwerp
Belgium

Anna Birna Almarsdóttir
Clinical Pharmacology
Institute of Public Health
University of Southern Denmark
Denmark

Morten Andersen
Centre for Pharmacoepidemiology
Department of Medicine
Karolinska Institutet
Sweden
and
Research Unit of General Practice
Department of Public Health
University of Southern Denmark
Denmark

Indranil Bagchi
Pfizer
United States

Nadia Barozzi
Healthy4Life
Basel
Switzerland

Pia Bastholm Rahmner
Medical Management Centre
Department of Learning, Informatics, Management and Ethics
Karolinska Institutet
Sweden

Ria Benko
Department of Clinical Pharmacy
Faculty of Pharmacy
University of Szeged
Hungary

Kathleen Bennett
National Centre for Pharmacoeconomics
St James's Hospital
Ireland

Marion Bennie
Institute of Pharmacy and Biomedical Sciences
University of Strathclyde
Scotland
and
Information Services Scotland,
NHS National Services Scotland, United Kingdom

Ulf Bergman
Department of Clinical Pharmacology
Karolinska Institutet
Karolinska University Hospital
Sweden

Kevin Blake
Best Evidence Development Service
Human Medicines Research and Development Support Division
European Medicines Agency
United Kingdom

Hege Salvesen Blix
WHO Collaborating Centre for Drug Statistics Methodology
Department of Pharmacoepidemiology
Norwegian Institute of Public Health
Norway

Colin Bradley
Department of General Practice
University College Cork
Ireland

Nicky Britten
University of Exeter Medical School
United Kingdom

Stephen Byrne
School of Pharmacy, University College Cork
Ireland

Stephen Campbell
Centre for Primary Care
Institute of Population Health
and
Patient Safety Translational Research Centre
Institute of Population Health
University of Manchester
United Kingdom

Matthias Cavassini
Service of Infectious Disease
Centre hospitalier universitaire vaudois
and
University of Lausanne
Switzerland

Jennifer Celio
Community Pharmacy
School of Pharmaceutical Sciences
Universities of Geneva, University of Lausanne
Switzerland
and
Community Pharmacy
Department of Ambulatory Care & Community Medicine
University of Lausanne
Switzerland

Samuel Coenen
Department of Epidemiology and Social Medicine (ESOC)
Department of Primary and Interdisciplinary Care (ELIZA) and
Vaccine & Infectious Disease Institute (VAXINFECTIO)
University of Antwerp
Belgium

Shane Cullinan
University College Cork
Ireland

Petra Denig
Clinical Pharmacy and Pharmacology
University of Groningen, University Medical Center Groningen
The Netherlands

Fabrizio De Ponti
Pharmacology Unit
Department of Medical and Surgical Sciences
University of Bologna
Italy

Mirko Di Martino
Department of Epidemiology
Lazio Regional Health Service, Roma
Italy

Monique Elseviers
Centre for Research and Innovation in Care
Faculty of Medicine and Health Sciences
University of Antwerp
Belgium

Irene Eriksson
Centre for Pharmacoepidemiology
Department of Medicine
Karolinska Institutet
Sweden
and
Department of Healthcare Development
Stockholm County Council
Sweden

Andrew Gilbert
School of Pharmacy and Medical Sciences
University of South Australia
Australia

Brian Godman
Department of Laboratory Medicine
Karolinska Institutet
Sweden
and
Strathclyde Institute of Pharmacy and
Biomedical Sciences, University of Strathclyde,
Glasgow, United Kingdom

Jean-Pierre Grégoire
Faculty of Pharmacy
Laval University
Canada
and
Population Health and Optimal Health Practices
Research Unit
CHU de Québec Research Centre
Canada

Flora Haaijer-Ruskamp
Clinical Pharmacy and Pharmacology
University of Groningen, University Medical Center Groningen
The Netherlands

Jesper Hallas
Clinical Pharmacology
Institute of Public Health
University of Southern Denmark
Denmark

Donald Han
Pfizer
United States

Dorte Gilså Hansen
Research Unit of General Practice
Institute of Public Health
University of Southern Denmark
Denmark

Hanne Herborg
Pharmakon
Danish College of Pharmacy Practice
Denmark

Mikael Hoffmann
The NEPI Foundation
Linköping University
Sweden

Thomas Hofmarcher
Department of Economics
Lund University
Sweden

Kathleen Holloway
World Health Organization Regional Office for South-East Asia
India

Dyfrig Hughes
Centre for Health Economics & Medicines Evaluation
Bangor University
United Kingdom

Vu Thi Thu Huong
Pharmacy Department, E Hospital, Hanoi, Vietnam and
Administration Medical Services, Ministry of Health, Hanoi
Vietnam

Luisa Ibáñez
Foundation of the Catalan Institute of Pharmacology (FICF)
Spain

Saira Jan
Department of Clinical Pharmacy Management
Horizon Blue Cross Blue Shield of New Jersey
United States and
Clinical Professor
Rutgers State University of New Jersey, Piscataway
New Jersey
United States

Bengt Jönsson
Stockholm School of Economics
Sweden

Roberta Joppi
Pharmaceutical Drug Department
Azienda Sanitaria Locale of Verona
Italy

Maarit Jaana Korhonen
Department of Pharmacology
Drug Development and Therapeutics
University of Turku
Finland

Janet Krska
Medway School of Pharmacy
Universities of Greenwich and Kent
United Kingdom

Xavier Kurz
Pharmacovigilance Division
European Medicines Agency
United Kingdom

Hye Young Kwon
Institute of Health and Environment
Seoul National University
South Korea

Laurent Laforest
PharmacoEpidemiology Lyon (PEL),
HESPER Unit, Claude-Bernard University-Lyon1
France

Irene Langner
AOK Research Institute (WIdO)
Germany

Hubert G.M. Leufkens
Division of Pharmacoepidemiology and Clinical
Pharmacology
Utrecht Institute for Pharmaceutical Sciences
Utrecht University
The Netherlands

Tatiana Chama Borges Luz
René Rachou Research Center
Oswaldo Cruz Foundation
Brazil

Sean MacBride-Stewart
Prescribing and Pharmacy Support Unit
NHS Greater Glasgow and Clyde
United Kingdom

Lorenzo G. Mantovani
Department of Statistics
School of Medicine
University of Milano
Italy

Jaana E. Martikainen
Research Department
Social Insurance Institution (Kela)
Finland

Maria Matuz
Department of Clinical Pharmacy
Faculty of Pharmacy
University of Szeged
Hungary

Frank May
Drug and Therapeutics Information Service,
Repatriation General Hospital, Daw Park,
South Australia
School of Pharmacy, Faculty of Health and
Behavioural Sciences, University of Queensland,
Australia

Giampiero Mazzaglia
Scientific and Regulatory Management Department
Human Medicines Evaluation Division
European Medicines Agency
United Kingdom

Stuart McTaggart
National Health Service for Scotland
United Kingdom

Juan Merlo
Unit for Social Epidemiology
Faculty of Medicine
Lund University
Skåne University Hospital
Sweden

Jocelyne Moisan
Faculty of Pharmacy
Laval University
Canada
and
Population Health and Optimal Health Practices
Research Unit
CHU de Québec Research Centre
Canada

Peter Mol
Medicines Evaluation Board
The Netherlands
and
Department of Clinical Pharmacy and Pharmacology
University Medical Centre Groningen
University of Groningen
The Netherlands

Luigi Naldi
Unità Complessa di Dermatologia
Azienda Ospedaliera Papa Giovanni XXIII and Centro
Studi GISED (Italian Group for Epidemiologic Research in
Dermatology)
Italy

Martin Neovius
Clinical Epidemiology Unit Department of Medicine
Karolinska Institutet
Sweden

Antje Neubert
Department of Paediatric and Adolescent Medicine
University Hospital Erlangen
Germany

Evalill Nilsson
The Research and Development Department of Local
Health Care
Östergötland Region
Sweden

Hedvig Nordeng
Pharmaco-Epidemiology and Drug Safety Research Group
School of Pharmacy
University of Oslo
Norway

Claudia Garcia Serpa Osorio-de-Castro
Department of Medicines Policies and Pharmaceutical
Services (NAF)
Sergio Arouca National School of Public Health
Oswaldo Cruz Foundation
Brazil

David O'Sullivan
University College Cork
Ireland

Carlo Piccinni
Pharmacology Unit
Department of Medical and Surgical Sciences
University of Bologna
Italy

Elisabetta Poluzzi
Pharmacology Unit
Department of Medical and Surgical Sciences
University of Bologna
Italy

Lisa Pont
Australian Institute of Health Innovation
Macquarie University
Australia

Anton Pottegård
Clinical Pharmacology
Institute of Public Health
University of Southern Denmark
Denmark

Emanuel Raschi
Pharmacology Unit
Department of Medical and Surgical Sciences
University of Bologna
Italy

Marit Rønning
WHO Collaborating Centre for Drug Statistics Methodology
Norwegian Institute of Public Health
Norway

Elizabeth Roughead
School of Pharmacy and Medical Sciences
University of South Australia
Australia

Debra Rowett
Drug and Therapeutics Information Service
Repatriation General Hospital, South Australia
Australia

Marie-Paule Schneider
Community Pharmacy
School of Pharmaceutical Sciences
Universities of Geneva, University of Lausanne
Switzerland
and
Community Pharmacy
Department of Ambulatory Care & Community Medicine
University of Lausanne
Switzerland

Gisbert W. Selke
AOK Research Institute (WIdO)
Germany

Alesha Smith
School of Pharmacy
University of Otago
New Zealand

Jens Søndergaard
Research Unit of General Practice
Institute of Public Health
University of Southern Denmark
Denmark

Henrik Toft Sørensen
Department of Clinical Epidemiology
Aarhus University Hospital
Denmark

Paul Spivey
Independent international pharmacy consultant

Douglas T. Steinke
Manchester Pharmacy School
University of Manchester
United Kingdom

Henrik Støvring
Department of Public Health, Biostatistics
Aarhus University
Denmark

Katja Taxis
Department of Pharmacy
Unit of Pharmacotherapy and Pharmaceutical Care
University of Groningen
The Netherlands

Richard Torbett
European Federation of Pharmaceutical Industries and Associations (EFPIA)
Belgium
and
IMT Institute of Advanced Studies
Italy

Janine Traulsen
Department Pharmacy
Section for Social and Clinical Pharmacy
University of Copenhagen
Denmark

Gianluca Trifirò
Department of Biomedical and Dental Sciences and Morphofunctional Imaging
University of Messina
Italy
and
Department of Medical Informatics
Erasmus Medical Center
Rotterdam, Netherlands

Cara Usher
National Centre for Pharmacoeconomics
St James's Hospital
Ireland

Yoleen van Camp
Centre for Research and Innovation in Care (CRIC)
Faculty of Medicine and Health Care
University of Antwerp
Belgium

Robert Vander Stichele
Heymans Institute of Pharmacology
Ghent University
Belgium

Eric Van Ganse
PharmacoEpidemiology Lyon (PEL)
HESPER Unit, Claude-Bernard University-Lyon1
and
CHU-Lyon
France

Vera Vlahović-Palčevski
Department of Clinical Pharmacology
University Hospital Center Rijeka
Croatia
and
Department of Pharmacology
University of Rijeka Medical Faculty
Croatia

Sabine Vogler
WHO Collaborating Centre for Pharmaceutical Pricing and Reimbursement Policies
Health Economics Department
Gesundheit Österreich GmbH/Geschäftsbereich ÖBIG – Austrian Public Health Institute
Austria

Mia von Euler
Department of Clinical Science and Education
Karolinska Institutet
Södersjukhuset
Sweden

Bernard Vrijens
WestRock Healthcare
Belgium
and
University of Liège
Belgium

Björn Wettermark
Clinical Pharmacology and Centre for Pharmacoepidemiology
Department of Medicine
Karolinska Institutet
Sweden
and
Department of Healthcare Development
Stockholm County Council
Sweden

Nils Wilking
Department of Oncology
Skåne University Hospital Lund/Malmö
Sweden

Ulla Wilking
Department of Oncology-Pathology
Karolinska Institutet
Sweden

Ian C.K. Wong
Centre for Safe Medication Practice and Research
The University of Hong Kong
China
and
Research Department of Practice and Policy
UCL School of Pharmacy
London, United Kingdom

Ksenia Zagorodnikova
North-Western State Medical University n.a. I.I.Mechnikov
Russia

Helga Zoëga
Centre of Public Health Sciences
Faculty of Medicine
University of Iceland
Iceland

Acknowledgements

The editors are indebted to the members of the advisory board for their input into the creation of this book. They particularly want to express their gratitude to the 100 authors for their willingness to share their specific expertise in drug utilization research. After being read internally by the editorial board members, the chapters were critically reviewed by 73 external reviewers. Their valuable contribution is highly appreciated.

For the organization of editorial board meetings, the editors are grateful for the financial support of:

- Heymans Foundation, Ghent University, Ghent, Belgium
- Karolinska Institutet, Stockholm, Sweden
- ISPE, the International Society for Pharmacoepidemiology

Advisory board

Reviewers

Silvia Alessi-Severini
College of Pharmacy
Faculty of Health Sciences
University of Manitoba
Canada

Claire Anderson
School of Pharmacy
University of Nottingham
United Kingdom

Anthony J. Avery
Division of Primary Care
University of Nottingham
United Kingdom

Kathleen Bennett
National Centre for Pharmacoeconomics
St James's Hospital
Ireland

Hege Salvesen Blix
WHO Collaborating Centre for Drug Statistics Methodology
Department of Pharmacoepidemiology
Norwegian Institute of Public Health
Norway

Maurizio Bonati
Department of Public Health
Mario Negri Institute for Pharmacological Research
Italy

Alison Bourke
Real World Evidence Solutions
IMS Health
United Kingdom

Stephen Campbell
Centre for Primary Care
Institute of Population Health
University of Manchester
United Kingdom

Li-Chia Chen
School of Pharmacy
University of Nottingham
United Kingdom

Milan Čižman
Department of Infectious Diseases
Ljubljana University Medical Centre
Slovenia

Antonio Clavenna
Laboratory for Mother and Child Health
Department of Public Health
Mario Negri Institute for Pharmacological Research
Italy

Giovanni Corrao
Department of Statistics and Quantitative Methods
University of Milano-Bicocca
Italy

Kees de Joncheere
Department of Essential Medicines and Health Products
World Health Organization
Switzerland

Lolkje T.W. de Jong-van den Berg
Department of Pharmacoepidemiology and
Pharmacoeconomics
University of Groningen
The Netherlands

Dominique J. Dubois
Health Economics & Patient Reported Outcomes Research
PHARMED
Belgium

Daniel Eriksson
Quantify Research
Sweden

Jurij Fürst
Department for Medicinal Products
Health Insurance Institute of Slovenia
Slovenia

Helga Gardarsdottir
Department of Clinical Pharmacy, Division of Laboratory
Medicines and Pharmacy
University Medical Center Utrecht
The Netherlands

Mugdha N. Gokhale
Department of Epidemiology
Gillings School of Global Public Health
University of North Carolina at Chapel Hill
United States

Peter Groenewegen
NIVEL, Netherlands institute for health services research
The Netherlands

Jolanta Gulbinovič
Department of Pathology, Forensic Medicine and Pharmacology
Vilnius University
Lithuania

Jesper Hallas
Clinical Pharmacology
Institute of Public Health
University of Southern Denmark
Denmark

Linda Härmark
Netherlands Pharmacovigilance Centre Lareb
The Netherlands

Kevin Haynes
Government and Academic Research
HealthCore, Inc.
United States

Eibert R. Heerdink
Division of Pharmacoepidemiology and Clinical Pharmacology
Utrecht Institute for Pharmaceutical Sciences
The Netherlands

Hans Hogerzeil
Faculty of Medical Sciences
University Medical Centre Groningen
The Netherlands

Katrin Janhsen
Department of Community Health
University of Applied Sciences
Germany

Kristina Johnell
Aging Research Center
Karolinska Institutet and Stockholm University
Sweden

Roberta Joppi
Pharmaceutical Department
Local Health Authority of Verona – Veneto Region
Italy

Raul Kiivet
Department of Public Health
University of Tartu
Estonia

Niek Klazinga
Department of Social Medicine
Academic Medical Centre
University of Amsterdam
The Netherlands

I fan Kuo
College of Pharmacy
Faculty of Health Sciences
University of Manitoba
Canada

Synnöve Lindemalm
Department of Clinical Science, Intervention and Technology
Karolinska Institutet
Sweden

Marie Lindquist
Uppsala Monitoring Centre
Sweden

Annemiek Linn
Department of Communication Science
University of Amsterdam/Amsterdam School of Communication Research (ASCoR)
The Netherlands

Cecilia Stålsby Lundborg
Department of Public Health Sciences
Karolinska Institutet
Sweden

Nello Martini
Accademia Nazionale di Medicina
Italy

David Morgan
Department of Sociology
Portland State University
United States

Vicki Osborne
Drug Safety Research Unit
United Kingdom

Claudia Garcia Serpa Osorio-de-Castro
Department of Medicines Policies and Pharmaceutical Services (NAF)
Sergio Arouca National School of Public Health
Oswaldo Cruz Foundation
Brazil

Byung-Joo Park
Department of Preventive Medicine
Seoul National University College of Medicine
South Korea

Ken Paterson
Faculty of Medicine
University of Glasgow
United Kingdom

Lisa Pont
Centre for Health Systems and Safety Research
Australian Institute of Health Innovation
Macquarie University
Australia

Colin Richman
Rx-info Ltd.
United Kingdom

Jane Robertson
Clinical Pharmacology
School of Medicine and Public Health
Faculty of Health and Medicine
University of Newcastle
Australia

Leena K. Saastamoinen
Research Department
Social Insurance Institution (Kela)
Finland

Mònica Sabaté Gallego
Foundation of the Catalan Institute of Pharmacology (FICF)
Spain

Angela Patricia Acosta Santamaría
Faculty of Medicine
Pontificia Universidad Javeriana
Colombia

Emilio J. Sanz
Department of Physical Medicine and Pharmacology
University of La Laguna
Spain

Junko Sato
Pharmaceuticals and Medical Devices Agency
Japan

Karin Schenck-Gustafsson
Department of Medicine
Cardiac Unit
Centre for Gender Medicine
Karolinska Institutet
Sweden

Gisbert W. Selke
Wissenschaftliches Institut der AOK (WIdO)
Germany

Catherine Sermet
IRDES (Institute for Research and Information in Health Economics)
France

Ingrid Sketris
College of Pharmacy
Dalhousie University
Canada

Janet Sluggett
Quality Use of Medicines and Pharmacy Research Centre
Sansom Institute for Health Research
University of South Australia
Australia

Til Stürmer
Department of Epidemiology
Gillings School of Global Public Health
University of North Carolina at Chapel Hill
United States

Karolina Andersson Sundell
Section for Epidemiology and Social Medicine
Department of Public Health and Community Medicine
Sahlgrenska Academy
University of Gothenburg
Sweden

Petra A. Thürmann
Institute of Clinical Pharmacology
Helios Klinikum Wuppertal
University Witten/Herdecke
Germany

Lesley Tilson
National Centre for Pharmacoeconomics
St James's Hospital
Ireland

June Tordoff
School of Pharmacy
University of Otago
New Zealand

Ilse Truter
Drug Utilization Research Unit, Department of Pharmacy
Nelson Mandela Metropolitan University
South Africa

Liset van Dijk
NIVEL, Netherlands Institute for Health Services Research
The Netherlands

Floortje van Nooten
Health Economics and Outcomes Research
Astellas
The Netherlands

Agnes Vitry
Quality Use of Medicines and Pharmacy Research Centre
Sansom Institute for Health Research
University of South Australia
Australia

Jiří Vlček
Department of Social and Clinical Pharmacy
Faculty of Pharmacy
Charles University in Prague
Czech Republic

Bernard Vrijens
WestRock Healthcare
Belgium
and
University of Liège
Belgium

Lynn Weekes
NPS MedicineWise
Australia

Barbro Westerholm
The Swedish Parliament
Sweden

Tommy Westerlund
Social Medicine
Institute of Medicine
Sahlgrenska Academy
University of Gothenburg
Sweden

Eva Wikstrom-Jonsson
Department of Medicine
Karolinska Institutet
Sweden

Catherine Will
Department of Sociology, School of Law, Politics and Sociology
University of Sussex
United Kingdom

Yea-Huei Kao Yang
School of Pharmacy
Institute of Clinical Pharmacy and Pharmaceutical Sciences
National Cheng Kung University
Taiwan

Leah Zullig
Department of Medicine
Duke University
United States

About the companion website

This book is accompanied by a companion website:

www.wiley.com/go/elseviers/drug_utilization_research

The website includes:

- References and further reading
- A large version of Figure 34.2
- Appendix to Chapter 11

PART 1
Introduction

CHAPTER 1

Introduction to drug utilization research

Björn Wettermark[1], Monique Elseviers[2], Anna Birna Almarsdóttir[3], Morten Andersen[1], Ria Benko[4], Marion Bennie[5], Irene Eriksson[1], Brian Godman[6], Janet Krska[7], Elisabetta Poluzzi[8], Katja Taxis[9], Robert Vander Stichele[10] & Vera Vlahović-Palčevski[11]

[1]*Centre for Pharmacoepidemiology, Department of Medicine, Karolinska Institutet, Sweden*

[2]*Centre for Research and Innovation in Care, Faculty of Medicine and Health Sciences, University of Antwerp, Belgium*

[3]*Clinical Pharmacology, Institute of Public Health, University of Southern Denmark, Denmark*

[4]*Department of Clinical Pharmacy, Faculty of Pharmacy, University of Szeged, Hungary*

[5]*Institute of Pharmacy and Biomedical Sciences, University of Strathclyde, United Kingdom*

[6]*Department of Laboratory Medicine, Karolinska Institutet, Sweden*

[7]*School of Pharmacy, Universities of Greenwich and Kent, United Kingdom*

[8] *Pharmacology Unit, Department of Medical and Surgical Sciences, University of Bologna, Italy*

[9]*Department of Pharmacy, Unit of Pharmacotherapy and Pharmaceutical Care, University of Groningen, The Netherlands*

[10]*Heymans Institute of Pharmacology, Ghent University, Belgium*

[11]*Department of Clinical Pharmacology, University Hospital Center Rijeka, Croatia*

KEY POINTS

- Drug utilization research can be defined as 'an eclectic collection of descriptive and analytical methods for the quantification, the understanding and the evaluation of the processes of prescribing, dispensing and consumption of medicines, and for the testing of interventions to enhance the quality of these processes'.
- The discipline may be seen as the bridge between pharmacoepidemiology and health services research. It is also closely connected to clinical pharmacology, with the principal aim of drug utilization research being to facilitate the safe and effective use of medicines in populations.
- Research in drug utilization began to develop in the 1960s. Some pioneering studies focused on assessing differences in drug utilization between countries or regions. Other studies focused on factors influencing the prescribing patterns of physicians.
- The eclectic nature of drug utilization research requires expertise in a broad range of research methodologies. Part 2 of the book provides guidance on a wide range of quantitative and qualitative methods used in drug utilization research.
- The numerous applications of drug utilization research are illustrated in Part 3, which include sections on comparative drug utilization research, drug utilization and health policy, drug utilization in specific populations and therapeutic areas, determinants of drug utilization, adherence and drug utilization research, the role of drug utilization within the field of pharmacoepidemiology and the assessment and improvement of the quality of medicine use.

Room for improvement in drug utilization

Medicines play an important role in the provision of optimal care and have a major impact on health. During the last decades of the 20th century, new medicines have markedly decreased mortality, shortened hospitalization duration and improved quality of life for millions of people [1,2]. However, it is also important to recognize the negative consequences of drug therapy and the emerging problem of inappropriate drug use, with issues ranging from increased morbidity and mortality to excessive medicalization, polypharmacy, adverse drug reactions (ADRs) and increased antimicrobial resistance.

Drug Utilization Research: Methods and Applications, First Edition. Edited by M. Elseviers et al. © 2016 John Wiley & Sons, Ltd.
Published 2016 by John Wiley & Sons, Ltd.

The economic consequences associated with inappropriate drug use are considerable. The average treatment cost for a single ADR in Germany has been estimated at approximately €2250, equating to €434 million per year [3]. Drug-related hospital admissions have been assumed to account for more than 4% of the total health expenditure in Great Britain [4]. In the United States, the incremental expenditure related to inappropriate use of medicines in the community-dwelling elderly was estimated at $7.2 billion in 2001, and these costs are likely to have increased over time [5]. Other researchers have suggested that for every dollar spent on medications, one additional dollar is needed to correct problems caused by inappropriate use of medicines [6].

The extent of inappropriate use of medicines may be even greater in low- and middle-income countries. Common problems include overuse of drugs such as antibiotics and antidiarrhoeals, polypharmacy and the prescribing of inappropriate drugs (e.g. those with limited efficacy or an uncertain safety profile). In many of these countries, up to 60–80% of health problems are self-medicated and poor adherence to doctors' prescriptions is common [7].

Medicines are also important from an economic perspective. Internationally, there is increased scrutiny of pharmaceutical expenditures, and medicines have been the most rapidly growing cost component in ambulatory care in most countries [8–13]. Challenges in financing drugs may be an even greater concern in low- and middle-income countries, where medicines can account for up to 60% of total health care spending [14]. The reasons behind the increasing expenditure on medicines include demographic changes, the continued launch of new expensive medicines, rising patient expectations and stricter clinical targets [9,15,16].

The history of drug utilization research

The emerging problems of rising expenditure and inappropriate use of medicines clearly demonstrate the need for drug utilization research, a cross-disciplinary and multiprofessional science that aims to describe and understand the use of medicines in society. Research in drug utilization began to develop in the 1960s. The pharmaceutical industry early on expressed the need for drug utilization data that could be used to monitor the performance of its representatives, serve as a basis for marketing and define areas for future drug development and research. This laid the basis for the development of large, commercial databases capable of tracking the prescribing and sales of medicines; Intercontinental Marketing Services (IMS) was one of the pioneers [17]. At the same time, concern about pharmaceutical expenditures stimulated the development of public statistics on drug use, independent of those produced by pharmaceutical companies for marketing purposes. These statistics were initially compiled to allow informed financial, administrative and reimbursement decisions, but they were also valuable for research, assessment of the quality of prescribing and quantification of the risks and benefits of drug use in the population. The extent and nature of these early databases varied substantially between countries; in the beginning, they were mostly based on data collected from wholesalers or health authorities. In recent decades, technical development has facilitated the establishment of large databases in many countries across the world.

The pioneering drug utilization studies in Europe focused on assessing differences in drug utilization between countries or regions [18–21]. Other studies focused on factors influencing the prescribing patterns of physicians [22–24]. In 1969, the World Health Organization (WHO) organized its first meeting on Drug Consumption in Oslo, where researchers expressed the need for a common medicines classification system and for a technical unit of comparison in drug utilization studies [19]. As a result, scientists, mainly from Northern European countries, came together in an informal group and developed a new unit of measurement, initially called the 'agreed daily dose', but subsequently named the 'defined daily dose' (DDD) [20,21,25]. In 1975, the Norwegian agency Norsk Medisinaldepot published a list of DDDs of medicines registered in Norway, which were classified according to the European Pharmaceutical Market Research Association (EPhMRA) code, with the addition of two chemical subgroups. The invention of the Anatomical Therapeutic Chemical (ATC) classification system and the DDDs enabled cross-national comparisons of drug utilization and was of key importance for the future development of the discipline [25].

In 1976, a small group of scientists active in these areas established the informal Drug Utilisation Research Group (DURG). For approximately 20 years the WHO Regional Office for Europe served as the group's secretariat, and, consequently, the DURG was often referred as the 'WHO-DURG'. From 1993, the relationship between the and a standard set of indicators to describe core aspects of prescribing and dispensing [47]. The first International Conference on Improving the Use of Medicines (ICIUM), held in Chiang-Mai, Thailand, in 1997, systematically reviewed the interventions in developing countries [47]. Considerable research gaps in the understanding of safe and effective medicines use were identified, and it was suggested that more research should be directed to promoting the rational use of medicines across multiple settings, including hospitals, the private sector and the community. A number of key areas were also identified for future research, such as interventions to improve the use of antibiotics and antimalarial drugs, methods to assess the impact of drugs and therapeutic committees and the impact of financial incentives on drug utilization patterns.

Over the years, drug utilization research has continued to grow, and a Medline search run in 2015 using the term 'drug utilization' gave more than 20 000 hits. In addition, several thousand drug utilization studies can be found under other search terms related to the prescribing, dispensing and consumption of medicines. Although there has been an explosion in the availability of data and the development of methods, the research questions raised by EuroDURG in 1969 are still relevant in summarizing the important aims of drug utilization research.

It is also important to acknowledge the commonalities in the development of drug utilization research and pharmacoepidemiology. In 1985, the first International Conference on Linked Databases was held in the United States. The name of the conference was subsequently changed to the International Conference on Pharmacoepidemiology (ICPE), and, in 1989, during the fifth conference in Minneapolis, the International Society for Pharmacoepidemiology (ISPE) was officially launched. Many drug utilization researchers joined the society, and drug utilization studies constituted a large proportion of the presentations at all annual conferences. In 2006, a special interest group in Drug Utilization/Health Service Research (SIG DUR/HSR) was formed within ISPE with the aim of creating a global forum for discussion and cooperation between drug utilization researchers in different continents. EuroDURG merged with ISPE and became the European branch of the special interest group. In 2012, EuroDURG, in collaboration with ISPE SIG DUR/HSR, decided to develop *Drug Utilization Research: Methods and Applications* for use by researchers, academics and policymakers active in the field.

Definition and delineation

In 1977, the WHO defined drug utilization research as 'studies on the marketing, distribution, prescription and the use of drugs in a society, with special emphasis on the resulting medical, social and economic consequences' [48]. However, this definition does not fully capture the depth and breadth of drug utilization, and, in 2008, a more extensive one was proposed in the textbook *Pharmacoepidemiology and Therapeutic Risk Management* [37]:

> Drug Utilization Research is an eclectic collection of descriptive and analytical methods for the quantification, the understanding and the evaluation of the processes of prescribing, dispensing and consumption of medicines, and for the testing of interventions to enhance the quality of these processes.

Drug utilization research focuses on various medical, social and economic aspects of drug use. Medical consequences include the risks and benefits of drug therapy, while social aspects can be related to inappropriate use. Economic issues deal with the cost of medicines and treatment for patients and society. These areas are described in Box 1.1.

The WHO definition of drug utilization places the research area close to a number of related research fields. The greatest commonality lies with pharmacoepidemiology, which is defined as 'the study of the utilization and effects of drugs in large numbers of people' [49]. The main difference between drug utilization research and pharmacoepidemiology is that the latter focuses to a greater extent on the assessment of quantitative risks (and, recently, also benefits) of drug treatment in cohorts of patients, mostly followed in databases. Drug utilization research, on the other hand, focuses on the quantity and quality of medicine use in different countries, regions and settings, and the explanatory factors behind these patterns (Figure 1.2).

Another way to describe the difference between the two research fields has been suggested by Bergman: 'While drug utilization studies employ various sources of information focusing on drugs, e.g. wholesale and prescription registers, the term "epidemiology" implies that pharmacoepidemiological studies are population based, and link health events to drug exposure' [50]. Over time, the distinction between the two terms has diminished, and they are sometimes used interchangeably. This interplay between the two fields is illustrated in a bibliometric study on the scope and range of drug

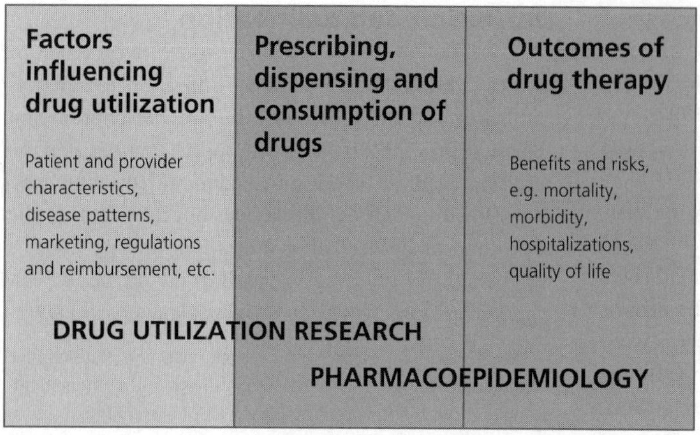

Figure 1.2 Traditional descriptions of drug utilization research and pharmacoepidemiology.

utilization research abstracts presented at the International Conference on Pharmacoepidemiology [51].

The current definition of drug utilization research illustrates the broad nature of the field, which includes both quantitative and qualitative studies. It also emphasizes that intervention studies aimed at improving drug utilization are an important part of the discipline. Thus, it links drug utilization research to health services research. The latter has been defined as 'a multidisciplinary field of inquiry, both basic and applied, that examines the use, costs, quality, accessibility, delivery, organization, financing, and outcomes of health care services to increase knowledge and understanding of the structure, processes, and effects of health services for individuals and populations' [52]. Consequently, drug utilization research may be seen as the bridge between pharmacoepidemiology and health services research (Figure 1.3).

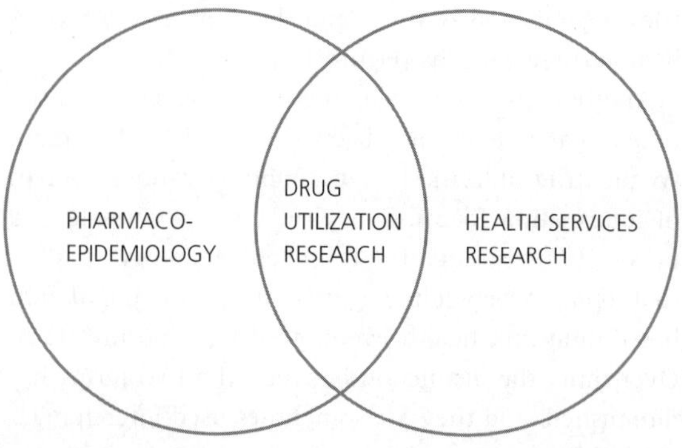

Figure 1.3 Drug utilization research as a bridge between pharmacoepidemiology and health services research.

Drug utilization research is also connected to the discipline of clinical pharmacology. Researchers in this field study pharmacokinetics (what the body does to the drug) and pharmacodynamics (what the drug does to the body). The original aims of clinical pharmacology were to develop new medicines and to determine the balance between drug benefit and risk in clinical trials. In recent years, the scope of clinical pharmacology has widened to include exploration of drugs as therapeutic agents and assessment of the beneficial and adverse effects of the use and the deliberate misuse of drugs [53]. Clinical pharmacology has a strong focus on pharmacovigilance activities, such as the reporting, collecting and evaluation of ADRs; however, clinical pharmacologists are also engaged in promoting rational drug use through medical education, drug information centers, therapeutic drug monitoring services and drug and therapeutic committees.

While clinical pharmacology studies the 'absolute' efficacy of a drug in clinical trials under ideal conditions, drug utilization research and pharmacoepidemiology study the 'real-world' effectiveness of medicines and attempt to identify and quantify risks that are difficult to observe or assess in clinical trials or spontaneous reporting systems. Furthermore, drug utilization research includes assessment of the appropriateness of drug use and expenditure.

There are a number of other scientific disciplines that share relationships with drug utilization research, as shown in Table 1.1. The interplay with some of these disciplines is further described in Part 3, Section G.

Table 1.1 Scientific disciplines related to drug utilization research.

Discipline	Definition	Commonalities of interest	Reference
Clinical pharmacology	Scientific discipline that involves all aspects of the relationship between drugs and humans. Its breadth includes the development of new drugs, the application of drugs as therapeutic agents, the beneficial and adverse effects of drugs in individuals and society and the deliberate misuse of drugs	Studies of the beneficial and adverse effects of drugs in society	Birkett et al. 2010 [53]
Clinical pharmacy	Branch of pharmacy in which pharmacists provide patient care that optimizes the use of medication and promotes health, wellness and disease prevention	Drug utilization studies are important tools in optimizing the use of medicines in society	ACCP 2008 [54]
Health services research	A multidisciplinary field of inquiry, both basic and applied, that examines the use, costs, quality, accessibility, delivery, organization, financing and outcomes of health care services in order to increase our knowledge and understanding of the structure, processes and effects of health services for individuals and populations	Analyses of the use, costs, quality, accessibility, delivery, organization, financing and outcomes of medicines in society Intervention studies to promote rational use of drugs	IOM 1995 [52]
Health technology assessment	Research that systematically examines the short- and long-term consequences, in terms of health and resource use, of the application of a health technology, a set of related technologies or a technology-related issue	Analyses of the medical, organizational, economic and societal consequences of drug utilization	Henshall et al. 1997 [55]
Outcomes research	Study of the end results of health services taking patients' experiences, preferences and values into account	Analyses of the outcome of drug therapy for patients and society	Clancy & Eisenberg 1998 [56]
Pharmacoeconomics	Description and analysis of the costs of drug therapy to health care systems and society	Descriptive and analytical studies of expenditure on medicines	Bootman et al. 2005 [57]
Pharmacoepidemiology	Study of the utilization and effects of drugs in large numbers of people	Descriptive and analytical studies of drug utilization	Strom 2012 [49]
Pharmacovigilance	The science and activities relating to the detection, assessment, understanding and prevention of adverse effects or any other drug-related problems	Surveillance of side effects related to the use of medicines Drug utilization studies may provide denominator of drug exposure	WHO 2002 [58]
Therapeutic risk management	Strategies to ensure that the benefits of a particular drug outweigh its risks in general practice	Analyses of the appropriate use of medicines and interventions to promote rational use of drugs	Hirst et al. 2006 [59]

Skills needed to be a drug utilization researcher

The eclectic nature of drug utilization research requires expertise in a broad range of research methodologies (Box 1.2).

Given the wide range of methods used and the breadth of research expertise needed in drug utilization research, it is important to recognize the multidisciplinary and multiprofessional nature of the area and the need to involve multiple stakeholders from different perspectives, including health care providers, regulators, payers, pharmaceutical companies and the general public. Furthermore, many studies require input from experts in other disciplines, such as health economists and behavioural scientists.

Areas of inquiry in drug utilization research reflected in this book

The ***methodology section*** (Part 2) provides guidance on the wide range of methods used in the field. The principal aim of drug utilization research is to facilitate the

Box 1.2 Skills needed to be a drug utilization researcher following the definition of drug utilization research.

An eclectic collection of descriptive and analytical methods for the quantification...
- Classification systems (ATC and others)
- Measurement units (DDD, expenditure, prescriptions, etc.)
- Analysis of individual usage patterns (persistence, switching, etc.)
- Biostatistical methods (descriptive statistics, sampling, significance, correlation, regression analyses, etc.)
- Epidemiological study designs (ecological studies, cohort studies, case–control studies, case-crossover studies)
- Epidemiological terminology (prevalence, incidence, exposure, outcome, relative risk, odds ratio, bias, confounding, etc.)

...the understanding...
- Qualitative methods (in depth interviews, focus group discussions, observations, etc.)
- Purposive sampling and triangulation
- Approaches to the generation and analysis of qualitative data (phenomenology, grounded theory, qualitative content analysis and narrative analysis, etc.)
- Consensus methods (Delphi and nominal group techniques, consensus development conferences)

...and the evaluation...
- Evaluation techniques
- Single user-focused evaluation versus scientific research evaluation
- The four hierarchical levels of evaluation, including the measurement of reactions to, learning from, behaviour towards and results of interventions (Kirkpatrick's evaluation model)

...of the processes of prescribing, dispensing and consumption of medicines...
- Content and validation of databases derived from medical records or pharmacy dispensing systems
- Data collection from patients (questionnaires, interviews, electronic monitoring devices, etc.)
- Prescribing and reimbursement regulations
- Principles of clinical pharmacology (rational use of drugs, guidelines, critical drug evaluation, etc.)

...and for the testing of interventions...
- Implementation research (how to design and carry out interventions)
- Quasiexperimental study designs (controlled before-and-after studies, time series analyses)
- Cluster randomized trials

...to enhance the quality of these processes
- Quality standards for the prescribing, dispensing and consumption of medicines
- Quality assessment tools
- Quality indicators (terminology, requirement, validation, use, etc.)
- Development techniques for successful interventions and implementation programmes

safe and effective use of medicines in populations. This may be achieved in a variety of ways. Descriptive drug utilization studies can be used to stimulate discussions on potential over- or underuse of medicines. Prescribing patterns may be compared with current recommendations and guidelines to identify areas for improvement. Analytical studies may be conducted to explore factors potentially influencing patterns of drug prescribing, dispensing or consumption. Qualitative studies are also needed to gain an understanding of the perceptions of prescribers, pharmacists and patients.

The ***applied drug utilization research sections*** (Part 3) are designed to illustrate recent developments in drug utilization research from different perspectives. The chapters are grouped under the following headings:

- Section A: Comparative drug utilization research
- Section B: Drug utilization and health policy
- Section C: Drug utilization in specific populations
- Section D: Drug utilization in specific therapeutic areas
- Section E: Determinants of drug utilization
- Section F: Adherence and drug utilization research
- Section G: The role of drug utilization within the field of pharmacoepidemiology
- Section H: Assessment and improvement of the quality of medicine use

Section A on ***comparative drug utilization research*** explores studies comparing drug utilization patterns across geographical areas, between health settings (primary care practices and hospitals) and over time (e.g. exploring seasonality in drug use). Comparative drug utilization research relates to theories of benchmarking (i.e. the process of establishing best practices through comparison of performance). There are multiple, diverse reasons for the variation in clinical practice, reflecting personal, organizational and system levels. The desire to compare different countries was one of the main reasons for the development of drug utilization research. In addition to comparisons across geographical areas, comparative drug utilization research may be conducted across different health care settings or different populations. Examples of comparative studies exploring drug utilization in relation to various patient, prescriber and health care system characteristics are also presented.

Section B on ***drug utilization and health policy*** focuses on how policymakers and other key stakeholders shape pharmaceutical policy and how drug utilization research contributes to this process. Health policy has been defined as the conscious attempt by public officials or executives entrusted with public funds, including those working in health authorities, health insurance agencies or managed care organizations, to achieve certain objectives through a set of laws, rules, procedures and incentives [60]. Pharmaceutical policy debates issues of unmet need, access to medicines, pricing, cost containment, irrational use of medicines, innovation and services provision. This is growing in importance, given ever-increasing pressure on resources through changes in demographics, the continued launch of new premium-priced drugs to address areas of unmet need and financial concerns in a number of countries.

Section C on ***drug utilization in specific populations*** describes drug utilization research in three distinct populations across the life span, from conception until the end of life. There is a specific focus on pregnancy, children and the elderly, since drug use in these groups is often associated with considerable risks and inappropriate use. These chapters give an overview of frequently used medications in these populations. Specific methodological issues that have to be considered when assessing medication use in these populations are also discussed.

Section D on ***drug utilization in specific therapeutic areas*** explores drug utilization studies of antibiotics as an example of acute therapy, cardiovascular and neuropsychiatric medicines as examples of medicines for chronic use, and biologicals and cancer drugs as emerging topics in drug utilization research. The section includes discussions around the main directions of drug utilization research and provides examples of drug utilization studies conducted in the given therapeutic areas.

Section E on ***determinants of drug utilization*** describes the key influences on utilization, starting with health systems/policies, followed by prescriber perspectives (exploring the role of the prescribers and factors influencing their behaviour) and ending with a chapter on patient perspectives. The use of medicines is determined by a complex range of interrelated factors, including individual patients' beliefs in medicines, differences in the practices of prescribers/suppliers and health systems/policies and international influences.

Section F on ***adherence and drug utilization research*** explores recently emerged interest in adherence within the drug utilization domain. Adherence to medicines refers to taking medication as prescribed, starting from prescribing and the initiation of treatment, through the implementation of the correct dose regimen and finishing with discontinuation. In this section, the use of diverse methodologies and data sources for adherence research is explored and determinants of nonadherence and interventions to improve adherence are discussed.

Section G on the ***role of drug utilization within the field of pharmacoepidemiology*** examines the role of drug utilization research in risk management, pharmacovigilance, outcome research and pharmacoeconomics. In these areas, drug utilization research expertise contributes to a number of key issues, including drug safety and effectiveness, pharmaceutical expenditure and drug policy strategies. These aspects of drug utilization are described across five chapters, taking into account the views of both the researcher and the regulator.

Finally, Section H on ***assessment and improvement of the quality of medicine use*** explores current strategies for assessing and improving medicines use. From an overview of existing quality indicators in a specific conceptual framework, it evolves to describe academic detailing and other interventions already tested for the improvement of prescribing and the implementation plans by which these interventions and quality indicators are put into action. Additionally, behavioural change, key to any attempt to enhance the quality of prescribing and dispensing, is discussed, as is the need to consider a realistic approach to the evaluation of interventions designed to enhance drug utilization.

To summarize, the aim of this book is to provide the reader with a toolkit containing the various methods used within drug utilization research, to give examples of various applications of research and to demonstrate how drug utilization studies help shape health policy and clinical practice internationally.

PART 2
Methodology

CHAPTER 2

Study designs in drug utilization research

Björn Wettermark[1], Mirko Di Martino[2] & Monique Elseviers[3]

[1]*Clinical Pharmacology and Centre for Pharmacoepidemiology, Department of Medicine, Karolinska Institutet, Sweden*

[2]*Department of Epidemiology, Lazio Regional Health Service, Roma, Italy*

[3]*Centre for Research and Innovation in Care, Faculty of Medicine and Health Sciences, University of Antwerp, Belgium*

KEY POINTS

- Drug utilization studies can be conducted using a wide variety of study designs. Researchers must select the most appropriate method for answering the questions they want to investigate.
- Research methods in drug utilization can broadly be categorized as either quantitative or qualitative.
- Quantitative descriptive studies are studies that identify patterns or trends in drug utilization without making inferences about causal associations.
- Quantitative analytical studies are studies designed to reach causal inferences about hypothesized relationships. They aim to gain a deeper understanding of the explanatory factors behind patterns of drug prescribing, dispensing or consumption.
- A variety of study designs can be used to evaluate interventions, including quasiexperimental designs (uncontrolled or controlled before-and-after studies and interrupted time series) and experimental designs, such as randomized controlled trials.

Introduction

Drug utilization studies can be conducted using a wide variety of study designs. All methodologies have their advantages and limitations, and researchers must select the most appropriate method for the questions they want to investigate. The choice of method and the way in which it is implemented will largely be determined by the research questions, but it is important to acknowledge that it is also influenced by ethical principles and many practical considerations, including the type of data available, the budget and the knowledge and skills of those undertaking the research. Sometimes, the appropriate strategy includes a combination of different methods. This chapter describes some important study designs in drug utilization research and provides examples of studies that have used them. Further guidance may be found in various handbooks on epidemiology, pharmacoepidemiology and health services research (see website).

Quantitative and qualitative research

Research methods in drug utilization can broadly be categorized as either quantitative or qualitative. ***Quantitative research*** deals with things that can be measured in quantities. It gathers data in numerical form, which can be put into categories or in rank order and measured in various units. Quantitative methods can be used to measure, explain, predict or generalize observations. Quantitative research usually starts with the data collection, which should be based on a predefined hypothesis or theory. Usually, the data collected requires verification, validation and recording before analysis can take place. Associations and differences between variables may be studied by using different statistical methods.

Qualitative research refers to the examination, analysis and interpretation of observations for the purpose of discovering underlying meanings and patterns

Drug Utilization Research: Methods and Applications, First Edition. Edited by M. Elseviers et al.
Published 2016 by John Wiley & Sons, Ltd.

Table 2.1 Key features of quantitative and qualitative drug utilization research.

Characteristics	Quantitative research	Qualitative research
Objective	To measure prescribing, dispensing or consumption of medicines in populations	To gain in-depth understanding of the prescribing, dispensing or consumption of medicines
Examples of research questions around patient adherence	How many patients do not redeem their first prescription? Which are the most important factors associated with poor adherence to medication? How often do patients use different tools to assist adherence?	To explore the perspectives of patients regarding factors perceived as barriers to medication adherence To provide an in-depth understanding of general practitioners' beliefs about patient adherence
Confidence level	Conclusive, with a specific degree of certainty and generalizability	Explorative
Tools	Surveys, analyses of existing databases	Focus groups, in-depth interviews, content analyses
Participants	Total data or statistically representative samples of the population studied, recruited through random selection	Small groups of information-rich subjects (physicians, patients or other stakeholders), recruited purposively or through snowballing
Results	Phenomena are described numerically, with appropriate statistical measures	Phenomena are described in a narrative fashion. Themes may be identified
Strengths	Hypotheses may be confirmed. Results can be inferred for the population	Allows for in-depth understanding. Can generate hypotheses to be tested quantitatively
Weaknesses	Limited possibilities to provide deeper insight into phenomena	Findings cannot be quantified and inferred for the population

of relationships [1]. Qualitative researchers gather information that is not in numerical form through methods including focus-group discussions, open-ended questionnaires, in-depth interviews and observations. Such studies may be used to explore the perceptions of prescribers, dispensers and patients in dealing with medicines. Consequently, they are extremely important in gaining a deeper understanding of various phenomena in drug utilization.

Basic differences between quantitative and qualitative study designs, with examples of research questions around patient adherence, are illustrated in Table 2.1.

Quantitative and qualitative methods can complement each other, when used together. Combining methodologies allows to generate statistical evidence from collected data and to provide a deeper understanding of the obtained statistical results. As an example, a qualitative interview study could be helpful in understanding prescribing patterns observed in a quantitative study. Qualitative studies may also be valuable as a first step in the development of questions subsequently used in quantitative surveys. For further reading on qualitative methods, see Chapter 13.

Observational studies: from descriptive to analytical approaches

Quantitative observational studies are conducted in a 'real-life' situation, without any experimental set-up. Research activities are limited to the interpretation of data obtained from observations, and the researcher does not influence the factors under study. Quantitative observational drug utilization studies may be either descriptive or analytical.

Descriptive studies are studies identifying patterns or trends in drug utilization that do not allow for inferences to be drawn about causal associations. They often represent the first scientific studies conducted in new areas of enquiry. A fundamental element of descriptive reporting is a clear, specific and measurable definition of the condition or therapy under investigation. Like a good newspaper article, good descriptive reporting answers the five basic 'W' questions: Who?, What?, Why?, When? and Where?, as well as a sixth: So what? [2]. Descriptive drug utilization studies may, for example, be used to delineate trends in the pattern of drug use in a defined setting over a defined period of time. Such studies can be used to provide denominator data (the number of patients or a specific patient population exposed to specific drugs within a given time period) for use in calculating rates of reported adverse drug reactions. They could also be used in estimating disease prevalence, estimating drug expenditures, planning drug acquisition, importation, production and distribution and assessing the quality of the prescribing, dispensing, and use of medicines. These studies are also valuable in the assessment of patient-, provider-, and system-related barriers to treatment, especially in settings without universal drug coverage.

Analytical studies are studies designed to reach causal inferences about hypothesized relationships. They aim to gain a deeper understanding of the explanatory factors behind patterns of drug prescribing, dispensing and consumption. They may also be conducted to analyse the positive or negative effects of therapy. Analytical studies require a design that will permit an evaluation of the causal effect association between exposure and outcome. ***Case–control studies*** and ***cohort studies*** contain control groups and can be referred to as analytical studies. Case–control studies investigate phenomena that happened in the past, starting from a group of cases where the effect is present and controls where it is absent and going back to the cause(s). In contrast, cohort studies start from the cause and follow a cohort prospectively over time to study the effect(s). In traditional pharmacoepidemiological studies focusing on the safety or effectiveness of therapy, the outcome event is the occurrence of disease. In drug utilization studies, the event of interest is most often the prescribing, dispensing or use of a drug or a change in drug use patterns, including discontinuation and switching. Some drug utilization studies, however, address the consequences of drug use. For further reading on the interplay between pharmacoepidemiology and drug utilization research, see Chapters 1 and 38–42.

Figure 2.1 provides an overview of study designs, ranging from descriptive observations to analytical studies. Most designs can be applied to analyses at different levels of data aggregation, from individual patient data over different categories of health care units to aggregate data on entire populations/nations. Examples of studies are given later in this chapter and in Part 3.

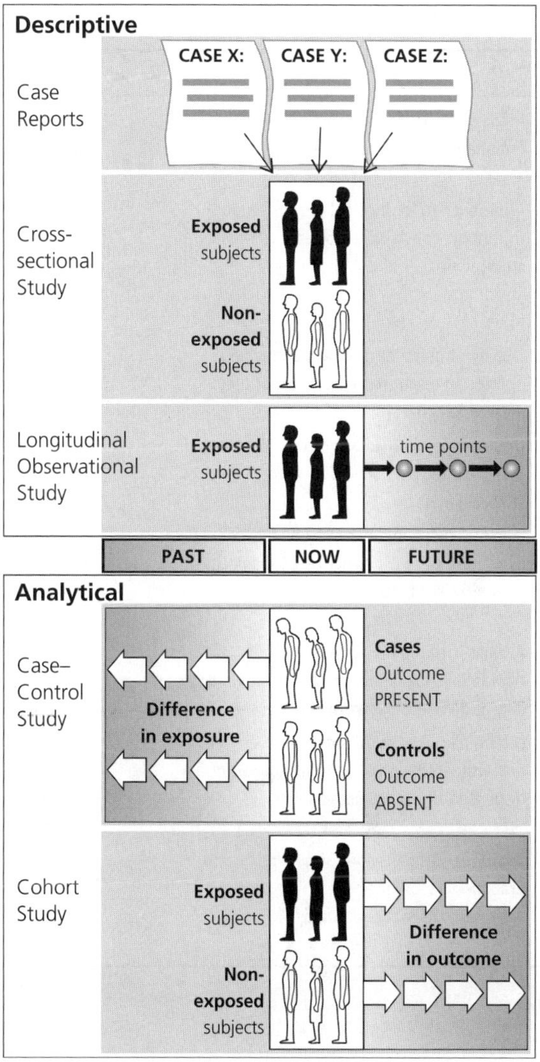

Figure 2.1 Overview of quantitative study designs in drug utilization research.

Study designs for descriptive drug utilization studies

Descriptive studies consist of two major groups: those dealing with individual observations and those that relate to populations [2]. Studies presenting data for individual cases (patients or practices) are case reports or case series, while cross-sectional studies and longitudinal observational studies examine populations.

The *case report* is the least publishable unit in medical literature. Such a study might present drug consumption

Table 2.2 Examples of cross-sectional studies in drug utilization research.

Title	Design	Country
Medication use in pregnancy: a cross-sectional, multinational web-based study [6]	Pregnant women and mothers were asked about their medicine use through an anonymous online questionnaire	Europe, North and South America and Australia
Adherence to local guidelines for venous thromboprophylaxis: a cross-sectional study of medical inpatients in Argentina [7]	Venous thromboprophylaxis was investigated in patients admitted to two university hospitals using data from filled prescriptions, medical records and interviews with chief physicians	Argentina
Quality of prescribing in Belgian nursing homes: an electronic assessment of the medication chart [8]	Inappropriate under- and overprescribing were investigated using medical records for nursing home residents	Belgium
Medication use in adults living in Brasilia, Brazil: a cross-sectional, population-based study [9]	Adults received structured interviews in their homes about their use of medicines during the last week	Brazil
Doctor's injection prescribing and its correlates in village health clinics across 10 Provinces of Western China [10]	Prescriptions were collected from a large number of village clinics in different provinces to assess levels and determinants of injection use	China
Antibiotic prescribing in paediatric populations: a comparison between Viareggio, Italy and Funen, Denmark [11]	Aggregate drug dispensing data for antibiotics were compared between the two countries, stratified by age	Italy and Denmark
Differences in drug utilisation between men and womens: a cross sectional analysis of all dispensed drugs in Sweden [12]	Systematic analysis of the differences between all men and all women in the prevalence of dispensed drugs for 50 pharmacologic groups in ambulatory care	Sweden
Attitudes and behaviour of general practitioners and their prescribing costs: a national cross sectional survey [13]	A postal survey was sent to general practitioners to investigate the relationship between prescribing costs and attitudes towards prescribing decisions	England

in a single patient or the prescribing pattern at an individual clinic. Examples of case reports in drug utilization research include studies presenting drug prescribing over time in a single practice [3] and examinations of reforms promoting rational use of drugs or low prices for generics in an individual country [4,5].

Cross-sectional studies, also referred to as prevalence studies, describe the utilization of drugs in a given population at a given point in time. Data on drug prescribing, dispensing or consumption are also collected, and utilization patterns may be presented by geographical area or patient age or sex (Table 2.2). These designs can also be applied in studies presenting prescribing patterns in relation to diagnoses or conditions. It is important, however, to acknowledge that since these studies lack information on whether the factor of interest precedes or follows the effect, they may not be used to draw any conclusions on cause and effect. Cross-sectional studies are relatively inexpensive and easy to perform. They can be conducted using either individual-level or aggregated data and can be executed using databases or surveys. For further reading on data sources, see Chapters 3 and 4.

Longitudinal observational studies involve repeated observations of the same variables over time. These may be used to study trends in drug utilization, such as whether the prescribing of inappropriate drugs has changed. Such studies may either examine the same group of people

Table 2.3 Examples of longitudinal observational studies in drug utilization research.

Title	Design	Country
Utilisation of antihyperglycaemic drugs in ten European countries: different developments and different levels [14]	Annual sales of insulin and oral antidiabetic agents were compared between countries using defined daily doses (DDDs)/1000 inhabitants per day as the volume measure	10 European countries
Utilization of anti-Parkinson drugs in Australia: 1995–2009 [15]	Prescription trends were analysed over time by sex, age and type of prescriber	Australia
Impact of socioeconomic status on the use of inhaled corticosteroids in young adult asthmatics [16]	Associations between socioeconomic status and antiasthmatic treatment among young adults were investigated through the linkage of different registers	Denmark
Trends in the prescription of antidiabetic medications in France: evidence from primary care physicians [17]	Changes in patient characteristics and trends in prescribing of antidiabetic drugs over time were investigated	France
Psychotropic drug use among Icelandic children: a nationwide population-based study [18]	A nationwide study on the paediatric population, calculating prevalence and incidence of use by year and psychotropic drug group	Iceland
Trends in antibiotic use among outpatients in New Delhi, India [19]	Seasonal trends in antibiotic use were assessed using structured patient exit interviews at private retail pharmacies, public sector facilities and private clinics	India
National trends in long-term use of antidepressant medications: results from the US National Health and Nutrition Examination Survey [20]	Duration of antidepressant use and correlates of long-term use were assessed using data from six cross-sectional surveys, as a representative sample of the general population in the United States	United States
Four-year trends of inappropriate proton pump inhibitor use after hospital discharge [21]	A retrospective review of the medical records and pharmacy prescription database of a large regional insurance carrier. The frequency of inappropriate proton pump inhibitor use was calculated at discharge each year	United States

over time (closed cohort) or be designed as repeated cross-sectional studies, in which an independent sample is collected repeatedly to represent the population for that time period (open/dynamic cohort). Examples of the two different approaches are given in Table 2.3.

Study designs for analytical drug utilization studies

Analytical studies aim to gain a deeper understanding of the explanatory factors behind utilization patterns or the effectiveness or safety of medication use.

The analytical studies providing the greatest evidence are cohort studies and case–control studies. These designs offer advantages over the cross-sectional and longitudinal observational studies by introducing a clear temporal dimension between the exposure and the outcome (disease occurrence or drug utilization). The major differences between cohort and case–control studies lie in the selection of study subjects and in the assessment of the effect in the future (cohort study) versus the cause(s) in the past (case–control study). In a cohort study, subjects are selected based on their exposure and are followed prospectively over time, whereas in a case–control study, subjects are identified on the basis of the presence or absence of the outcome and the exposure prior to the event is investigated looking back into the past (Figure 2.1). In drug utilization research, cohort and case–control studies can be used to evaluate the impact of different factors influencing drug prescribing, dispensing or consumption. They are also commonly used in traditional pharmacoepidemiological studies to evaluate the positive or negative effects of medication use.

In a ***cohort study***, subjects are included on the basis of exposure (or lack of exposure). Basically, cohort studies are studies in which exposed and non-exposed subjects are followed over a period of time to investigate the effects of the exposure. More traditional pharmacoepidemiological studies focusing on safety and effectiveness will prospectively investigate the effect of drug exposure on the development of disease. In more specific drug utilization research, the effect of exposure to an influencing factor (e.g. information campaigns, frequent hospitalizations) on drug utilization patterns in subsequent years can be prospectively studied to determine whether there is an association (Figure 2.1). Nowadays, most cohort studies are conducted using data from existing data sources. In this approach, subjects are followed over time, from exposure to outcome, but all of the data (including baseline and follow-up data) are extracted from databases.

Cohort studies are particularly suitable for examining rare exposures. Other benefits include the potential to monitor multiple outcomes. Consequently, this study design could be a suitable choice in adherence research to assess factors associated with discontinuation, switching or combination of therapy. Cohort studies also allow the measurement of the absolute risk of being initiated on a drug after a given exposure (e.g. hospitalization for a specific disease). Examples of cohort studies in drug utilization research are found in Table 2.4.

In a ***case–control study***, subjects are included on the basis of having the outcome of interest or not. Previous exposure to the factor of interest may then be compared retrospectively between those with (i.e. cases) and without (i.e. controls) the study outcome. Traditional pharmacoepidemiological studies will select diseased (cases) and non-diseased (controls) subjects and will investigate previous exposure to a particular drug in both groups. In drug utilization research, subjects can be included on the basis of whether or not they have (or had) been prescribed/dispensed the drug of interest. An investigation of previous exposure to the factor of interest will then reveal whether there is an association between drug utilization and previous exposure (Figure 2.1). Case–control studies are suitable for studying rare utilization patterns

Table 2.4 Examples of cohort studies in drug utilization research.

Title	Design	Country
Advertising of antihypertensive medicines and prescription sales in Australia [22]	Cohort study investigating the relationship between advertising of antihypertensive medicines and prescription sales	Australia
Benzodiazepine use among older adults with chronic obstructive pulmonary disease: a population-based cohort study [23]	Cohort study describing patterns of benzodiazepine use among older adults with chronic obstructive pulmonary disease	Canada
Impact of BMI and BMI change on future drug expenditures in adults: results from the MONICA/KORA cohort study [24]	Cohort study using data from health surveys to assess the impact of baseline body mass index (BMI) and BMI change on drug utilization and expenditures over 10 years	Germany
Drug treatment in patients with newly diagnosed unprovoked seizures/epilepsy [25]	Cohort study using clinical data from a disease registry linked to drug dispensing data to analyse drug treatment in patients diagnosed with unprovoked seizures	Sweden
Family history of cardiovascular disease and influence on statin therapy persistence [26]	Cohort study analysing discontinuation of statin treatment in relation to family history of cardiovascular disease	Sweden

Table 2.5 Examples of case–control studies in drug utilization research.

Title	Design	Country
The association between prescription change frequency, chronic disease score and hospital admissions [27]	Case–control study assessing the association between prescription changes frequency (PCF) and hospital admissions and comparing the PCF to the chronic disease score	The Netherlands
Aspirin may prevent cholangiocarcinoma: a case–control study from the United Kingdom [28]	Case–control study comparing previous aspirin and nonsteroidal antiinflammatory drug use in patients with cholangiocarcinoma and controls	United Kingdom
Medication regimen complexity and hospital readmission for an adverse drug event [29]	Case–control study comparing the complexity of the discharge medication regimen in patients with a hospital readmission and controls within 30 days after discharge	United States
Extent of uncontrolled disease and associated medical costs in severe asthma – a PHARMO study [30]	Nested case–control study using data on drug dispensing and hospitalizations to identify treatment-related lack of effectiveness	The Netherlands
Inappropriate benzodiazepine use in older adults and the risk of fracture [31]	Nested case–control study comparing the proportion of 'inappropriate' benzodiazepine use, according to the Beers criteria, between fracture patients and controls	The Netherlands
Drug–drug interactions among elderly patients hospitalized for drug toxicity [32]	Nested case–control study analysing the association between hospital admission for drug toxicity and the use of an interacting medication in the preceding week	United States

when researchers specifically search for people with the drug and include them in the study. This was a common strategy when there were no databases available. Today, most case–control studies are conducted using existing data sources, and often within well-defined cohorts; the latter are referred to as ***nested case–control studies***.

Another benefit of case–control studies is the possibility of investigating associations between multiple exposures and drug utilization patterns. Results in case–control studies are presented as odds ratios (ORs), and data collected in a case–control study cannot be used to calculate absolute risks after an exposure, since the sampling fraction is not known. Examples of case–control studies are found in Table 2.5. All these studies have a traditional pharmacoepidemiological focus, analysing the effectiveness and safety of drugs. In theory, the same design could be applied using drug prescribing as the outcome, but in reality these studies are scarce in the literature.

Experimental and quasiexperimental study designs in drug utilization research

In contrast with observational studies, the main characteristic of an experimental study design is the planned introduction of an experimental factor with the intention of studying the effects of this intervention. In drug utilization research, interventions may range from educational outreach visits in general practice to media alarms or reimbursement restrictions. A variety of study designs can be used to evaluate interventions, including randomized controlled trials (RCTs) and quasiexperimental designs (uncontrolled or controlled before-and-after studies and interrupted time series, ITS) [33,34].

The ***randomized controlled trial (RCT)*** has the highest degree of evidence, as it is intended to avoid bias through a randomized selection of the exposed and the non-exposed group, controlled exposure to the experimental factor and a parallel evaluation of the effect of the exposure in the exposed and non-exposed groups. Randomization may be conducted either for individuals or for groups of subjects; the latter design is referred to as a 'cluster RCT'. Cluster RCTs may be conducted in studies of interventions that cannot be directed towards selected individuals (e.g. interventions targeted at primary care practices, including many physicians). The disadvantages of cluster RCTs include their greater complexity in terms of design and analysis and the large number of participants they require, in order to provide high statistical power. Some examples of RCTs designed to evaluate the effect of interventions are given in Table 2.6.

Intervention studies with a quasiexperimental design differ from RCTs in the time sequence of the observations. While in an RCT the exposed and non-exposed groups are studied in the same time frame, intervention studies have a before-after design, with baseline measurements before the intervention and a second set of observations after it. Before-and-after observations can be performed using repeated cross-sectional or cohort study designs (with one data collection at baseline and another after the intervention) or in a longitudinal way (with consecutive measurements before and after the intervention period, in an ITS design).

Uncontrolled before-and-after studies compare drug utilization patterns in a particular setting before and after an intervention has taken place [33]. Any observed differences in utilization are assumed to be explained by the intervention. It is a weak design, since it does not control for secular trends or the impact of other factors influencing drug utilization at the same time as the intervention is carried out. Consequently, a number of uncontrolled before-and-after studies overestimate the effects of interventions [43]. Uncontrolled before-and-after studies should therefore be avoided, and the results of such studies need to be interpreted with caution.

Table 2.6 Examples of intervention studies in drug utilization research. RCT, randomized controlled trial; ITS, interrupted time series; CBA, controlled before-and-after study.

Title	Design	Country
Randomised controlled trial of effect of feedback on general practitioners' prescribing in Australia [35]	RCT	Australia
Changes in use of antidiabetic medications following price regulations in China (1999–2009) [36]	ITS	China
Intensive community pharmacy intervention had little impact on triptan consumption: a randomized controlled trial [37]	RCT	Denmark
Impact of restricted reimbursement on the use of statins in Finland: a register-based study [38]	ITS	Finland
The influence that electronic prescribing has on medication errors and preventable adverse drug events: an interrupted time-series study [39]	ITS	The Netherlands
Can a multifaceted educational intervention targeting both nurses and physicians change the prescribing of antibiotics to nursing home residents? A cluster randomized controlled trial [40]	Cluster RCT	Sweden
Can mass media campaigns change antimicrobial prescribing? A regional evaluation study [41]	CBA	England
A randomized trial assessing the impact of a personal printed feedback portrait on statin prescribing in primary care [42]	RCT	United States

Controlled before-and-after studies are conducted by adding a group not exposed to the intervention to control for other factors influencing the prescribing pattern. These can include seasonal variations in disease patterns, the introduction of new drugs and changes in treatment policies, the marketing activities of pharmaceutical companies and changes in regulatory policies [33]. Appropriate pre- and post-intervention periods are selected and the change in performance is compared between the intervention and control (Figure 2.2a). This study design can be useful in cases where multiple interventions are combined and it is difficult to assign the intervention to a particular point in time. Some examples of studies are presented in Table 2.6.

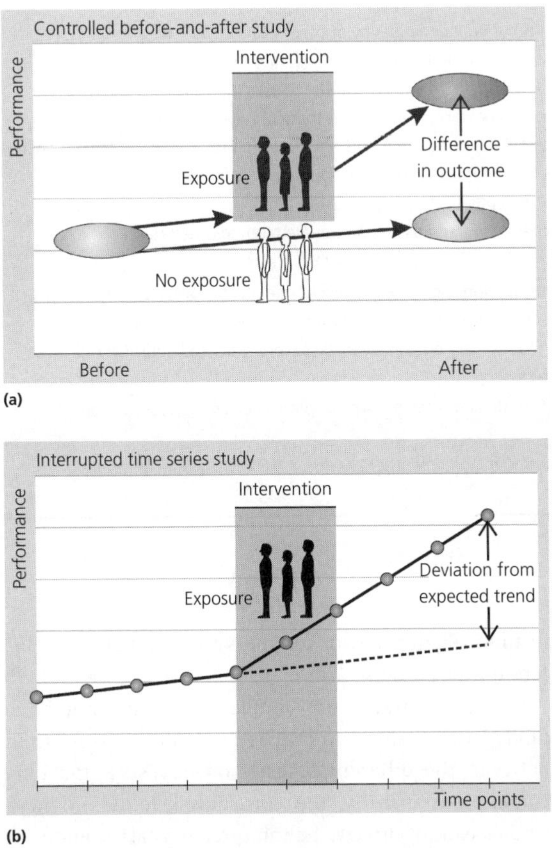

Figure 2.2 Principles of (a) a controlled before-and-after study and (b) an interrupted time series (ITS) study.

The controlled before-and-after design provides stronger evidence than the uncontrolled version. It is important to acknowledge, however, the difficulties in finding comparable control groups in reality. Even in well-matched control groups, performance at baseline can differ. It is also likely that those who participate in an intervention are more motivated than those who decline, and so are likely to change their behaviour to a greater extent. Consequently, controlled before-and-after studies should also be interpreted with caution. A helpful tool for drug utilization researchers in assessing and planning these studies is the criteria for high methodological quality of controlled before-and-after studies recommended by the Cochrane Effective Practice and Organisation of Care (EPOC) [44,45]. These criteria are summarized in Table 2.7.

An ***interrupted time series (ITS)*** is the strongest quasiexperimental design for evaluating the effects of interventions, since it aims to determine whether an intervention has a greater effect than the underlying trend [33]. Data are collected at multiple points in time before and after the intervention to adjust for the underlying trend (Figure 2.2b). The ITS design is particularly useful for drug utilization studies evaluating the effects of interventions for which it is difficult to identify an appropriate control group. These include dissemination of drug formularies, safety warnings and mass media campaigns. Some examples of studies applying this design are presented in Table 2.6.

Segmented regression analysis of ITS data allows the statistical quantification of the effect of the intervention directly and over time; instantly or with delay; and transiently or long-term. It also allows the question of whether factors other than the intervention could explain the observed changes to be determined [46]. An ITS analysis requires data to be collected regularly over time, with a sufficient number of measurement points before and after the intervention, and organized at equal time intervals. Routinely available prescribing data from medical records, dispensing data from pharmacies and claims data from reimbursement agencies are all suitable for ITS, since they are independently collected over a long period of time. For further information on ITS in drug utilization research, see Wagner et al. [46]. The Cochrane EPOC has established a number of criteria for quality assessment of these studies, which are presented in Table 2.7 [44,45].

Table 2.7 Cochrane EPOC quality criteria for controlled before-and-after studies and interrupted time series (ITS) designs. Data from http://epoc.cochrane.org/sites/epoc.cochrane.org/files/uploads/datacollectionchecklist.pdf (last accessed 18 November 2015).

Category	Criteria for high quality
Controlled before-and-after study	
a) Baseline measurement	Performance or patient outcomes measured before the intervention, and no substantial differences present across study groups
b) Characteristics of study and control	Characteristics of study and control providers are reported and similar
c) Blinded assessment of primary outcome(s) (protection against detection bias)	Stated explicitly that primary outcome variables were assessed blindly OR outcome variables are objective
d) Protection against contamination	Allocation by community, institution or practice and unlikely that control group received the intervention
e) Reliable primary outcome measure(s)	Two or more raters with agreement ≥90% or $\kappa \geq 0.8$ OR outcome assessment is objective
f) Follow-up of professionals (protection against exclusion bias)	Outcome measure for ≥80% of professionals
g) Follow-up of patients	Outcome measures for ≥80% of patients
Interrupted time series	
Protection against secular changes	
a) The intervention is independent of other changes	The intervention occurred independently of other changes over time
b) There are sufficient data points to enable reliable statistical inference	At least 20 points are recorded before the intervention and the authors have done a traditional time series analysis (ARIMA model) OR at least three points are recorded pre- and post-intervention and the authors have done a repeated measures analysis OR at least three points are recorded pre- and post-intervention and the authors have used ANOVA or multiple t-tests and there are at least 30 observations per data point
c) Formal test for trend	Formal test for change in trend using appropriate method is reported
Protection against detection bias	
d) Intervention unlikely to affect data collection	Reported that intervention itself was unlikely to affect data collection, e.g. sources and methods of data collection were the same before and after the intervention
e) Blinded assessment of primary outcome(s)	Stated explicitly that primary outcome variables were assessed blindly OR outcome variables are objective
f) Completeness of data set	Data set covers 80–100% of total number of participants or episodes of care in the study
g) Reliable primary outcome measure(s)	Two or more raters with agreement ≥90% or $\kappa \geq 0.8$ OR outcome assessment is objective

Other study designs for drug utilization research

The ***ecological (correlation) study*** is a kind of observational study design that examines associations between exposure and outcome in populations, rather than individuals [47]. Ecological studies in drug utilization research can be used to compare data on dispensed or prescribed drugs with, for example, morbidity or mortality, either for different areas/groups at a certain point in time (Figure 2.3) or for the same population at different times (Figure 2.4).

Ecological studies are simple to conduct but have limited value, since no individual linkage is conducted between the different datasets on exposure and outcome. Consequently, the correlations found in these studies cannot directly be interpreted as associations at the level of the individual. Hypotheses about causation from such studies should preferably be tested in more advanced analytical drug utilization studies or RCTs.

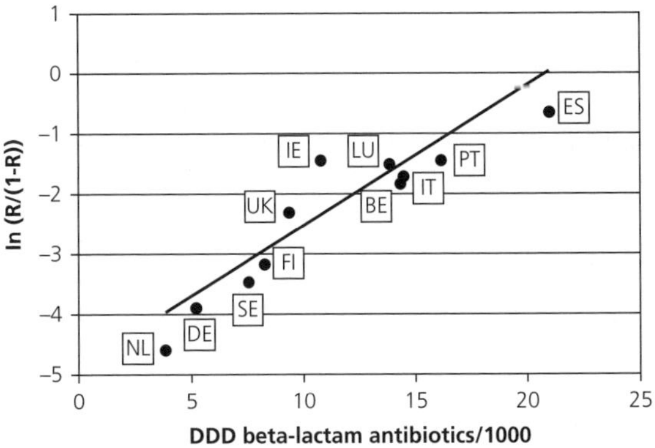

Figure 2.3 Ecological study comparing outpatient sales of antibiotics with resistance to penicillin among invasive isolates of *Streptoccus pneumoniae* patterns in 11 European countries [39]. Antimicrobial resistance data are from 1998–99 and antibiotic sales data are from 1997. DDD, defined daily dose; BE, Belgium; DE, Germany; FI, Finland; IE, Ireland; IT, Italy; LU, Luxembourg; NL, The Netherlands; PT, Portugal; ES, Spain; SE, Sweden; UK, United Kingdom.

Source: Bronzwaer et al. 2002 [48]. Copyright 2002 Centers for Disease Control.

Some examples of ecological studies in drug utilization research are presented in Table 2.8.

Validation studies generate evidence that observed utilization patterns are a good presentation of 'true' drug consumption. Such studies can either validate the drug exposure as recorded in a database or a survey or use the drug utilization data to validate other clinical information. Validation studies may be conducted through linkage between data on drug exposure collected from different sources, such as by combining prescription records with patient reported data. Since all datasets on drug utilization have their limitations, such studies are urgently needed.

Assessment of validity requires a decision on which method of determining drug utilization should be considered 'true' or the 'gold standard'. The agreement between other methods and the gold standard may be described in terms of sensitivity and specificity. Sensitivity is the ability of a given method to correctly classify an individual as using a drug, while specificity is the ability of a method to correctly classify an individual as drug-free (Figure 2.5). A method's positive predictive value (PPV) is the percentage of patients classified as having the drug who actually use the drug.

Poor sensitivity may indicate that patients are receiving drugs that cannot be detected using the method under investigation (i.e. patients actually using the drug are not identified). This can occur when patients borrow drugs from relatives or purchase drugs over the Internet. Problems of poor specificity may indicate that many patients do not actually take the drugs they are prescribed or dispensed.

A common problem in validation studies is to decide what would be the golden standard. Examples

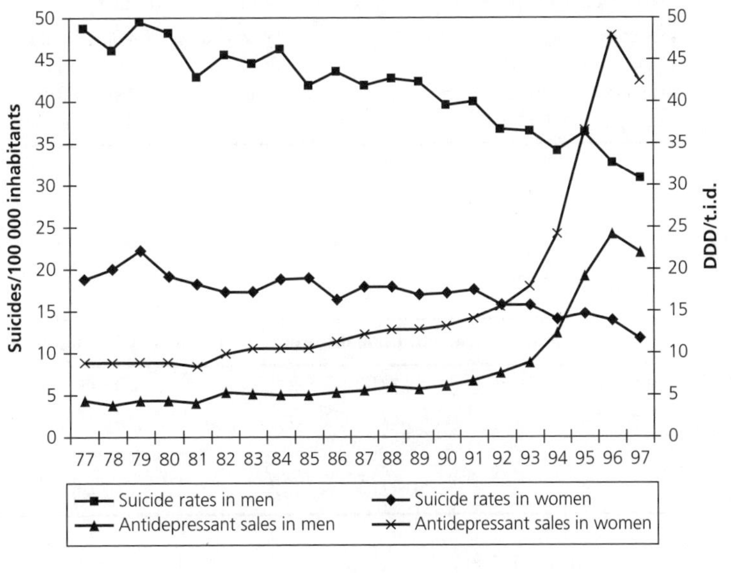

Figure 2.4 Ecological study comparing suicide rates with antidepressant sales rates in men and women 15 years of age and older in Sweden from 1977 to 1997. DDD/t.i.d., Defined Daily Doses per 1000 inhabitants per day.

Source: Carlsten et al. 2001 [49]. Reproduced with permission from John Wiley and Sons.

Table 2.8 Examples of ecological studies in drug utilization research.

Title	Design	Country
Antidepressant utilization and suicide in Europe: an ecological multi-national study [50]	Trends of antidepressant sales and suicides were compared over time, adjusted for gross domestic product, alcohol consumption, unemployment and divorce rates	29 European countries
The effect of universal influenza immunization on antibiotic prescriptions: an ecological study [51]	Changes in rates of influenza-associated respiratory antibiotic prescriptions before and after universal immunization were compared between provinces	Canada
Gender equity and contraceptive use in China: an ecological analysis [52]	Association between indicators and women's contraceptive use were compared across provinces	China
Trends in coronary heart disease mortality and statin utilization in two European areas with different population risk levels: Stockholm and Sicily [53]	Time trends in cardiovascular morbidity were compared with statin utilization in two regions	Italy and Sweden
Bisphosphonate use and increased incidence of subtrochanteric fracture in South Korea: results from the National Claim Registry [54]	Registry data on fractures were compared with utilization patterns of bisphosphonates over time	South Korea
Association between respiratory prescribing, air pollution and deprivation, in primary health care [55]	Prescribing patterns were compared cross-sectionally between different clinics in relation to their deprivation index	United Kingdom
What was the immediate impact on population health of the recent fall in hormone replacement therapy prescribing in England? Ecological study [56]	Time trends in hormone replacement therapy (HRT) prescribing were compared with hospital admissions, incidence and mortality from breast cancer, colorectal cancer and hip fracture	England
Association between unemployment rates and prescription drug utilization in the United States, 2007–2010 [57]	Prescription sales of different drugs over time were compared with labour statistics in different states to examine the association between unemployment and utilization	United States

	Patients using the drug	Patients NOT using the drug
Test positive	a (TP)	b (FP)
Test negative	c (FN)	d (TN)
	Sensitivity:	Specificity:
	a/ (a+c)	d/ (b+d)

Figure 2.5 Calculation of sensitivity and specificity in drug utilization studies. TP, true positive; FP, false positive; FN, false negative; TN, true negative.

of validation studies in drug utilization research include a comparison between a prescription registry and questionnaires in measuring psychotropic drug exposures among elderly Finns [58] and a comparison between a registry-based assessment and parental-reported use of asthma drugs in Swedish adolescents [59]. Validation studies may also be used in the development of quality indicators. This is further described in Chapter 12.

The ***case-population design*** may provide, albeit approximately, early estimates of the magnitude of the risk of rare adverse drug reactions [60]. Particularly when a new drug is released for marketing, its safety regarding the risk of rare adverse events is substantially unknown. In a case-population study, cases are collected using different possible approaches, such as spontaneous reporting and hospital admissions, and related to the population of a specific area (at the regional or national level). The distinctive feature of this methodology is that the control group is not a set of individuals specifically selected for the purposes of the study but an aggregated *comparator* consisting of population data [61]. With respect to the two-by-two table, for the control group, cells b and d are expressed not in terms of number of individuals but in person-time units, the latter representing the sum of exposed (PT_E) and not-exposed (PT_{NE}) time in the source population (Table 2.9).

Under the null hypothesis (no association between exposure and event), and in the absence of selection bias, the ratio of exposed to not-exposed cases (a/c) is not expected to differ from the ratio of exposed person-time to not-exposed person-time (PT_E/PT_{NE}) in the source population. The 'case-population' OR can be estimated as follows: $[(a/c)/(PT_E/PT_{NE})]$.

The case-population design was used in a study by Roujeau et al. [62] investigating the risk of toxic epidermal necrolysis (TEN) related to the use of cotrimoxazole, carbamazepine, phenobarbital, piroxicam and allopurinol. The authors identified all cases of TEN occurring in France from 1981 to 1985. The sales data for each drug, expressed in defined daily doses (DDDs), made it possible to estimate the exposed person-time in the general population. In all cases, the ORs computed by means of the case-population approach and sales data showed a significant association between exposure to the study drug and occurrence of TEN and were roughly of the same order of magnitude as the corresponding relative risks subsequently estimated with an actual control group [63,64].

Table 2.9 Two-by-two table for case-population studies.

	Diseased (cases)	Population (person-time)
Exposed	a	PT_E
Not exposed	c	PT_{NE}
Total	n	PT_{POP}

Prescription sequence symmetry analysis may be useful as a screening tool for unknown adverse drug reactions. The study design is strictly based on drug utilization patterns and can be performed with a small amount of resources. This method was first used by Hallas [65] in order to determine whether there was evidence of depression provoked by beta-blockers. All new users of both beta-blockers and antidepressants during a predefined period were identified. If beta-blockers did not cause depression, this particular population would show equal numbers of people starting each drug first. A depression-provoking effect of beta-blockers would generate an excess of persons starting beta-blockers first; that is, a nonsymmetrical distribution of prescription orders. The Hallas study provided clear evidence against a causal association between beta-blockers and antidepressant use (rate ratio = 1.09; 95% confidence interval (CI): 0.95–1.26).

Prescription sequence symmetry analysis has since been repeatedly used to confirm or reject suggested associations across various therapeutic areas [66,67]. An interesting application of this study method was recently published by Lai et al. [68], who attempted to provide information on the potential risks of sulpiride treatment of schizophrenia. These authors performed analyses to test associations between sulpiride (index drug) and adverse events suggested or confirmed in other antipsychotics, including extrapyramidal syndromes, metabolic syndromes (such as hyperglycemia), hyperprolactinemia and cardiac arrhythmias (Figure 2.6). Among 1680 total incident sulpiride users, 568 had also been prescribed an anticholinergic agent, with 367 in the 'index → marker' group and 201 in the 'marker → index'

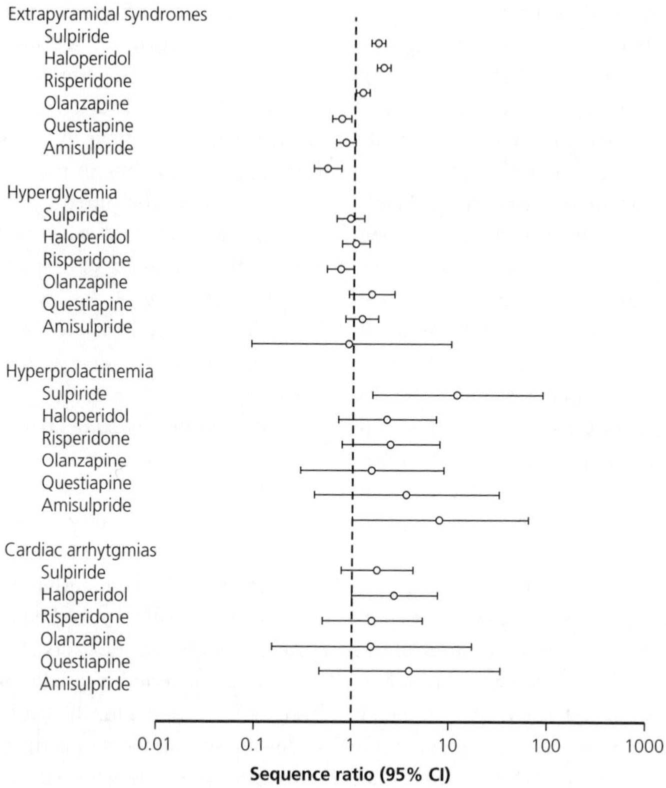

Figure 2.6 Adverse events of sulpiride and other antipsychotics.

Source: Lai et al 2014 [68]. Copyright: © 2014 Lai et al.

group. The results, based on anticholinergic use as a signal of extrapyramidal syndromes, found sulpiride significantly associated with this adverse event, with risk only slightly lower than haloperidol but higher than risperidone. With regard to nonsulpiride drugs, results were largely consistent with previous studies, proving the validity of the prescription sequence symmetry analysis methodology.

Reporting drug utilization studies

Finally, when reporting results from drug utilization research studies, it is important to follow good practice for reporting. A number of guidelines that were developed in the field of epidemiology can be applied in drug utilization research, including Strengthening the Reporting of Observational studies in Epidemiology (STROBE) [69], Consolidated Criteria for Reporting Qualitative Research (COREQ) [70], the Reporting of Studies Conducted using Observational Routinely Collected Data (RECORD) statement [71], the ENCePP Guide on Methodological Standards in Pharmacoepidemiology [72] and the ISPE Guidelines for Good Pharmacoepidemiology Practices (GPP) [73].

CHAPTER 3

Primary data collection for drug utilization research

Tatiana Chama Borges Luz[1] & Evalill Nilsson[2]

[1]*René Rachou Research Center, Oswaldo Cruz Foundation, Brazil*

[2]*The Research and Development Department of Local Health Care, Östergötland Region, Sweden*

KEY POINTS

- Primary data are original data that, for specific research purposes, have never previously been gathered or been structured to be accessible to research, whether in a particular way or at a certain point in time.
- Primary data collection for drug utilization research can involve both individuals (e.g. patients, physicians, pharmacists) and documents (e.g. prescriptions, medical records, dispensing records). Data are collected mostly through standardized structured questionnaires and forms designed for data extraction and abstraction.
- Standardized structured questionnaires are an established set of questions used to capture a variety of self-reported observations from individuals. These instruments are less prone to interviewer bias and are efficient with regards to time, acceptance and cost.
- To be used as patient-reported outcome measures regarding perceived health status, functional status or health-related quality of life, such questionnaires must, in addition to standard requirements concerning validity and reliability, meet requirements regarding responsiveness and clinical significance.
- There are many techniques available for the administration of questionnaires: in person, by telephone, by post or online, depending on, among other things, the amount and type of information needed, the target population and financial constraints.
- This chapter covers the main advantages and disadvantages of various data sources, instruments and techniques that should be taken into account when proposing and conducting drug utilization research.

Introduction

Drug utilization research aims to describe patterns of drug utilization at various levels of the health care system, whether national, regional, local or institutional, and to evaluate drug use at a population level, linking drug utilization data to figures on morbidity, treatment outcome and quality of care, with the ultimate goal of assessing the rationality of drug therapy [1].

Due to the wide scope of drug utilization research, a considerable variety of data sources can be used. These can generally be classified as ***primary data sources*** or ***secondary data sources*** [2–4]. Primary data sources are original data collected directly by an investigator conducting research for a particular purpose [2,3]. Secondary data sources encompass already-collected data that have not (usually) been generated for a specific research purpose, but can be adapted to the analysis of a new research question [3,4]. Data collected for research differ significantly from data collected for non-research purposes [5], because the former rely on the use of the scientific method to generate and/or test hypotheses and provide analysable results.

The primary and secondary data available for drug utilization research vary from country to country. In general, these data are obtained from sales registries, procurement records, warehouse drug records, prescriptions, medical records, dispensing records, pharmacy

Drug Utilization Research: Methods and Applications, First Edition. Edited by M. Elseviers et al.
Published 2016 by John Wiley & Sons, Ltd.

stock records and health professionals, as well as from the patients themselves. More than one source may be suited to the investigation of a given research question.

Regardless of the data source chosen, it is necessary for the investigator to define their research method, the study population and the data collection instruments. Measures to limit potential bias and confounding should be employed to ensure the study's quality and validity [6].

This chapter defines basic concepts and terminology around primary data sources and discusses some theoretical and practical aspects that underlie data collection for drug utilization research purposes. It also discusses basic concepts of patient-reported outcome measures (PROMs).

Identifying primary data sources for drug utilization research

'Data' is the plural form of 'datum', which means a collection of items of information or a body of observations recorded directly from empirical facts [7,8]. Primary data are, then, original data that, for specific research purposes, have never previously been gathered or structured to be accessible to research, whether in a particular way or at a certain point in time [2,4].

Primary data collection can involve both individuals (e.g. patients, physicians, pharmacists and other stakeholders participating in drug utilization process, such as relatives, regulators or third-party payers) and documents (e.g. prescriptions, medical records, dispensing records and laboratory data). Each source of information has strengths and limitations that should be taken into account when planning and evaluating a particular study. The features of some of these sources and a few points to consider when utilizing them are presented in this section.

Patient-reported data

Patients are drugs' end users, and their perspectives on the use and the outcomes of drugs are therefore unique and crucial. Several aspects of the process of drug utilization should be investigated from the user's point of view, including adherence to medication regimen and information on factors that might relate to drug effects; aspects related to access to drugs, affordability problems and other barriers to use; and information on consumption of over-the-counter (OTC) drugs, drugs taken intermittently for symptom relief and medications bought without a prescription. Studies that collect information directly from the patient also have the potential to generate a contextual understanding of users' experiences and how they interpret them [9].

As with all person-reported data, patient self-reports are subject to recall bias [10,11], misinterpretation or misinformation, reporting bias and nonresponse [12]. However, careful development of the questions will help prevent these issues from becoming a problem (see later).

There are situations where proxy respondents are necessary substitutes, notably for older persons with cognitive impairment or other chronic debilitating conditions and for younger children. In these situations, information from proxies may be more reliable and valid than that given by the users themselves. However, issues to consider regarding use of proxies include the 'proxy effect' (under-reporting due to lack of knowledge) and the 'saliency principle' (over-reporting those events the proxy considers to be most relevant).

Health care providers-reported data

Health care providers, especially physicians, nurses and pharmacists, can provide useful information on the understanding of health care practices and the settings in which care is delivered, as well as on the process of medicine use. From these professional perspectives, it is also possible to gather information on experiences, knowledge, attitudes, opinions and behaviours related to pharmacotherapy and patients. When using health professionals as information sources for research purposes, however, the possibility of the 'Hawthorne effect' should be considered: the knowledge that we are under study often influences our behaviour [8].

Physicians can provide relevant information about factors underlying prescribing behaviour and other important topics, such as adherence to guidelines and sources adopted for drug information. They can vary in their pharmacological decision-making according to their specialty, training, experience and tradition, as well as regulations in their place of work [13,14]. Personal characteristics, such as age and sex, can also influence prescription practices [13,14]. Data obtained from physicians may highlight various aspects related to care and pharmacotherapy, such as the patient–physician relationship, communication skills, awareness of drug cost and continuity of care. It is noticeable, however, that physicians are often recognized as a professional group from which it is difficult to obtain high response rates, especially in surveys, which can introduce bias and uncertainty in study results [15–19]. There is some evidence that using monetary incentives and recorded delivery/registered mail are effective strategies by which to obtain excellent response rates when surveying physicians [17].

Nurses are another professional group that can be viewed as an appropriate study population for drug utilization research, given their direct level of patient contact and their collaborative relationship with physicians. Questions regarding medication storage, preparation and administration can be evaluated from the nurses' perspectives and practices [20]. In countries that have legislation giving prescriptive authority for selected drugs to nurses, it is also possible to evaluate variation in their prescribing patterns and the reasoning behind their therapeutical choices [21].

Over the years, the pharmacy profession has evolved from its traditional drug-focused basis to a more patient-focused outlook. As such, pharmacists, as part of the health care team, are another potential study population for drug utilization research, providing valuable information around medication-related problems, dispensing practices and the pharmacist–patient relationship. Authors such as Braund et al. [22], Pedersen et al. [23], Schommer & Gaither [24], Hughes et al. [25] and Worley et al. [26] have published evidence on these topics, and there are many other examples in the literature. In some countries, pharmacists are also authorized to prescribe medication, and this practice too can be the subject of investigation, as in Hutchison et al. [27].

Prescriptions, medical records and dispensing records

In many countries across Europe and North America, there has been a considerable increase in the use of nationwide electronic systems for the storage of prescriptions and medical records [28,29]. In many other parts of the world, however, handwritten documents are still used, or, where there is an electronic system, it is only for local data input. Nevertheless, prescriptions and medical records are useful, alternative and complementary primary data sources for drug utilization research.

These sources can be used, for instance, to evaluate aspects of health provision and drug use, information on prescribing habits and other aspects related to patient care. Rigour and objectivity in the use of these sources are necessary in order to ensure accuracy of information and maintenance of quality standards in the data collection process.

Prescriptions are instructions written by a medical professional that authorize a patient to be provided a medicine or treatment. These documents are also a communication medium between prescribers and pharmacists. Prescriptions permit the study of national/regional/local variation in prescribing practices, facility-prescribing patterns and physicians' preferences regarding treatment [30]. Several research projects are currently being conducted with these type of data [31–34]. Data from paper-based prescriptions are subject to many limitations for research purposes, notably, inaccuracy, illegibility and incompleteness [35,36].

Medical records provide useful information on individuals' treatment, medical history and clinical profile [37]. Information contained in hospital and ambulatory care records may be used as the sole source of data or in tandem with other sources. However, the data contained in these documents are recorded in a non-standardized manner by a large variety of health care professionals, as they are not designed for research purposes [38]. Further, patient-reported information is often lacking, or is limited to the reporting of the main presenting symptom(s). When clinical information is stigmatized (e.g. sexual history, alcohol or drug use) or difficult to assess systematically in primary care settings (e.g. depression), it is often underreported in the medical record [37]. Data from medical records may also be limited by illegibility, incompleteness or inaccuracy [37].

Dispensing records may also be a source of data in drug utilization research, providing information on drug(s) prescribed and their dose(s), the number of items per prescription, cost and the quantity of medications dispensed (i.e. the number of items prescribed that were actually supplied). These data may be obtained from records kept at pharmacies [39]. Again, such data may be limited by illegibility, incompleteness or inaccuracy.

Collecting valuable primary data in drug utilization research

The crude primary data are the core of any study, but their successful utilization depends largely on how they are collected and managed. The research question precedes the type of data required. The data source must be chosen carefully to ensure that it can address the study question, that it has a sufficient number of observations and that it provides all the variables needed (e.g. exposures, confounders, outcomes) [5]. It is also important to bear in mind that primary data collection can be quite time-consuming and expensive [2].

Before starting a new data collection, it should first be determined whether a suitable data source already exists [29]. For drug utilization research purposes, for instance, secondary data (usually) stored in electronic databases is considered the best choice to answer a variety of questions [40]. However, such data are not available for all populations worldwide, and they do not always contain complete drug exposure information, including initiation date, discontinuation date and reason for discontinuation [41]. Further limitations include a lack of information on whether the drug is actually taken (see Part 3, Section E).

In many research situations, the only way to obtain the necessary information is by means of a new data collection. In other situations, primary data collection may be needed to enhance the extent and the quality of information already available in automated registers. Bias and other factors that could distort information from register-based data can be evaluated through comparison with data obtained directly from self-reports and medical records [42–46].

A variety of quantitative (e.g. cross-sectional, case–control, cohort) and qualitative (e.g. in-depth interviewing) techniques is available for the collection of primary data [3,4]. To ensure validity through minimization of bias and confounding, it is important to consider the type of data required for research purposes, the strategies to be used to gather the data, what kinds of expertise, skills and staffing are necessary and the time and financial resources needed [47].

Harwood et al. [47–52] propose six iterative and reciprocal practical steps for implementing and collecting quality primary data, as summarized in Table 3.1.

Table 3.1 Practical steps in the collection of quality primary data.

Step	Scope	Implementation
Define a clear purpose for collecting data	Clarify the need to collect primary data and the types of data required for a particular research project (this step can be revisited many times before data collection begins)	Acknowledge personal motivation for taking on the study Gather other perspectives from key stakeholders Write a clear, concise and informed problem statement Create a list of research purpose options, focused on realistic goals or purposes
Select the most feasible data collection mode	Select the best possible strategy that allows the most accurate and unbiased data in support of the study's findings and conclusions to be obtained	Consider: • The study's purpose: related to the degree to which statistically accurate research estimates are needed • The study's complexity: related to expected data needs (depending on study population, study instruments and how the collected data will be managed and stored) • Available resources: monetary, physical and intellectual capital, such as funding; staffing; materials, incentives and equipment; expertise and expert services; time; physical space in which to carry out the work • Target population: related to literacy, hearing abilities, cultural expectations and language barriers • Research team: related to the ability to carry out data collection tasks
Develop protocols for collecting data	Establish a tailored, written protocol for the study, avoid collection bias	Study data collection mode details carefully Map out the general planned workflow of all data collection activities Create and maintain a working/day-to-day protocol manual
Design forms and instruments	Determine the key principles behind designing high-quality data collection forms	Review the study's purpose and concepts List the main concepts to be measured Seek existing measurement items and instruments in order to locate question items that might be adapted/used Write new items, if necessary Organize items to enhance the natural flow and improve response accuracy Pre-test the instrument

Step	Scope	Implementation
Train the personnel for data collection	Manage activities related to staffing that occur prior to and during data collection	Hire the right personnel: take into account their particular experience, skills, expertise, attitudes and behaviours Train the staff on the study's purpose and quality assurance for assigned tasks Monitor the staff for adherence to protocols and quality control of data collection Conduct a pilot study
Manage collected data	Format and prepare data, control data quality, secure data and finalize a data file for analysis	Format: format data for use by analytic software for either quantitative or qualitative research approaches Prepare: precode, code and enter data into a data file Control: train the staff and set up procedures to check for errors and to ensure data quality Secure: secure data to protect participants and study data Finalize: create a final and locked data file that can be copied and used for analysis

Instruments and forms for primary data collection in drug utilization research

Quality control for primary data collection is built into the study design [4,6]. The investigator must establish *a priori* means by which to collect accurate and precise data on drug utilization and other relevant information required for the investigation. A qualitative approach is an option for drug utilization research, in which interview guides are frequently used for data collection (for more information, see Chapter 13). Another methodological option is to adopt a quantitative approach, collecting data by way of standardized structured questionnaires and using forms designed specifically for data extraction and abstraction [37,50,53]. This section will focus mainly on instruments used for quantitative studies.

Data extraction and abstraction

Data extraction is the process of reviewing and transferring documents for a specific research data collection form. Data abstraction is the process of reviewing source materials in order to summarize and interpret their meaning in the context of the research purpose. Several situations involve both abstracting and extracting data activities. Blood pressure values, for instance, are extracted from the chart and transferred to a research data collection form. Physician notes on disease symptoms and treatment, on the other hand, may be reviewed, summarized and abstracted on the same data collection form [50].

Obtaining data from these processes offers advantages such as accessibility, cost and flexibility [54]. On the other hand, there may be variations in data collection processes and interpretation, especially when multiple investigators are involved. These problems can be minimized with rigorous training of the abstractors/extractors and by the use of a standardized extraction/abstraction protocol, or by masking the investigators to the study hypotheses: double-review of the first 10 charts abstracted, in addition to a monthly double-review and simultaneous data collection and cleaning [37,50,55].

Structured questionnaires

Structured questionnaires are an established set of questions designed to elicit responses that can be converted into measures of the variables under investigation [8,56]. These instruments capture a variety of individuals' self-reported observations and can contain specific measures designed to capture complex constructs that cannot be measured directly, such as knowledge, attitudes, emotion and cognition [57,58]. The advantages of a structured questionnaire are that the researcher controls the theme and format of the data collection, it is less prone to interviewer bias and it is efficient with regards to time, acceptance and cost [4,53,59]. However, structured questionnaires do not allow any adaption of the questions to the context of a particular individual, and they are thus subject to some criticism for not being sufficiently individual-centred [60].

Designing a questionnaire requires the development of a set of statistically valid and reliable questions by which to measure and quantify the phenomena under study [57,61]. An ideal questionnaire should be clear, unambiguous and logically structured, so that it keeps the respondent interested and cooperative [56,61].

With respect to questionnaire formatting, the questions can be closed or open-ended, with participants responding in their own words. Mixed questions can also be employed [53]. Open-ended questions are preferred when there is a large number of possible answers or it is important to capture all of the details in the information provided [58,62,63]. It is also possible to use open-ended questions to capture numerical information, such as age, weight and height.

Closed questions contain either binary (yes/no) response options, mutually exclusive multiple response options or more than one response option (e.g. 'tick all that apply'). It is also possible to add an option that allows the respondent to present an answer that is not already included (e.g. 'other:___'). Data may exist at different levels, as either nominal (reflecting qualitative differences in the construct being measured) or ordinal (e.g. using fixed choice response formats options that imply a ranked order, like in Likert-type response scales) responses. For more information on this, see Chapter 9.

The question stem (i.e. the statement or question to which a response is sought) should focus on a single construct and should contain fewer than 20 words, in order to be easy to understand and interpret. It is also recommended that the questions should be written in a socially and culturally sensitive manner, avoiding definite terms such as 'always', 'none' or 'never' and abbreviations or complex terminology. They should also be nonjudgmental and unbiased [63]. The wording of the questions and the number and order of response categories can influence the responses obtained, and should be carefully tested [62,63]. Several textbooks on how to develop questionnaires are available [64,65].

In order to allow for meaningful comparisons across studies, it is recommended that standardized pre-tested questions and validated and reliable instruments be used [4,66]. Today, several hundreds of questionnaires are available for free online, or for purchase for a license fee. These are especially useful for information on topics such as basic demographic data, common health problems/disease symptoms, health-related behaviours (e.g. alcohol consumption, smoking and diet) and health and quality of life. Since some topics range from very simple constructs, such as pain intensity, to more complex ones, such as health-related quality of life, questionnaires correspondingly vary from single- to multi-item, and even multi-domain, instruments. The more advanced instruments, which use more or less complex algorithms to yield different kinds of summary scores, are often referred to as 'scales'.

Box 3.1 Key points to consider during the evaluation of an instrument.

- Validity: the extent to which the instrument measures the construct(s) it is intended to measure.
- Reliability: the degree of internal consistency (i.e. the logical relation between items) and the repeatability with which the instrument measures the attribute it is designed to measure (i.e. the results are the same for repeated measurements under similar conditions).
- Respondent and administrative burden: the questionnaire should be easy to use and to respond to.
- Availability of electronic versions of the questionnaire (if applicable).

It is important to note that many of these instruments are context-specific, so the simple translation of a questionnaire may lead to misinterpretation due to cultural and language differences. Therefore, it is recommended, when using instruments developed in other countries or cultural contexts, to simultaneously carry out a cross-cultural adaptation and validation [67]. For a review on how to perform a cross-cultural adaptation of questionnaires, see Epstein et al. [67]. Some general points to consider during the evaluation of an instrument are presented in Box 3.1 [57,68,69].

Questionnaires in drug utilization research

Specifically with respect to drug utilization research, there is no standardized methodology for measuring drug utilization, and data on the reliability and validity of questionnaires are scarce in the literature [70,71].

Questionnaire design in drug utilization is an object of concern, since it may lead to different estimates of drug exposure [70,71]. In their systematic review of the evidence regarding the effect of questionnaire design on the recall of pharmacological treatments, Gama et al. [70] identified four core methodological problems, all of which require careful questionnaire design to ensure unbiased evaluations: the acute versus chronic nature and the severity of a disease; the number of drugs available for a single condition; the number of drugs that include the same active ingredients; and the varying complexity of treatment regimens. Some key strategies by which to handle threats to the validity of questionnaire design in drug utilization studies are presented in Box 3.2, while a range of question types is summarized in Table 3.2 [59,72].

Box 3.2 Strategies for handling threats to the validity of questionnaire design in drug utilization research.

- Definition of what constitutes a drug: the definition must be clear, or else some drugs (e.g. contraceptives, analgesics, natural products and products for topical use) may not be reported by respondents.
- Types of question: questions involving indication for use and drug-specific questions increase the prevalence estimates for drug utilization compared to open-ended questions.
- Recall period: there is no consistency in the literature regarding the ideal recall period. Some authors recommend a 2-week (14–15 days) period, to enable comparison across studies regarding prevalence estimates of medicine utilization.
- Drug packaging and prescriptions: asking for the drug packaging or prescriptions is a way of validating data on drug utilization.
- Memory aids: when drug names and indications or pictures are used as memory aids, recall of drug utilization is improved.

Table 3.2 Formats, examples and advantages of common questions in drug utilization research.

Format	Description	Example[a]	Advantages
Open-ended questions	The expected response is in the respondent's own words	Could you tell me about any unusual symptoms that occurred after you took your medicines? Describe the symptoms in your own words. How did they affect your day-to-day life?	Allows participant's expression of their feelings and experiences. These questions are useful for narrative, qualitative information
Category questions	The response options are a set of mutually exclusive categories. The respondent can select only one response	Thinking about the cost of the medicines prescribed to you in the past 30 days (please, tick the one that best matches your answer): • I did not have a completed prescription, because it was too expensive • I skipped doses to make the drug last longer • I took smaller doses to make the drug last longer • I did not have financial problems in getting my prescription • I did not need any medication	Allows participant's choice among a set of options. These questions are useful for getting a sense of the participant's general attitude. They are easily understood and quick to complete
List options	The response options are not mutually exclusive. The respondent can select more than one response	Has a doctor or nurse ever told you that you have (please, tick all that apply): • hypertension • arthritis • high cholesterol • atherosclerosis • congestive heart failure • back pain • pulmonary disease	Allows participant's choice among a set of options. Easily understood and quick to complete
Rating scales (e.g. Likert scale)	The response options represent the respondent's attitudes, beliefs and experiences of a topic	Currently, cost savings are the only aim of International Non-Proprietary Name prescribing (please, tick the box that best matches your answer): Strongly agree / Agree / Neutral / Disagree / Strongly disagree	Allows participant's choice among a ranked option from a list often on a 5- or 7-point scale. These questions are good for participants who can understand linear scales

[a] Question examples extracted and adapted from Chaipichit et al. [73], Luz et al. [74], Van Bever et al. [75] and Piette et al. [76].

Questionnaires for patient-reported outcomes

This section describes the specific requirements of a questionnaire if it is to be used for the measurement of patient-reported outcomes and how to develop a measurement strategy. Patient-reported outcomes are important for gaining knowledge about a patient's views of the outcomes of treatment. Although the term 'outcome' is very broad, in the context of outcomes of medical treatments it usually denotes changes in self-reported health status, health-related quality of life, symptoms or functional ability, as they pertain to the treatment in question. Furthermore, it may also include satisfaction with the care or with the treatment received [77].

PROMs are used to capture patient-reported outcomes in a systematic way. A PROM is usually a self-administered valid and reliable structured questionnaire. Although the established validity and reliability of a questionnaire is always important, there are additional aspects to take into account when using it as a PROM. First, a PROM must provide evidence of acceptable responsiveness; that is, it must be able to detect relevant changes in health status, health-related quality of life, symptoms or functional ability after treatment. The response alternatives in the questionnaire must allow the respondent to describe not only pronounced but also more subtle improvements and deteriorations. Furthermore, the distribution of responses should be even, in order to avoid floor and ceiling effects (too many respondents scoring near the bottom or top, respectively, hampering variance in the data). Second, the results must be capable of interpretation in a clinically meaningful way. That is, it is not enough for a change to be statistically significant: it must also be perceived as noticeable and important to both patients and clinicians. It is helpful to establish the minimum change in the scale score of a health measure that can be recognized as an improvement for the patient group under study, both in reality and statistically [78].

PROMs are commonly divided into two main types – generic and disease- or symptom-specific measures – according to their purpose. Disease-specific instruments may be more responsive than generic, supposedly because they target the health aspects directly subjected to the treatment in question [79,80]. Generic instruments, on the other hand, have the potential to identify unanticipated health problems, and furthermore give the possibility of comparing health impact across patient groups [79].

Two of the best known generic instruments used as PROMs today are the EQ (EuroQol)-5D [81–83] and the SF (Short Form)-36/RAND-36 [84]. The EQ-5D is a short instrument that provides a summary index originally intended to be used for health economic evaluations. Items were chosen to reflect common health problems experienced by patients and, therefore, relevant treatment goals (outcomes) for health care providers. The EQ-5D also contains a numeric rating scale (0–100) that measures general health, sometimes called the EQ-5D VAS (Visual Analogue Scale). The SF-36/RAND-36 is a multidomain instrument with eight subscales, reflecting the World Health Organization (WHO)'s definition of health as physical, mental and social well-being and functional ability. It is also possible to calculate an index value analogue to the EQ-5D index from the SF-36 (called the SF-6D), also to be used for health economic evaluations [85]. For more information, see Chapter 42.

Although it is impossible to give any general recommendations on which questionnaire (whether generic or disease-specific) to use as the PROM of choice, since its suitability will vary with the context, matching the intended outcomes of interest with an adequate PROM is crucial [82]. Guidance is available for the selection of measurement instruments [86–88]. A systematic approach, consisting of several steps, such as that suggested by Snyder [88], is preferable, as it ensures the validity of the measurements (see Box 3.3).

The field of drug research and development has been a forerunner in the use of PROMs, especially in clinical trials. Today, PROM use is expanding into product safety evaluations and effectiveness research. This expansion is not without its challenges. An increased use of PROMs requires implementation of larger patient-reported outcome programmes, which may be costly and logistically advanced. The issue of bias (due to missing data from the very ill or hard-to-reach patients) must be better addressed. Furthermore, to facilitate comparisons, some standardization of measurements would be desirable [89,90].

Box 3.3 Strategies to ensure the validity of measurements.

- Choose relevant health outcomes. Use existing research and clinical knowledge to identify domains of interest.
- Develop a conceptual framework based on the identified domains, outlining all relevant relationships.
- It may be necessary to choose multiple PROMs in order to cover all targeted domains. In instances where a suitable PROM is not available, adaptations of related PROMs may be necessary, or, as a last resort, a new questionnaire may have to be developed. Do not rely on the fact that a PROM is said to measure a specific domain; always examine and evaluate all the items individually. Aim at receiving a balance between patient- and clinician-reported data and generic and disease-specific PROMs.
- Deviations from the optimal strategy may be necessary to ensure feasibility (e.g. prioritizing only some of the identified domain or substituting a longer and more precise PROM for a shorter one). A good way to enhance feasibility is to involve patients in the choice of PROMs and the creation of the measurement strategy.

Modes of primary data collection for drug utilization research

Another challenge for researchers is to choose among different modes of data collection. Interview is one of the most frequently used techniques in both quantitative and qualitative research [37,53]. The interview can be administered in person or by phone. Another mode is the self-administered questionnaire, via post or online [53]. The technique chosen depends on the amount and type of information needed, the target population, investigator time, financial constraints and whether test properties have been established [63]. Table 3.3 summarizes some useful information on modes of data collection for drug utilization research purposes.

Table 3.3 Modes of data collection: advantages and disadvantages.

	Advantages	Disadvantages
In-person interview (also called 'face-to-face interview')	Presence of the interviewer, who can hold the responder's attention, clarify questions, etc. Lengthy, complex instruments are easier to administer in a face-to-face interaction in which the interviewer can clarify questions, present visual aids, probe responses and assess respondent fatigue Minimizes nonresponse Maximizes the quality and completeness of the data collected	Requires trained interviewers Provides limited time in which to supply an answer Privacy issues: respondents may adjust their answers to survey items in order to report socially appropriate or desirable responses Difficult to monitor for quality High costs
Telephone interview	Cost-effective compared to in-person interview High response rates High item completion rates Opportunity to probe the respondent to get more complete answers Faster delivery of data compared to face-to-face interview	Requires trained interviewers Proliferation of cell phones makes it difficult to reach potential responders Legislative restrictions Increasing reluctance to participate in telephone surveys among the general public
Self-administered questionnaire (including Web-based)	Generally less expensive compared to in-person or telephone interviews Can be distributed in person, by post or online If administered via the Internet, the answers are entered directly into the database Respondents are more likely to report sensitive or illegal behaviour than in in-person or telephone interviews	Respondents/proxies must be able to read and write (and, in some cases, have access to a computer and the Internet) Special care must be taken with how the questions are worded and how the questionnaire is formatted: the questionnaire must be completely self-explanatory Acquiescence response bias Can be time-consuming and inconvenient for research goals Susceptible to misunderstandings and nonresponse bias Requires correct postal/email addresses for each participant May require a telephone helpline

Ethical considerations

Most types of primary data collection require the approval of an institutional review board/research ethics committee to ensure the adequate protection of human subjects and institutions [91–93].

The central ethical issues are to protect the rights, welfare and anonymity of research subjects and to ensure the scientific quality of the ongoing investigation. Concerns about respect for autonomy, nonmaleficence, justice and confidentiality should also be considered. In order to protect human subjects, informed consent is required from all research participants. The informed consent must emphasize the voluntary nature of participation in the research and that the participant's decisions will be based on an adequate understanding of what the research entails [91,93,94].

In studies involving data extraction/abstraction from documents (e.g. prescriptions, medical records, dispensing records, etc.), it is not always possible to obtain the direct consent of participants. In such cases, authorization for access to the data is given by the responsible institution. Several works addressing the ethics of health research are available [91–93].

Conclusion

When the available evidence is limited, conflicting or uncertain, the collection of primary data may be considered for drug utilization research. Many potential sources of primary data are available, and there are therefore a number of factors to consider when deciding which will be used and how much data should be collected.

This chapter discussed the main advantages and disadvantages of various data sources, instruments and techniques that should be taken into account when proposing and conducting drug utilization research.

CHAPTER 4

Secondary data sources for drug utilization research

Irene Eriksson[1] & Luisa Ibáñez[2]

[1]Centre for Pharmacoepidemiology, Department of Medicine, Karolinska Institutet, Sweden

[2]Foundation of the Catalan Institute of Pharmacology (FICF), Spain

KEY POINTS

- Data useful for drug utilization studies are routinely gathered for administrative purposes and as part of patient care. Drug utilization researchers can answer a wide range of questions using secondary analyses of aggregate- and individual-level drug utilization data.
- Aggregate-level data, such as sales data, can be used to describe and forecast drug utilization and expenditure and to evaluate the impact of pharmaceutical policies and interventions. Cross-national comparisons of drug utilization and ecological studies can be performed based on analyses of aggregate-level data.
- Secondary analyses of individual-level data, including electronic health records, pharmacy dispensing and reimbursement databases, as well as patient registries and population health survey data, are performed frequently in drug utilization research. Individual-level data can be used to estimate the incidence, prevalence and duration of drug use and to follow drug utilization patterns over time.
- Linking records from different data sources allows a more comprehensive patient and prescriber profile to be built, enabling researchers to study the appropriateness of drug use and factors potentially influencing drug utilization. Record linkage can also help complete drug exposure histories across different health care settings.
- Data quality is of importance in database analyses of drug utilization. Before conducting analyses of secondary data, the drug utilization researcher should obtain a thorough knowledge of the unique characteristics of the data source and weigh the strengths and limitations of its use in answering the research questions of interest.

Introduction

Large amounts of data useful for drug utilization studies are routinely gathered for administrative purposes and as part of patient care. These are called ***secondary data*** as, unlike primary data (see Chapter 3), they are collected for purposes other than answering specific research questions. Secondary data analyses have been conducted in drug utilization research for decades, and, given the improving quality of collected data and methodological advances in database analyses, they will continue to play an important role in the future.

To provide an overview of different processes leading to the generation of drug utilization data, it may help to discuss them in the context of the pharmaceutical supply chain, beginning with the manufacturer and concluding with the patient (see Figure 4.1). Most drugs are provided to hospitals and community pharmacies either directly from the manufacturer or through wholesalers. At this step, aggregate-level data on sales (from the manufacturer/wholesaler/pharmacy) or purchases (from the purchaser/payer; e.g. data on acquisition of drugs by hospitals and community pharmacies) are collected. ***Aggregate-level data*** reflect the total amount of drugs in a system and carry no information on how these drugs are distributed among individuals. Once the drugs reach the pharmacy, drug dispensing data at the individual level may become available

Drug Utilization Research: Methods and Applications, First Edition. Edited by M. Elseviers et al.
Published 2016 by John Wiley & Sons, Ltd.

(in some countries, however, drugs may also be purchased by medical practices for onward distribution to patients, thereby bypassing pharmacies). ***Individual-level data*** provide information about individual patients. For those dispensed drugs that are reimbursed, payers collect reimbursement claims data for administrative purposes relating to billing. Health care providers are another important source of data on drug utilization – information on drugs prescribed to patients is documented in ambulatory care and in hospitals using either paper or electronic health records (EHRs). Health care providers may also report information on selected drugs to patient registries. Finally, patients themselves can provide information on drugs they take, although patient-reported data have so far rarely appeared in databases, with the exception of some patient registries and population health surveys.

This chapter gives an overview of secondary data sources used in drug utilization research: sales data, EHRs, pharmacy dispensing databases, reimbursement data, patient registries and population health survey data. It also provides examples of drug utilization studies based on analyses of secondary data.

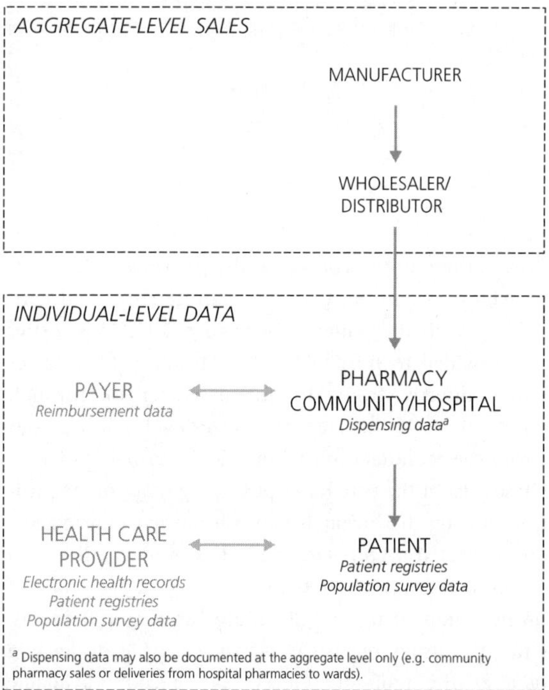

Figure 4.1 Drug utilization data in the pharmaceutical supply chain.

Sales data

Sales data provide information about sales of drugs from manufacturers or wholesalers to community and hospital pharmacies and nonpharmacy outlets with permission to sell or supply drugs. The main data elements collected are the drug name and the amount sold. Both prescription and over-the-counter (OTC) drugs are usually included in the sales statistics, but it may not be possible to distinguish between the two. Furthermore, aggregate sales data can also be obtained from pharmacies (prescription and OTC drugs) and grocery stores (OTC drugs).

Sales data have been used in drug utilization research for decades. In the 1970s, when no other readily available databases existed, manufacturers collected detailed sales data, which were eventually made available to researchers, who used them to study drug utilization. In 1975, Bergman the et al. published a paper describing utilization of insulin and oral antidiabetic drugs in Northern Ireland, Norway and Sweden [1], and, in the following year, the Nordic Council on Medicines produced the Nordic Statistics on Medicines using the Anatomical Therapeutic Chemical (ATC) classification system and the defined daily dose (DDD) methodology [2]. These two publications are examples of early drug utilization studies conducted based on secondary data (see Chapter 1 for more about the history of drug utilization research). The ATC classification system and the DDD as a measuring unit have since been used frequently to convert and standardize drug quantity data (e.g. packages, tablets, injection vials, bottles), readily available in sales data, into crude estimates of clinical exposure to drugs (see Chapter 6 for a detailed description of the ATC/DDD methodology) [3].

Most countries keep records of drug sales, often collected at a national level. These data can be obtained from health authorities [4,5] and from private companies such as IMS Health, a well-known commercial source of drug utilization data [6]. An overview of European secondary data sources performed by the Pharmacoepidemiological Research on Outcomes of Therapeutics by a European ConsorTium (PROTECT) indicates that aggregate sales data are widely collected across Europe [4,5]. In the United States, the IMS National Sales Perspectives database documents sales data for prescription drugs, OTC products and some self-administered diagnostic products. Data collected include volume of dollars and quantities moving from manufacturers into various outlets within all states. In Canada, the IMS CompuScript database contains data on prescriptions sold from approximately two-thirds of all Canadian retail pharmacies. Sales data (collected by authorities or by companies such as IMS Health) may be the only secondary source available to studies conducted in regions where other databases are not yet established or not accessible.

While sales data are crude and can only give an overview of total drug utilization and trends over time, they are useful for a number of applications within drug utilization research. Examples of studies based on sales data include assessment of the impact of pharmaceutical policies and interventions [7], cross-national comparisons of drug utilization [8,9], forecasting of drug utilization and expenditure [10], estimation of denominators by which to calculate the incidence of adverse drug reactions [11,12] and descriptive analyses of drug utilization, including OTC drug use [13]. Furthermore, sales data can be used in ecological studies to measure drug use within a certain geographical area, as in studies of opioid prescription sales and overdoses [14], antidepressant sales and suicide rates [15] and antibiotic use and resistance [16].

Electronic health records

Health care providers document a wide range of information, both for administrative purposes and as part of patient care. A patient health record usually contains information about the patient and health care provider, services provided (including the date, setting and reason for seeing the patient) and drugs prescribed. It may also document the outcome of care and treatment. Historically, patient records were kept in paper form, but in recent decades more and more data have been stored electronically. Today, EHRs comprise many components that work together to capture, create, share, maintain and store an accurate and complete patient health record (see Table 4.1) [17]. However, using EHRs for research requires implementation of a system for structured data capture, as well as functions to ensure the accuracy and completeness of data collected. These features have been lacking, impeding the use of EHRs in research [18].

Table 4.1 Examples of administrative and clinical data recorded in electronic health records (EHRs).

Administrative data	Clinical data
Demographic data (e.g. patient name, sex, date of birth, address)	Diagnoses, physical examination and assessment, diagnostic and laboratory tests and reported findings
Unique patient identifier (e.g. health insurance number)	Procedures performed for diagnostic, exploratory or definitive treatment
Legal data (e.g. consent for health care services signed by the patient)	Recommendations, treatment plans and progress notes
Data relating to the payment of fees for services provided (e.g. source of payment, health care insurance number, registration dates)	Drugs prescribed (e.g. drug name and code, prescription date, dosage instructions; for hospital EHRs, date and time of drug administration and administered dose)
Data on the doctor or other health care professional providing services to the patient (e.g. name, qualifications)	Patient medical history (e.g. past and present illnesses and medication use, family medical history, social history and habits, including risk factors (e.g. smoking and alcohol consumption)) Nursing notes (e.g. blood pressure measurement, height and weight) Additional health information (e.g. fitness, vaccinations, immunizations, OTC medication, other health care resources used (e.g. osteopathy))

While the adoption of EHRs across health care settings may so far have been hampered by usability issues [19] and the cost of implementation and maintenance [20], it can be seen that governmental policies and incentives [21] stimulate the use of health information technology and will continue to do so in the future [22]. While EHRs are already increasing in use across wealthier countries, their adoption is expected to rise in low- and middle-income countries as they gain experience from pilot EHR implementation programmes [23].

Primary care practices may use EHR systems to generate patient prescriptions, thereby automatically documenting every drug prescribed to patients within the practice. Prescription data documented in EHRs therefore reflect the behaviour of the prescriber rather than the patient, who may or may not fill the prescription at a pharmacy [24,25], and indeed may not actually take the medication even if the prescription is filled. Since EHRs are usually contained within a given primary care practice or hospital, they may therefore provide incomplete drug utilization histories for patients who receive care from multiple prescribers located in different practices and health care settings, as well as for patients who change health care providers. It follows that inaccuracy in the assessment of a true denominator may make the calculation of incidence and prevalence figures difficult. While health care providers can record information on risk factors, such as body mass index (BMI), smoking and alcohol consumption, these data may often be missing, and their recording can be heavily influenced by health care policies and incentives. Furthermore, it has also been noted that sicker patients may have more complete EHR records [26]. Some information (e.g. dosing instructions and clinical notes) is usually recorded as free text, and special techniques (e.g. natural language processing) are required to process this. Consequently, secondary analyses of EHR data can pose a number of methodological challenges.

Despite these limitations, EHR-based databases represent an important source of drug utilization data, particularly for researchers interested in studying prescribing patterns. Drug data in primary care EHRs contain information on drugs prescribed to patients, while hospital EHR data may include additional information on the administration of drugs, such as infusion start and end times, interruptions and the total administered dose [27]. Furthermore, EHRs may contain a wealth of clinical information, including diagnoses, procedures, laboratory data, lifestyle habits and family history, giving the opportunity for more elaborate drug utilization studies to be conducted, as well as studies of drug effectiveness, safety and cost in the real world [28].

The value of clinical information stored in EHRs has long been established. In the late 1980s, researchers witnessed the creation of the first primary care EHR-based research databases in the United Kingdom, where general practitioners play a gatekeeper role in the health care system [29–31]. Nowadays, there are a number of such databases there, including the Clinical Practice Research Datalink (CPRD) (previously known as the General Practice Research Database, GPRD) [32], The Health Improvement Network (THIN) [33] and QResearch [34].

Examples of EHR-based research databases in other countries include the Integrated Primary Care Information (IPCI) Database in the Netherlands [35], the Skaraborg Primary Care Database in Sweden [36], the Electronic Medical Record Administrative data Linked Database (EMRALD) in Canada [37], the Health Search Database [38] and Pedianet [39] in Italy and the Base de datos para la Investigación Farmacoepidemiológica en Atención Primaria (BIFAP) database [40] in Spain. National research networks that bring together information from EHRs also exist in the United States, such as the American Academy of Family Physicians National Research Network (DARTnet) [41], the Centricity Healthcare Users Research Network (CHURN) [42] and the Veterans Health Information Systems and Technology Architecture (VistA) [43]. Examples of drug utilization studies based on some of these data sources are provided in Table 4.2.

While EHRs in hospitals are becoming more and more common, there are relatively few published studies based on hospital EHR data (see selected examples in Table 4.3) [47]. As EHRs are typically implemented in stages, some hospital information may be documented on paper and some stored electronically, making data

Table 4.2 Examples of drug utilization studies based on primary care electronic health record-based research databases.

Data source	Study
Clinical Practice Research Datalink (United Kingdom)	Opioid prescribing for cancer pain during the last 3 months of life: associated factors and 9-year trends in a nationwide United Kingdom cohort study [44]
The Health Improvement Network (United Kingdom)	Trends in depression and antidepressant prescribing in children and adolescents: a cohort study in The Health Improvement Network (THIN) [45]
Centricity Health Care User Research Network (United States)	Antidepressant medication use for primary care patients with and without medical comorbidities: a national electronic health record (EHR) network study [42]
Integrated Primary Care Information (The Netherlands)	Use of tiotropium Respimat Soft Mist Inhaler versus HandiHaler and mortality in patients with COPD [46]

Table 4.3 Examples of drug utilization studies based on hospital electronic health record (EHR) data.

Data source	Study
Hospital EHR data (Karolinska University Hospital, Stockholm, Sweden)	Extraction of electronic health record data in a hospital setting: comparison of automatic and semi-automatic methods using anti-TNF therapy as model [48]
Hospital EHR data (Ajou University Hospital, Seoul, South Korea)	A quantitative method for assessment of prescribing patterns using electronic health records [49]
Hospital EHR data (the National Eye Centre, Singapore)	Trends in age-related macular degeneration management in Singapore [50]

completeness an issue. Furthermore, EHR systems often vary from hospital to hospital, and sometimes several systems are implemented within a single hospital (e.g. neurology and oncology clinics may not use the same system to document data), which poses a barrier to collecting data at a the population level and restricts analyses to data from a single hospital, or a number of hospitals that use the same EHR system [27].

Data from hospital EHRs can be integrated into research databases alongside other data and made available to analysts and researchers. Examples of such databases include the Cerner Health Facts Database [51], the Premier Perspective Database [52] and the Pediatric Health Information System [53], all in the United States. EHR data can also be integrated across specialties, such as in the IMS LifeLink Electronic Medical Record Database, which is based on EHR data from participating general practitioners and specialists [54,55].

Pharmacy dispensing data

Data on dispensed drugs are documented in pharmacies for both administrative and clinical reasons (e.g. to monitor for drug–drug interactions). Pharmacy dispensing databases, unlike the reimbursement data discussed in the next section, normally register all dispensations of prescription drugs regardless of the drug's reimbursement status.

In the case of a community pharmacy dispensing database, recorded drugs are prescription drugs that have been dispensed to patients in ambulatory care. Drugs dispensed in hospitals would typically not be included in the database. Documented drug data usually include the name of the dispensed drug (brand and International Nonproprietary Name (INN)), ATC code, pharmaceutical form, strength, amount dispensed, dates of prescribing and dispensing, total cost, reimbursed cost and patient cost. Dispensing databases may include unique patient identifiers, as well as information on the patient's age, sex and place of residence. Some information about the prescriber (specialty and practice location, e.g. primary care or hospital clinic) may also be present [56]. Some databases (e.g. the Prescribed Drug Register in Sweden) also record information on dosage instructions, but these are typically documented as unstructured free text, and text mining techniques would thus be required in order to extract useful information [57].

Pharmacy dispensing databases also exist in hospitals, although hospital pharmacy databases often limit the documentation of data to the amounts of drugs dispensed to individual wards, with no information on how these drugs are distributed to individual patients. The Hospital Pharmacy Audit of IMS Health is an example of hospital pharmacy dispensing data that also can be linked with individual-level NHS Hospital Episode Statistics data [58].

Individual-level pharmacy dispensing data may be considered the best secondary data source available for the study of drug utilization in patients, as it generally documents all drugs prescribed and dispensed regardless of the reimbursement status and irrespective of who the prescriber is (see Table 4.4 for examples of drug utilization studies based on pharmacy dispensing data). As the patient has to come to a pharmacy to fill the prescription, these data are one step closer to estimating actual drug exposure than are prescribing data from EHRs. However, if the patient has alternative ways of obtaining medications (e.g. drugs purchased abroad, drugs dispensed outside a pharmacy (such as in long-term care facilities), free drug samples), these will not be captured in the database. Furthermore, uncertainty around whether or not the patient will take the received drug as indicated always remains: even if a drug is dispensed, it may not be taken by patient, or it may be taken but not as indicated (see Chapter 36).

Table 4.4 Examples of drug utilization studies based on pharmacy dispensing data.

Data source	Study
Prescribed Drug Register (Sweden)	Differences in drug utilisation between men and women: a cross-sectional analysis of all dispensed drugs in Sweden [59]
Danish National Prescription Registry (Denmark)	Use of exenatide and liraglutide in Denmark: a drug utilization study [60]
PHARMO Record Linking System (The Netherlands)	Prescribing of rosiglitazone and pioglitazone following safety signals: analysis of trends in dispensing patterns in the Netherlands from 1998 to 2008 [61]
Community pharmacy dispensing data (Gisborne, New Zealand)	Allopurinol use in a New Zealand population: prevalence and adherence [62]

In some countries, aggregate drug utilization data, derived from individual-level pharmacy dispensing records, are made publicly available. For example, the National Board of Health and Welfare in Sweden (based on data from the Prescribed Drug Register) and the Danish State Serum Institute (based on data from the Register of Medicinal Product Statistics) publish drug utilization statistics online. Statistics reported include volume sold, both in total (number of DDDs) and per 1000 inhabitants per day, and total number of users. These data can be aggregated by a number of pre-specified variables, including age, sex and region.

Reimbursement data

Health care services are funded and delivered differently around the world. Health care delivery and financing can be simplified as a transfer of resources: the provider transfers health care resources to patients, and patients or third-party payers (public or private) transfer financial resources to the provider. The third-party payer collects revenue from the population it covers, and the collected funds are used to pay for health care services provided [63]. In some countries, prescription drugs are funded only for selected groups of the population (e.g. the elderly) [64,65], and a combination of public and private prescription drug plans is used for other population groups. Third-party payers, both public and private, collect reimbursement claims data in order to keep track of what services are provided and how they are reimbursed. The funding mechanism defines what is reimbursed, and consequently what is documented in the records of the payer.

Drug reimbursement data typically contain unique identifiers for the patient, prescriber and pharmacy dispensing the drug, the drug name (brand and INN) and ATC code, the strength, dosage form, quantity dispensed, dates of prescription and dispensation and number of days supplied, as well as reimbursement-related information, such as patient copayment and total drug cost. In some countries (e.g. Hungary), reimbursement data also include information on indication, as an ICD code is written on prescriptions and electronically registered when the drug is dispensed to the patient [66]. The presence of unique patient and prescriber identifiers allows researchers to link information on patients (e.g. age, sex, socioeconomic and clinical data) and prescribers (e.g. age, sex, academic and professional credentials, specialty and practice location) that is typically stored in separate databases [67]. Similarly, unique pharmacy identifiers may be used to retrieve information about a particular pharmacy (e.g. community/hospital pharmacy, location).

Reimbursement data have been used for secondary research purposes for decades (see Table 4.5 for examples of drug utilization studies based on reimbursement data). They are deemed highly accurate for information on the utilization of reimbursed drugs dispensed to insured patients. Like pharmacy dispensing databases, reimbursement data capture drugs prescribed by multiple prescribers; however, drugs documented in the database are limited to those that are reimbursed. Reimbursement data share the limitations of pharmacy dispensing databases (see previous section). Additionally, changes in copayment may lead to distortions of information on exposure; for example, drugs that cost less than a copayment may not be recorded (e.g. in Finland). The population captured in reimbursement databases is limited to insured individuals only, and thus the generalizability of studies conducted using reimbursement data may not be absolute [68]. Furthermore, in countries with a lack of insurance coverage continuity (e.g. the United States), patient medical histories may be fragmented, as patients move in and out of systems as their insurance eligibility changes [69]. However, in some countries,

Table 4.5 Examples of drug utilization studies based on reimbursement data.

Data source	Study
Pharmanet (Belgium)	Exposure of the elderly to potential nephrotoxic drug combinations in Belgium [71]
Estonian Health Insurance Fund database (Estonia)	Off label use of prescription medicines in children in outpatient setting in Estonia is common [72]
Manitoba Health administrative data (Canada)	Ten years of antipsychotic prescribing to children: a Canadian population-based study [73]
Health Insurance Review and Assessment Service database (South Korea)	Utilization of evidence-based treatment in elderly patients with chronic heart failure: using Korean Health Insurance claims database [74]
Medicare Part D data (United States)	Geographic variation in outpatient antibiotic prescribing among older adults [75]
Pharmaceutical Benefits Scheme (PBS) reimbursement data (Australia)	Australian population trends and disparities in cholinesterase inhibitor use, 2003 to 2010 [76]
National Health Insurance Research Database (Taiwan)	A retrospective study on the usage of cough and cold medications in viral respiratory tract infections in Taiwanese children [77]
IMS LifeLink Health Plans Claims Database (United States)	Long-term patterns of use and treatment failure with anticholinergic agents for overactive bladder [78]

insurance coverage can be close to 100% of the population (e.g. South Korea, Japan, Taiwan), increasing the generalizability [70].

Given these limitations, analyses of reimbursement data pose a number of methodological challenges. These data are nonetheless a great source of information on drug utilization in routine clinical practice. Reimbursement data have been used to describe drug utilization patterns and assess the appropriateness of drug use [71–77], to assess factors influencing drug utilization, to study the safety and effectiveness of drugs in clinical practice [78] and to evaluate the effect of health policy interventions, such as reimbursement restrictions [79].

Patient registries

A patient registry is an organized system that collects uniform data to evaluate specified outcomes for a population defined by a particular disease, condition or exposure, and that serves predetermined scientific, clinical or policy purposes [80]. Based on the population selection criteria, patient registries can be classified into two types: disease registries (patients diagnosed with a certain condition, e.g. rheumatoid arthritis) and drug or product registries (patients exposed to pharmaceutical products, e.g. TNFα inhibitors). Patient registries can be set up and maintained by health care professionals and academic researchers (e.g. the national Swedish Multiple Sclerosis Registry [81] and the British Society for Rheumatology Biologics Register [82]) or by manufacturers (e.g. the Global Registry on Long-Term Oral Antithrombotic Treatment in Patients with Atrial Fibrillation, GLORIA-AF) [84,85]. Alternatively, post-marketing registries can be established by regulatory agencies to monitor the appropriateness of prescribing of new drugs (e.g. the registries of the Italian Medicines Agency) [86].

Information collected in a patient registry is defined by the registry's purpose and scope. It usually includes data reported by health care providers (e.g. patient sociodemographic characteristics, diagnoses, laboratory tests, procedures and prescribed drugs) and by patients (e.g. patient-reported outcomes, including quality-of-life measures). Data on drugs can include indication, drug name, classification code, dose and dosing regimen, route of administration, prescription, start and end dates, reasons for discontinuation (if the drug treatment is stopped) and information on adverse events. Data can either be collected as primary data or imported from an existing electronic database, such as a pharmacy dispensing database or EHR. Data collection typically starts at the baseline visit, with continued longitudinal recording during the process of routine patient care. Registries may also include patient and health care provider identifiers, thereby allowing for record linkage.

In drug utilization research, data from patient registries have been used to describe drug utilization patterns over time [87], to assess variations in drug use [88] and to monitor drug safety and effectiveness [89–93]. For more information about patient registries, see Chapter 29.

Secondary analysis of population health survey data

Data on drug utilization can also be gathered as part of a population health survey or a data collection system run by a government statistical agency in order to obtain information about the health status and behaviour of a population for the purpose of informing policymakers. Population health surveys collect a wide range of information, including data on drug utilization. Collection methods range from self-administered questionnaires to in-person interviews and home medication reviews of medicine cabinets (see Chapter 3). The nature of the survey data requires that researchers performing secondary analyses recognize potential sources of error associated with survey sampling, data collection, nonresponse and missing data [94]. Population health surveys have the advantage of being able to quantify the use of drugs actually consumed by patients, including OTC drugs and herbal supplements, as well as other patient-reported data, such as reasons for not filling prescriptions [95,96].

In the United States, the National Center for Health Statistics (NCHS, part of the Centers for Disease Control and Prevention (CDC)) conducts a number of health surveys, including the National Health and Nutrition Examination Survey (NHANES), the National Ambulatory Medical Care Survey (NAMCS) and the National Hospital Ambulatory Medical Care Survey (NHAMCS). NHANES utilizes a computer-assisted personal interview approach that includes questions on dietary supplement and prescription medication use in addition to a physical medical examination [97]. Secondary analyses of the NHANES data have been performed in order to study prescription and OTC drug utilization across different populations [98–100]. NAMCS and NHAMCS collect information about the provision and use of physician services and hospital outpatient and emergency department services, respectively. NAMCS and NHAMCS data reflecting the prescribing behaviour of surveyed doctors have also been used in drug utilization studies [101–104].

Similar data collection systems exist in other countries. The statistical office of the European Union, Eurostat, implemented the first wave of the European Health Interview Survey (EHIS) in 17 European countries between 2006 and 2009 [105]. The survey collected data on health status, health care use (including self-reported data on prescription and OTC drugs and dietary supplements) and health determinant variables from the population of the European Union. The EHIS data have been used in a number of drug utilization studies [106,107]. Studies based on secondary analyses of population health survey data from other countries, such as Mexico [108] and Australia [109], have also been published.

Record linkage in drug utilization research

Drug data alone can be sufficient to allow studies of drug utilization. For example, if sales data or individual-level pharmacy dispensing or reimbursement data are used, a general overview of drug utilization, including uptake, market share and utilization trends, can be provided. Further, the observed patterns can be evaluated within the context of implemented health policies and interventions. Individual-level pharmacy dispensing and reimbursement data may also contain basic patient-specific information, such as age, sex and place of residence, thus enabling analyses of drug utilization across different patient characteristics. EHR databases gather both administrative and clinical information, which can be helpful in analyses of prescribing patterns. Similarly, patient registries and population surveys usually go beyond collecting drug utilization data exclusively, giving researchers the opportunity to address various questions using a single data source.

However, explaining drug utilization patterns and assessing the appropriateness of drug use often requires more extensive data on patients and prescribers: information that is typically stored in separate databases. Records from different data sources are typically linked in such cases, in order to obtain a more comprehensive patient (or prescriber) profile. Record linkage can also help complete drug exposure histories across health care settings. Importantly, record linkage facilitates more elaborate studies, which can generate knowledge about explanatory factors underlying observed drug use patterns, identify patient and prescriber characteristics that determine drug use and evaluate the benefits and adverse effects of drug use in clinical practice, as well as related economic consequences.

The term ***record linkage*** was first proposed by Dunn in 1946 to describe the process of assembling a person's records of principal events in life into a unique volume [110]. Since then, several methods of record linkage have been proposed and refined, and linkage of administrative data and health records has become common practice in observational research [111–113]. For example, out of 515 published pharmacoepidemiology and drug utilization studies using data from the Nordic prescription databases, 356 (69%) used record linkage between the prescription database and at least one additional data source [114]. Examples of data sources that can be linked to drug data include census data (education, income, occupation), EHRs, reimbursement data, registers (birth, cause of death, cancer, pathology), biobanks and health surveys, to name just a few [115].

Techniques used in record linkage can be classified into two types: deterministic and probabilistic. Deterministic record linkage involves exact one-to-one character matching of linkage variable(s); studies using Nordic data would typically make use of a unique patient identifier that allows linkage of data sources [114]. Probabilistic methods involve calculation of linkage weights based on all observed agreements and disagreements between the data values of the matching variable(s). Typically, personal identification information, such as the names and addresses of subjects, is used. Probabilistic record linkage methods are often relied upon when creating and maintaining research data repositories [116] that assemble individual-level information from sources such as EHRs, laboratory tests, imaging results, pharmacy databases and reimbursement data.

Privacy, confidentiality and security

Use of individual-level data for secondary purposes raises concerns around privacy, confidentiality and security. 'Privacy' refers to the right of individuals to keep information about themselves from being disclosed to others and to be free from surveillance or interference from other individuals, organizations and the government [117]. 'Confidentiality' refers to the issue of how personal data may be held and used by an organization that collects it, what other secondary uses may be made of it and when the permission of the individual concerned is required for such uses [118]. 'Security' can be defined as the procedural and technical measures required to prevent unauthorized access, modification, use and dissemination of data stored or processed in a computer system, as well as to prevent any deliberate denial of service and to protect the system in its entirety from physical harm [119].

Policymaking in both developed and developing countries plays a role in making high-information content available for public health purposes while ensuring protection of privacy [120]. Legislative bodies in the European Union, the United States and other countries have passed laws to regulate the use of identifiable information. The EU General Data Protection Regulation (GDPR) is expected to come into effect in 2018 [121]. In the United States, the Health Insurance Portability and Accountability Act (HIPAA) outlines rules to protect the privacy of individually identifiable health information and to set national standards for the security of electronic protected health information [118,122,123].

While regulations state unambiguously that individually identifiable health information must be protected, the definitions concerning what constitutes de-identified data and what rules regulate the use of such data for secondary purposes are vague [124]. The GDPR, for example, states that the principles of data protection should not apply to anonymous data. However, it is not completely clear what 'anonymous data' mean. The HIPAA elaborates on what is considered de-identified data (18 specific variables need to be removed to render data de-identified) and specifies that de-identified data represent minimal risk and as such are not protected.

However, even the most elaborately de-identified datasets may retain identifiable information, and concerns over the current de-identification standards have been expressed [125]. The volume of data collected today, and the level of detail it contains, is unprecedented, and the notion that de-identifying data in itself protects privacy is outdated. The possibility of re-identifying individuals from such de-identified data has been demonstrated [126], and it may be that it is no longer possible to create truly de-identified or anonymized datasets [127]. Furthermore, striving to achieve a high level of de-identification may limit the utility of the data for research purposes. The ultimate level of de-identification is aggregate-level data, from which the identity of the patient cannot be ascertained. However, the utility of aggregate data for more elaborate analyses is limited. Efforts should therefore be made to ensure that data re-identification does not occur (e.g. by requiring a signed data use agreement that includes provisions on re-identification).

Data quality

Secondary data sources are of value to researchers and decision-makers only if they contain high-quality data [128]. 'Data quality' can be defined as the totality of features and characteristics of a dataset that bear on its ability to satisfy the needs resulting from its intended use [129]. Components of data quality include accuracy and validity, reliability, completeness, legibility, timeliness and accessibility [130]. The value of a database in epidemiological research can be assessed by determining the completeness of registration of individuals (e.g. the proportion of individuals who are correctly classified as exposed), the comprehensiveness of the information registered (e.g. variations in coding, incompleteness in coding of variables collected or of variables not collected, proportion of missing data), the size of the data source (population coverage), the registration period, accessibility, availability and cost, the data format (e.g. available age categories) and record linkage (the presence of unique identifiers) [131].

Before conducting secondary analyses of administrative or clinical data, the researcher should be familiar with the process of data generation and with the context and health care environment in which the data were collected. As errors can arise at different stages of the data collection process (e.g. coding, entering, transferring, editing and extraction of data) and the presence and influence of these errors may change over time, knowledge of the validity of the data is required before a research project is carried out [68]. Familiarity with the unique data characteristics of each dataset and experience in using analytic techniques specific to large volumes of data are essential. Quality assessment results may be available either from the database holder or from published articles [132]. Hence, a literature search for validation studies of the data source can be helpful. In recent years, there have been a number of studies performed to assess the validity of data recorded in secondary data sources [33,133,134]. This can be done by comparing the variable of interest with an external source, preferably one considered the gold standard (see Chapter 2) [135,136]. Furthermore, when analysing secondary data, researchers often rely on algorithms to identify patients with various diseases or exposures. It is therefore advisable that validation studies of these definitions are also carried out. If no studies assessing the validity of data have been conducted, the researcher should consider performing one, although inevitably this will have cost/resource implications.

The European Network of Centres for Pharmacoepidemiology and Pharmacovigilance (ENCePP) Guide on Methodological Standards in Pharmacoepidemiology points out the importance of quality control (ensuring that the defined standards on study quality assurance procedures are followed) during and after data collection [137]. The Guidelines for Good Database Selection and Use in Pharmacoepidemiology Research also discuss quality and validation procedures [132]. Extended information on the rules, procedures, roles and responsibilities involved in quality assurance and quality control for observational studies is available in the US Food and Drug Administration (FDA) guidelines [138].

CHAPTER 5

Classification systems for drugs and diseases

Marit Rønning[1] & Stuart McTaggart[2]

[1]*WHO Collaborating Centre for Drug Statistics Methodology, Norwegian Institute of Public Health, Norway*

[2]*National Health Service for Scotland, United Kingdom*

KEY POINTS

- Classification and terminology systems are important for standardizing the way that information is recorded and enable information to be aggregated, allowing meaningful comparisons.
- A basic principle of a good classification system is that there is only one code for each medicinal product. This allows drug utilization data to be aggregated without a single product being counted more than once.
- The Anatomical Therapeutic Chemical (ATC) system meets this principle and is the standard for international comparisons of drug utilization, although other systems may be widely used within individual countries.
- Proper knowledge of the benefits and limitations of any classification system is crucial to appropriately analysing and interpreting drug utilization data.
- All classification systems must be updated regularly, and reference to the version used should always be given when data are published.

Introduction

If drug utilization studies are to be reliable, they will have to adhere to strict methodological standards, the most basic of which continue to be the use of a common drug classification system and of an international unit of measurement

D. Capellá, 1993 [1]

The need for validated drug classification systems in drug utilization research has been evident since the very beginning of the era, in the late 1960s. The main conclusion from one of the first studies was that in order to measure drug use, it is essential to have both a classification system and a unit of measurement [2]. A drug classification system represents a common language for describing the range of drugs available in a country or region and is a prerequisite for national and international comparisons of drug utilization data, which have to be collected and aggregated in a uniform way [3].

Electronic health records (EHRs) can provide information on the context of drug use, and disease classifications are included in some of the prescription databases now available for drug utilization research. Additionally, the increased use of record linkage in drug utilization studies in recent years requires that researchers also have knowledge of the various medical terminology/classification systems used in these databases, most of which have separate categories for medicinal substances.

This chapter will briefly describe various drug classification systems and other classification systems relevant for drug utilization research. The Anatomical Therapeutic Chemical (ATC) system will be discussed in most detail, as this is the preferred classification system in drug utilization studies [1,3].

ATC

Brief history: caretakers and decision-makers

The ATC classification system was developed as a tool for drug utilization research in the 1970s by Norwegian researchers in close collaboration with the then newly formed Drug Utilization Research Group (DURG)

Drug Utilization Research: Methods and Applications, First Edition. Edited by M. Elseviers et al.
Published 2016 by John Wiley & Sons, Ltd.

network (see Chapter 1). International interest in the ATC classification (and the defined daily dose (DDD) unit; see Chapter 6) quickly grew, largely through the work of the DURG network. In the early 1980s, the system was recommended by the World Health Organization (WHO) as the international standard for drug utilization studies and in 1982 the WHO Collaborating Centre for Drug Statistics Methodology (WHOCC) was established, tasked with the responsibility of coordinating the development and use of the ATC/DDD system. In 1996, the WHOCC was recognized as a global centre responsible for maintaining the system and establishing new entries in the ATC classification. The centre, located at the Norwegian Institute of Public Health, works in close collaboration with an international expert group appointed by the WHO headquarters in Geneva. All decisions regarding new ATC codes, new DDDs and changes to the system have to be approved by this expert group (the International Working Group for Drug Statistics Methodology). New entries in the ATC classification are assigned based on requests from users, so coverage of new drugs and drugs used in different countries is user-dependent. The application form for new ATC codes is available on the centre's website (www.whocc.no) [4].

Structure

In the ATC classification system, active chemical substances are classified in a hierarchy of five levels. The first level comprises 14 main anatomical/pharmacological groups (Table 5.1), each of which is divided into pharmacological or therapeutic subgroups (second level). The third and fourth levels are chemical, pharmacological or therapeutic subgroups and the fifth level is the chemical substance (see Box 5.1 for an example) [5,6].

The ATC classification is not strictly an anatomical therapeutic chemical classification, as the name may indicate. Pharmacological groups exist at all levels in the hierarchy, some of which have been there from the very beginning. However, in the last couple of decades, the number of pharmacological groups has increased, mainly at the expense of therapeutic and chemical groups. For the chemical substance, International Nonproprietary Names (INNs) are preferred. If INNs are not assigned, United States Adopted Names (USANs) or British Approved Names (BANs) are usually chosen (see later in this chapter).

Table 5.1 ATC system main groups.

ATC first level	Name
A	Alimentary tract and metabolism
B	Blood and blood forming organs
C	Cardiovascular system
D	Dermatologicals
G	Genitourinary system and sex hormones
H	Systemic hormonal preparations, excluding sex hormones and insulins
J	Antiinfectives for systemic use
L	Antineoplastic and immunomodulating agents
M	Musculoskeletal system
N	Nervous system
P	Antiparasitic products, insecticides and repellents
R	Respiratory system
S	Sensory organs
V	Various

ATC, Anatomical Therapeutic Chemical.

Box 5.1 Classification of metformin in the ATC.

The complete classification of metformin illustrates the structure of the ATC code:

A	Alimentary tract and metabolism (first level, anatomical main group)
A10	Drugs used in diabetes (second level, therapeutic subgroup)
A10B	Blood glucose-lowering drugs, excluding insulins (third level, pharmacological subgroup)
A10BA	Biguanides (fourth level, chemical subgroup)
A10BA02	Metformin (fifth level, chemical substance)

Thus, in the ATC system, all plain metformin preparations are given the code A10BA02.

Classification principles and challenges

New chemical entities

When an application for marketing authorization has been submitted for a new medical substance, an ATC code can be assigned. Most new entries are easy to add into the existing classification structure. For some new medicines, however, it may be a challenge to find an appropriate classification reflecting the new mechanism of action/new indication, as the general classification structure was assigned many decades ago. The challenge for the caretakers of the classification is to keep a stable classification system over time with as few changes as possible and still to have a system in which new therapeutic and pharmacological principles can find an appropriate place. Further, some promising medicines with new mechanisms of action may show themselves to be not so promising after a while and be withdrawn from the market. To avoid the creation of too many specific ATC groups containing only one or two substances, some new drugs are classified in general groups initially and then reclassified into more specific groups when they have confirmed their place in drug therapy.

Medicines with several uses

Medicinal substances are classified according to their main therapeutic use on the basic principle of *only one ATC code* for each medicinal product (as defined by route of administration and, in some cases, strength). In many ATC main groups, pharmacological groups are assigned on the second, third and fourth level, allowing drugs with several therapeutic uses to be included without specifically considering the main indication. An example is calcium channel blockers, which are classified in the pharmacological group C08 (Box 5.2), avoiding the need to consider whether the main indication is coronary heart disease or hypertension.

Medicinal substances quite frequently have several ATC codes for various routes of administration with different therapeutic uses; for example, prednisolone in single-ingredient products has eight different ATC codes based on different indications for systemic and various local application formulations. A few medicinal substances have different ATC codes for different strengths of pharmaceutical formulation, such as finasteride tablets. A low-strength tablet for treatment of baldness is classified under D11AX *Other dermatologicals,* while the high-strength tablet for benign prostatic hypertrophy (BPH) is classified under G04C *Drugs used in BPH.* The challenge occurs when a medicinal product (same strength and route of administration) is approved and used for two or more equally important indications and the main therapeutic use differs from one country to another. In such cases, the main indication is decided by the International Working Group for Drug Statistics Methodology on the basis of available literature and a qualified assumption of the most prevalent indication worldwide. Such drugs are usually only given one code, which may be a problem for users in countries where other uses are predominant. An example of a recurrent classification problem is the classification of sildenafil tablets in similar strengths, which are used for both erectile dysfunction and pulmonary arterial hypertension. Despite requests from users proposing two ATC codes, sildenafil is still only classified in G04BE *Drugs for erectile dysfunction,* following the principles for ATC classification.

Box 5.2 Classification of verapamil.

C	Cardiovascular system
C08	Calcium channel blockers
C08D	Selective calcium channel blockers with direct cardiac effects
C08DA	Phenylalkylamine derivatives
C08DA01	Verapamil

Combination products

The classification of combination products is a challenge in any classification system. In the ATC system, products containing two or more active ingredients are regarded as combinations and given codes different from those of the plain (one active ingredient) products. As for plain medicinal products, combinations are in general classified according to their main use. The most commonly used principle is that the main ingredient in the combination be identified and the combination be given a separate fifth-level code in the same fourth level as this ingredient (e.g. R06AA02 *diphenhydramine* and R06AA52 *diphenhydramine, combinations*). On this principle, different combination products sharing the same main active ingredient are given the same ATC code. In recent years, and as more rational combinations have been marketed, it has been more common to assign separate third or fourth levels for combinations and to make the fifth-level code specific for all active ingredients (e.g. C09DX01 *valsartan, amlodipine and hydrochlorothiazide*). How specific and 'visible' a combination appears in the ATC classification will to some extent depend on the need for a detailed classification from a drug utilization point of view.

The principles for ATC classification are further described in the annually updated *Guidelines for ATC Classification and DDD Assignment* [5], available on the ATC/DDD section of the WHOCC website [4].

Use and misuse of the ATC/DDD classification

ATC codes are included in many national and international drug catalogues as a common language for the grouping of medicines. Use of the ATC/DDD system allows standardization of drug groups and a stable drug utilization measure to enable comparisons of drug use between countries, regions and other health care settings and to examine trends in drug use over time. The system has been used in national and international drug utilization studies with various aims since the early 1970s. This is the purpose for which it was developed, and it is with this purpose in mind that all decisions about ATC codes and DDDs are made. Consequently, using the system for other purposes can be inappropriate. Health authorities in some countries are basing reimbursement and pricing decisions on ATC codes and DDDs. This is not a recommended use of the system, simply because the necessary considerations for such use are not taken into account when assigning ATC codes and DDDs [5].

Implementation and maintenance of the ATC/DDD system

As already described, medicinal substances are classified according to their main therapeutic or pharmacological use on the basic principle of *only one ATC code* for each medicinal product (as defined by route of administration and, in some cases, strength). This is an important principle for the ATC classification as it allows aggregation of data in drug utilization studies without a single medicinal product being counted more than once. It is strictly handled by the caretakers so that users in different countries are able to classify the same pharmaceutical product (defined by active ingredient(s), route of administration and strength) in the same way. For monitoring and comparison of drug use internationally, it is important to ensure that the data retrieved are comparable; in other words, that ATC groups from different countries have the expected content. In order to achieve this, it is of vital importance that the ATC code is correctly linked to each medicinal product package in the national medicinal products registry. The number of DDDs per package should be calculated for each medicinal product package, and this information should be added to the national medicinal products registry [7]. As new entries (ATC and DDDs) are added and a few changes are made every year, the registry is updated annually and a strict version control is implemented [8]. This is done by competent authorities at the national level, as implementation and update at an international level would require enormous resources. Besides, national knowledge of the methodology is crucial in order to use and interpret the data appropriately. Updated information about new entries and changes is available on the ATC/DDD section of the WHOCC website [4], alongside a complete and updated list of all assigned ATC codes and DDDs [6]. Proper reference to the ATC/DDD version used is important when publishing drug utilization data [9].

ATCvet

The ATC classification for veterinary medicinal products, ATCvet, was developed by the Nordic Council on Medicines and was taken over by the WHOCC in 2001. New entries and changes in the classification system are decided by the WHOCC in collaboration with a European expert group (ATCvet Working Group). The ATCvet is based on the same principles as the ATC for humans and is kept as close to the human system as possible. In many cases, an ATC code already exists and the ATCvet code is created by placing the letter 'Q' in front of it (e.g. the ATCvet code for ampicillin is **Q**J01CA01). ATCvet codes will always have a Q as the first letter and will consist of eight characters (letters and numbers), compared to the seven characters of the ATC code. Specific ATCvet codes are created for drugs that are only used in veterinary medicines or where indications differ from those for similar human products. Further information about the ATCvet classification is available in annually updated ATCvet publications [10,11] and on the ATCvet section of the WHOCC website [12]. The ATCvet classification is used in many catalogues of veterinary medicines in Europe. It is also used in the European Surveillance of Veterinary Antimicrobial Consumption (ESVAC) project of the European Medicines Agency (EMA), which collects information on how antimicrobial medicines are used in animals across the European Union [13].

Other drug classification systems

EphMRA

The ATC classification system was originally based on the same main principles as the Anatomical Classification developed by the European Pharmaceutical Market Research Association (EphMRA) and the Pharmaceutical Business Intelligence and Research Group (PBIRG).

In this system, drugs are classified in a hierarchy of three and sometimes four levels, mainly according to their indications and use. Many of these are quite similar to the ATC structure, but in many cases less detailed. There are no specific codes for the active ingredient (fifth level in the ATC). Unlike the ATC classification, EphMRA classifies ***medicinal products***. It is possible to find products with the same active ingredient, route of administration and strength in several different classes; for example, naproxen tablets can be classified in M1A (antirheumatics, nonsteroidal), N2B (nonnarcotics and antipyretics) and G2X1 (gynaecological antispasmodics). Despite a similar structure at the higher levels, the ATC classification and the EphMRA classification developed separately for many years. Since the early 1990s, the caretakers of the two systems have met annually to discuss classification problems and to harmonize when possible. The purposes of the two systems differ, as the primary objective of the EphMRA classification is to satisfy the marketing needs of the pharmaceutical companies. A complete harmonization is therefore neither feasible nor an aim. There are many differences between the two classification systems, and a direct comparison is sometimes difficult due to their different natures and purposes. This means that data prepared using the ATC classification cannot be directly compared with data prepared using the EphMRA system. An annually updated comparison booklet on the two systems is available on the EphMRA website [14]. The EphMRA classification system is used by Intercontinental Medical Statistics (IMS) in producing marketing research statistics for the pharmaceutical industry globally. These data are commercially available to anyone and are sometimes used by drug utilization researchers. Awareness of the differences between the two systems is particularly important in such applications. In some settings, and on the EphMRA website, the system is referred to as the 'ATC classification', and this has caused confusion among users over the years. Further details of the EphMRA classification systems are available on EphMRA's official website (www.ephmra.org) [15].

AHFS Pharmacologic-Therapeutic Classification System

The American Hospital Formulary Service (AHFS) classification was developed and is maintained by the American Society of Health-System Pharmacists, the national professional association that represents pharmacists who practice in inpatient, outpatient, home care and long-term care settings. In the United States, and to some extent Canada, the classification has been the foundation for organizing drug formularies since 1959. It allows the grouping of drugs with similar pharmacologic, therapeutic and/or chemical characteristics in a four-level hierarchy. There are 31 main classes (the first levels are given in Table 5.2).

Table 5.2 AHFS Pharmacologic-Therapeutic Classification System main classes.

AHFS class number	AHFS class description
4:00	Antihistamine drugs
8:00	Antiinfective agents
10:00	Antineoplastic agents
12:00	Autonomic drugs
16:00	Blood derivatives
20:00	Blood formation, coagulation and thrombosis agents
24:00	Cardiovascular drugs
26:00	Cellular therapy
28:00	Central nervous system agents
32:00	Contraceptives (foams, devices)
34:00	Dental agents
36:00	Diagnostic agents
38:00	Disinfectants (for agents used in objects other than skin)
40:00	Electrolyte, caloric and water balance
44:00	Enzymes
48:00	Respiratory tract agents
52:00	Eye, ear, nose and throat (EENT) preparations
56:00	Gastrointestinal drugs
60:00	Gold compounds
64:00	Heavy metal antagonists
68:00	Hormones and synthetic substitutes
72:00	Local anaesthetics
76:00	Oxytocics
78:00	Radioactive agents
80:00	Serums, toxoids and vaccines
84:00	Skin and mucous membrane agents
86:00	Smooth muscle relaxants
88:00	Vitamins
92:00	Miscellaneous therapeutic agents
94:00	Devices
96:00	Pharmaceutical aids

Some of the main classes (e.g. 16:00 and 60:00) only have a first level, while others continue down the hierarchy, with more granularity the further they go. There are no specific codes for active ingredients (see also Table 5.4).

Table 5.3 British National Formulary (BNF) classification main chapters.

Code[a]	Chapter title
01	Gastrointestinal system
02	Cardiovascular system
03	Respiratory system
04	Central nervous system
05	Infections
06	Endocrine system
07	Obstetrics, gynaecology and urinary tract disorders
08	Malignant disease and immunosuppression
09	Nutrition and blood
10	Musculoskeletal and joint diseases
11	Eye
12	Ear, nose and oropharynx
13	Skin
14	Immunological products and vaccines
15	Anaesthesia
18	Preparations used in diagnosis
19	Other drugs and preparations
20	Dressings
21	Appliances
22	Incontinence appliances
23	Stoma appliances

[a] Chapters above 15 are pseudochapters not specifically listed in the printed BNF. Many of the products are included in appendices to the BNF [19].

Because of the structure of the AHFS classification system, and because its main use is not in drug utilization studies, there are several cases in which a drug can have multiple classes, either by indication, mechanism of action or route of administration. All classes are considered equally valid for a single drug, even though in the printed AHFS Drug Information [16], due to space constraints, a choice has been made as to which classification the drug monograph is printed under. All other valid classes will have cross-references to the 'print class'. There are no specific codes for combination products; they inherit all the classifications of the individual ingredients.

The AHFS Pharmacologic-Therapeutic Classification System may be licensed from the American Society of Health-System Pharmacists. Changes to the classification are published each year, together with the release of the annually updated edition of the printed AHFS Drug Information [16]. For further details of the AHFS classification systems, see the official AHFS website (www.ahfsdruginformation.com) [17].

Table 5.4 Classification hierarchy of celecoxib in four different classification systems.

Classification system	Level	Level (code)	Level (name)
ATC	First	M	Musculoskeletal system
	Second	M01	Antiinflammatory and antirheumatic products
	Third	M01A	Antiinflammatory and antirheumatic products, nonsteroids
	Fourth	M01AH	Coxibs
	Fifth	M01AH01	Celecoxib
EphMRA	First	M	Musculoskeletal system
	Second	M1	Antiinflammatory and antirheumatic products
	Third	M1A	Antirheumatics, nonsteroidal
	Fourth	M1A3	Coxibs, plain
			(no specific code for celecoxib)
AHFS	First	28:00:00:00	Central nervous system agents
	Second	28:08:00:00	Analgesics and antipyretics
	Third	28:08:04:00	Nonsteroidal antiinflammatory agents
	Fourth	28:08:04:08	Cyclooxygenase-2 (COX-2) inhibitors
			(no specific code for celecoxib)
BNF	Chapter	10	Musculoskeletal and joint diseases
	Section	1001	Drugs used in rheumatic disease and gout
	Paragraph	100101	Nonsteroidal antiinflammatory drugs
	Subparagraph	1001010	Nonsteroidal antiinflammatory drugs
	Drug	1001010AH	Celecoxib
	Product	1001010AHAA	Celecoxib[a]
		1001010AHBB	Celebrex[b]
	Preparation	1001010AHAAAAAA	Celecoxib_Cap 100 mg
		1001010AHBBAAAA	Celebrex_Cap 100 mg

[a] Generic.

[b] Brand.

BNF codes

BNF codes are widely used within prescribing databases and for drug utilization studies in the United Kingdom. They are based upon the British National Formulary (BNF) [18], which provides monographs for drugs available within the United Kingdom and guidance on their clinical use, arranging the information into numbered chapters, sections, paragraphs and subparagraphs. This numbering system forms the basis of the BNF codes produced by NHS Prescription Services (part of the NHS Business Services Authority in England), which has extended the classification to produce specific codes that identify chemical substances, products and preparations, as well as products that are prescribed but not listed in the BNF [19].

The classifications system of the BNF codes is not dissimilar to the ATC classification [4,5] in that drugs are arranged into a hierarchy based upon therapeutic use, pharmacology or chemical similarity. Preparations listed within multiple areas of the printed BNF are given a single BNF code based upon their principal therapeutic use. If a particular section of the printed BNF ceases to exist because of changing therapeutic practice and the discontinuation or withdrawal of products, the original BNF codes are maintained to ensure the integrity of historical data. As a result, the BNF codes available and their associated descriptions will diverge over time from the classification in the printed BNF. Table 5.3 shows the therapeutic chapters of the BNF, while Table 5.4 shows the BNF hierarchy for celecoxib.

Therapeutically equivalent preparations, such as branded and generic versions of the same drug, have separate distinct BNF codes. This may be problematic if one wishes to aggregate data based on chemical substance, formulation and strength, and where the dataset does not include more granular information that would allow this. However, as can be seen from Table 5.4, the only difference between the BNF codes for the generic and branded preparation is in characters 10 and 11. Aggregation could therefore be done based upon characters 1–9, representing the chemical substance, characters 12 and 13, representing the formulation and strength, and characters 14 and 15, representing the 'equivalent' (a brand or generic marker) [20].

Drug nomenclature/substance names

The INN is a unique generic name that is globally recognized and is public property [21]. The INN system was initiated in 1950 by the World Health Assembly, and the first list of names was published in 1953. The cumulative INN list now includes around 7000 names, and this number is growing by 120–150 every year. The WHO issues INNs in several languages (English, Latin, French, Russian, Spanish, Arabic and Chinese), on the advice of experts from the WHO Expert Advisory Panel on the International Pharmacopoeia and Pharmaceutical Preparations. The aim of the INN system is to provide health professionals with a unique and universally available name by which to identify each pharmaceutical substance. This is important for the clear identification, safe prescription and correct dispensing of medicines to patients and for communication and exchange of information between health professionals and scientists worldwide. INNs should be the preferred drug names within classification systems, as they are in the ATC system. The use of nonproprietary or generic names is normally required by national or, as in the European Union, international legislation. As a result of ongoing collaboration, national generic names such as USANs [22] and BANs [23] are today, with rare exceptions, identical to INNs. Important examples of divergent names are paracetamol (USAN: *acetaminophen*) and epinephrine (BAN: *adrenaline*).

Other classification systems relevant for drug utilization research

ICD codes

The International Classification of Diseases (ICD) is a system of diagnostic codes for classifying diseases and other health problems. The ICD is published by the WHO and used worldwide in morbidity and mortality statistics, drug reimbursement systems and automated decision support in health care [24]. The ICD is revised regularly to reflect advances in health and medical science, and is currently in its tenth revision. ICD-10 was adopted by WHO member states from 1994 and has been translated into 43 languages.

ICD-10 includes categories relating to medicinal substances, but in the context of adverse outcomes, and often in quite broad terms (Tables 5.5 and 5.6). ICD-10 does not include codes suitable for recording and classifying drug treatments received, and so its use in drug utilization studies will normally be in conjunction with other datasets and drug classification systems; for example, investigating rates of adverse events as compared to total exposure to a therapeutic group. A mapping to drug classification systems such as the ATC is being discussed.

Table 5.5 International Classification of Diseases (ICD) categories relating to medicinal product use.

Code range	Description
T36–T50	Poisoning by drugs, medicaments and biological substances
X40–X49	Accidental poisoning by and exposure to noxious substances
Y40–Y59	Drugs, medicaments and biological substances causing adverse effects in therapeutic use

Table 5.6 International Classification of Diseases (ICD) code Y40 and subgroups from the chapter 'Complications of Medical and Surgical Care'.

Y40	Systemic antibiotics (excludes: antibiotics, topically used (Y56.–); antineoplasticantibiotics (Y43.3))
Y40.0	Penicillins
Y40.1	Cephalosporins and other β-lactam antibiotics
Y40.2	Chloramphenicol group
Y40.3	Macrolides
Y40.4	Tetracyclines
Y40.5	Aminoglycosides
	Streptomycin
Y40.6	Rifamycins
Y40.7	Antifungal antibiotics, systemically used
Y40.8	Other systemic antibiotics
Y40.9	Systemic antibiotics, unspecified

The WHO is currently undertaking revision towards the ICD-11, which is expected to be finalized in 2017. For the first time, the WHO is calling on experts and users to participate in the revision process through a Web-based platform [25].

SNOMED

The Systematized Nomenclature of Medicine (SNOMED) started in 1965 with the Systematized Nomenclature of Pathology (SNOP), developed by the College of American Pathologists, and later extended into other medical fields. SNOMED CT (clinical terms) was developed in 1999 by merging, expanding and restructuring two terminologies: SNOMED Reference Terminology (SNOMED RT) and the Read codes version 3 or Clinical Terms Version 3 (CTV3), developed by the British NHS (see next section for more on Read codes). Since 2007, SNOMED CT has been owned and maintained by the International Health Terminology Standards Development Organisation (IHTSDO) in Denmark [26].

SNOMED CT provides a core general terminology for use in various clinical settings and for exchange of data from EHRs. The terminology contains more than 311 000 active concepts, organized into different hierarchies. Each concept is represented by an individual number, and several concepts can be used in combination to describe a complex condition. *Clinical finding/disorder* and *procedure/intervention* are examples of main levels in SNOMED CT. *The substance* and *pharmaceutical/biologic product* are the main levels where drugs will be included. The *pharmaceutical/biologic product* hierarchy was introduced as a top-level hierarchy in order to distinguish drug products from their chemical constituents (substances). It contains multiple levels of granularity, used to support a variety of purposes, including electronic prescribing and formulary management. The levels of drug product concepts represented in the International Release of SNOMED CT include Virtual Medicine Product (VMP; e.g. Lisinopril 20 mg tablets), Virtual Therapeutic Moiety (VTM; e.g. Lisinopril) and Product Category (a group of products with a similar mode of action). At the national level (e.g. US and UK), drug extensions have been developed to represent Actual Medicinal Products (AMPs). A brand name and manufacturer are added to these (e.g. Zestril 20 mg tablets, Astra Zeneca), along with the pack sizes available.

SNOMED CT is a multinational, multilingual terminology. Revisions to the international version are released twice a year. IHTSDO works to provide explicit links (cross-maps) to health-related classifications and coding schemes in use around the world, including diagnosis classifications such as ICD-10. Additional cross-maps are under development or consideration. In January 2014, 25 countries were members of IHTSDO. For further reading about SNOMED CT, see the IHTSDO website (www.ihtsdo.org) [27].

Read codes

Read codes are the principal clinical terminology used within primary care in the United Kingdom. They were developed in the 1980s by Dr James Read, a general practitioner; today, version 2 of the codes is in most widespread use. The terminology covers most information that needs to be recorded about a patient, including history, symptoms, laboratory tests, operations and

Table 5.7 Read code hierarchy.

Level	Read code	Preferred term
First	G...	Circulatory system diseases
Second	G3...	Ischaemic heart disease
Third	G30...	Acute myocardial infarction
Fourth	G301...	Anterior myocardial infarction NOS
Fifth	G3011	Acute anteroseptal infarction

procedures (codes beginning 0–9) and diagnosis (codes beginning A–Z). There is also a drug dictionary (codes beginning a–z), which as in other systems, is arranged into chapters based upon therapeutic use and goes to the level of individual medicinal products.

The relationship between codes and the information that they represent is built into the codes themselves, and this hierarchy can be used like a classification system. An example is shown in Table 5.7. It is important to be aware that similar terms may exist in different chapters of the Read code hierarchy in order to fulfil different purposes, such as:

- Acute pharyngitis: H02 – Respiratory disease chapter;
- Sore throat strep: A340 – Infectious disease chapter;
- Sore throat symptom: 1C9 – Symptoms chapter.

Additionally, some hierarchies may contain codes for terms that indicate the absence of a symptom or finding, such as:

- Backache symptom: 16C;
- No backache: 16C1.

This is particularly the case for symptoms and history hierarchies, so a high-level search that does not consider underlying codes for negative findings may return cases that do not have the criteria of interest.

The recording of information using Read codes is seldom done by trained clinical coders, so where there are similar terms in different chapters, incorrect codes may be selected. In addition, coding may not be done to the greatest possible level of detail; for example, someone might simply code to *G30...Acute myocardial infarction*, rather than being more specific.

The Read code source dataset includes relevant mappings to the Office of Population Censuses and Surveys Classification of Interventions and Procedures (OPCS-4) for operations and procedures and to the ICD-10 for diagnoses [28].

Read version 2 is now a deprecated terminology standard, and SNOMED CT is the preferred terminology for new clinical systems and is likely to be incorporated into existing clinical systems in the next few years. Tables providing mappings between Read and SNOMED CT are available.

Linkage of classification systems

Much work is currently underway in the area of mapping between different drug and disease classification systems. This is an important but large and difficult task. Although often developed for similar purposes, different classification systems often have very different structures and levels of detail, and cover different drugs and conditions. Hence, one-to-one or complete mappings are almost never entirely possible. Implementation in health technology platforms is a challenge in such cases. Furthermore, the data retrieved and the results obtained may vary according to the classification system used and whether it is native to the drug data or has been achieved via a map between classification systems.

CHAPTER 6

Measurement units of drug utilization

Hege Salvesen Blix

WHO Collaborating Centre for Drug Statistics Methodology, Department of Pharmacoepidemiology, Norwegian Institute of Public Health, Norway

KEY POINTS

- Information on aggregated drug use is important to understanding international differences in utilization. The Anatomical Therapeutic Chemical (ATC)/defined daily dose (DDD) system was developed with the aim of improving drug use and is a useful tool for presenting drug utilization statistics.
- DDD is a global standardized metric that provides a fixed unit of measurement independent of price, currencies, package size and strength and allows trends in drug consumption to be assessed and comparisons between countries and population groups to be performed.

Introduction

Aggregated data are a combination of separate datasets collected into a whole and presented as, for example, total use in a given country. Most countries do not have access to large registries containing patient-level data on prescribed or dispensed drugs. In these settings, aggregate data collected from wholesalers, pharmacies, hospitals or other settings may be useful for drug utilization studies. In order to measure drug use with aggregated data, assess volumes dispensed/prescribed to individual patients and compare drug use across countries, a global standardized metric is needed. When designing a drug utilization study, it is important to look into several methods of measurement, including costs, the weight of active ingredients, numbers of packs or tablets, numbers of prescriptions and defined daily doses (DDDs). Sometimes it is valuable to use more than one type of measurement, as this will provide other angles that can help us understand drug use better. In this chapter, the concept of DDDs, recommended by the World Health Organization (WHO) as a standard for drug utilization studies, is described. Other aggregate measures of drug utilization relevant for researchers are also described, and some practical examples are presented.

DDD: definition and general considerations

In order to deal with the limitation of traditional units of measurement, such as cost or number of units, a technical unit of measurement called the DDD was developed for use in drug utilization studies. The DDD concept is an integrated part of the WHO Anatomical Therapeutic Chemical (ATC) classification system [1]. The basic definition is:

> The DDD is the assumed average maintenance dose per day for a drug used for its main indication in adults.

Only *one* DDD is assigned per ATC code and route of administration. The DDD provides a fixed unit of measurement, independent of price, currencies, package size and strength.

The DDD reflects one global average dose: a compromise based on a review of the available information on recommended doses used in various countries. Drug consumption data presented in DDDs give a rough estimate of consumption and allow comparison of trends in drug consumption, both between countries and population groups and over time.

The DDD does not necessarily reflect the recommended or prescribed daily dose (PDD) in a given country. Drug

Drug Utilization Research: Methods and Applications, First Edition. Edited by M. Elseviers et al.
Published 2016 by John Wiley & Sons, Ltd.

use may differ according to cultural and ethnical differences, national guidelines and therapy traditions. In clinical practice, doses are individualized for patients and patient groups according to characteristics such as age, ethnic differences, type and severity of disease and pharmacokinetic features. It is crucial that researchers applying DDDs in drug utilization studies are aware of their advantages and disadvantages and are able to relate their results to clinical practice, and interpret them in this light.

Box 6.1 Example of DDD assignment in drug X with two indications.

> Drug X is classified in N06AX. It is approved for major depression with the dose recommendation 40 mg once daily. It is also approved for stress urinary incontinence with the dose recommendation 80 mg (40 mg twice daily). Because Drug X is assigned an ATC code in N06AX *Other antidepressants*, the DDD will be assigned according to doses given for depression: DDD = 40 mg.

Principles of DDD assignment

The WHO Collaborating Centre for Drug Statistics Methodology (WHOCC) in Oslo is responsible for the handling and maintenance of the DDDs in the ATC/DDD system. All DDDs are approved by the WHO International Working Group for Drug Statistics Methodology (see Chapter 5).

Information about DDDs is included in the ATC/DDD guidelines in separate paragraphs for each drug group. In this way, the guidelines provide in-depth information regarding DDDs. It is therefore important to consult the guidelines when looking into new drug utilization areas [1].

DDDs are assigned to single substances and to combination products. Only DDDs for single substances are published in the ATC/DDD index; the DDDs for fixed combinations are described in the guidelines and appear in a separate list for combined products [1,2].

DDDs are not established for topical products, sera, vaccines, antineoplastic agents, allergen extracts, anaesthetics or contrast media. There are different reasons for this for different drug groups, but the main one is that variations in dosages are too wide. For such drug groups, other measurements are recommended.

The DDD is valuable for measuring aggregated use in a whole population. Therefore, DDDs are assigned following marketing authorization approval. They are assigned on request: the WHOCC must be provided with sufficient information about the drug by the party requesting a DDD. Worldwide, there are still many drugs that do not have a DDD, simply because the WHO is not aware of their existence. The process for assigning a DDD, both for an old product and for a new one, takes some time; first, the DDD has to be decided by the WHO Expert group; then, sufficient time must be provided for objections to be raised; finally, the DDDs are published. Since the ATC/DDD index is only published once a year, it can take more than a year before an official DDD is available for a new medicine that has been registered on the market. While waiting for an official DDD, researchers may assign a local one. It is recommended that they report explicitly that a local DDD has been used and enumerate its value.

Plain products

Plain products contain one active ingredient. The ATC code reflects the main indication for the active ingredient and the average adult dose used for this indication is decisive for the DDD (see Box 6.1). If two indications that fit into the same ATC code have different recommended dosages, the indication regarded to be the main one, and which has the most patients, will be decisive for the DDD.

DDDs are given in terms of amounts of active ingredients according to the declared strength of the product: g, mg, mcg, mmol and U (unit). The duration of treatment is usually not considered when assigning a DDD. The maintenance dose is normally used, because this will give a better picture of drug use in the population, especially for drugs used in chronic disease.

Severity of illness has to be taken into consideration, since severe diseases often require different doses. An example is antibiotics: these are often given in higher doses in hospitals, due to the severity of infections, but by far their main use is in primary care, and therefore the DDD for antibiotics is based on use in moderately severe infections.

Combination products

DDDs are assigned for combination products on the principle that the combination is one daily dose,

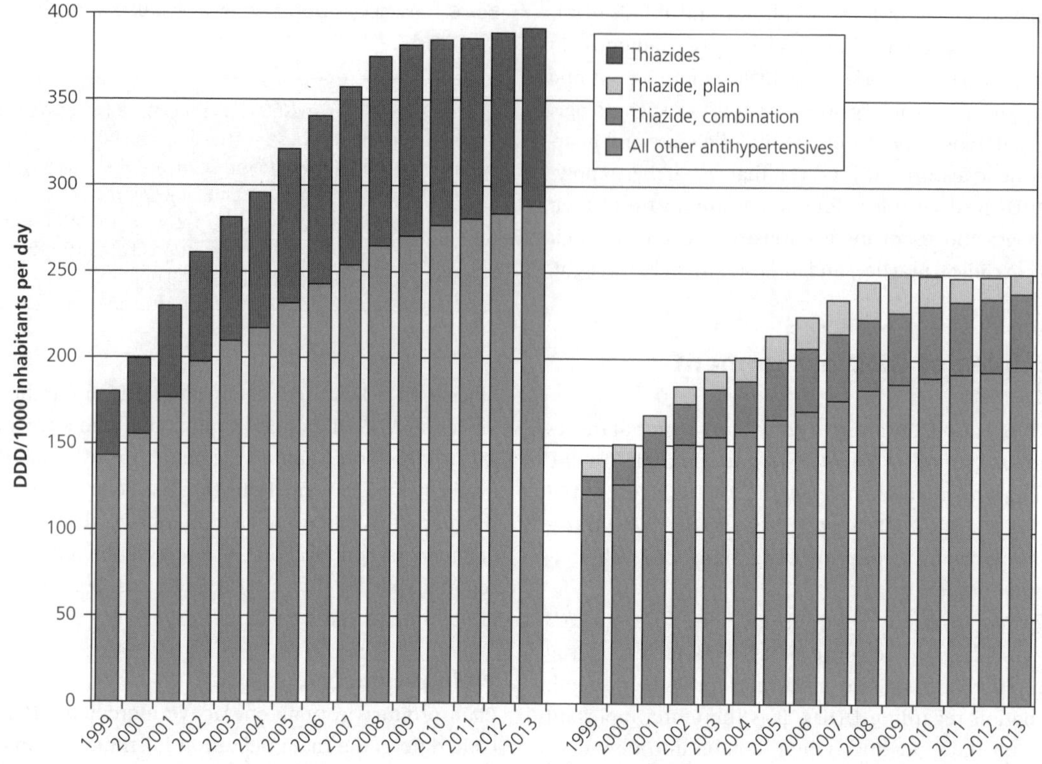

Figure 6.1 Use of antihypertensives. (a) Consumption in a country where only plain products are marketed (if a patient needs two antihypertensives, they must take two products). (b) Consumption in a country where combinations pills (e.g. thiazides combined with other antihypertensives, such as ACEIs or ARBs) are available. For colour details, please refer to the colour plates section.

regardless of the number of active ingredients it includes. Some of the main principles are described in the guidelines [1]. If a combination is given an ATC code naming a single ingredient, the DDD for the combination will often be equal to the DDD given for the single ingredient. For combination products where a DDD cannot for some reason be given in terms of amount of active ingredient, the UD (unit dose) is used. For example, one tablet equals 1 UD; if the dosage for the combination is two tablets a day, the DDD will be 2 UD.

Combinations are challenging for the interpretation of drug utilization statistics. When a patient is treated with two single-ingredient products, their consumption is measured by counting the DDDs of each single ingredient separately. Combined products are designed to ease patient adherence and/or to maximize patient safety. Some diseases are treated with several drugs (e.g. hypertension, human immunodeficiency virus (HIV)); if combinations are available on the market, it is likely that they will be prescribed more frequently than two or more single-ingredient products. In countries where combination products are used frequently, the usage in DDDs will appear to be lower than in countries where only single-substance products are used. This may cause problems in understanding the statistics (e.g. for historical and cross-national comparison) and is a challenge for the interpretation of data (see Figure 6.1).

When presenting consumption by drug group, it is necessary to be familiar with the availability of products, local guidelines and therapeutic practice. Changes in patterns must be explained with this in mind; if they are not, incorrect conclusions may be drawn (see Figure 6.2).

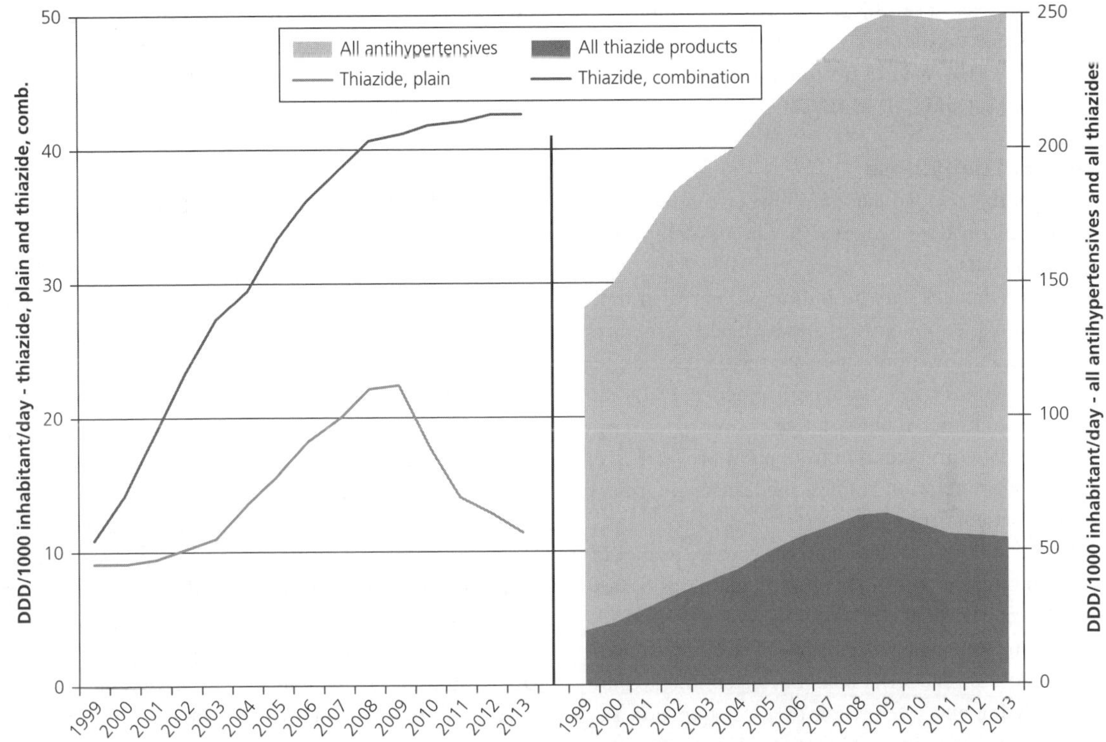

Figure 6.2 The use of antihypertensives in Norway increased from 141 DDD/1000 inhabitants/day in 1999 to 250 in 2013. National guidelines recommended thiazides as first-line therapy for hypertension for new users in 2004–09. This was connected to reimbursement rules, which contributed to an increased use of plain thiazides in the same period. When looking only at products containing thiazides (purple area), one might assume that thiazide (ATC code C03A) use was decreasing, but after 2009, use of plain thiazides decreased, while combinations containing thiazides (ATC codes C09BA and C09DA) increased. (Source: Norwegian drug wholesaler statistics).

Alterations and misuse of DDDs

Recommended dosages can change over time, so it is sometimes necessary to make alterations to DDDs. However, changes are kept to a minimum, because too many alterations would be disadvantageous for long-term drug utilization studies. DDDs are routinely reviewed 3 years after assignment. Moreover, the WHO International Working Group for Drug Statistics Methodology may review DDDs on request.

It is important to bear in mind that the DDD is an international compromise that will often differ from the actual therapeutic dose. To use the DDD as a standard dose for rational drug therapy is wrong.

Several published studies have used DDDs as the measurement unit of utilization. Often, there are no references either to the WHO ATC/DDD or to a specific ATC/DDD version [3] (see Chapter 5). In other studies that use the term 'DDD', it turns out on closer examination that the researchers have invented their own theoretical dose and given it that name [4]. It is important always to refer to the official ATC/DDD methodology and to state the specific version being used when reporting drug use in DDDs [5].

Other aggregate measures for prescribing

Measuring prescribing is challenging, and no aggregate measure is perfect for all purposes. Measures can vary with the drug/drug group in question, drugs available, setting, guidelines, health systems, reimbursement programmes, population, age, sex and so on. Some studies have tried to validate and compare DDDs with other measurement units, including packages [6], estimated prevalence of drug users [7], minimum marketed dose [8], equipotential dose and average daily dose [8], average daily quantities [9], equivalents and percentages of the British National Formulary (BNF) [10], days of treatment [11,12], daily prescribed dose [12] and PDD [8,13–17].

Prescribed daily dose

The PDD is the average daily amount of a drug that is actually prescribed to patients. It can be determined from clinical data.

Prescribed dosages vary by indication, between individuals and population groups and by health structures and settings. Furthermore, there are regional variations according to culture and therapeutic practice. PDDs can be determined from a representative sample of prescriptions. Such data can be drawn from point prevalence or longitudinal prescription studies, medical or pharmacy records or patient interviews.

The fact that PDDs can differ from one country to another may be due to differences in approved indications or dosages and local guidelines. This should always be considered when making international comparisons. Large discrepancies between PDD and DDD should be taken into account when analysing and interpreting drug consumption statistics. For example, for antiinfectives, PDDs may vary according to the severity of the infection and to antibiotic resistance patterns in the area [18]. Another example is prescription patterns for antipsychotics in schizophrenia [19].

It should be noted that the PDD does not necessarily reflect actual drug consumption. Some prescribed medications are not dispensed, and patients do not always take all the medications they are dispensed. Specially designed studies are required to measure actual drug intake at the patient level. These are further described in Part 3, Section F.

Other drug utilization metrics

Costs and common physical units (e.g. grams, kilos, litres), numbers of packs or tablets and numbers of prescriptions have all been used to quantify aggregated drug consumption. In some areas, these have been found to be valuable [6]; in others, they have not [20]. These units can be applied only when the use of one drug or well-defined product is evaluated. When assessing the use of drug groups, dissimilarities in factors like product availability, pack size and potency will influence the results. How drugs are administered may help decide which method of measurement can be used. For example, drugs used in course doses can be counted by counting packs as a proxy for users or courses. For drug groups not assigned DDDs, other measurements may be an option.

The counting of tablets can be used, but the strengths of tablets vary, which means that low-strength preparations contribute relatively more than high-strength preparations, while short-acting preparations will often contribute more than long-acting preparations. However, for substances where a fixed daily regimen is used (e.g. one tablet a day), the counting of tablets may be an option (see Figure 6.3).

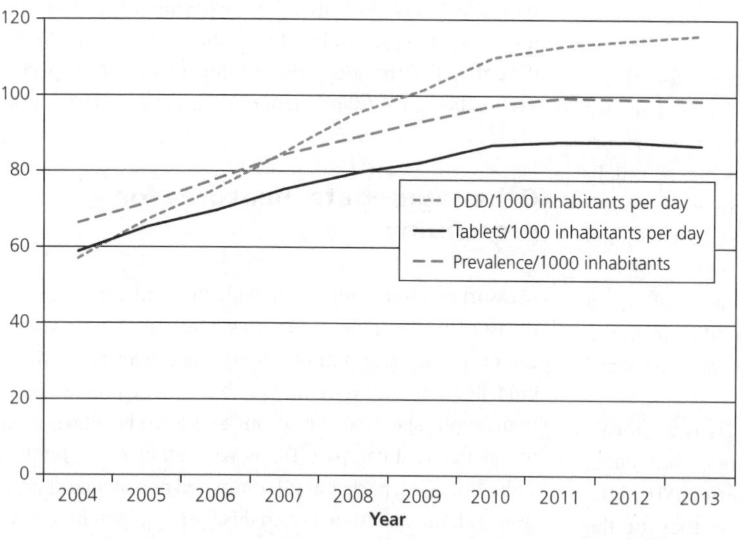

Figure 6.3 Use of statins (C10AA) in Norway, 2004–13, by DDDs/1000 inhabitants per day, number of tablets/1000 inhabitants per day and prevalence/1000 inhabitants per year. For statins, the assumption is that the patient takes one tablet every day, regardless of strength (in real life, patients start and stop dosages, but for aggregate measurements this gives an estimate). An increase is seen for both measurements. The higher increase in DDDs is due to the use of higher strengths of statin over time. The true annual prevalence of users (number of individuals dispensed statins per year) is drawn from the NorPD (Norwegian Prescription Database).

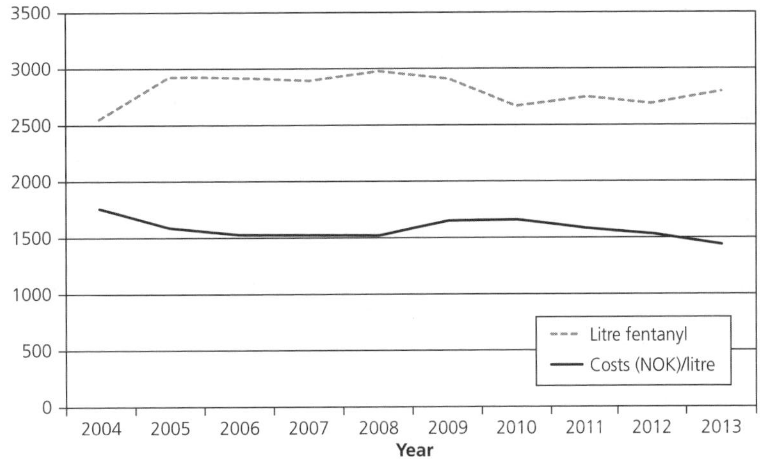

Figure 6.4 Use of fentanyl (N01AH01) solution for injection/infusion, measured in volumes (litre) and costs (Norwegian kroner, NOK (1 NOK = €0.12, June 2014)) per year. Fentanyl is used to provide analgesic anaesthesia. The dosage is individualized, and no DDDs are assigned, but by using volume and costs, surveillance over time may be performed.

For liquid pharmaceuticals such as mixtures, infusions, injections and eye drops, the amount in volume can be used as a measurement. For example, if we want to assess the amount of anaesthetic used in a hospital, data can be presented in volumes over time (see Figure 6.4).

Counting of packages has been used as an add-on measure in studies of antibiotic use. This can be of great value in countries were the pack size is fitted to recommended course lengths and when there are changes in pack size or increases per unit over time. For example, in Belgium, the counting of packages was added to DDD measurements in order to allow better understanding of changes in prescription patterns [6].

Counting of prescriptions can be of great value in the evaluation of the clinical use of drugs. In Sweden, national targets are set for antibiotic use in outpatients. Numbers of prescriptions/1000 inhabitants, together with DDD/1000 inhabitants, are for benchmarking against targets [21]. Numbers of prescriptions do not give a good expression of total use unless total amounts of drug per prescription are also considered.

Drug use can be expressed in terms of costs (see Figure 6.4). However, international comparisons based on cost parameters can be misleading and of limited value in the evaluation of drug use, due to price differences between alternative preparations and different national cost levels. Long-term studies are also difficult, due to fluctuations in currency and changes in prices. Drug expenditure may be even more difficult to use as a volume measure in the hospital sector due to different rebates and special price agreements.

Weight in grams can be a practical measure in several cases. For example, if we want to study the effect of total drug exposure on the environment, we might measure the use of drugs (e.g. hormones or hormone-like substances and antimicrobials) in humans, animals and food production [22,23]. Such studies require data collection from humans, animals, water sewage, soil samples and so on. In this setting, weight in grams can mirror a country's drug burden and can guide health authorities in their work against possible adverse drug effects on the population level and the emergence of antimicrobial resistance. For example, if you want to measure dermatological products like ointment, lotions and creams, weight in grams (of drug formulation) may be suitable (see Figure 6.5).

Use of drugs in animals

The One Health Initiative [24] argues that humans, animals and the ecosystem are inextricably linked. This becomes particularly obvious when looking at the field of antimicrobial resistance. While legislation is in place concerning residues of veterinary medicinal products in food-producing animals, in order to ensure the protection of consumers against possible harmful exposure, few countries have surveillance systems in the veterinary field that can present aggregated measures for drug use. One major obstacle is the lack of a proper unit of measurement, which it is more complicated to establish in the veterinary field due to the large variations between species. The few countries able to present total

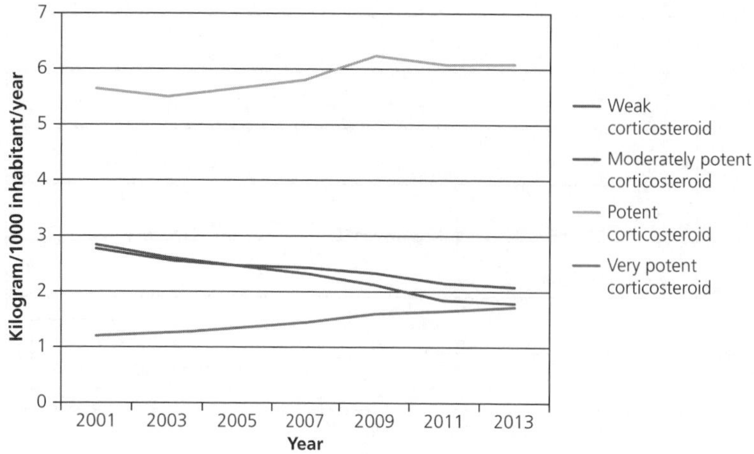

Figure 6.5 Use of corticosteroids in dermatology, measured as kilograms of topical preparations. In Norway, increased use of potent and very potent topical corticosteroids is observed over time, while use of weak and moderately potent corticosteroids is decreasing.

human and animal drug use have used weight as the unit of measurement.

The Danish government has monitored the use of medicines in food-producing animals since 2000, using animal defined daily doses (ADDs) for each species and age group [25]. In 2010, the European Surveillance of Veterinary Antimicrobial Consumption (ESVAC) project was initiated, aiming to collect information on antimicrobials in the veterinary field in the European Union [26]. In this project, consumption data are measured by weight of active ingredient and linked to the animal demographics in each country through a population correction unit (PCU). The PCU is a proxy for the size of the animal population. Drug use in food-producing animals needs to be measured in terms of impact on human health. Drug dosages vary a lot between species (due to differences in animal size, pharmacology and pharmacokinetics), so more sophisticated methods of measuring aggregated drug use are required in the veterinary field.

How to report aggregated drug use

Aggregated data on drug utilization can be used as a tool for health administration, quality assurance, development of guidelines and provision of feedback to prescribing doctors, preferably in combination with therapy discussions identifying areas for improvement. In most countries, DDDs are used as volume measures in these datasets. There are many examples across the world [27–37].

Drug use varies between institutions, and discussion around the variability in prescribing patterns between hospitals has the potential to create awareness of rational prescribing. It is important to keep in mind that the DDD is assigned according to the assumed average daily use. In various settings, drugs are used differently according to indication, severity, comorbidity and patient population. Particularly in children and the elderly, DDDs may be inappropriate (see later). This may lead to difficulties in interpreting DDD data for practising physicians.

There are four main settings to address: total use, which includes all settings, and use in ambulatory care, hospitals and nursing homes. The reporting of drug use should be expressed according to the population exposed.

Total use and ambulatory care

The ATC/DDD methodology is suitable for addressing total aggregated use, and especially use in ambulatory care. Total aggregated drug consumption figures and use in ambulatory care are commonly presented as numbers of DDDs per 1000 inhabitants per day (DDD/1000 inhabitants/day). For example, if the use of a drug is measured as 50 DDDs/1000 inhabitants/day in a given country, this indicates that around 5% of the population can receive a certain treatment daily. It is an estimate, but when a drug is used continuously and the DDD mirrors the recommended doses, the estimate is good. Drug exposure has also been given as DDDs/day. For example, if a drug is measured as 150 000 DDDs/day, this indicates it has 150 000 daily users. Sometimes, better estimates can be given by adjusting for sex and age or by limiting the use to a target population (e.g. for oral contraceptives the denominator is females below 45 years of age, while for mixtures of antibiotics the denominator is children below 10 years of age).

Other indicators that have been used are DDDs/patients (to estimate dosages given or volumes dispensed per patient), DDDs/insured person (for reimbursement databases) and DDDs/1000 practice population/day (to compare general practitioners' (GP) offices). For further reading on how to compare prescribing between primary care practices, see Chapter 15.

Hospitals

DDDs are widely used to measure drug use in the hospital setting [38–42]. Often, discrepancies are seen between assigned DDDs and the dosages used in hospitals [14–16]. Some researchers have tried to deal with these discrepancies by designing more accurate measures to fit their purpose (e.g. PDDs, average daily quantities (ADQs) [9], hospital-adjusted defined daily doses (haDDDs) [15]). These measures are valuable for drug utilization studies comparing regions or practices within a country, but are generally of limited value for comparisons between different health systems.

Several denominators have been used in hospitals, but currently there is no global standardized definition. The examples in Table 6.1 underline the importance of always reporting the definition of a selected denominator.

Table 6.1 Two common denominators and some possible definitions.

Denominator	Definitions
Bed days	**Definition 1:** A bed day is a day during which a patient is confined to a bed and stays at the hospital overnight. Day cases (patients admitted for a medical procedure or surgery in the morning and released before the evening) should be excluded.
	Definition 2: Bed days are calculated by subtracting the admission date from the discharge date and deducting total leave with and without permission days. A same-day patient is allocated 1 bed day.
Patient days	**Definition 1:** Each day represents a unit of time during which the services of the institution or facility are used by a patient; thus, 50 patients in a hospital for 1 day would represent 50 patient days
	Definition 2: Patient days are the number of days for which inpatients (excluding newborns in the nursery) are hospitalized. The day of admission, but not the day of discharge, is counted as a patient day. If both admission and discharge occur on the same day, this is counted as 1 patient day.
	Definition 3: A patient day denotes lodging facilities provided and services rendered to one inpatient between the census-taking hours on two successive days. Synonymous terms: inpatient day, inpatient service day, census day, bed occupancy day.

Several indicators include the DDD in the calculation of drug use. A commonly used indicator in hospitals is DDD/100 bed days, which reflects the percentage of patients using a specific drug or drug group in a particular hospital. For example, 60 DDD/100 bed days indicates that 60% of patients will be given a certain treatment. This gives an estimate that is easy to understand and is therefore valuable in discussions with doctors about their prescribing. Other denominators have been used besides bed days; the most common are shown in Table 6.2. Combined use of different denominators may add variety to resource indicators and increase our understanding of drug use in hospitals.

Variations in drug use in hospitals can be explained by the type of hospital/ward, different specialties, types of patient, comorbidities and so on. Various risk-adjustment measures have been used to account for these variations (e.g. case mix index) [43].

Other methods of measuring drug use in hospitals include days of therapy (DOT), which calculates each drug given (e.g. three antibiotics given over 2 days equals $3 \times 2 = 6$ DOT) and length of therapy (LOT), which measures exposure time (e.g. three antibiotics given over 2 days equals 2 LOT) [44].

In hospitals, antimicrobial stewardship programmes involve, among other things, the monitoring of antibiotic use. If the ATC/DDD system is not incorporated in the administrative system, it can be calculated manually (see Box 6.2).

Table 6.2 Common indicators used to measure exposure to drugs in hospitals.

Measure	Definition	Comments
DDD/1000 inhabitants/day	DDD divided by total population per day	Used to compare hospital use between countries. Does not take into account health structure or number of hospital patients
DDD/100 bed days	DDD divided by number of occupied bed days	Used to compare hospital use between wards, hospitals and countries. Definitions of bed days may differ and the measure is sensitive to changes in hospital resource indicators
DDD/1000 patient days	DDD divided by number of patient days	Used to compare hospital use between wards, hospitals and countries. Definitions of patient days may differ and the measure is sensitive to changes in hospital resource indicators
DDDs/100 discharges	DDD divided by number of discharges	Used to compare hospital use between wards, hospitals and countries. Definitions of discharge may differ and the measure can be affected by changes in length of stay and case mix
DDD/100 admissions	DDD divided by number of admissions	Used to compare hospital use between wards, hospitals and countries. Definitions of admission may differ (e.g. patients transferred between hospital units can account for multiple admissions) and the measure can be affected by changes in length of stay and case mix

DDD, defined daily dose.

Box 6.2 Example of DDD calculation from sales figures.

Total sales of ciprofloxacin 0.25 g tablets equal 320 packs. One pack contains 50 tablets. The DDD for ciprofloxacin tablet is 1 g.

$$\frac{\text{No packs} \times \text{tablets in pack} \times \text{strength}}{\text{DDD value}} = \text{DDDs}$$

$$\frac{320 \text{ packs} \times 50 \text{ tablets/pack} \times 0.25 \text{ g/tablet}}{1\text{g/DDD}} = 4000 \text{ DDDs}$$

Thus, 4000 DDDs have been sold.

For antibiotics, a freely available programme, the AMC Tool (previously the ABC Calc tool), can be downloaded [45]. The AMC Tool was developed to calculate antimicrobial consumption. It computes antimicrobial consumption data (provided as numbers of packages) into numbers of DDDs by using the updated ATC/DDD index. The AMC Tool can calculate DDD/100 bed days and DDD/1000 inhabitants/day. The European Centre for Disease Prevention and Control (ECDC) reports comparisons of hospital use of antimicrobials by the indicator DDD/1000 inhabitants/day [46].

When comparing drug use in hospitals, both within-country and across borders, the presentation of data is important for a meaningful understanding of observed trends. As such, there is a need to develop optimal measurements that can account for differences in type of hospital, type of patient, activity and case mix and how hospitals are organized within a health system [38,47].

Long-term care institutions

Drug statistics using the ATC/DDD methodology have been used routinely in clinical practice in the Nordic countries to ensure quality of care in nursing homes. Patients in this setting are often fragile and very old, and they use many drugs. Due to age, morbidity and polypharmacy, these patients are highly sensitive to adverse drug reactions. It is therefore important to focus on rational pharmacotherapy in this population. Methods used for the measurement of drug use in hospitals can also be used in long-term care institutions. Often, comparisons are easier, since the patients are more uniform and the flow of patients is more stable than in a hospital setting. Drug utilization research in long-term care institutions is not common, but antibiotics, psychotropics and inappropriate drugs have been studied [48–53]. There is a need for increased surveillance in this area.

DDDs for special population groups

DDDs are normally assigned based on use in adults, and the ATC/DDD methodology has been criticized because it can be difficult to interpret data from drug utilization studies in special patient groups. Other kinds of measures could be used, but since the ATC/DDD methodology has been used successfully for drug use comparisons, there has been a call for the development of similar methods that allow comparison between special populations, such as children, the elderly and patients with renal impairment [54,55]. The WHO International Working Group for Drug Statistics Methodology has acknowledged these challenges, but at present only the generic (adult) DDDs are established. Work is ongoing to make more information available regarding the use of correction factors for various patient groups and settings. The first special population group to be addressed will be that in paediatric hospital settings. The plan is to develop correction factors for different age groups to be used in paediatric hospital wards.

CHAPTER 7
Individual-level drug utilization analyses

Jesper Hallas[1], Henrik Støvring[2] & Anton Pottegård[1]
[1]*Clinical Pharmacology, Institute of Public Health, University of Southern Denmark, Denmark*
[2]*Department of Public Health, Biostatistics, Aarhus University, Denmark*

KEY POINTS

- We present a selection of analytical templates that can be uniformly applied to describe use of all drugs and all drug classes. All of these templates require data on the individual's drug dispensing histories.
- These templates include epidemiological measures of frequency, such as prevalence and incidence rate, as well as duration of use. We also present survival analysis, waiting-time distribution and Lorentz curves as a tool for drug utilization studies.

Introduction

The introduction of gross-volume statistics in the 1970s was an immensely important development in the toolbox for analysing drug utilization. These statistics were based on aggregate data on drug sales or dispensing (see Chapter 6), but carried no further information on how the drugs were distributed among users. As important as the aggregate statistics were, they also had their obvious limitations. If, for example, an increase in overall consumption was observed, it was difficult to know whether this was caused by an increased number of users, intake of higher doses by a constant number of users, a shift towards more long-term use or any combination of these. A good example is the striking increase in the use of proton pump inhibitors (PPIs) observed over the last decades. Analyses of individual-level drug dispensing data have revealed that it was mainly explained by a shift towards more long-term use [1].

With the advent of large databases recording drug use at the level of individual patients, it became possible to consider the patient as the unit of analysis, and thereby provide more detailed measures of drug use than the crude aggregate amounts. However, the complexity and sheer volume of individual-level prescription data are overwhelming (e.g. the National Danish Prescription Database has in the order of 53 million prescription recordings per year, corresponding to nearly 10 per inhabitant) and it is thus vital to structure and target analyses. In this chapter, we present some of the templates available for structured analyses of individual-level data sources.

General principles

One important problem that permeates all work with individual-level statistics is the surprising dynamics of drug use. From a clinical viewpoint, it would seem reasonable to assume that drugs like statins, low-dose aspirin, antihypertensives or insulin would be used indefinitely once initiated. However, not only are these drugs discontinued by a surprisingly large proportion of users, but there is evidence that they are often used intermittently, with interspersed periods on and off them (see Chapter 36). Any attempt to analyse individual-level drug use patterns should take these potential dynamics into account.

It is also important to make a distinction between individual-level statistics and quality indicators. The templates for individual-level statistics presented in this chapter are generic; that is, they are applicable to all drugs and all therapeutic classes, and they may uniformly be applied to these. The quality of usage for a drug class is not considered *a priori* in an analysis of individual-level statistics, although the output of such an

Drug Utilization Research: Methods and Applications, First Edition. Edited by M. Elseviers et al. © 2016 John Wiley & Sons, Ltd.
Published 2016 by John Wiley & Sons, Ltd.

analysis may provide important clues to quality problems. Analyses of quality indicators have quality of prescribing as their primary goal, and they are always tailored to the particular therapeutic area (see Chapters 12 and 43). For example, a template for analysing the quality of asthma treatment would not be relevant for an analysis of antibiotic use.

Another important point is that the individual-level statistics are just as dependent on a sensible classification of drugs as are the aggregate statistics. Although the hierarchical Anatomical Therapeutic Chemical (ATC) classification was primarily developed for aggregate statistics, it has proven immensely useful for individual-level statistics as well. The defined daily dose (DDD) methodology is also useful for individual-level statistics, although to a lesser degree (see Chapters 5 and 6) [2].

Epidemiological measures

Prevalence proportion

From an epidemiological viewpoint, the prevalence proportion (or point prevalence proportion) can be defined as the proportion of a population that is afflicted by a disease (or some other trait) at a given point in time. The prevalence proportion ranges from 0 to 1, or equivalently from 0 to 100%. The prevalence proportion of drug use is defined in a similar manner. A statement such as '3.6% of the Danish population used antidiabetics on 1 January 2014' uses a measure of prevalence proportion.

The typical measure from the aggregate statistics, the therapeutic intensity, can be construed as a crude measure of prevalence proportion. The therapeutic intensity of PPI use was 55 DDD/1000 inhabitants/day in Denmark in 2012 [3]. This implies that the amount sold was sufficient to treat 5.5% of the Danish population with 1 DDD each day in 2012. If all users of PPIs on average ingest 1 DDD per day when using the drug, then the therapeutic intensity is exactly equal to the prevalence proportion.

As simple as it seems, it is surprisingly difficult to estimate the point prevalence of drug use even from individual prescription data. The underlying problem is that prescriptions are redeemed on certain dates, occasionally with little information on how long they should be consumed for. Since nearly all drugs are used in irregular patterns by individual users, with periods spent on and off them, it is in practice difficult to distinguish between intermittent use and continuous use with irregular dispensings.

Nearly all approaches to estimating the point prevalence proportion have the same format: a period of usage is assigned to all prescriptions and the numerator in the prevalence proportion is the number of subjects who have a prescription with a period of usage covering the date of interest. How the periods of usage are assigned to prescriptions varies. If such data are available, it is possible to assign the period of usage on the basis of the legend duration or the dispensed quantity and prescribed dose [4]. Other options include assigning a constant period to each prescription, assuming a constant use of, say, 1 DDD or one tablet or assuming other fixed amounts of daily drug use [5]. These possibilities are illustrated in Figure 7.1. Noncompliance is frequent, and one should not blindly trust the legend duration as indicating the period of usage for a prescription. Usually, a minor allowance is made for irregular drug intake, minor noncompliance or stockpiling by adding a so-called 'grace period' to the calculated duration of a prescription [6,7]. If a prescription is redeemed after the expiry of the assigned duration – including the grace period – of a prescription for the same drug then a new episode is commenced.

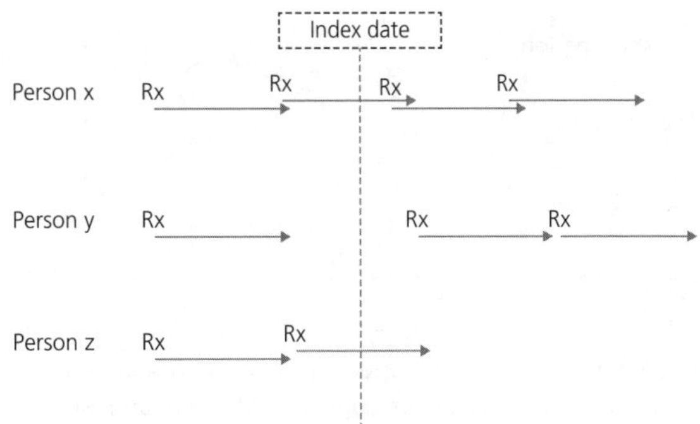

Figure 7.1 Methods for estimating prevalence proportion. A fixed index date is chosen and all subjects who have a prescription whose period of usage covers this date are considered users on that day. The period of usage may be assigned by different assumptions (e.g. a legend duration, a fixed period or a constant daily use). Person x and person z are both users on the index date, but person y is not, having a gap between two episodes.

Unless there are good reasons to choose differently, single prescriptions and the last prescription within an episode should be assigned durations using the same rules as for prescriptions that are in the middle of an episode [8]. For cohort studies, using different rules for single prescriptions or for the last prescriptions in an episode entails the risk of immortal time bias [9], since classifying these prescriptions as 'single' or 'last' is dependent on the future – in this case, on the absence of new prescriptions to follow.

Point prevalence estimates are surprisingly robust towards the durations assigned to single prescriptions, at least if these periods are not too short [10]. If a long duration is specified, then the assigned periods for a chain of prescriptions will overlap in most chronic users, and only the last prescription might extend beyond the patient's actual use. On the other hand, if a too-short period is assigned then the treatment will apparently consist of an alternating series of short intervals on and off the drug. Thus, for a drug that is typically used chronically, a generous grace period should be assigned to each prescription when determining point prevalence. These points are illustrated in Figure 7.2.

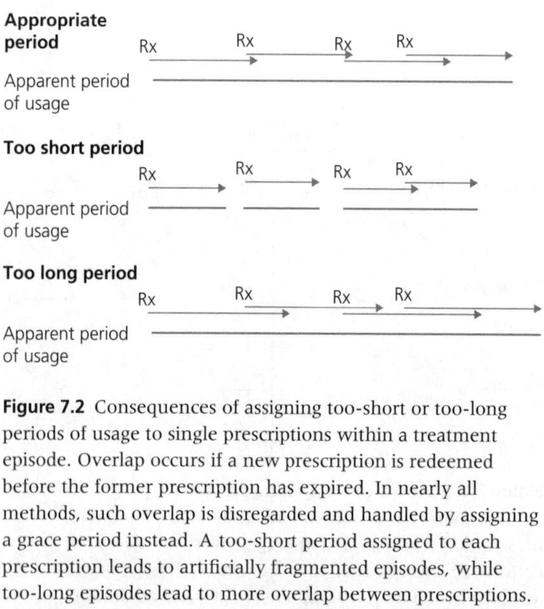

Figure 7.2 Consequences of assigning too-short or too-long periods of usage to single prescriptions within a treatment episode. Overlap occurs if a new prescription is redeemed before the former prescription has expired. In nearly all methods, such overlap is disregarded and handled by assigning a grace period instead. A too-short period assigned to each prescription leads to artificially fragmented episodes, while too-long episodes lead to more overlap between prescriptions. As overlap is disregarded, it only affects the duration of the last prescription within the episode, which extends beyond the true period of usage.

Period prevalence

The most common prevalence measure provided in publicly available statistics based on individual-level data is the period prevalence proportion, typically presented as a 1-year prevalence. For example, in the Danish national prescription database, the 1-year prevalence of PPI use was 9.1% in 2012 [3]. This implies that of 1000 people alive and resident in Denmark in January 2012, 91 would redeem a prescription during 2012.

While this measure seems fairly intuitive and is much simpler to calculate than the point prevalence proportion, it is problematic from a theoretical viewpoint. The period prevalence represents an indeterminate mixture of prevalent and incident users; that is, of people who were already users of PPIs from the beginning of the year and people who become new users during the year [11]. Thus, a high period prevalence might represent a high rate of new users (e.g. for antibiotics), a high number of persistent users (e.g. for insulin) or both (e.g. for nonsteroidal antiinflammatory drugs, NSAIDs).

Incidence rate

The incidence rate is determined straightforwardly as a count of new users divided by the person time at risk for becoming a new user. A statement such as '1.2% of the Danish population started using PPIs in 2013' employs the concept of incidence rate. The technically correct version of the same statement would be that 'in Denmark in 2013, 1.2 new users emerged per 100 years of follow-up'.

Establishing a person as a new user of a drug usually requires a run-in period, in which the person does not redeem prescriptions for the drug in question. Otherwise, an intermittent user or a regular user with long intervals between prescriptions might be falsely classified as a new user. The appropriate length of this run-in period varies according to therapeutic area, but requiring run-in periods of more than 2–3 years rarely has a major impact on the labelling of new users [12]. Individual-level migration data are also required to establish a person as a new user, since otherwise it is not possible to distinguish a genuinely new user from a person migrating into the population who was already a user at the time of migration.

The exact, cumulative person time at risk of becoming a drug user can be calculated from census data on individuals' births, deaths and migrations. The time at risk should not include follow-up for people who are already treated, as they are not at risk of becoming new users [13]. Thus, prevalent and past users should be removed from the pool. If a drug is rarely prescribed, a reasonable approximation for the time at risk is to use census data alone; that is, to ignore information on current and past drug use in the calculation of person time at risk.

Duration

The duration of drug use is also of strong interest in individual-level statistics. For example, there have been a number of disturbing reports on early discontinuation of drugs prescribed for the secondary prevention of myocardial infarction or stroke [14–16]. A calculation of duration may thus serve as a screening tool for persistence problems (see Chapter 36). We present here three different methods of estimating duration: the prevalence/incidence relationship, the Kaplan–Meier method and the waiting-time distribution (WTD).

According to epidemiological theory, the average duration of a disease can be estimated by a simple equation:

$$d = \frac{p}{(1-p)\times i}$$

where d is duration, p is point prevalence and i is the incidence rate of the disease [17].

This equation may also be applied to calculate durations of drug use, which in some settings is advantageous. First, it can be used to estimate very long durations even if only data from, say, a single calendar year are available. The key requirement is that the incidence and cessation rates are stable over an extended period of time. Second, provided that the incident users are classified correctly, there is no need to account for migration in or out of the population. Third, the equation applies equally well whether the reason for stopping the treatment is planned discontinuation, switch to another drug, nonpersistence, cure or death. Fourth, the processing is very simple, and less dependent on assumptions than, for example, the Kaplan–Meier approach.

When this approach is applied, some surprisingly short durations emerge (e.g. 6.4 years for insulin) [11]. These short estimates are not unique [18], and they have several possible explanations (e.g. the majority of insulin users have type 2 diabetes and may not need the drug permanently or have a high mortality) [19,20]. For nearly all drugs, we find a surprisingly high proportion of users who apparently only redeem one prescription [11]. Obviously, these users have a strong impact on the average duration.

There are a number of caveats to these duration estimates:

- There can be inherited problems from using biased prevalence proportion or incidence rate estimates as input.
- They only apply to equilibrium states. If, for example, the incidence rate is rising, then the duration will be biased downward.
- They are biased downward by heterogeneity in the prevalence proportion and incidence rate of drug use in the underlying population [17].
- They do not apply to any real population of users. For example, we might formally estimate the average duration of insulin use to be 10.4 years for 25-year-olds in 2012. This seems peculiar on a couple of counts: 25-year-olds do not continue to be 25 for 10.4 years and 2012 lasted only 1 year. However, its interpretation is equivalent to that of life-table techniques: a newborn child experiencing the same age-specific mortality as the present population will not relive the present year again and again.

As an alternative to using the prevalence/incidence relationship, duration may be estimated using the Kaplan–Meier technique. This entails the identification of a number of new users, who are followed until their treatment apparently stops (emigration and death are treated as either censoring or competing events). The chain of prescriptions that belong to the current treatment episode may be identified using the same techniques as are used to determine the point prevalence of drug use; that is, assigning periods of usage to single prescriptions under different assumptions and using grace periods. In contrast to the estimates based on the prevalence/incidence relationship, the Kaplan–Meier estimates do apply to real populations of users and can estimate other parameters besides average duration. On the other hand, they often require several years of data, including data on migration.

Some Kaplan–Meier analyses have shown disturbingly poor persistence for antithrombotic drugs prescribed to prevent relapse of stroke or myocardial infarction [14,16]. One important caveat should be considered. Drug survival analyses based on the Kaplan–Meier technique are remarkably sensitive to assumptions about grace periods and how usage periods are assigned to prescriptions [16,21]. In particular, if too short periods are employed, many drug users who are moderately noncompliant will have gaps between prescriptions that exceed the allowed limit and will be deemed to have stopped treatment temporarily. It is usually wise to assign a long period to each prescription. If the true period of usage for each prescription is shorter, it will have no consequence for the calculated persistence, except for the last prescription in a treatment episode, which might be assigned a period that exceeds the true period of usage. Too short periods, on the other hand, will lead to false early discontinuations and overly pessimistic drug survival results. Generally, it is wise to include sensitivity analyses for different choices of grace periods.

Drug survival analyses are often comparative; that is, they analyse persistence for competing therapeutic alternatives. There are several examples of new drugs that have claimed advantages over older alternatives but, surprisingly, show a much shorter persistence [22–24].

WTD is the distribution of individual waiting times from the beginning of a time window until an individual's first prescription occurs within that window. Typically, the WTD distribution will have an initial peak at the beginning of the window, which reflects drug users continuing their treatment from the preceding period (i.e. prevalent users). Towards the end of the observation window, the WTD will level off and reach a more or less constant level, corresponding to the underlying rate of treatment initiation (i.e. incident users). In its simplest form, the WTD is thus constructed by identifying the first prescription redemption for each person within an observation window and then plotting these redemptions in a histogram against time since start of window (Figure 7.3).

After the initial peak caused by prevalent users, the constant level towards the end of the observation window consists of incident users, and consequently this part of the distribution can be used to study the incidence rate (e.g. its magnitude, trend and seasonality) [25]. The right 'tail' of the WTD is not always declining or constant (e.g. if the incidence rate of new treatments is rising). The area at the left of the histogram above this level must therefore correspond to users already in treatment at the beginning of the interval (i.e. prevalent users). Based on the histogram, it is thus possible to estimate the number of incident and prevalent users, respectively, and estimates of the population incidence and prevalence can in turn be directly obtained, provided the corresponding total population size is known (Figure 7.3). In practice, this approach involves defining a cut-off point after which the WTD is deemed to have reached its plateau level of incident use [26].

The WTD was first introduced by Hallas et al. in 1997 [26] to avoid using run-in periods in estimations of incidence and prevalence. We described how the WTD

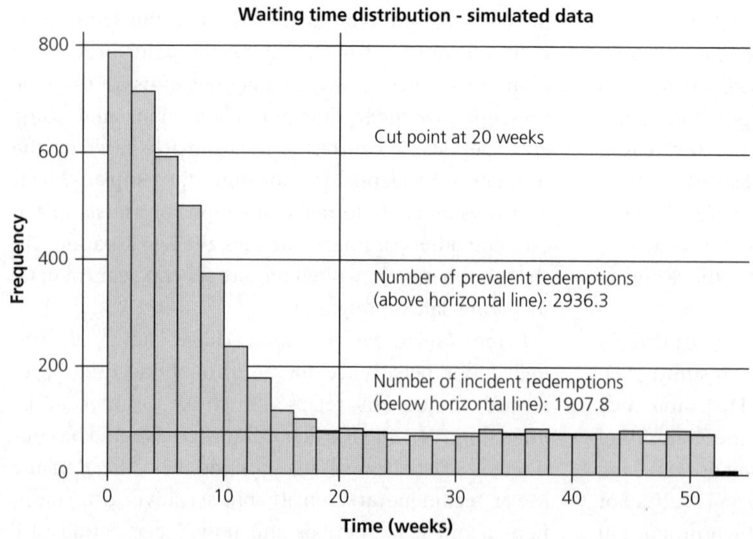

Figure 7.3 Hypothetical waiting-time distribution (WTD) for a simulated population of 100 000 people, where the true prevalence is 3% and the true incidence is 2 per 1000 person years. The estimated prevalence in this example would be 2.94% (found as 2936.3/100 000) and the estimated incidence would be 1.99 per 1000 person years (i.e. 1907.8/(100.000 – 2936.3 – 1907.8/2)).

is useful for visual inspection of important characteristics of drug use, particularly for determining duration of usage after a prescription. Støvring and Vach formalized the method by introducing parametric probability distributions for the two compartments of the WTD [27]. The model allows estimation of incidence and prevalence by the ordinary statistical method of maximum likelihood without having to first choose a cut-off point. As a consequence of the formalization, the method directly provides valid confidence intervals and test statistics for its parameters. It further allows formulation of an extended model for all subjects under observation, not just those with observed prescription redemptions. Subjects will then contribute either an observed first redemption in the time interval or a right-censored observation. The approach was formulated in detail and validated by simulation [27], but apart from a few studies [28,29] it has not seen widespread use in its parametric form. An example of its application is shown in Figure 7.4. The simulation studies indicated that the method approximately requires a doubling in sample size to maintain precision in incidence and prevalence estimates of situations where the actual status, incident or prevalent user is directly observed for each individual.

In the usual situation, where a drug is used intermittently by some users, the WTD will be made up of three components: prevalent users, intermittent users and truly new users. This will manifest itself by a long tail of the right part of the histogram, which may mean that the distribution does not reach the nearly constant level within the observation window, which is needed to estimate the incidence rate. It has been suggested that the WTD is then useful for detecting the presence and

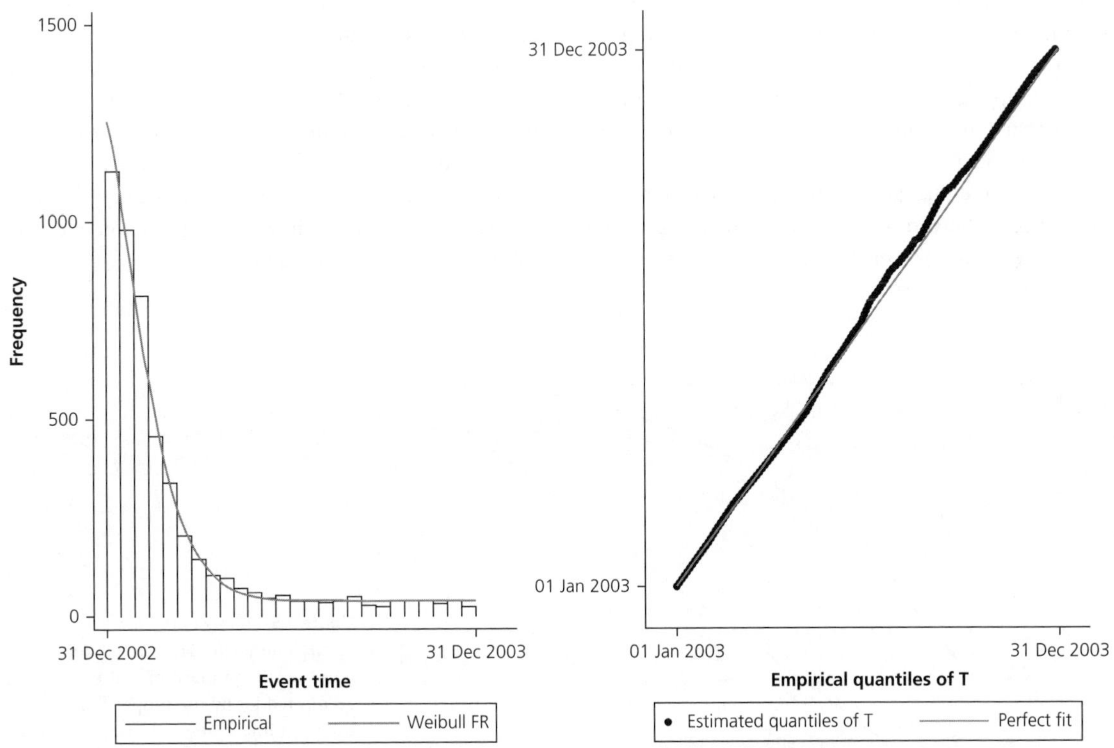

Figure 7.4 Observed and fitted WTD for insulin users, County of Funen, Denmark, 2003 (n = 491 691). Left: observed and expected frequencies; right: quantile–quantile. Corresponding estimates of prevalence and incidence are 8.12 (95% CI: 7.84; 8.41) per thousand and 2.16 (1.97; 2.37) per thousand person years, respectively. 'Weibull FR' refers to the declining distribution for prevalent users being modelled by a Weibull forward recurrence distribution; that is, the gap times between subsequent prescription redemptions of individuals are assumed to follow a Weibull distribution.

Source: Hallas & Støvring 2006 [11]. Reproduced with permission from John Wiley and Sons.

possibly the duration of intermittent usage patterns (see, for example, the WTD for antiulcer treatment presented in the original paper by Hallas et al. [26]), although formal analyses are complicated by the fact that the components no longer have distinctly different shapes.

Other measures

Lorenz curves

The Lorenz curve is an analytical tool, first used in the field of economics, that may be used to assess skewness in drug consumption [11]. To construct a Lorenz curve for a given drug, all users of that drug within a pre-specified time window (e.g. a year) are identified and ranked in descending order of total amount of drug (e.g. in DDD) dispensed within the window. A graph is produced, displaying which percentile of the users (x axis) accounts for a particular percentile of the total amount of redeemed DDDs (y axis). An example, showing the Lorenz curve for methylphenidate users, is depicted in Figure 7.5. The Lorenz curve allows for a direct visual inspection of the degree of skewness in drug consumption.

From the resulting graph, the Gini coefficient can be calculated. The Gini coefficient is a measure of the inequality seen in the Lorenz curve, with a value of 0 expressing complete equality and a value of 1 expressing complete inequality. The Gini coefficient is the area between the actual Lorenz curve (the curved line in Figure 7.5) and the Lorenz curve for a drug with complete equality (the diagonal line in Figure 7.5) divided by 0.5 (representing the proportion of the total area of the graph that is above the diagonal line). The Gini coefficient for the Lorenz curve in Figure 7.5 is 0.49.

Other descriptive parameters derived from the Lorenz curve include the 'n-percentile' (the proportion of drug use accounted for by the top n% of heavy users). For example, in Figure 7.5, the 1-percentile is 6.1% and the 50-percentile is 84.4%. As another example, a Danish drug utilization study on the use of sumatriptan, an antimigraine drug, produced a Lorenz curve that displayed a 5-percentile of 50% (i.e. 5% of users used 50% of the total drug prescribed volume), indicative of a very skewed drug consumption [30].

Average daily dose

In many prescription databases (e.g. the Nordic prescription databases [31]), the dose instructions are not recorded in a structured format. While measures of DDD used per 1000 inhabitants per day are suggested as aggregate measures of drug use in society [32], individual-level drug data allow for an evaluation of the distribution of doses among subjects.

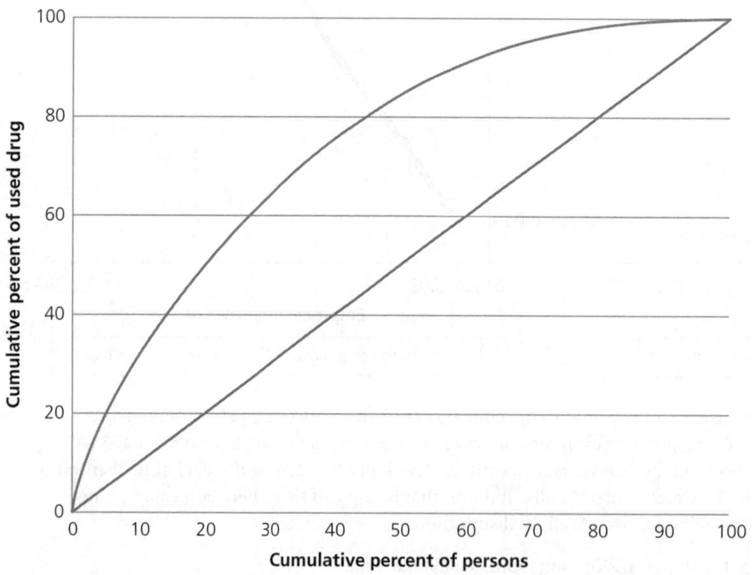

Figure 7.5 Lorenz curve for methylphenidate. The curved line indicates the proportion of drug use accounted for by the proportion of the most intensive users. The diagonal line indicates a completely homogenous drug use, with all users taking the same amount.

Source: Pottegård et al. 2012 [36]. Reproduced with permission from European Journal of Clinical Pharmacology.

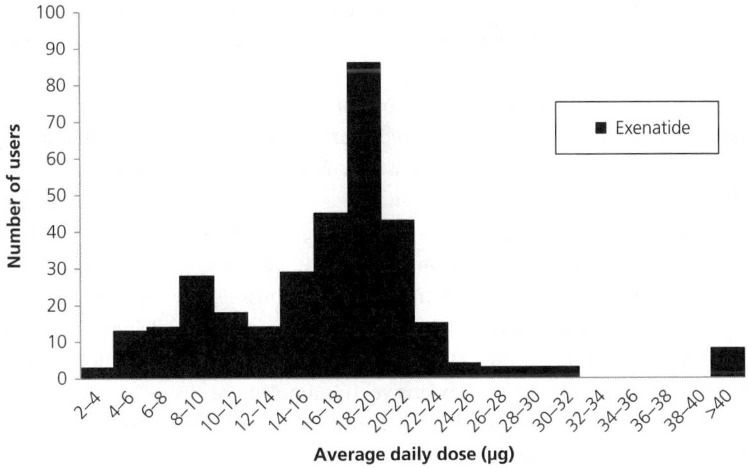

Figure 7.6 Average daily dose among Danish users of exenatide in 2012, calculated as a moving average of the up to four last prescriptions leading up to the last prescription in 2012.

Source: Pottegård et al. 2014 [33]. Reproduced with permission from European Journal of Clinical Pharmacology.

When dose instructions are not available, the average dose used can be calculated for a single subject as follows. The amount of drug used per day in a period between two dispensings is calculated as the amount of active drug substance redeemed at the first prescription divided by the number of days between the two prescriptions. The average dose used is then calculated as a moving average of the drug used per day in the last, say, three periods, weighed by the length of each period. For a patient redeeming 30 tablets of 20 mg, 30 tablets of 40 mg and 30 tablets of 20 mg of a given drug, each with a 30-day interval, the average dose used would be 20 mg/day by the end of the first interval and 30 mg/day (not 40 mg/day!) by the end of the second interval.

The estimated daily dose can be displayed graphically, either as a distribution of doses for users of a drug (as shown in Figure 7.6 for the antidiabetic exenatide [33]) or as a temporal trend of doses used (as shown in Figure 7.7 for the ADHD drug methylphenidate [34]).

Strengths and limitations of individual-level statistics

The strength of the analytical templates presented here is their wide applicability: they can be processed meaningfully on nearly all drugs or drug classes with little or no adaptation. The output of these analyses can give

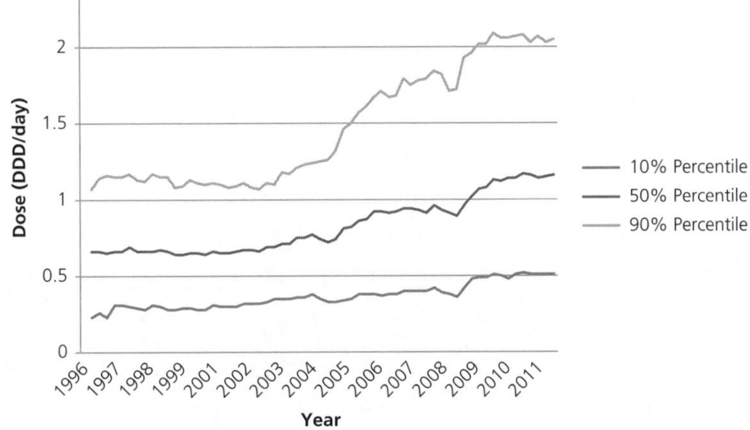

Figure 7.7 Development in doses of methylphenidate among Danish children aged 6–12 years. The dose distribution was estimated as the moving average of daily doses among all users of methylphenidate over time.

Source: Pottegård et al. 2013 [34]. Reproduced with permission from European Journal of Clinical Pharmacology.

very generic clues to problematic usage and prescribing behaviours (e.g. an unexplained skewness in doses). However, their wide applicability is also to some extent their limitation: if the intention is to capture problematic prescribing within a well-defined therapeutic field, it is usually wise to tailor the analysis specifically to that field.

Another potential limitation is the extent to which these measures are dependent on health care structure (e.g. reimbursement practice or in-hospital dispensing). Our description is based on a typical Western European model, with a strong primary care acting as gatekeeper, little in-hospital dispensing, extensive reimbursement, universal coverage of a health plan and a full account of a geographically defined, stable population. However, as our description is founded on very general epidemiological concepts, it is widely robust towards differences in health care structures. A good example is the WTD. Some health plans do not allow a single dispensing of medication for more than 1 month's supply. Obviously, this will affect the shape of the WTD (towards a steeper initial decline), but the parameters estimated from the graphs (e.g. incidence rate, prevalence proportion and duration) will not be affected, all other thing being equal. Some data sources (e.g. American MEDICAID databases) have very unstable populations, with a large proportion leaving or entering the cohort every year [35]. In such situations, great care should be taken to account for censoring. It is difficult to give general rules as to how health care structure might affect specific measures, but a good piece of advice is to be very well acquainted with the data source that is used for analyses.

CHAPTER 8

Measurement of drug expenditure

Sabine Vogler[1] & Jaana E. Martikainen[2]

[1]*WHO Collaborating Centre for Pharmaceutical Pricing and Reimbursement Policies, Health Economics Department, Gesundheit Österreich GmbH/Geschäftsbereich ÖBIG – Austrian Public Health Institute, Austria*

[2]*Research Department, Social Insurance Institution (Kela), Finland*

KEY POINTS

- Pharmaceutical expenditure can be used to measure the economic importance of various medicines.
- Pharmaceutical expenditure is medicine price multiplied by volume. Both price and volume components are influenced by a range of policy measures.
- Data gaps related to pharmaceutical expenditure exist for most countries. National databases usually don't include pharmaceutical expenditure data from the inpatient sector or on (outpatient) medicines not funded by public payers.
- It is of key importance to know the definitions and specifications of national pharmaceutical expenditure data before analysing and comparing them.
- Medicines prices can be indicated at different price types and may include (usually confidential) discounts.

Introduction

Pharmaceutical expenditure provides a measure of the economic importance of medicines. It is affected by both volume and price and is used in national and cross-national statistics and for pharmaceutical policy analyses. However, there is a lack of comparable data for this major indicator, particularly for low- and middle-income countries. As a result, major questions remain unanswered: How much do countries spend on medicines, and has this increased? How are expenditures funded (e.g. public funding through taxes or health insurance contributions, private funding via out-of-pocket payments or private insurance) and what is the relevance of their components? Worldwide, the most up-to-date data are available only for the years 2005 and 2006, following a World Health Organization (WHO) study in 2011 [1].

The availability and quality of data on pharmaceutical expenditure are better in high-income countries. Major repositories of pharmaceutical expenditure data are the Organisation for Economic Co-operation and Development (OECD) Health Data [2] and Eurostat Health database [3], which cover only most high-income and a few middle-income countries. Clear definitions guide countries when they populate these databases. Efforts have been made to develop international standards and definitions in the field of health accounting. For instance, the OECD, Eurostat and WHO cooperated in the collection of health expenditure data based on the System of Health Accounts (SHA) methodology, which led to the launch of the Joint OECD–Eurostat–WHO Health Accounts Data Collection [4,5] and resulted in the SHA 2011 publication (see Box 8.1) [6]. Still, methodological challenges related to pharmaceutical expenditure remain, and in-depth knowledge and understanding are required for the collection, analysis and comparison of pharmaceutical expenditure data.

Large variances exist in pharmaceutical expenditure between different countries and regions of the world, due to differences in the size and wealth of these countries and regions: according to a WHO publication in 2011, pharmaceutical expenditure per capita in 2005/06 (most recent data available) ranged from USD7.61/EUR5.5 in low-income countries to USD431.6/

Drug Utilization Research: Methods and Applications, First Edition. Edited by M. Elseviers et al.
Published 2016 by John Wiley & Sons, Ltd.

Box 8.1 System of Health Accounts (SHA) – a global standard by which to comparably record health expenditure.

The first SHA, which proposed a framework for the systematic description of financial flow related to health care, was presented by the OECD in 2000. In 2003, a WHO/World Bank/US Agency for International Development (USAID) Producers Guide for producing national health accounts with specific applications in low- and middle-income countries was published. With the goal of producing a global standard in health accounting, a formal collaborative effort between the OECD, Eurostat and WHO was agreed in 2006 to oversee the revision of the SHA Manual. This resulted in the updated manual *A System of Health Accounts, 2011 Edition* [5], published by the three organizations.

The SHA 2011 tracks all health spending in a given country over a defined period of time regardless of the entity or institution that financed and managed that spending. It aims at generating consistent and comprehensive data on health spending in a country, which can contribute to evidence-based policymaking.

The core accounting framework is organized around a triaxial system for the recording of health care expenditure, namely classifications of the functions of health care, health care provision and financing schemes, in order to address three basic questions:

- What kinds of health care goods and services are consumed?
- Which health care providers deliver these goods and services?
- Which financing scheme pays for these goods and services?

The nearly 500-page textbook provides definitions, classifications, concepts and guidelines for compilers.

Source: Data from OECD, Eurostat, WHO. *A System of Health Accounts.* OECD Publishing, 2011 [5].

EUR315.0 in high-income countries, with considerable variation between income groups. On average, 24.9% of total health expenditure was spent on medicines, ranging from 7.7 to 67.6% in the around 120 countries surveyed [1].

Total pharmaceutical expenditure in the OECD countries was approximately USD800 billion/EUR582 billion in 2011 (latest available year) [7]. Even within the OECD countries, most of them high-income, wide variations exist: At almost USD1000/EUR730, the United States spent far more on medicines than any other OECD country on a per capita basis (Figure 8.1). On average, spending in medicines accounted for almost one-sixth (17%) of all health expenditure in 2011, making medicines the third largest spending component after inpatient (hospital) and outpatient (ambulatory) care (Table 8.1) [7].

Table 8.1 Variation in total and public pharmaceutical expenditure in EU member states, 1990, 1995, 2000, 2005, 11. Includes all 28 EU member states, except Croatia and Malta (no data available).

Source: Data from OECD Health Data 2013 (for OECD countries) [2] and Eurostat (for non-OECD countries) [3].

	Total pharmaceutical expenditure in the outpatient sector (in billion euros)					Total pharmaceutical expenditure as a share (%) of current health expenditure				
	1990	1995	2000	2005	2011	1990	1995	2000	2005	2011
Austria	1.1	1.5	2.5	3.3	3.8	10	10	10	13	12
Belgium	1.9	2.9	n.a.	5.1	6.0	16	18	n.a.	17	16
Bulgaria	n.a.	n.a.	n.a.	0.6	n.a.	n.a.	n.a.	n.a.	34	n.a.
Cyprus	n.a.	n.a.	n.a.	0.2	n.a.	n.a.	n.a.	n.a.	22	n.a.
Czech Republic	0.2	0.7	0.9	1.8	2.3	24	28	25	26	20
Denmark	0.7	1.0	1.3	1.7	1.8	8	9	9	9	7
Estonia	n.a.	n.a.	0.1	0.1	0.2	n.a.	n.a.	23	24	22
Finland	0.7	1.0	1.5	2.1	2.3	10	14	16	17	14
France	14.6	18.5	23.9	31.7	36.2	17	15	17	17	16
Germany	15.4	23.9	28.8	36.1	41.4	15	13	14	16	15
Greece	0.4	1.2	2.0	4.0	5.4	15	16	20	22	29
Hungary	0.0	0.4	n.a.	2.3	2.6	n.a.	27	n.a.	31	34
Ireland	0.3	0.4	0.9	2.0	2.5	13	12	15	17	18
Italy	11.0	13.7	20.5	25.0	23.6	21	21	23	21	17
Latvia	n.a.	n.a.	n.a.	0.2	n.a.	n.a.	n.a.	n.a.	23	n.a.
Lithuania	n.a.	n.a.	n.a.	0.4	0.5	n.a.	n.a.	n.a.	34	26
Luxembourg	0.1	0.1	0.2	0.2	0.2	15	12	11	10	9

	Total pharmaceutical expenditure in the outpatient sector (in billion euros)					Total pharmaceutical expenditure as a share (%) of current health expenditure				
	1990	**1995**	**2000**	**2005**	**2011**	**1990**	**1995**	**2000**	**2005**	**2011**
Netherlands	1.9	2.8	3.9	5.9	6.8	10	12	12	11	10
Poland	n.a.	n.a.	n.a.	4.3	5.7	n.a.	n.a.	n.a.	30	24
Portugal	0.8	1.6	2.4	3.3	3.1	25	24	22	22	19
Romania	n.a.	n.a.	n.a.	1.2	2.2	n.a.	n.a.	n.a.	28	30
Slovakia	n.a.	n.a.	0.6	1.1	1.5	n.a.	n.a.	35	33	29
Slovenia	n.a.	n.a.	n.a.	0.5	0.6	n.a.	n.a.	n.a.	22	20
Spain	3.7	6.4	9.7	15.1	17.2	19	20	22	21	18
Sweden	1.1	2.1	3.0	3.6	4.4	9	13	15	14	13
United Kingdom	7.4	12.5	16.0	19.4	n.a.	14	16	15	13	n.a.

Total pharmaceutical expenditure in the outpatient sector = pharmaceuticals and other medical nondurables dispensed to outpatients according to System of Health Accounts (SHA) classification.

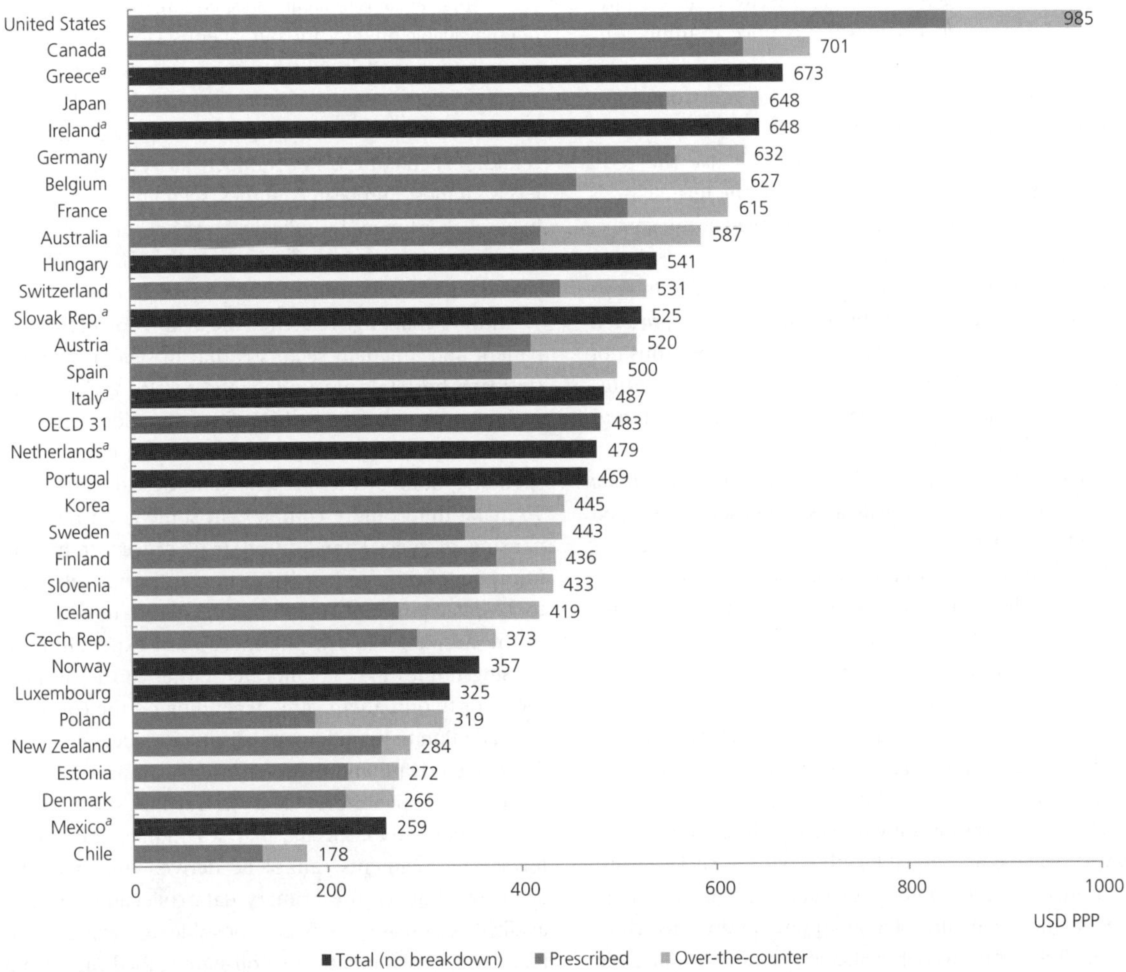

Figure 8.1 Pharmaceutical expenditure per capita, 2011 (latest available year). OECD31: 31 of the 34 OECD countries covered; USD PPP: United States Dollar Purchasing Power Parities. For colour details, please refer to the colour plates section.

[a]Includes medical non-durables

Source: Organisation for Economic Co-operation and Development 2013 [6]. Reproduced by permission of OECD Publishing.

The aim of this chapter is to present methodological considerations related to the measurement, analysis and comparison of pharmaceutical expenditure. We first present relevant definitions and highlight the importance of the underlying context. We then look at issues of pricing and of volume. We conclude by discussing methodological challenges to the measurement of pharmaceutical expenditure.

Definitions and perspectives

The OECD Glossary defines expenditures as 'the values of the amounts that buyers pay, or agree to pay, to sellers in exchange for goods or services that sellers provide to them or to other institutional units designated by the buyers' [8].

In simpler words, ***expenditure*** is price multiplied by volume.

The term ***cost*** is sometimes used as a synonym for expenditure(s); the term ***expenses*** is also used, but to a lesser extent. In this section we will use the term 'expenditure'. Sometimes, confusingly, the term 'cost' is used as synonym for 'price'; this is, however, not correct in economic terminology.

Price is the value component of expenditure. In general, it is defined as 'the value of one unit of a product, for which the quantities are perfectly homogeneous not only in a physical sense but also in respect of a number of other characteristics' [8]. For medicines, different price types are applied (see later).

Related to medicines, different measures of ***volume*** refer to the amount of medicines dispensed, prescribed or sold (see later).

To correctly interpret pharmaceutical expenditure, it needs to be understood which medicines, or further related goods, are covered by the data.

In many statistics, data refer only to public expenditure, with information on private pharmaceutical expenditure missing. For instance, data include prescription-only medicines (i.e. those medicines which require a medical prescription) and reimbursable medicines (i.e. medicines whose costs are fully or partially funded by public payers, such as a national health service or social health insurance). Pharmaceutical expenditure data often do not include spending for nonprescription medicines (over-the-counter (OTC) medicines) or nonreimbursable medicines, since they are typically derived from databases run by public payers and data on nonprescription and nonreimbursable medicines are owned by private market players (e.g. wholesalers, commercial publishing companies) and are not publicly available. In statistics, this distinction is usually summarized under the headings 'public' and 'private' pharmaceutical expenditure. Ideally, private pharmaceutical expenditure includes all out-of-pocket payments: the costs of both nonprescription and nonreimbursable medicines, as well as patient copayments on medicines (i.e. a contribution to reimbursable medicines through a fixed prescription fee or a percentage copayment on the price of the medicine).

In some databases (e.g. in the OECD Health Data), pharmaceutical expenditure data may include certain nonpharmaceuticals, such as medical devices, as medical nondurable goods (see also Figure 8.1).

Another caveat is that data on spending for medicines are often available only for the outpatient sector, due to different financing models: whereas public payers' spending on medicines in the outpatient sector is reported in the national reimbursement databases, hospital (or inpatient) pharmaceutical expenditure is not routinely surveyed at national levels. In most European countries, spending on medicines in hospitals is funded by individual hospital budgets [9], and data on medicine prices and consumption are usually not shared outside the hospital or the hospital group.

Another challenge related to the distinction of the outpatient and inpatient sectors is that in several national statistics, hospitals are understood to also include outpatient departments [10,11]. Thus, inpatient pharmaceutical expenditure data, where available, may include spending for medicines prescribed in these departments. To make things more complex, in some countries, dispensing of special medication (e.g. cancer or human immunodeficiency virus (HIV) medication) is restricted to hospital pharmacies, even for patients not residing in the hospital. Finally, pharmaceutical expenditure in nursing homes may be allocated either to the hospital sector or to outpatient care, depending on the country.

In addition to the traditional distinctions between public versus private and outpatient versus inpatient pharmaceutical expenditure, data on further subsegments may be required for specific analyses. In many cases, data for specific segments cannot be derived from national databases, but require primary data collection. In most available databases, it is not possible to separate, for instance, the expenditure of off-patent medicines from the expenditure of on-patent medicines or the expenditure of medicines prescribed by general practitioners in primary care from the expenditure of medicines prescribed by specialists working in outpatient care.

In one of its standard publications, *Health at a Glance*, the OECD defines the indicator 'pharmaceutical expenditure' as follows: 'Pharmaceutical expenditure covers spending on prescription medicines and self-medication, often referred to as over-the-counter products. In some countries, the data also include other medical nondurable goods (adding approximately 5% to the spending). The expenditure also includes pharmacists' remuneration when the latter is separate from the price of medicines. Pharmaceuticals consumed in hospitals are excluded (their inclusion would add another 15% to pharmaceutical spending approximately). Final expenditure on pharmaceuticals includes wholesale and retail margins and value-added taxes' [7]. This long definition highlights that pharmaceutical expenditure includes several perspectives and units of measurements.

Price-related units of pharmaceutical expenditure

In this section, we will discuss the typical price types applied in the outpatient and the inpatient sectors. We will also address how pricing and reimbursement policies in both sectors impact medicine prices.

Outpatient sector

Price components as a result of pricing policies

Outpatient medicine prices are expressed by the following components: the ex-factory price (price set at the level of the manufacturer); the pharmacy purchasing price/wholesale price (price at the level of the wholesaler; this includes the remuneration for the wholesaler); and the pharmacy retail price (price at the level of the pharmacy; this includes the remuneration for the wholesaler and the pharmacist). The pharmacy retail price may be net (excluding taxes such as the value-added tax or a pharmacy tax) or gross (including these taxes). Figure 8.2 lists the price types related to the various stakeholders in the system.

In countries with a publicly funded pharmaceutical system (e.g. all EU member states; see Box 8.2 for background information on the organization and funding of pharmaceutical systems), prices tend to be regulated at all price levels, at least for those medicines which are fully or partially funded by the public payers (so-called reimbursable medicines) [10].

In Europe, prices for reimbursable medicines are usually set by the state at the ex-factory price level, but a few countries (e.g. Finland, the Netherlands, Sweden, the United Kingdom) set the price at the wholesale level (pharmacy purchasing price) [12,13]. In several countries, the prices of

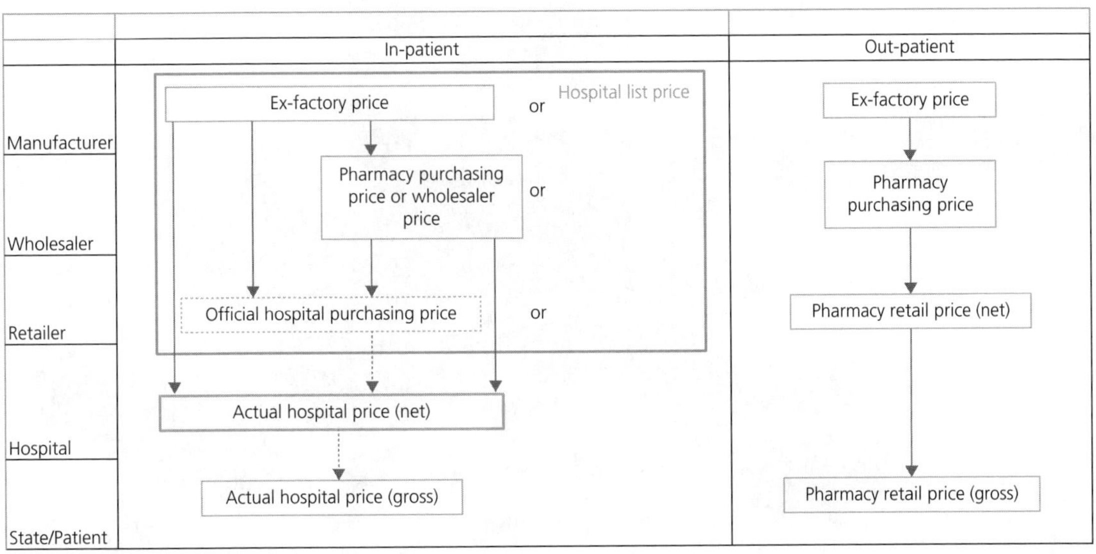

Figure 8.2 Build-up of medicine prices in the inpatient versus the outpatient sector.

Source: Vogler S, Habl C, Leopold C, Mazag J, Morak S, Zimmermann N. PHIS Hospital Pharma Report. Vienna: Pharmaceutical Health Information System (PHIS), 2010 [8]. Source: Reproduced by permission of Dr Dr Sabine Vogler.

Box 8.2 Organization and funding of pharmaceutical systems.

In most countries, the pharmaceutical system is split into two sectors: a public and a private. In the public sector, medicines are provided to eligible patients for free or against a modest copayment in public sector facilities. These medicines are procured by the state. The state selects which medicines are provided in the public sector (such medicines are typically put on an 'essential medicines list'). In the private sector, patients have to purchase medicines fully out-of-pocket from private retailers (e.g. private pharmacies). There is no public (co-)funding for these medicines.	In European countries and some other high-income countries (e.g. Canada, Australia, New Zealand), the distinction between the public and private sectors is not always clear, and the terms 'public sector' and 'private sector' are not applied. In these countries, medicines are usually supplied through private channels (private wholesalers, private pharmacies), but they are largely publicly funded: the state either pays the full price or pays most of the price (i.e. patients have to co-pay). Thus, the organization of these pharmaceutical systems is apparently private, but funding is predominantly public.

reimbursable medicines are statutorily set (i.e. based on a legal act such as a law or decree). Prices can also be negotiated between the state (typically represented by the reimbursement authority) and the manufacturer. Sometimes, a combination of both procedures is applied [14,15].

Different methods of setting an (ex-factory) price can be applied. One frequently used approach is external price referencing, whereby price(s) in other countries are used to derive a benchmark or reference price by which to set the price of a new product [10]. As of 2014, 25 out of the 28 EU member states (all but Denmark, Sweden and the United Kingdom) applied external price referencing, at least as a supportive tool, for new medicines in the outpatient sector (see Figure 8.3) [16–18].

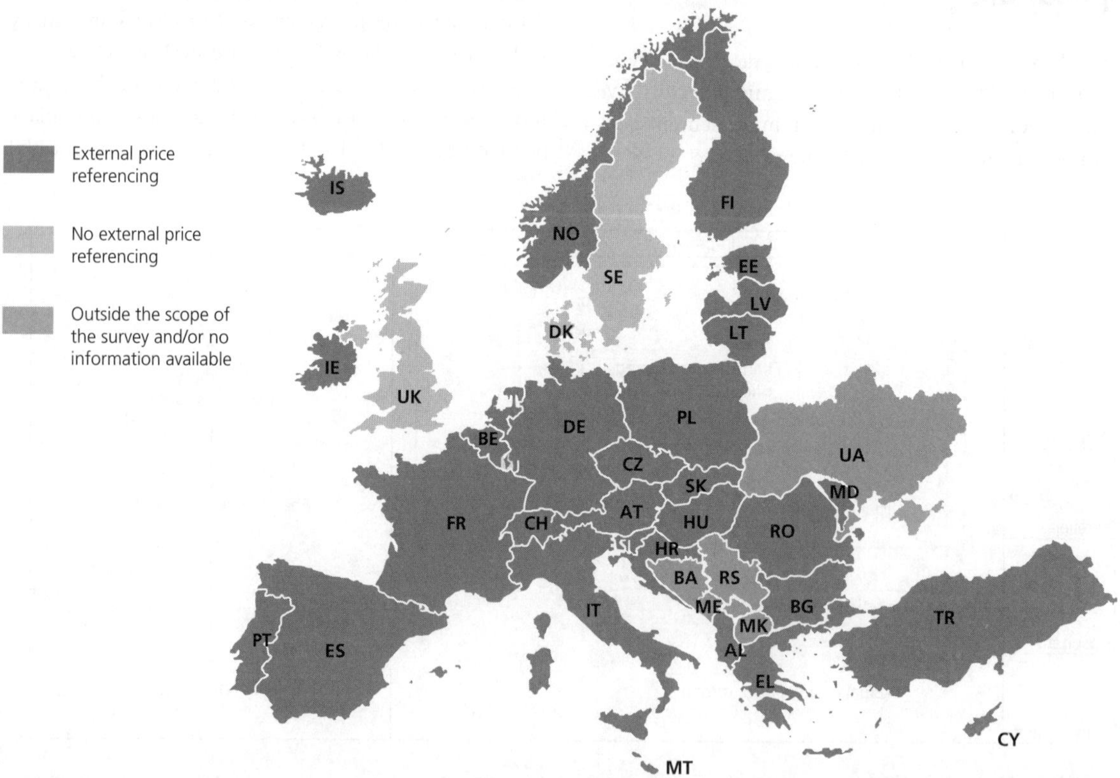

Figure 8.3 External price referencing applied as pricing policy in the 28 EU member states, Albania, Iceland, Moldova, Norway, Switzerland and Turkey. For colour details, please refer to the colour plates section.

Source: Data from [15] and [16].

Various methodological approaches can be employed in external price referencing (Box 8.3): generic medicine prices can be set a specific percentage lower than the price of the originator ('generic price link'), competition mechanisms can be used to decrease prices, or a mixture of the two approaches can be employed [11,19–21].

Pharmacy purchasing and retail prices can be set through regulations stipulating maximum remuneration to wholesalers and pharmacies, as well as further retailers. Wholesale remuneration is statutorily regulated in most EU countries (all except Denmark, Cyprus, Finland, the Netherlands, Sweden and the United Kingdom), and pharmacy remuneration is regulated in all but one EU member state (it is liberalized in the Netherlands). Remuneration is usually regulated for reimbursable and/or prescription-only medicines, but in some European countries it covers all medicines [22–24]. Wholesale and pharmacy remuneration can take the form of fixed mark-ups/margins or regressive schemes. The design of wholesale and pharmacy remuneration influences pharmacy purchasing prices and pharmacy retail prices. Several European countries have opted for regressive wholesale and pharmacy margin schemes, whose proportional remuneration decreases as the price of the medicine increases. The share of the price attributable to wholesalers and to pharmacies tends to be higher for low-price medicines in regressive margin schemes. However, pharmacy remuneration may also be designed independently of the price, such as by granting a fee for service, as in the Netherlands or the United Kingdom, or by using a combination of price- and performance-oriented remuneration [11–13,23–25].

Box 8.3 Methodologies applied in external price referencing.

There is great variation in the methodology used in external price referencing between different European countries (data for all EU member states plus Norway, as of November 2010).

1. ***Methodology related to reference countries in the basket:*** The most common methodology is to have fewer than 10 countries in the basket; six countries have between 10 and 20 countries in their basket and four countries (Austria, Belgium, Malta and Slovakia) have more than 20. Slovakia has the maximum number of countries (n = 26) in the reference basket, and Luxembourg has the fewest (country = 1).
2. ***Methodology related to the reference price:*** The most commonly used approach is to take the average of the prices of the countries in the basket. Bulgaria, Greece and Norway define the average of the three lowest prices as their reference price, whereas Hungary, Luxembourg, Poland and Romania take the lowest price in their basket.
3. ***Methodology related to accessing the medicine price data:*** The majority of countries have some kind of agreement with manufacturers so that they will report price changes to public authorities. In addition, competent authorities check the manufacturers' reported prices. Austrian Social Insurance legislation provides for a public health institution, which runs a medicines price service (Pharma Price Information), to check the prices on a random basis.
4. ***Methodology related to price reviews:*** The frequency of reviewing prices differs between countries: some (e.g. Portugal) review prices on a quarterly basis, while others do not review prices regularly at all.

Changes related to the methodology of external price referencing, particularly related to the countries in the baskets, have occurred frequently in recent times, as a response to the global financial crisis.

Source: Data from [15] and [16].

The price of a medicine may be increased by duties and taxes, which are known to account for a considerable part of medicine prices in middle- and low-income countries [26–28]. In European countries, only value-added tax is applied to medicines. In most European countries, the value-added tax rate on medicines is lower than the normal rate for goods and services (standard value-added tax rate). When comparing pharmaceutical expenditure between countries, it is strongly advised to check whether data are indicated with or without taxes (i.e. gross or net).

Price databases often publish one or two price type(s). The other price types can be calculated taking into account relevant taxes and the statutory wholesale and pharmacy remuneration schemes. For the unregulated segments (e.g. nonreimbursable medicines or areas without regulated wholesale mark-up), medicine prices at other price types can, at best, be calculated based on estimated average margins, which are often not published and are therefore difficult to assess.

Relevance of reimbursement

When medicines are funded by public payers (e.g. national health services, social health insurance), there is a strong link between pricing and reimbursement. From the perspective of public payers, and also from a public health and equity perspective, the ***reimbursed***

price or ***reimbursement price*** is of key relevance. This refers to the maximum amount covered by public payers [29]. In European countries, the term 'reimbursement price' is usually not explicitly indicated, except in Austria, where the term 'sickness fund price' is used. In other countries, the reimbursement price can be derived from the medicine price, usually the pharmacy retail price, by deducting the percentage copayments incurred by consumers. Many European countries (all EU member states except Austria, Germany, Italy, the Netherlands and the United Kingdom [12,25]) ask the patient to copay a specific percentage of the medicine price. For instance, if the pharmacy retail price is €100 and the reimbursement rate is 80% then the reimbursement price amounts to €80. In this case, patients are required to copay €20, plus a prescription fee, if applicable. The percentage copayment/reimbursement often depends on the therapeutic value of the medicine or the seriousness of the disease that the medicine will treat and/or on the socioeconomic status of the patient.

A particular reimbursement price is called the ***reference price***, which is applicable in a reference price system. A reference price system, more a reimbursement than a pricing policy, should be distinguished from an external price referencing policy. An external price referencing policy compares international prices and is used when prices are set. A reference price system is a form of internal price referencing and is used to define the maximum price for reimbursement. In a reference price system, identical or similar medicines (e.g. originator medicines and generics) are clustered to a reference group, and a public payer defines the maximum amount (reference price) used as a basis for reimbursement for all medicines in the group [21,29]. A reference price group can be clustered according to the molecule, the class or the therapeutic group [30]. If a patient purchases a medicine that is more expensive than the reference price, they are required to pay the difference between the reference price and the pharmacy retail price, plus any further copayments (e.g. in Portugal, the percentage copayment is also applicable to the reference price [31]). As of 2014, 22 EU member states had a reference price system in place [18].

The ***tender price*** can be considered another type of reimbursement price. In many low- and middle income countries, medicines are centrally procured via tendering. This is also the case for specific high-cost medicines (e.g. blood factors) in European countries, particularly in the inpatient sector [9]. The price achieved – the tender price – is published. Tendering in the outpatient sector is a known strategy for bringing generic prices for public payers down in some European countries (e.g. preferential pricing) [32].

Discounts and rebates

Published price databases and price lists typically give the official prices (so-called 'list prices'). In practice, actual prices for many products in European countries are lower than the list prices, due to discounts, rebates and various arrangements between the pharmaceutical industry, wholesalers or pharmacies and public payers. The provisions of these arrangements are usually kept confidential.

Discounts and rebates can be granted between the actors along the supply chain (e.g. from wholesalers to pharmacies or from pharmacies to consumers). Legal provisions may specify the maximum amount of discount and rebate granted among market players. In France, for example, pharmacies are permitted to obtain a maximum discount of 2.5% on the pharmacy purchasing price (wholesale price) for reimbursable medicines from wholesalers; the limit is 17% for reimbursable generics [33].

The importance of discounts and rebates to public payers has increased in recent years. According to a survey of public authorities and payers [34], discounts and rebates were granted by pharmaceutical companies in the outpatient sector in 21 and in the inpatient sector in 25 of 31 surveyed European countries. The most common discounts or similar arrangements are price reductions and refunds linked to sales volume, but price-volume and risk-sharing agreements are also in place. A mix of various types of discounts and rebates is common. Risk-sharing and further managed-entry agreements, which attempt to manage uncertainty, are on the rise in several European countries, including the United Kingdom (patient access schemes), Italy, Poland and the Baltic States [35,36].

Discounts and rebates to public payers may also be granted by distribution actors. As of 2014, discounts arrangements, clawback schemes and similar financial contributions by pharmacists to public payers were in place in 14 of 30 European countries (all 28 EU member states, Norway and Switzerland) [24]. These can be calculated as a specific share of the price per dispensed medicine or per sales volume, with specifications for low-turnover and/or rural pharmacies.

The confidential character of discounts and rebates, and the resulting distortion of transparency related to medicine prices, is an important challenge and limitation in price-comparison studies (see later), and has major policy implications given the widespread use of external price referencing. Since countries will refer to the list prices indicated in the price databases instead of the actual discounted prices, they can risk overpaying. Discounts and rebates have been offered by industry to public payers in order to avoid statutory cuts of list prices, but this is likely to prevent a transfer of possible savings from price cuts to reference countries.

Inpatient sector

Price components as a result of pricing und procurement policies

In contrast to the outpatient sector, pharmacy retail prices are not applicable to the inpatient sector (Figure 8.2). Hospitals are usually directly supplied by the pharmaceutical industry or by wholesalers [9,37]. Thus, the 'official hospital price' is the only relevant official price type in hospitals; it generally corresponds to the ex-factory price or, in the case of delivery by a wholesaler, to the pharmacy purchasing price (wholesale price) or the 'tender price'.

Discounts and rebates

In the hospital sector, discounts and rebates are substantial. This is particularly true for medicines whose competitors have come on to the market or which are used for long-term treatment that continues in outpatient care. In some European countries, even cost-free medicines are permitted, and hospitals can obtain medicines at a price of €0 per unit. While large discounts and rebates are granted for high-volume medicines, in order to facilitate treatment initiation in hospitals, hospitals appear to have little headroom to negotiate price reductions for medicines to which no therapeutic alternatives are available [9,38]. This pattern suggests the need to bridge the gap between the outpatient and inpatient sectors, which results from a dual financing system in most European countries: medicines used in inpatient and in outpatient care are financed by different payers. This might incentivize payers to shift costs to the other sector [9].

Price data sources

Assessing price data is a challenge. According to the European Transparency Directive [39], EU member states have to publish price data for reimbursable medicines. In addition, there are a few commercial providers that offer price data, usually for big countries.

Since many countries require access to international price data, as they apply external price referencing [16,40], competent authorities in some European countries have established their own price collection systems (see also Box 8.3). One of these is the Pharma Price Information (PPI) service of the Austrian Health Institute. Based on Austrian General Social Insurance Law, PPI was established to support the Austrian Pricing Committee at the Austrian Federal Ministry of Health, but it also offers price data to third parties, including researchers (for a fee) [41].

With the support of a European Commission grant (2009–13), a European database (Euripid) has been established which takes data from and provides data to competent authorities of EU member states [42]. Since 2014, Euripid has continued as a member states collaboration.

Researchers working on drug utilization studies frequently use Intercontinental Marketing Services (IMS) data. IMS Health, a private information, services and technology provider, is known for the provision of sales data. IMS also provides price data for some countries, but this is not its core business.

In European countries with a publicly funded health care system (see Box 8.2), the prices (at all price types) of reimbursable medicines are identical throughout the country and can thus be accessed from national price lists. However, when prices vary (e.g. for the hospital sector, the OTC market and the large private sector of low- and middle-income countries), prices must be collected from individual health care providers. The WHO/HAI (Health Action International) Working Group has developed a methodology for assessing the availability and prices of medicines [26,43,44], which has allowed a database of survey findings to be built (http://www.haiweb.org/MedPriceDatabase).

Box 8.4 provides examples of research projects on medicine prices, some of them related to specific segments.

Box 8.4 Medicine price studies.

Various cross-national studies have compared the prices of medicines within a specific region or across a group of countries [17, 49–52].
Brekke et al. [53] compared prices in Norway to those in other countries in order to assess the impact of Norwegian pricing policies; they found that prices in Norway were among the lowest in Western European countries, both overall and for the on-patent and generics segments.
An OECD project [54] aimed to assess how OECD countries refer to 'value' when making decisions on reimbursement and the prices of new medicines by collecting the prices of 12 innovative products from 14 countries. The price of fingolimod, for example, a medicine used for multiple sclerosis, varied between USD2236/EUR1630 and USD2482/EUR1810 at market entry across the study countries.
Schulenberg et al. [55] looked at price data for angiotensin-converting enzyme (ACE) inhibitors in six Western European countries over the period 1991–2006 in order to analyse the impact of policy measures, and found that some measures (e.g. mandatory generic substitution, regressive pharmacy mark-ups and clawbacks) had been effective in reducing originator prices, whereas others had had an insignificant effect.
Some studies looked at the segment of off-patent medicines. They found large, smaller and sometimes no differences between the prices of on- and off-patent medicines, and identified a scope for reducing generic prices [19,56,57].
The prices of medicines used in hospitals were studied in the Pharmaceutical Health Information System (PHIS) project, which compiled information on pharmaceutical procurement, pricing and financing in 27 European countries. Detailed price information on both official list prices and actual prices in hospitals was gathered from five countries. Actual hospital prices proved to be lower than official list prices for medicines with therapeutic alternatives and for medicines intended to be continued in outpatient care. Discounts and rebates varied between therapeutic classes [9,38].

Volume-related units of pharmaceutical expenditure

Pharmaceutical expenditure is often expressed as expenditure per volume unit (for volume units, see Chapter 6). Commonly used approaches are expenditure per medicine user, per package and per a 'unit' of the pack (e.g. tablet, vial). A 'Standard Unit', used in some statistics (such as by IMS Health), is defined as the smallest dose of a product, equivalent to one tablet or capsule for an oral dosage form, one teaspoon (i.e. 5 ml) for a syrup and one ampoule or vial for an injectable product [45].

Expenditure per defined daily dose (DDD) is used in many statistics and studies. It must be kept in mind that the DDD is a measurement for drug utilization: DDDs are neither typically used doses nor are clinically equivalent doses. While DDDs are valuable measurements in drug utilization research, they are not considered suitable for comparing medicines for pricing, reimbursement and cost-containment decisions [46].

Approaches that include the outcome of a treatment (e.g. expenditure per cured patient) are seldom published.

Methodological challenges related to pharmaceutical expenditure

Overall challenges of pharmaceutical expenditure analyses and comparisons

In this chapter, we have already discussed several challenges related to the limitations in data availability and comparability:

- For some low- and middle-income countries, no (recent) data on pharmaceutical expenditure are available. Primary research is often required.
- Even for high-income countries, such as the European countries, getting access to comprehensive pharmaceutical expenditure data is a challenge. What is indicated in the standard databases as total pharmaceutical expenditure can refer, in practice, to outpatient pharmaceutical expenditure only. However, ignoring spending on the hospital sector in the context of European countries means that around a fifth of total pharmaceutical expenditure is not taken into consideration [22]. Private pharmaceutical expenditure also is a frequent data gap.
- Pharmaceutical expenditure data may be available from different sources, which implies variations in the underlying definitions and specifications.

Expenditure is affected by both volumes and prices of medicines. Thus, expenditure data are sensitive to variations in utilization and the product mix of medicines, as well as to changes in ex-factory, wholesale or retail prices. Given these data gaps and inconsistencies, researchers and policymakers are recommended to carefully check the scope and methodology of expenditure data.

As the number of patients or inhabitants has an effect on pharmaceutical expenditure, in cross-country comparisons data often need to be made comparable, such as by using pharmaceutical expenditure per patient or inhabitant. Another major challenge to pharmaceutical expenditure comparisons is the complexity of exchange rates. It must be ensured that all exchange rates are calculated using the same methodology (e.g. average monthly rate) and for the same date. Exchange rates will be discussed further in the next subsection, since they are related to the 'value' (price) component of pharmaceutical expenditure.

In this chapter, we have not discussed the challenges of time series analyses, such as breaks in series and retrospective adjustments of preliminary published data, because the methodological difficulties are the same as for time series analyses relating to other data (e.g. consumption data; see Chapter 10).

Challenges related to cross-national price comparisons

Cross-national medicine price comparisons can be used to compare the prices of individual products, the prices of medicine groups or the general price levels between countries, among other things. In all comparisons, the use of corresponding price types converted to common currency and comprehensive and representative products samples is crucial for a valid comparison.

The aim of the comparison defines what kinds of product are included in the analysis. When assessing the general price level, for instance, a large selection of products (i.e. a basket) representing the whole pharmaceutical market is required. The basket can include only medicines that are available in all countries under comparison, which can make product selection challenging. Even when a medicine is available in each country, there may be differences in package sizes, strengths, pharmaceutical forms, manufacturers and so on. Requiring complete matching of products often reduces the number of products available for the analysis, which can lessen the representativeness of the study. On the other hand, more flexible matching gives less precise results [47]. To make prices comparable, they must be measured per unit. Unit prices might either be prices per pack, per 'unit' of the pack (e.g. per tablet or vial), which may be challenging for some pharmaceutical forms, or per Standard Unit. A common approach is to compare prices per DDD. However, using DDD in price analyses can be controversial, as already mentioned.

Converting medicine prices to a common currency (euros or dollars) is necessary for accurate comparison. When doing this, it should be noticed that highly fluctuating currencies negatively impact the validity of the results, particularly in time-series analyses. Conversion can also be made by using exchange rates or purchasing power parities (PPPs). PPPs convert expenditure expressed in national currency into an artificial currency that aims to equalize the purchasing powers of different currencies by eliminating the differences in general price levels across countries [48]. PPPs are used for currency conversions on many statistics of the OECD and Eurostat. If medicines in the comparison are not equally consumed, which is usually the case, the price data should be combined with consumption data; that is, the prices should be weighted. A high-volume medicine should be given more weight than a medicine that is used by a few patients only. Typical consumption measures used in weighting are DDD and number of packages. The focus of the comparison determines whose volume data is used. If the study uses a basket that is weighted by the consumption data of one country, the comparison will show how much this basket would cost at the prices of that country. In cross-national price comparisons, relative price differences between countries are usually measured by using price indices (see Box 8.5) [47].

A data gap particularly relevant to cross-national price comparisons is the nonavailability of discounted price data, since they are usually confidential. Interpretations of price comparisons have to take this limitation of referring to list prices only into consideration.

Box 8.5 Price indices.

There are several price indices that can be used in cross-national price comparisons. The Laspeyres index uses the volume weights of the base country, the Paasche index uses the weights of the comparison countries and the Fisher index uses the geometrical mean of the Laspeyres and Paasche index numbers.

Danzon and Kim [47] compared medicine prices in eight high-income countries using all three of these indices. It turned out that the results were sensitive to the choice of index. A country's price level was lower if the evaluation was made using its own volume weights rather than those of a comparison country.

CHAPTER 9

Basic statistical methods in drug utilization research

Douglas T. Steinke[1] & Monique Elseviers[2]

[1]*Manchester Pharmacy School, University of Manchester, United Kingdom*

[2]*Centre for Research and Innovation in Care, Faculty of Medicine and Health Sciences, University of Antwerp, Belgium*

KEY POINTS

- The statistical approach to be used depends on the research question and the data collected.
- There are different tests for different types of variables, and they must be used appropriately.
- The process of statistics must be properly understood in order to interpret and critically evaluate its results.

Introduction

The purpose of this chapter is to review the basic concepts of statistics that are used in drug utilization research. We will not give details of the various statistical tests; the reader can find this information in a dedicated statistical textbook [1–4]. The chapter should be used to help inform statistical decisions and to review statistical methods that can be used for specific research questions.

The data given in Table 9.1, taken from a sample of hospitalized patients, will be used in the various examples in this chapter.

Why we need statistical methods in drug utilization and health services research

As drug utilization researchers, we supply health care providers and decision-makers with important new information that may contribute to the treatment of patients or to a change in practice. A good understanding of basic statistics will aid the researcher and clinician in:

- Evaluating the literature: Whether or not to believe the results presented.
- Applying study results to patient care: Applying evidence-based medicine to decisions about the care of individual patients.
- Interpreting information about drugs and equipment: Critically evaluating information given in reports, presentations and advertisements.
- Evaluating study protocols and articles: Critically evaluating literature submitted to peer review journals.
- Participating in research projects: Knowledge of statistical methods is indispensable when participating in research.

Use of population data versus sample data

Before starting an analysis of data, it is important to understand what kind of data we have. The question we should ask ourselves is, do we have data from the entire study population or data from a sample of that population?

Population data

Population-based statistics utilize the entire study population, and the results provide an accurate summary of that population. For the statistician, the main advantage

Drug Utilization Research: Methods and Applications, First Edition. Edited by M. Elseviers et al.
Published 2016 by John Wiley & Sons, Ltd.

Table 9.1 Patient characteristics for analysis.

ID	Age (years)	Sex	Ward	Number of medications	Antidiabetic medication	Anticoagulants	IV antibiotics	Care level	LOS (days)	QoL before	QoL after
1	88	M	Geriatrics	18	Met	Y	Y	2	21	6	4
2	59	F	Geriatrics	12	SU	Y	Y	2	14	4	2
3	83	F	Geriatrics	12	Met	Y	N	2	29	8	7
4	78	F	Geriatrics	16	SU	N	N	2	11	5	3
5	87	F	Geriatrics	5	Met	Y	N	2	1	9	5
6	82	F	Geriatrics	10	Met	N	N	1	48	3	3
7	89	F	Orthopaedics	12	Met	N	N	1	41	7	6
8	74	M	Orthopaedics	9	Met	N	Y	3	1	5	5
9	67	M	Orthopaedics	6	Met	N	Y	3	1	6	3
10	81	F	Orthopaedics	14	SU	N	Y	2	14	4	4
11	71	F	Orthopaedics	12	Met	N	N	1	4	7	4
12	86	M	Orthopaedics	11	Met	Y	N	2	7	5	5
13	86	M	Orthopaedics	5	Met	Y	N	1	16	8	4
14	55	M	Orthopaedics	9	Met	N	N	1	4	9	4
15	82	M	Orthopaedics	17	SU	N	N	1	8	6	6
16	55	M	Orthopaedics	13	SU	N	Y	3	12	4	4
17	79	M	Orthopaedics	11	SU	Y	Y	3	4	2	3
18	77	F	Vascular	8	SU	N	N	2	35	8	6
19	70	M	Vascular	16	Met	N	Y	2	17	6	6
20	53	M	Vascular	12	SU	Y	N	2	6	8	6
21	88	M	Vascular	11	SU	N	Y	2	16	6	6
22	67	M	Vascular	11	Met	Y	N	2	15	4	4
23	61	M	Vascular	14	SU	Y	N	2	15	9	6
24	87	F	Vascular	14	Met	Y	N	2	7	2	2
25	72	F	Vascular	17	Met	N	N	1	34	8	7
26	57	F	Vascular	18	SU	Y	N	2	3	9	7

IV, intravenous; LOS, length of stay; QoL, quality of life; Met, metformin; SU, sulfonylurea.

of population-based data is the lack of uncertainty in the results deriving from fluctuations in sample results and sampling errors. In drug utilization research, many examples using population-based data can be found. For example, several publications handle data from multiple nations in comparisons of antibiotic consumption based on complete national datasets of antibiotic prescriptions or sales data (see Chapter 14).

Sample data

Most medical knowledge, however, is still based on research performed in one or more ***samples*** selected out of the total population. Statistical methods that are used to make statements based on information gathered from samples drawn from a larger population fall into the category of inferential statistics. Here, the results of an inferential statistical analysis are 'inferred' back to the entire population [2]. For example, the English government can organize a health survey gathering data on a large sample of the English population and inferring the results to be representative for the entire population of England.

Sampling and selection bias

An important issue in sample design is what sampling procedure to use to select subjects. There are numerous possible methods, which differ in terms of cost, effort and the extent to which they are representative of the general population [5]. A random selection of the study population is highly recommended to avoid bias. A random sample is defined as one selected in such a way that every subject in the population has an equal and independent chance of being selected. If the sample is not representative of the larger population, the study results will be misleading. This is called ***selection bias***, which leads to systematic errors between the findings of the sample and the reality of the entire population.

Sample size

Another important issue that must be considered when using inferential statistics is the ***size of the sample population*** [6]. If a sample is too small to accurately represent the entire population, inaccurate estimates of the patient characteristics will be calculated and the inference will be inaccurate. Therefore, a sample-size calculation is used to ensure that inferential statistics give precise estimates of patient characteristics of the whole population. For comparative studies, the sample size greatly depends on the (predefined) type I and type II errors. A type I error arises if it is concluded from the sample study results that there is a statistical difference when in reality no difference exists. A type II error (power) is the opposite: it arises if it is concluded that no difference exists when in fact there is one. Power requirements, in particular, will determine the sample size. Sample size and power calculations are beyond the scope of this chapter, but details can be found in the literature [3].

Confidence interval

Even well-designed studies can give misleading results due to an extreme random variation in the sample. This means that if another sample of the same population is taken, the results will always be slightly different from those first calculated. Thus, results of a single sample are always subject to a degree of statistical uncertainty. Fortunately, the imprecision can itself be estimated, and may be presented as a ***confidence interval*** around the sample result. The most common is the 95% confidence interval (95% CI); this expresses that the real population result will lie within the limits of the confidence interval with a chance of 95%. In other words, out of 100 subsequent samples, 95 of the estimated CIs would be expected to encompass the true population mean. Confidence intervals can be calculated for most statistical results and are helpful for inferring sample results to the entire population [7,8].

Types of variables

To decide which statistical test to use, we need to know what kind of data we are working with [9,10]. A simple classification of data types is provided in Figure 9.1.

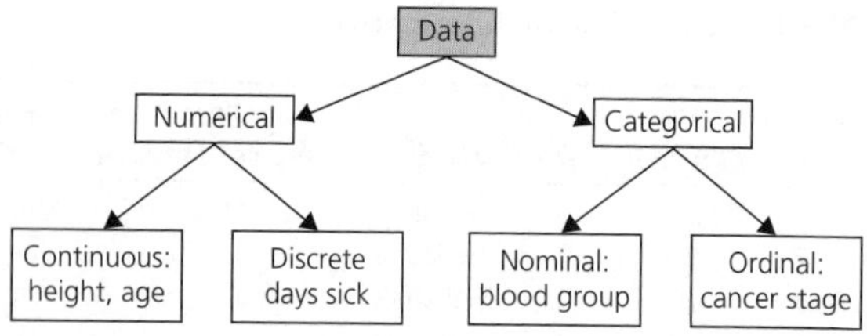

Figure 9.1 Data types.

The first decision is to differentiate between numerical (continuous or discrete) and categorical variables. A numerical variable is a series of numbers or counts (e.g. height, weight, age, sick days, drug expenditures or the number of days a drug was taken). A categorical variable is a variable that can be grouped into one of several, mutually exclusive, categories. There are two types of categorical variables, according to the ordering of the data within the group. Nominal variables do not have an order within the group (e.g. gender, blood type (A, B, O)). Ordinal variables, on the other hand, do have an order, which must be accounted for in the analysis. Examples of ordinal variables include cancer stage (stage 1, 2 or 3) and responses to a questionnaire (strongly agree, agree, disagree, strongly disagree). A variable is called dichotomous if it can only take two values (e.g. antibiotic treatment: yes/no). Dichotomous variables are most commonly measured using 1 and 0 as the two possible values.

Describing data with descriptive statistics

Once data collection is finished and the data have been recorded in a spreadsheet, the researcher can enjoy analysing the data, filling in tables and drawing graphs and figures. The first stage of analysis is to summarize the results [9]. Once the type of data is identified, summarizing is an easy task.

Description of numerical variables

Numerical variables may be summarized by using a measure describing the 'middle' (central tendency) and the 'spread' (variation) of the observations. Measures commonly used to describe the ***central tendency*** are the mean and the median. The arithmetic mean of a dataset is the average obtained by the sum of the values divided by the number of observations. The median is the 'middle-ranking' value obtained by ordering all the values (from the smallest to the largest) and selecting the one that appears in the middle. For the data in Table 9.1, age is a numerical variable with a mean of 74.4 years and a median of 77.5 years.

The ***spread*** of a numerical variable can be described using the standard deviation (SD), normally used with the mean, and the range or interquartile range (IQR), used with the median. The size of the SD depends on the number of observations of the sample, the mean and the distance to the mean of each observation in the sample. The range of values is preferentially mentioned as the interval between the lowest and the highest values. The IQR is the interval between the 25th and the 75th percentile of all ordered observations. Again using the example of age in Table 9.1, SD = 11.9, range = 53–89 and IQR = 67–85.

Description of categorical variables

Categorical variables may be summarized by counts, frequencies (%) or ratios. In Table 9.1, sex is a categorical variable and can be described as 14 males/12 females or 54% males/46% females or male/female ratio of 7/6.

Investigating the difference between the means and medians of numerical variables

Once the data have been summarized using descriptive statistics, comparisons can be made between variables to identify differences between groups [11]. An overview of statistical tests used for comparison is given in Figure 9.2. This section will use numerical variables from Table 9.1 to demonstrate how to use the appropriate statistical test.

Two-sample t-test for the difference between two independent groups

The most common application of statistical testing is in the comparison of two independent population parameters, such as the means of two subpopulations, using the ***independent or two-sample t-test***. This test compares the mean values of two groups. Let us compare the mean number of medications taken by patients in the geriatric and orthopaedic wards as presented in Table 9.1. The two groups are independent (the data are not matched) and the SDs are approximately similar for the geriatric and orthopaedic wards; the means (SD) are 12.2 (4.6) and 10.8 (3.5), respectively.

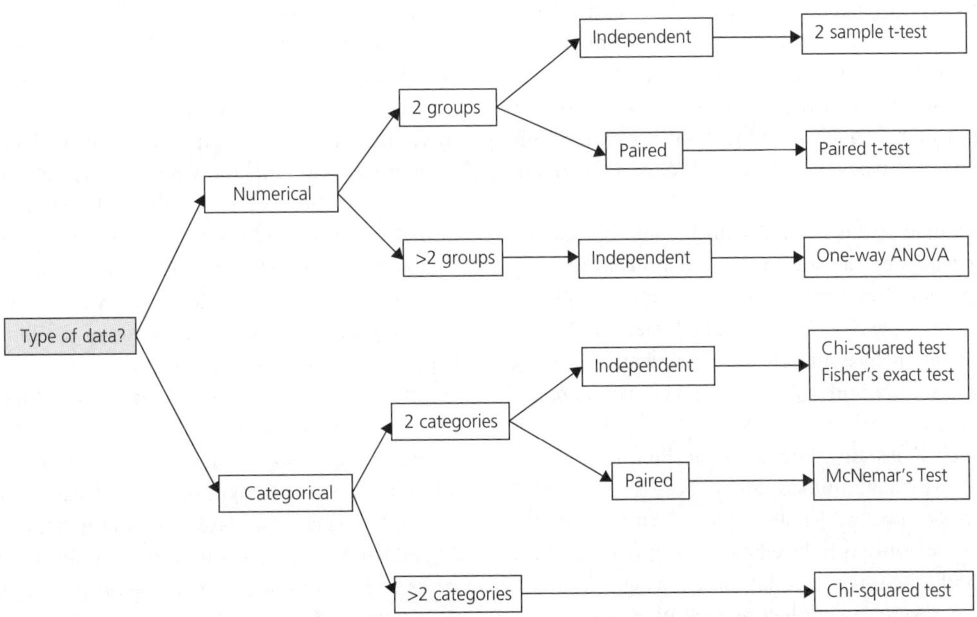

Figure 9.2 Flowchart for determining which standard statistical test is appropriate.

A two-sample t-test will determine whether the observed difference between both means can be considered as statistically significant. A p-value (or probability) is calculated using the mean, SD and population size of each group [11]. The p-value is usually compared to a threshold value, the significance level of the test (typically $\alpha = 0.05$). A researcher can calculate the p-value by hand, which is tedious, but there are several spreadsheet and statistical programmes that can do the calculation for us. With the independent two-sample t-test, we investigate the difference between two groups, starting from the null hypothesis that there is no 'real' difference between both. If the probability of obtaining the observed difference (or one that is more extreme) is less than 5% ($p < 0.05$), we have to reject the null hypothesis. In such a case, the data are more supportive of the alternative hypothesis: that the observed difference is a 'real' difference resulting from a systematic effect. In our example, the p-value is 0.503. Consequently, we cannot reject the null hypothesis and have to conclude that there is no significant difference between the number of medications taken in the two wards [12,13].

Paired sample t-tests for differences between paired data

For matched or paired data, similar tests can be used that account for the similarity of the groups. In this case, the data are not independent, but are derived from the same subjects (e.g. in a pre- or post-test) or from matched pairs of subjects in an experimental design (e.g. pairs of subjects matched for age and sex).

An example of this is quality-of-life data on patients measured before and after a surgical procedure (with a higher value indicating a worser quality of life), as provided in Table 9.1. The estimated means (SDs) of quality of life before and after the procedure in these data are 6.1 (2.2) and 4.7 (1.5), respectively. A paired t-test is used in this case to calculate a p-value of 0.00 014, which is usually written in the literature as $p < 0.001$ (a very small number). Since this p-value is <0.05 (i.e. there is only a probability of less than 5% that the observed difference is induced by chance), we reject the null hypothesis and accept that there is a significant difference in quality of life before and after the surgical procedure.

ANOVA test for the difference between three or more independent groups

The ***one-way analysis of variance (ANOVA) test*** is used to test whether there is a difference between three or more group means [14]. Let us compare the mean ages of patients hospitalized in the geriatric, orthopaedic and vascular wards, as presented in Table 9.1. The mean ages (SD) in years are 79.5 (10.7), 75.0 (11.9) and 70.2 (12.3), respectively. Using the ANOVA to test the significance of the difference in mean age, we obtain a p-value of 0.338. Consequently, we cannot reject the null hypothesis that the groups are not statistically different in age.

Nonparametric tests as an alternative for assessing the difference between numerical variables

Sometimes, numerical data are not well described using the mean, because the distribution is skewed (i.e. it is not a symmetrically distributed Gauss curve). The mean and median of this distribution are usually different, and this type of data needs special consideration when using statistical tests. The same is true for small samples (in general, smaller than 30), in which each outlier in the dataset will highly influence the test results when using standard statistical tests. So-called nonparametric tests are recommended in both these cases. The basic principle of a nonparametric test is to convert the data to ranks and use the ranks in the test, rather than the raw data [15].

Table 9.1 contains data on the length of stay of patients in various wards. Hospital length-of-stay data are considered skewed, with most people staying a short time but some staying a very long time. Therefore, the distribution has a long tail towards stays of longer lengths. To determine if there is a difference in the length of stay between the orthopaedic and vascular wards, we use the nonparametric counterpart of the independent t-test, namely the Mann–Whitney U test. The median length of stay for orthopaedic patients is 7 days, while that for the vascular ward is 15 days. To assess the difference between the groups, the raw data are first transformed into ranks (length of stay of 1 day receives rank 1; length of stay of 48 days receives the highest rank, of 26) and the statistical test is then performed on these ranks to give a p-value = 0.172. This p-value is greater than 0.05, so there is no statistically significant difference in length of stay between wards.

Table 9.2 Standard statistical tests and corresponding nonparametric tests for numerical variables.

Type of statistical analysis	Standard parametric test	Nonparametric test
Assessment of difference		
• between two paired datasets	Paired-sample t-test	Wilcoxon sign–rank test
• between two independent samples	Independent-sample t-test	Mann–Whitney U test
• between more than two independent samples	One-way ANOVA	Kruskal–Wallis test
Assessment of association		
• Relationship between two numerous datasets	Pearson correlation	Spearman rank correlation

As shown in Table 9.2, nonparametric tests are also available for other statistical analyses comparing groups of numerical variables (e.g. paired-sample t-test, one-way ANOVA). Each time, the same principle is used: performing the appropriate analyses on the ranks and not on the raw data.

Investigating the difference between proportions of categorical variables

The frequency or count of two categorical variables can be statistically tested using the ***chi-square test*** to compare proportions. When analysing the data, categorical variables can be input into a contingency table, with rows and columns representing each variable. Table 9.3a shows a contingency table and the results of a chi-square test for data from the example dataset. From the chi-square test, a p-value can be calculated to determine whether there is a significant difference between the expected and observed frequencies.

A contingency table is called a two-by-two table when each of the variables has only two categories (see Table 9.3b). In this case, and when a categorical variable has small numbers (an expected cell count <5), a chi-square test does not perform optimally; in such a case, the ***Fisher's exact test*** can be used to calculate the p-value instead (see Table 9.3b).

There are cases when the researcher would like to compare data that are paired and can be categorized. The ***McNemar's test*** is used in such cases as it allows us to compare dichotomous categorical data that come from the same individual subjects (e.g. results from before-and-after measurements). This situation is rare, but does occur; we should be prepared to identify and use the correct test in this situation. An example using the McNemar's test with data from the example dataset is found in Table 9.3c.

Table 9.3 Examples of contingency tables and statistical tests for categorical data.

Source: Based on data presented in Table 9.1.

(a) Number of subjects taking metformin or sulfonylurea by ward

	Metformin	Sulfonylurea
Geriatrics	4 (67%)	2 (33%)
Orthopaedics	7 (64%)	4 (36%)
Vascular	4 (44%)	5 (56%)

Chi-square p-value = 0.605. This probability is >0.05 and therefore the difference between wards is not significant

(b) Number of subjects with IV antibiotics by sex

	IV antibiotic use	
	Yes	No
Male	7 (50%)	7 (50%)
Female	2 (17%)	10(83%)

Because in this 2 × 2 table there is a cell with counts <5, the Fisher's exact test must be used. Fisher's exact test p-value = 0.110. This probability is >0.05 and there is no significant sex difference.

(c) Number of subjects with poor quality of life (score >5) before and after surgery

		Poor quality of life after surgery	
		Yes	No
Poor quality of life before surgery	Yes	10	6
	No	0	10

Because quality-of-life estimates, before and after, are matched observations derived from the same subjects and presented as dichotomous variables (poor quality of life: no/yes), the McNemar test must be used.

To calculate the p-value in a dataset with matched categorical data, a McNemar test is used to evaluate the discordant pairs of cells or those cells that do not agree 'before' and 'after'.

In this example, six patients went from poor to high quality of life and zero patients went from high to poor quality of life after surgery.

The Exact McNemar's test p-value = 0.031. This probability is <0.05 and therefore showing a significant improvement in quality of life after surgery. The Exact test was used because one of the cells has a zero count.

Understanding the notion of a risk calculation

In the dataset presented in Table 9.1, quality of life after surgery differed considerably between patients, with 10/26 still reporting a poor quality of life (the cut-off point for the definition of quality of life is here defined as 5, with higher scores indicating worse health). A researcher can investigate the factors related to poor quality of life. The outcome variable can be operationalized as a dichotomous variable with poor quality of life = 1 and good quality of life = 0. The factors of interest in the investigation include: (i) hospitalized in a vascular ward (yes/no), (ii) antibiotics IV (yes/no) and (iii) number of medications used (as numerical variable).

First, for each of these factors, we calculate whether there is a statistical difference between those with poor quality of life and those with good quality of life. Second, the magnitude of each risk factor is given, showing the contribution of each variable to having a poor quality of life. The appropriate tests and results are given in Table 9.4. For example, a chi-square test is used to calculate the p-value for ward and antibiotics (dichotomous variables). An independent sample t-test is used to calculate the difference between the mean number of medications (numerical variable). Hospitalization at a vascular ward shows a 16-times increase in the odds of having poor quality of life. The 95% interval does not contain '1', indicating that the increased risk is statistically significant. Receiving IV antibiotics shows a decreased odds of poor quality of life of 68% (1 − 0.32 = 0.68). However, the 95% CI does contain '1', so the decreased risk is not significant. The amount of medicines used seems to be associated with poor quality of life. Since number of medications is a numerical variable, OR = 1.27 means that for each additional medication, the odds of poor quality of life will increase by 27%. The 95% CI does contain '1', so the increased risk is not significant.

The risk is expressed as a ratio called the relative risk/risk ratio (RR) or odds ratio (OR), according to the study design (see Chapter 2) [16]. When there is no observed difference in risk between the two groups, the risk ratio will be 1. If the risk factor is more prevalent in the group of the studied outcome (here, those with a poor quality of life), an increased risk of OR > 1 will be observed. If the risk factor is less prevalent, a decreased risk of OR < 1 will be observed. The accompanying 95% CI of a risk ratio is again helpful when inferring sample results to the entire population. Inclusion of '1' in the 95% CI is equivalent to not being able to reject the null hypothesis of no association, meaning that an increased or decreased risk cannot be demonstrated.

Describing the relationship between two numerical variables using regression analysis

A linear regression analysis can be used to describe the strength of an association between two numerical variables [4,17]. An association between variables means that the value of one variable (the dependent variable) can be estimated, to some extent, by the value of the other one (the independent variable). To identify whether a relationship between two continuous variables exists, a scatterplot can be drawn. Additionally, a correlation coefficient (r) can be calculated, which gives the strength of the linear association between the variables and tells us whether this association is positive or negative. A correlation coefficient is a value between 1 and −1, where r = 0 means that there is no association. An example of a known positive correlation is that between height and weight: as height increases, so weight also increases. Different types of association between two variables are illustrated in Figure 9.3.

Table 9.4 Example of risk assessment: investigating risk factors related to having poor quality of life (>5) after surgery (based on data presented in Table 9.1).

	Comparative statistics			
	Poor quality of life			
	No (n = 16)	Yes (n = 10)	p-value of difference	OR (95% CI)
Hospitalized at vascular ward	2 (12.5%)	7 (70.0%)	0.003	16.33 (2.20–121.43)
Receiving antibiotics intravenously	7 (43.8%)	2 (20.0%)	0.216	0.32 (0.05–2.02)
Mean (SD) number of medications used	11.0 (3.7)	13.7 (3.2)	0.069	1.27 (0.97–1.65)

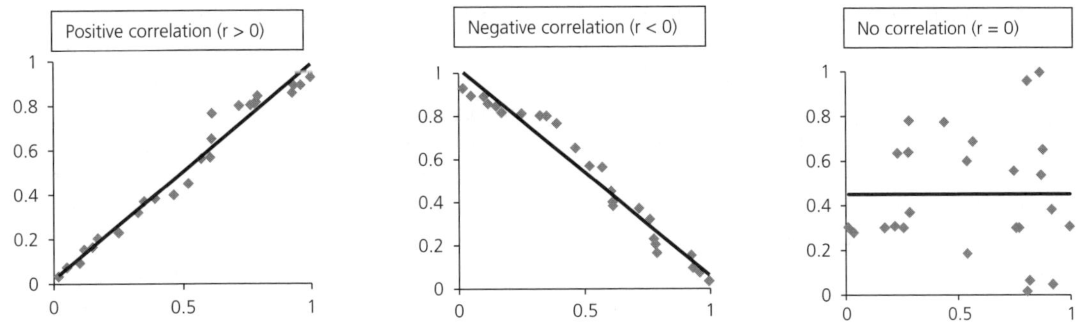

Figure 9.3 Scatterplots showing a positive, a negative and no correlation.

In Figure 9.3, a regression line is also shown. This line is estimated based on the method of least squares, resulting in a 'best-fitting' straight line that minimizes the sum of the squares of the vertical deviations between all the points of the scatterplot and the line. A linear regression will have the form Y = A + BX, where Y is the dependent variable (presented on the y-axis in the scatterplot) and X is the independent variable (presented on the x-axis). The intercept A is the value of Y when X is zero (i.e. the value of Y at which the regression line will cross the y-axis). The slope B can be interpreted as the change in Y given a unit change in X. If the slope is positive, Y will increase when X increases (a positive relationship and a corresponding positive correlation coefficient). If the slope is negative, Y will decrease when X increases (a negative relationship and a corresponding negative correlation coefficient). Figure 9.4 presents an example of the linear relationship between age and number of medications used in 107 patients. The scatterplot shows a statistically significant relationship (p-value < 0.001) between age and number of medications. The correlation coefficient (r = 0.49) indicates a positive correlation. The regression equation (y = 0.05x + 5.64) means that for each year of age, medication use increases by 0.05 units (or 0.5 per 10 years). The coefficient of determination ($R^2 = 0.24$) means that 24% of the variation in number of medications can be explained by age.

When describing the relationship between numerical variables, several additional points have to be considered:

- In previous examples, we talked about a linear relationship between two variables with a correlation coefficient as a measure of the strength of the linear association. It is always good 'statistical practice', however, to plot the data for a visual control of the model of the relationship, since not all relationships are well represented by a straight line. Many nonlinear associations between two variables exist, but their mathematical models will not be considered in this chapter.

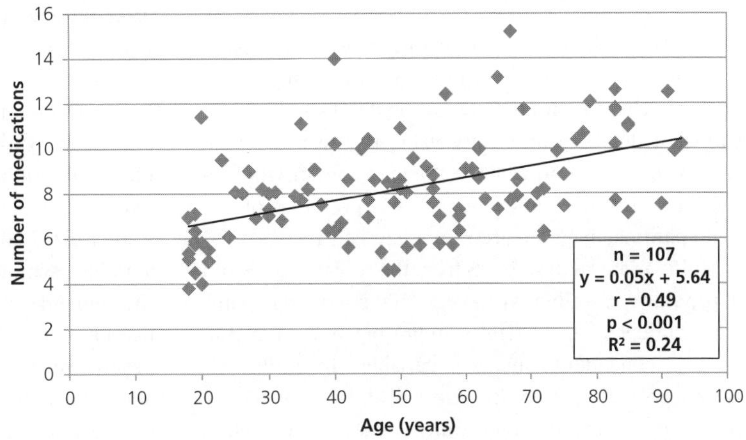

Figure 9.4 Scatterplot of the association between age and number of medications.

- For a regression analysis, a test of significance and a corresponding p-value can be calculated. We start from the null hypothesis that the slope (B) of the regression equation $Y = A + BX$ is zero. Obtaining a p-value < 0.05 means that we have to reject the null hypothesis and conclude that there are grounds to believe that there is a (positive or negative) correlation between variables X and Y (see the p-value in Figure 9.4).
- In regression analysis, calculating the square of the correlation coefficient (R^2) provides a result with an easy interpretation. This so-called 'coefficient of determination' gives the percentage of variation in the dependent variable (Y) that can be explained by the variation in the independent variable (X) (see Figure 9.4).
- An estimation of the relationship between two variables can be limited by various factors, including a small sample size, a skewed distribution of one of the variables and outliers in the data. To solve these problems, a nonparametric equivalent of the Pearson correlation should be used [15]. Here, again, the real values of both variables will be replaced by their ranks, which are used to compute the resulting Spearman rank correlation (see Table 9.2).
- Causal inferences should not be drawn from observational studies. A significant correlation between two variables does not necessarily mean that there is a causal relationship between the two variables [10].

Assessing the combined effect of explanatory variables in multivariate statistical analysis

This section will not explain the intricacies of regression modelling or give details of how to perform regression analysis. These topics take entire textbooks to cover in sufficient depth to be of any value to the researcher. However, this section will give the reader an insight into the basic principles and offer an interpretation of the main parameters of a regression analysis.

Multivariate analysis starts from the research question of the study. A study may have several potential explanatory independent variables indicating a relationship with a dependent outcome variable. In multivariate analysis, the combined effect of these explanatory predictors on the outcome can be assessed. The basic principle is to determine the separate and independent influence of each contributing variable on the outcome studied, taking into account that these 'contributors' are also intercorrelated [17,18].

Multivariate analysis produces a regression equation or a model, which is effectively a weighted combination of the explanatory variables. Apart from model-building, however, the analysis can also focus on one particular determining factor, while controlling for all others (so-called adjustment for confounding factors). In multivariate statistics, and regression analysis in general, the type and distribution of the outcome variable dictates the choice of an appropriate regression model. Two commonly used techniques are the multiple regression and logistic regression. In both, the explanatory variables can be either continuous or binary.

Multiple regression analysis with a continuous outcome variable

Multiple regression is used when the outcome studied is a numerical or continuous variable. For example, the outcome might be the number of drugs used or the cost of medications. The method is a combined regression analysis, as described previously. The regression equation will now have the form $Y = A + B_1X_1 + B_2X_2 + B_3X_3 + \ldots$, taking into account the slope of each contributing variable. Results are usually presented as B (unstandardized slopes) and corresponding beta (standardized) factors. Table 9.5 illustrates an example of a multiple regression analysis, using data from 8057 general practices in England, aimed at identifying the characteristics of practices that prescribe higher volumes of antibiotics [19]. The 'B' column gives the measure of the slope (with 95% CI) of the regression line for each of the variables included in the multiple regression equation, with the sign of the slope as an indication of the direction of the association (positive or negative). For example, a practice's patient morbidity index has a significant positive relation with the volume of antibiotic prescribing, while female gender shows a negative relation. The beta column gives the corresponding standardized coefficients. A larger beta means that the variable is more important in predicting variation in the dependent variable. For example, having a practice located in the north of England shows the highest positive relation and having a longer appointment duration shows the highest negative relation with the volume of antibiotic prescribing. The independent variables

Table 9.5 Example of multiple regression analysis, investigating the association between standardized antibiotic prescribing volume and practice characteristics in UK general practices.

Source: Data from Wang et al. [19].

	Unstandardized regression coefficient B (95% CI)	Standardized regression coefficient β
Practice characteristics		
Location		
North of England	0.07 (0.06 to 0.08)	0.17
Midlands	0.04 (0.03 to 0.05)	0.09
Longer appointment duration	−0.09 (−0.10 to −0.07)	−0.11
GP sex: female	−0.05 (−0.07 to −0.04)	−0.08
GP country of qualification: United Kingdom	−0.04 (−0.05 to −0.02)	−0.08
GP age: <45 years	−0.04 (−0.06 to −0.03)	−0.07
Training practice	−0.02 (−0.03 to −0.01)	−0.06
Patient characteristics		
Morbidity: limiting long-term illness	0.67 (0.57 to 0.77)	0.16
Ethnicity: white	0.15 (0.13 to 0.17)	0.15
All regression coefficients significant (p < 0.001)		
The model explains 17.2% of the variation in antibiotic prescribing		

GP, general practitioner.

included in the multiple regression equation explain 17.2% (R^2 = 0.172) of the variation in the volume of antibiotic prescribing.

Logistic regression analysis with a dichotomous outcome variable

Logistic regression is used when the dependent variable of interest is dichotomous rather than numerical. For example, the outcome might be the occurrence of a particular disease (yes/no) or mortality (yes/no). This statistical method is commonly used in drug utilization research, because the interpretation of the calculated estimates is easy to understand [1,3]. In the results table of a logistic regression analysis, the weighted effect of each variable in the model is expressed as an OR with corresponding 95% CI. Table 9.6 presents an example of a logistic regression analysis using data from a cross-sectional study investigating antipsychotic use in a nursing home population [20]. The dichotomous dependent variable studied is antipsychotic use (yes/no). In univariate analysis, separate ORs are given, along with corresponding 95% CIs. Here, each clinical characteristic shows a statistically significant association with antipsychotic use. In multivariate analysis, each OR can be interpreted as the association between variable and drug use, while controlling for remaining explanatory variables. Residents with dementia are 3.3 times more likely to use an antipsychotic; having insomnia gives an increased odds of 38%; and having hypertension gives a decreased odds of 34%. All are significant determinants of antipsychotic use, since '1' (OR = 1 means no increased or decreased risk) is not included in the 95% CI.

Table 9.6 Example of a logistic regression analysis investigating the clinical characteristics associated with antipsychotic drug use in a sample of 1730 nursing home residents, of whom 32.9% have at least one antipsychotic on their medication list.

Source: Azermai et al. 2011 [20]. Reproduced with permission from Cambridge University Press.

Characteristics	Univariate OR (95% CI)	Multivariate OR (95% CI)
Dementia	3.35 (2.70–4.15)	3.27 (2.61–4.09)
Insomnia	1.23 (1.01–1.51)	1.38 (1.10–1.73)
Depression	1.27 (1.03–1.57)	1.30 (1.03–1.65)
Age < 80 years	1.63 (1.29–2.06)	1.79 (1.38–2.33)
Incontinence	1.46 (1.19–1.80)	
Age ≥ 90 years	0.78 (0.63–0.97)	
Peptic ulcer	0.74 (0.58–0.94)	
COPD	0.68 (0.52–0.91)	0.67 (0.49–0.92)
Hypertension	0.63 (0.51–0.77)	0.66 (0.53–0.83)
Post-infarct	0.78 (0.62–0.99)	
Heart failure	0.63 (0.50–0.78)	
Glaucoma	0.52 (0.31–0.86)	

COPD, chronic obstructive pulmonary disease.

Study	Good adherence to drug therapy	Poor adherence to drug therapy	Odds ratio (random) (95% CI)	Weight (%)	Odds ratio (random) (95% CI)
Coronry Drug Project Research Group 1980[w1]	274/1813	249/882		27.53	0.45 (0.37 to 0.55)
β blocker heart attack trial (men) 1990[w2]	31/1037	4/57		5.11	0.41 (0.14 to 1.20)
β blocker heart attack trial (women) 1993[w3]	15/219	4/21		4.20	0.31 (0.09 to 1.05)
Canadian amiodarone myocardial infarction arrhythmia trial 1999[w8]	42/447	17/91		11.81	0.45 (0.24 to 0.84)
Cardiac arrhythmia suppression trial 1996[w4]	8/486	1/93		1.54	1.54 (0.19 to 12.46)
Physicians health study 1994[w16]	105/6864	90/4125		23.59	0.70 (0.52 to 0.93)
West of Scotland prevention study 1997[w17]	95/2420	40/873		19.54	0.85 (0.58 to 1.24)
University Group Diabetes Project 1970[w22] 1971[w18]	11/143	10/62		6.69	0.43 (0.17 to 1.08)
Total (95% CI)	13 429	6204		100.00	0.56 (0.43 to 0.74)

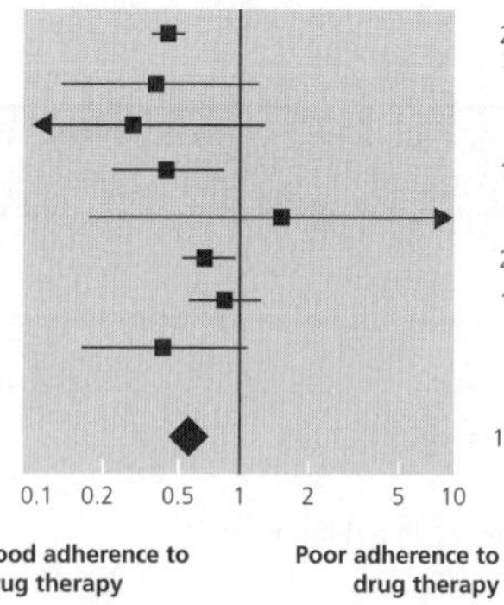

Total events: 581 (good adherence), 415 (poor adherence)
Test for heterogeneity: $\chi^2 = 14.34$, df = 7 (P = 0.05), $I^2 = 51.2\%$
Test for overall effect: Z = 4.23, P <0.0001

Figure 9.5 Forest plot of a meta-analysis of a systematic review investigating the risk of mortality associated with adherence to placebo medication.

Source: Simpson et al. 2006 [21]. Reproduced with permission from BMJ Publishing Group Ltd.

Summarizing the results of different studies in a meta-analysis

Many systematic reviews of the literature include a statistical meta-analysis to combine the results of several similar studies. A meta-analysis can be described as consisting of two analysis stages. First, for each included study, a similar summary of the results will be obtained or calculated. This summary can be the mean difference (numerical outcome variable) or a risk ratio (dichotomous outcome). Second, a weighted average of these separate results is obtained, where the weights relate to the sample size and the occurrence of the event in each study. If the results of the included studies show a heterogeneous pattern (e.g. when some studies have a decreased and others an increased OR), a correction factor will be included in the calculation [4].

The results of a meta-analysis are usually presented graphically in a forest plot. In Figure 9.5, such a plot shows the OR of each individual study (black boxes), with corresponding 95% CIs (whiskers). This systematic review investigated the risk of mortality associated with adherence to placebo medication [21]. For each selected study, the name of the trial, number of deaths in the good and the poor adherence group, weight of the study and OR (95% CI) are shown. The overall OR is calculated taking into account the size and the occurrence of the event in each study (presented as the study weight) and corrected for heterogeneity between the different ORs. The overall result is graphically presented by a diamond shape. The total OR (95% CI = 0.56 (0.43–0.74)) means that good adherence to placebo therapy reduced the risk of mortality by 44%. The result is significant, since '1' lies outside the borders of the 95% CI.

Conclusion

This chapter presented basic statistical methods offering some guidance to the correct interpretation of published statistical results. Before starting to perform your own statistical analysis, it is advisable to consult good statistical textbooks [1–4] and statistical research articles [10] for additional advice. The authors hope that the statistical exploration presented here will contribute to your making the right choices in your future statistical analyses. The first statistical question to be answered will always concern the nature or type of the data to be analysed. Do you focus on numerical or categorical data? Do your numerical data show a normal distribution? Once the choice of the appropriate statistical method has been made, a good statistical package will be instrumental to performing the analysis. After that, it is up to you to carefully and correctly interpret the results.

CHAPTER 10
Visualization of drug utilization data

Maria Matuz[1], Ria Benko[1] & Mikael Hoffmann[2]
[1]*Department of Clinical Pharmacy, Faculty of Pharmacy, University of Szeged, Hungary*
[2]*The NEPI Foundation, Linköping University, Sweden*

KEY POINTS

- Static and interactive visualization can help both the researcher and their audience to understand, analyse and present recorded data.
- Basic principles and recommendations must be respected in order to communicate the desired message in an effective way.
- Visualization is not an exact science; there are often many solutions. Several alternative graphs should be considered before choosing the one that best suits the data, the objectives of the visualization and the audience/readership.
- Despite the importance and relevance of graphs, suboptimal presentation and consequent misunderstanding of data are still present in the scientific literature. It is also common that correctly visualized data (e.g. boxplots) are not properly interpreted.

Introduction

Visualization can be described as the process of structuring data, focusing on one or several specific messages in order to help understand, analyse and present recorded data [1,2]. It is thus an important tool for communicating a data-rich message about, for instance, drug utilization.

There are two main reasons for visualizing datasets in research – to explore and to present data. The goal of presenting data is to communicate the research as effectively as possible by telling a story. The exploration of data is about understanding the dataset, but also about generating ideas and new hypotheses through data analysis in order to test them on another set of data. Static graphs and figures are a traditional way of solving both tasks. New software has simplified the process of generating and modifying static graphs and figures. In addition, software for interactive visualizations has made it easier to analyse datasets and communicate the findings (e.g. on a website).

Visualization is not an exact science. There is rarely a single right answer or best solution. There are nevertheless basic principles and recommendations that ought to be respected in order to communicate the desired message in an effective way [3,4]. This chapter focuses mainly on these basic principles for presenting data through static graphs in printed literature and traditional lectures.

The overall aim is to give advice not only on how to choose a relevant graph, but also on how to design it so as to make it as easy as possible to understand. In addition, it introduces some basic considerations around using interactive visualization techniques as an exploratory tool and as a means of communicating results interactively with other scientists and with decision-makers.

Basic principles of visualization

Graphs are tools used to encode information that will be decoded by the reader. Visual variables (attributes/cues) play a pivotal role in understanding graphs. The power of visualization comes from the ability to present data in a new and more informative way; that is, to represent them with the aim of informing the researcher [2].

Prior to conscious attention, both perceptual and cognitive processing occur. This is called ***preattentive processing***, a period of 200–250 milliseconds during which information is detected [5]. Basic knowledge on how the human visual system reacts to different visual cues

Drug Utilization Research: Methods and Applications, First Edition. Edited by M. Elseviers et al. © 2016 John Wiley & Sons, Ltd.
Published 2016 by John Wiley & Sons, Ltd.

makes it possible to have specific information 'pop out' in an illustration, whether static (e.g. traditional graphs) or interactive.

Cleveland and McGill were among the first to measure people's ability to carry out elementary perceptual task in decoding quantitative information [6,7]. They asked subjects to judge the relative magnitude between two values encoded with particular visual variables (e.g. length, angle, size and 2D position) and found that certain variables were efficient and accurate in estimating the difference, while others were not.

As an example, in visually encoding quantitative variables, only length and 2D position are highly effective. Therefore, line charts (2D position) or bar charts (2D position and length) should be used if actual values are important. Other attributes, such as area and colour hue, are less effective in representing actual quantitative values, as they are only able to show that one value is higher or lower; the exact difference is hard to judge [8]. Later, Mackinlay refined and extended the ranking of perceptual tasks to categorical data [9].

Basic (static) graphical display of findings

This section focuses on one of the main purposes of visualization: to communicate research findings once data analysis has been completed.

As the brain comprehends static graphics more easily than words or numbers [10,11], good graphics are an important part of academic publications, including those on drug utilization. Despite the importance and relevance of graphs, suboptimal presentation is still present in the scientific literature [11], and misinterpretation of correctly visualized data is frequent; both can hinder effective communication of findings. On the basis of existing literature, we will now attempt to provide the fundamentals of graphical display, focusing on drug utilization data. Before we begin, we should mention a couple of the important pioneers in the field, Edward Rolf Tufte and John Wilder Tukey, who published landmark books on data visualization [12–14].

Variable types in drug utilization research

As the optimal method of data visualization depends on the type of variable and on what we want to show, it is important to understand the two general groups of

Table 10.1 Classification of common drug utilization variables.

	Categorical variables	
Numerical variables	**Nominal**	**Ordinal**
Defined daily dose (DDD) per 1000 inhabitants per day (DID)	Anatomical Therapeutic Chemical (ATC) groups/subgroups	Educational status
Daily therapeutic cost	Geographical location	Age groups
Time	Sex (dichotomous)	Risk groups (yes/no)
Patient age	Presence of event (e.g. therapy discontinuation)	
Prevalence of drug use		
Number of drugs		
Number of drug users		
Length of therapy		

variables (see Chapter 9). Some frequently used drug utilization variables are classified in Table 10.1.

Numerical or quantitative variables have values that describe a measurable quantity as a number. They answer questions such as 'How many?' or 'How much?'.

Categorical or qualitative variables have values that describe a 'quality' or 'characteristic' of a data unit (i.e. values are often not numerical). They answer questions like 'What type?' or 'Which category?'. When observations can take a value that can be logically ordered or ranked, we call the variable ***ordinal***; when values cannot be organized in a logical sequence (i.e. they have no 'natural' order), we call the variable ***nominal***.

However, the distinction between variable types is not rigid, as one may transform a numerical variable into a categorical one by 'categorizing' the data. The two most common ways of categorizing data are:

1. Equal distribution of data values (e.g. 10-year age groups – see also Figure 10.4).
2. Equal number of data points per category (e.g. ordering drug utilization variables into quartiles or percentiles).

One should keep in mind, however, that categorization of data often entails information loss. For example, defining 'polypharmacy' by the usual cut-off value of five chronic drugs will place a patient with five drugs and a patient with fifteen in the same category (see Table 10.2).

To enhance the educational value of this chapter, we have set up a sample dataset. Let's imagine a small island with 30 inhabitants, all of whom used drugs in the previous year (inhabitants = patients). Hypothetical values for a set of different variables are summarized in

Table 10.2 Characteristics of island inhabitants (n = 30).

No.	Age	Age group	Gender	BMI category	Sport activity	Number of chronic drugs	PP	Number of DDDs/year dispensed	OAD	Diabetic treatment type	Length of OAD therapy (months)	Event
1	53	50–59	Male	Normal	Regularly	3	Non PP	523	No	No		
2	45	40–49	Male	Normal	Regularly	4	Non PP	1036	No	No		
3	71	70–79	Male	Underweight	Occasionally	3	Non PP	856	No	No		
4	69	60–69	Male	Obese	Occasionally	10	PP	7900	Yes	Met + Ins	13	CEN
5	54	50–59	Male	Obese	Occasionally	7	PP	1158	No	No		
6	45	40–49	Male	Obese	Regularly	5	PP	2159	No	No		
7	41	40–49	Male	Normal	Regularly	2	Non PP	658	No	No		
8	66	60–69	Male	Normal	Occasionally	8	PP	2536	Yes	Met + D	13	CEN
9	75	70–79	Male	Obese	Occasionally	7	PP	2896	No	No		
10	37	30–39	Male	Obese	Occasionally	3	Non PP	665	Yes	Met	2	ADD
11	29	20–29	Male	Overweight	None	6	PP	1100	No	No		
12	59	50–59	Female	Overweight	None	7	PP	2360	Yes	Met + D	10	ADD
13	55	50–59	Male	Normal	Regularly	1	Non PP	535	No	No		
14	54	50–59	Male	Normal	Regularly	0	Non PP	21	No	No		
15	50	50–59	Male	Normal	Occasionally	6	PP	2190	No	No		
16	49	40–49	Male	Overweight	None	4	Non PP	1023	Yes	Met	6	ADD
17	48	40–49	Male	Overweight	Regularly	2	Non PP	368	No	No		
18	22	20–29	Female	Overweight	Regularly	0	Non PP	14	No	No		
19	38	30–39	Female	Overweight	Regularly	3	Non PP	1205	No	No		
20	60	60–69	Female	Overweight	Regularly	10	PP	2635	Yes	Met + D	10	ADD
21	49	40–49	Female	Obese	Regularly	2	Non PP	1859	Yes	Met	8	CEN
22	48	40–49	Female	Obese	Occasionally	1	Non PP	226	No	No		
23	56	50–59	Female	Obese	None	8	PP	2158	Yes	Met + D	11	ADD
24	90	90–99	Female	Overweight	None	9	PP	1259	Yes	Met + Ins	13	CEN
25	85	80–89	Female	Overweight	Occasionally	8	PP	3158	No	No		
26	86	80–89	Female	Underweight	None	9	PP	5500	No	No		
27	53	50–59	Female	Underweight	None	5	PP	1957	No	No		
28	52	50–59	female	Overweight	Occasionally	8	PP	2513	No	No		
29	45	40–49	female	Normal	Occasionally	3	Non PP	356	No	No		
30	32	30–39	female	Normal	Occasionally	1	Non PP	429	No	No		

BMI, body mass index; OAD, oral antidiabetic drug; PP, polypharmacy; Met, metformin; Met + Ins, metformin and insulin; Met + D, metformin + DPP4 inhibitors; ADD, antidiabetic treatment discontinuation; CEN, censored.

Table 10.2. All graphics presented throughout this chapter – except those used to show trends and the forest plot – are based on this table.

Graphics for categorical variables

Categorical variables are usually visualized in either pie or bar charts.

Pie charts

In a pie chart, categories are represented by slices of a pie (see Figure 10.1). The area of each slice is proportional to the percentage of responses in the category (relative frequency of the category).

Pie charts are only effective for displaying the frequency distribution of a small number of categories (usually three to five) of a single variable. As the human ability to compare angles has its limitations, use of pie charts is discouraged if the number of categories is high or if we want to compare groups or changes [3,9,15].

Bar charts

Bar charts are one of the simplest ways of visualizing categorical data and their use is widespread in the scientific literature. The length of each bar is proportional to the absolute or relative frequency of the variable it represents. Importantly, the widths of the bars should

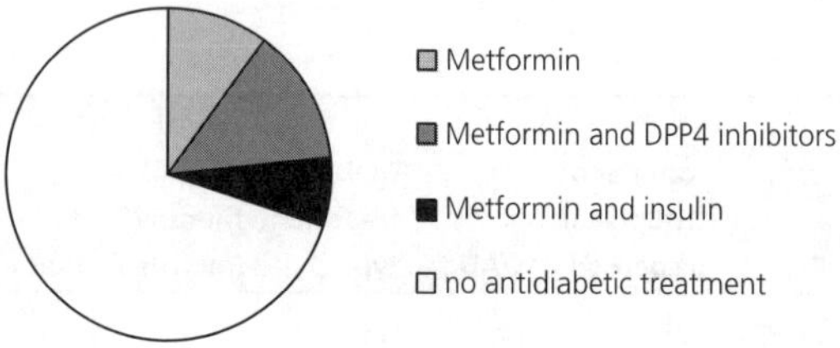

Figure 10.1 Pie chart showing the distribution of diabetic treatment types.

be equal [16]. Bar charts that display data vertically are also often called column charts.

Bar charts can be used as an alternative to pie charts, to show the frequency distribution of a single variable (see Figure 10.2a and 10.2b). Bar charts are also ideal for comparing the frequencies of different groups (i.e. for visualizing the results of crosstabs/contingency tables), see Figure 10.2c [17].

Bar charts are also widely used to communicate the average of numerical data (compare with Figure 10.9), which they often do not represent well (i.e. they poorly represent the distribution of data and are sensitive to outliers). Methodological experts advise avoiding bar charts in such cases [18]. For example, the mean number of dispensed defined daily dose (DDD) per year in the sample dataset (Table 10.2) would be 1708.4, but Figure 10.6 clearly shows that this is not a frequent value (the distribution is bimodal: lower and higher DDDs are dispensed more frequently).

Venn and Euler diagrams

Venn and Euler diagrams are used to present all logical relations between a finite set of data [16]. Due to their ease of interpretation and graphical simplicity, they are widely used in biomedical sciences. In drug utilization research, Venn and Euler diagrams can be used to describe comorbidities or concomitant drug therapies (although they are suitable only for two to four categories).

By definition all intersects (including empty zones) are shown on Venn diagrams, while Euler diagrams show only non-zero intersects (i.e. Euler and Venn diagrams are equivalent if all intersecting and nonintersecting areas exist; see Figure 10.3). Consequently, in many cases Euler diagrams are less complex than the corresponding Venn diagrams, which improves their overall readability [19].

A list of programmes capable of generating Venn or Euler diagrams, including a detailed comparison of their features, has been published [19]. Several of the programmes listed are able to adjust circle size according to set size (see Figure 10.3b).

Methods for displaying the interrelationships between categorical data (e.g. mosaic plots and chord diagrams (radial network diagrams)) and for displaying hierarchical data (e.g. tree maps) [3,4] are outside the scope of this chapter.

Graphics for numerical variables

Two key aspects in summarizing numerical data are the central tendency and the spread of its distribution. The central tendency of a distribution refers to the point around which most values are gathered (mean, median), while the spread refers to the dispersion of possible values; that is, how scattered the values are around the central tendency (e.g. minimum, maximum, quartiles, interquartile range (IQR), variance, standard deviation (SD)) [20]. The distribution of numerical variables can be illustrated by histograms or boxplots.

Histograms

A histogram shows the frequency distribution of a single numerical variable (e.g. age). To this end, the range of the numerical variable is discretized into a number of intervals (called bins). For each rectangle, the area is proportional to the frequency represented. Since bins usually have equal width, the height is proportional to the frequency represented (see Figure 10.4).

A histogram called a population pyramid can be used to represent the age distribution of a population (Figure 10.5), where age is plotted vertically and (a) frequency or (b) relative frequency is plotted horizontally. Such paired histograms can be used to compare two populations.

The main difference between histograms and bar charts is that in histograms a numerical variable is plotted, so there is no gap between the columns [16,21].

In order to visualize the shape of the distribution (e.g. symmetric, asymmetric, unimodal or bimodal), the

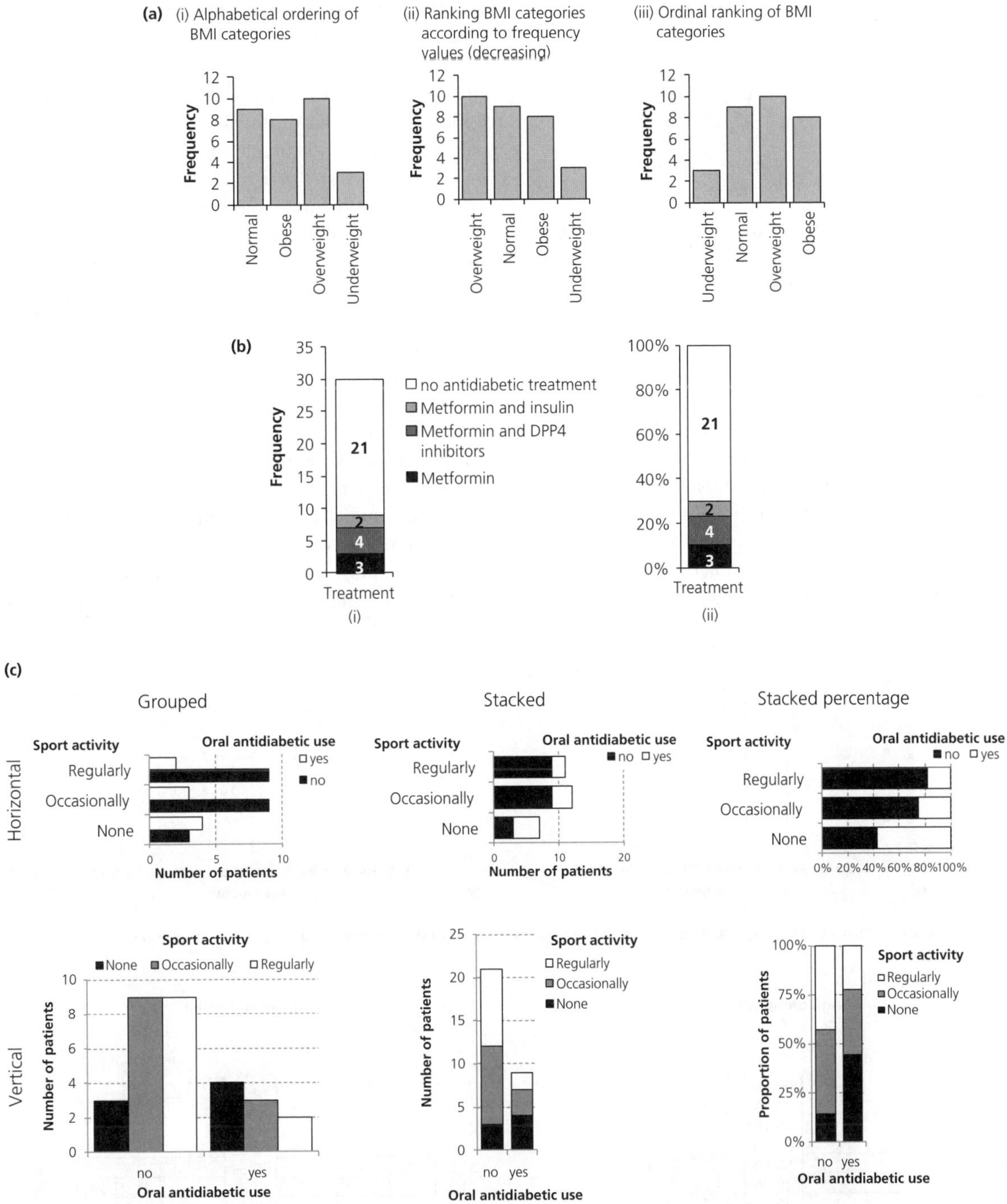

Figure 10.2 (a) Bar charts for a single variable (using one bar per category), presented in different orders. (b) Bar charts for (i) frequencies and (ii) the relative frequency of a single variable, using stacked bars. (c) Bar charts for comparison of the frequencies of different groups. BMI: Body Mass Index.

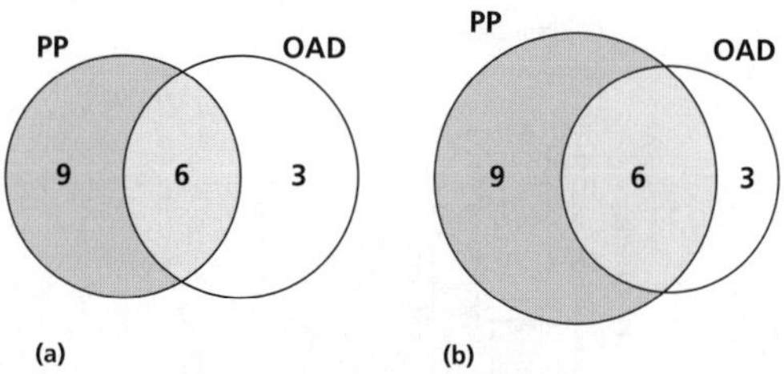

Figure 10.3 Venn diagrams (a, circle sizes are equal; b, circle sizes are proportional to the corresponding set size) showing the overlap between oral antidiabetic drug (OAD) use and polypharmacy (PP).

optimal density of bins should be found. There are several rules (e.g. Sturges' rule) [3] that might help in this, but in most cases plotting some meaningful alternatives is sufficient to find the optimal one. For example, in Figure 10.6, the number of dispensed DDDs among the inhabitants of the sample dataset (Table 10.2) is plotted with different bin widths; in panels (a) and (b), the bimodal distribution and the outlier can be identified, but in panel (c), they cannot.

Boxplots (box-and-whisker diagrams)

A boxplot is a very compact way of visualizing a numerical variable, as it represents both the summary statistics (including measures of central tendency) and the distribution of data [22,23]. Boxplots (see Figure 10.7) are able to visualize the minimum, maximum, median, lower (Q1, Q25 or lower hinge) and upper (Q3, Q75 or upper hinge) quartile, range and interquartile range (IQR or middle fifty, midspread or H-spread), which covers the central 50% of data. Additionally, to aid in the comparison of two datasets (to show the differences between medians), the 95% confidence interval (95% CI) of the medians can be illustrated by notches (see Figure 10.7c) [22,23].

The distribution of drug use among island inhabitants is shown in Figure 10.7. Asymmetric distributions can be recognized by the asymmetric median (i.e. the median is not in the middle of the box) and by asymmetric whiskers. Whiskers can be defined according to various criteria (e.g. Altman, Spear, Tukey), among which Tukey is the most widely used. In Tukey-style boxplots, the box represents the IQR, with whiskers extended to

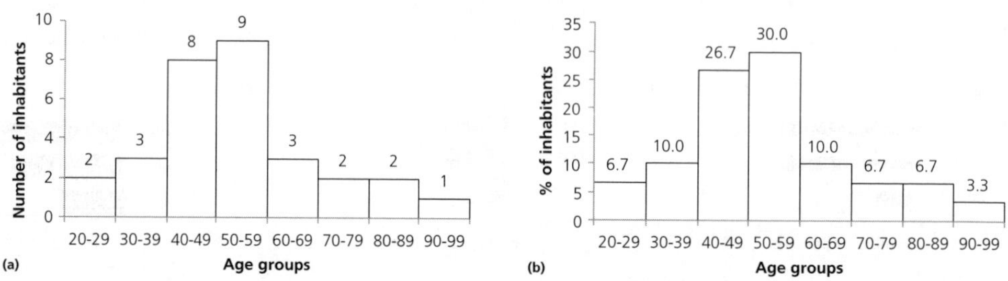

Figure 10.4 Histogram showing the age distribution of island inhabitants as (a) frequency and (b) relative frequency.

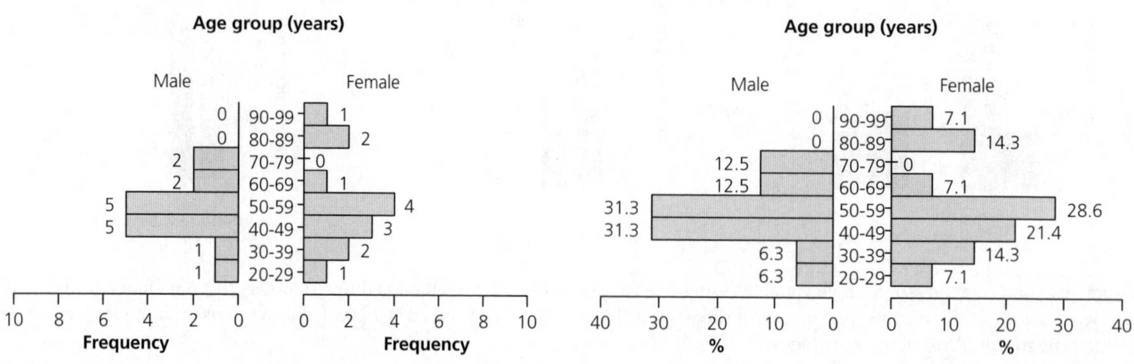

Figure 10.5 Population pyramid of island inhabitants.

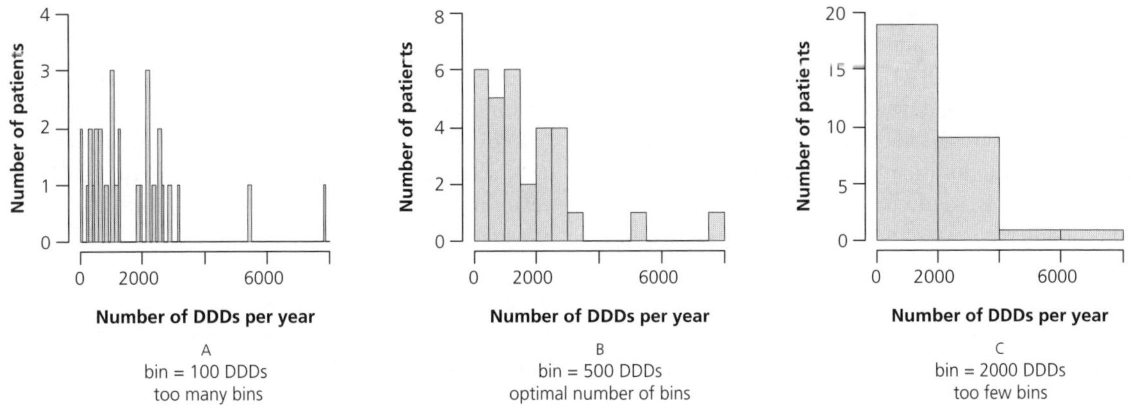

Figure 10.6 Histograms with different bin widths showing the distribution of drug use among island inhabitants. DDD: defined daily doses.

data points that are less than 1.5 × IQR (one step) away from the first or third quartile (i.e. box edges). Data points situated a further distance from the box edges, the so-called outliers, are independently highlighted. Some software (e.g. SPSS) differentiates between two kinds of outlier: outside values (outliers) and far-out values (extreme values).

As several boxplot characteristics (e.g. whisker position and outlier display) may differ between software, it is important to clearly label how a boxplot was constructed

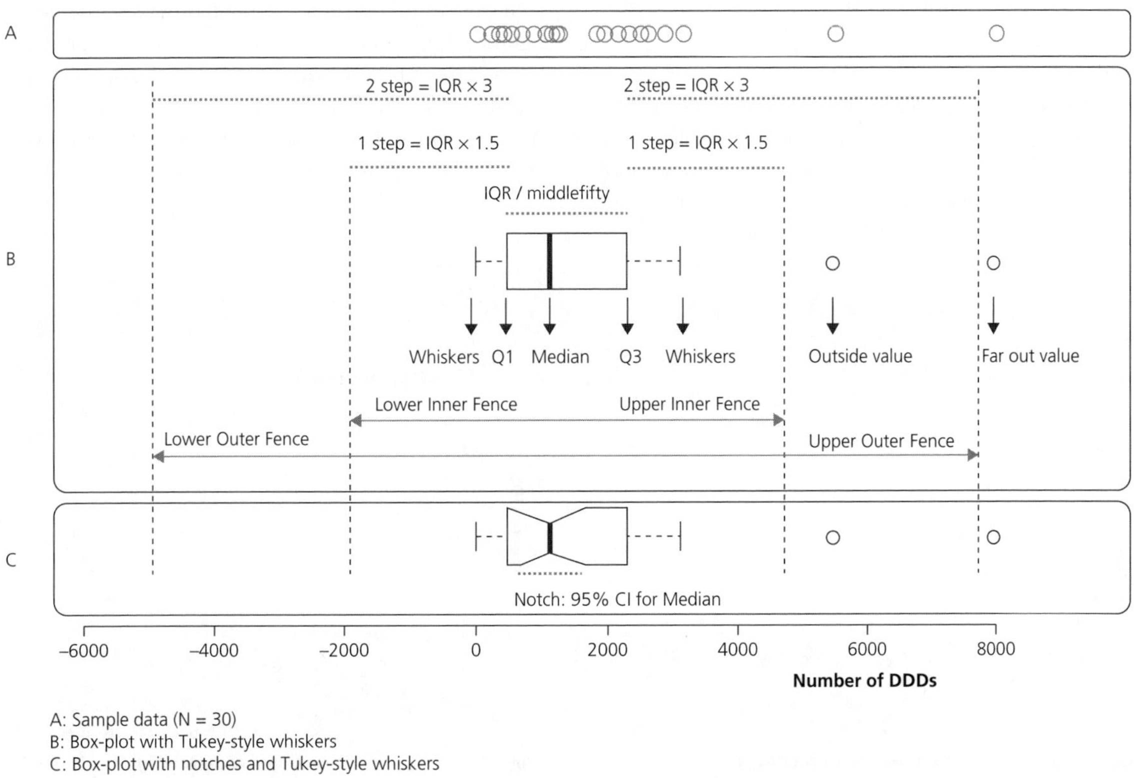

Figure 10.7 Boxplots showing the distribution of drug use among island inhabitants. (a) Sample data (n = 30). (b) Boxplot with Tukey-style whiskers. (c) Boxplot with notches and Tukey-style whiskers. IQR: interquartile range; DDD: defined daily dose.

(e.g. with Tukey-style whiskers). Also, as individual data points cannot be identified in boxplots, sample sizes should be reported [18,23].

A boxplot has the advantage of showing at least five statistical measures of the central tendency and spread of the data, with information on the form of the distribution. Boxplots are useful for comparing the distributions of different related numerical variables (e.g. number of drugs used by island inhabitants before and after an intervention) or for comparing two or more groups (e.g. number of drugs used by male and female island inhabitants).

Despite the obvious advantages of boxplots, their use is limited by the lack of easy means for generating them (e.g. spreadsheet software such as Excel cannot produce boxplots). Besides professional tools (SPSS, SAS, STATA, R), some free Web-based tools for creating customized boxplots are now available [22,24,25].

Further reading on alternatives to boxplots, such as beans plots and violin plots, which reveal additional details of the data distribution (e.g. bimodality), can be found in the literature [16,22].

Scatterplots

A scatterplot is the simplest way of visualizing the relationship between two numerical variables. Two numerical variables are displayed (one on the x-axis, one on the y-axis) in order to show patterns of correlation and clustering and to easily identify outliers (Figure 10.8). In distinguishing between two or more categories (e.g. oral antidiabetic use: yes/no), their values can be indicated using different plotting symbols or different colours [4,16]. The advantage of scatterplots is that individual values can be identified.

Information on more advanced methods such as pairwise scatterplot matrices (sploms – used to reveal correlations across a multivariate dataset) can be found in the literature [3,4].

Which graphic should be used to compare numerical data between different groups?

Figure 10.9 compares the chronic drug use of two patient groups using different chart types. This figure illustrates the importance of choosing the optimal diagram type and reporting the error bar type.

Use of bar charts with error bars is strongly discouraged, as they show only one arm of the error bar, which hinders overlap comparison. The bar also gives the impression that the mean is related to its height, rather than to the position of its top.

The mean-and-error scatterplot provides for meaningful comparison of groups. Since error bars may have different lengths according to the statistical property that they indicate (for the same data), the measure of uncertainty (e.g. SD, SE or CI), represented by the error bar, should be clearly stated (see Figure 10.9).

Since a boxplot visualizes five characteristics of a variable in a single diagram, it is among the most powerful ways of comparing groups.

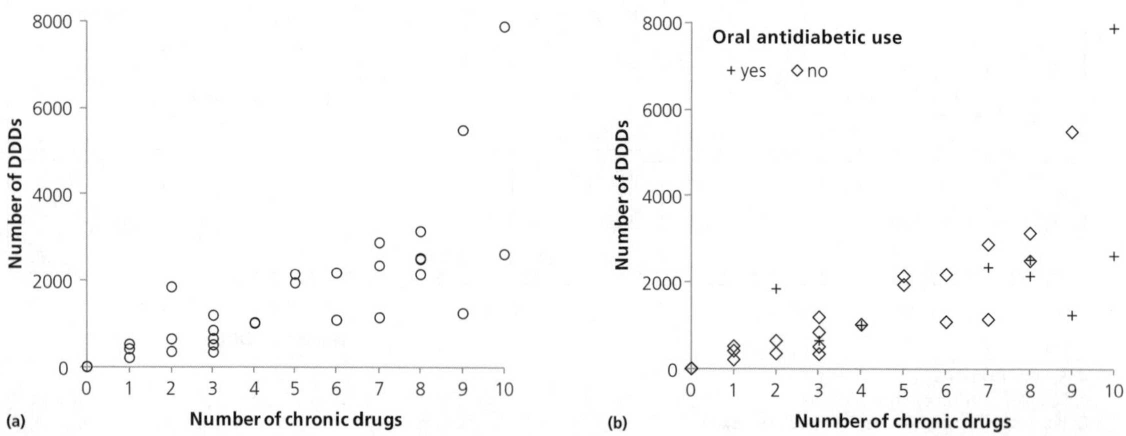

Figure 10.8 Scatterplots showing the relationship between the number of chronic drugs and the total annual drug use (in numbers of DDD) (a) in general and (b) according to oral antidiabetic use. DDD: defined daily dose.

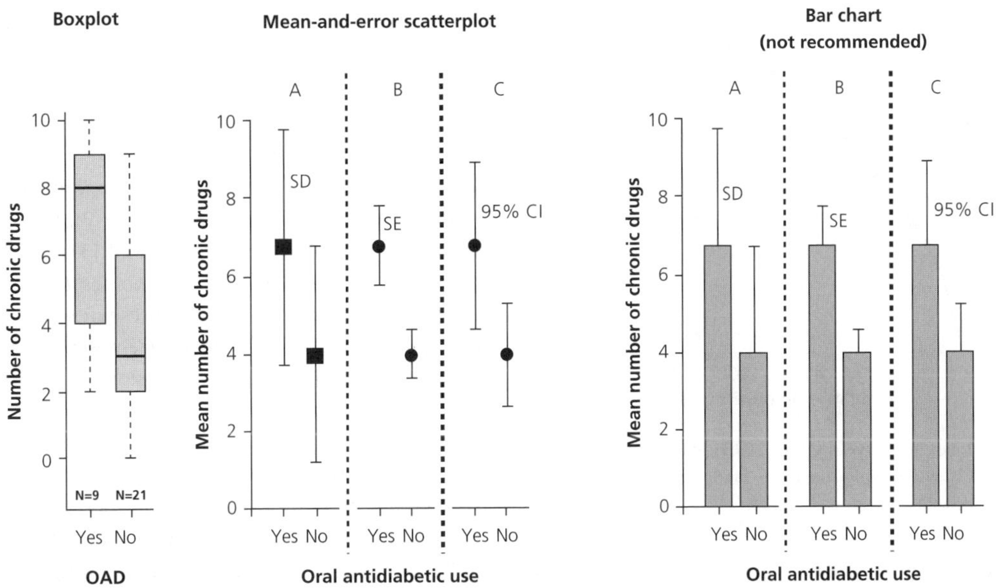

Figure 10.9 Comparison of groups using boxplots (with Tukey-style whiskers), mean-and-error scatterplots and bar charts. OAD: oral antidiabetic use.

Special diagrams used in drug utilization research

Pareto plots

Pareto plots combine a bar and a line chart. The bar chart represents the values (usually as relative frequencies) of individual categories (e.g. different patients or distinct drugs) in descending order, while the line chart represents the cumulative percentage or cumulative share. In the example presented in Figure 10.10, we can see that patient no. 4 alone is responsible for 15% of the drug consumption of the whole island, with a corresponding annual consumption of 7900 DDDs (see Table 10.2).

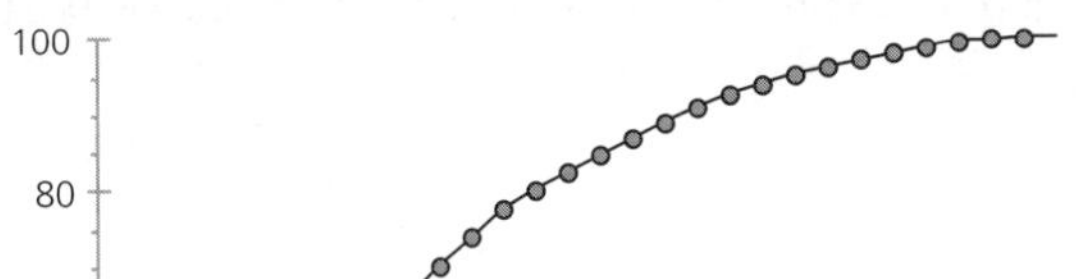

Figure 10.10 Pareto plot showing individual levels of drug exposure (see Table 10.2 column 9) of island inhabitants.

The DU90% (expressing the drugs responsible for 90% of the total volume) is commonly used in drug utilization research [26]. This measure can be visualized in a Pareto plot where the individual active agents of medicines are plotted on the horizontal axis as bars: the line (curve) will show the segment responsible for 90% of total drug use (see also Chapter 12).

Lorenz curves

Lorenz curves (named after a Swiss economist) were originally used in economics with the aim of describing skewness in income [27]. An adapted Lorenz curve was introduced to drug utilization research by Hallas [28] in order to reveal disparities in individual drug exposure. Lorenz curves are often used in drug utilization research to calculate the cumulative share of heavy users (e.g. the 1 or 5% of patients with the highest use) [28–30].

A Lorenz curve for the drug exposure of the island inhabitants is depicted in Figure 10.11. The

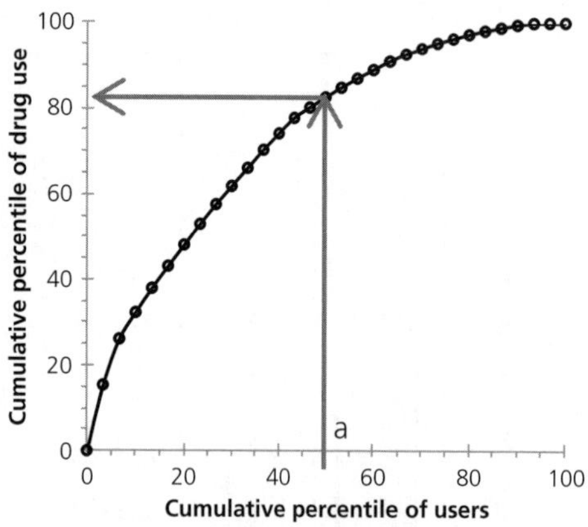

Figure 10.11 Lorenz curve showing individual-level drug exposure of island inhabitants. Point (a) shows the 50th percentile of users.

curve shows the cumulative proportion of drug use accounted for by cumulative percentiles of users, those with higher annual drug use being ranked first. Equal shares in drug use (if all inhabitants had used the same or a similar quantity of drugs) would be displayed as a diagonal line. As the curve deviates from this diagonal, it indicates the existence of quantitative differences in drug exposure. In the present example, the 50% of users with the highest consumption account for more than 80% of the total drug use.

The difference between the Pareto chart and the Lorenz curve is that on a Pareto chart individual items (patients, drugs) are plotted on the horizontal axis, while on a Lorenz curve the cumulative percentile of patients is placed there. For more information on Lorenz curves, see Chapter 7.

Forest plots (blobbograms)

Forest plots are usually used as a graphical representation of a meta-analysis (see Chapter 9), but they can be used for individual studies as well [31,32]. A forest plot presents a series of central values (relative risks (RRs) or odds ratios (ORs) – represented by markers) and their confidence intervals (represented by horizontal lines). The format and content of a forest plot is explained in a manuscript published by Schriger et al. [33]. Nice examples come from Swedish studies in which forest plots were used to visualize whether women are more or less likely than men to receive different antihypertensive drugs [34] or to show gender differences on the incidence of certain drug treatments (see Figure 10.12).

Kaplan–Meier curves

Kaplan–Meier curves are used to visualize 'survival' times (times to event). In medical research, they are often used to visualize survival after a patient is diagnosed with a particular illness (e.g. cancer). The 'event' need not necessarily mean death: it can be any event of interest. Hence, Kaplan–Meier curves are used across many (including nonmedical) disciplines [35]. In drug utilization research, they can be used to determine persistence of drug use in patient-level datasets. Figure 10.13 presents an example for the sample dataset

ATC	**Pharmacological group**	**PAT/1000PYs**	
		Men	Women
J02	Antimycotics	2,28	13,23
H03	Thyroid therapy	1,55	5,77
M05	Drugs for treatment of bone diseases	0,97	3,98
N06B	Psychostimulants	2,36	1,57
C01D	Vasodilators used in cardiac diseases	8,34	6,93
M04	Antigout preparations	2,71	1,44

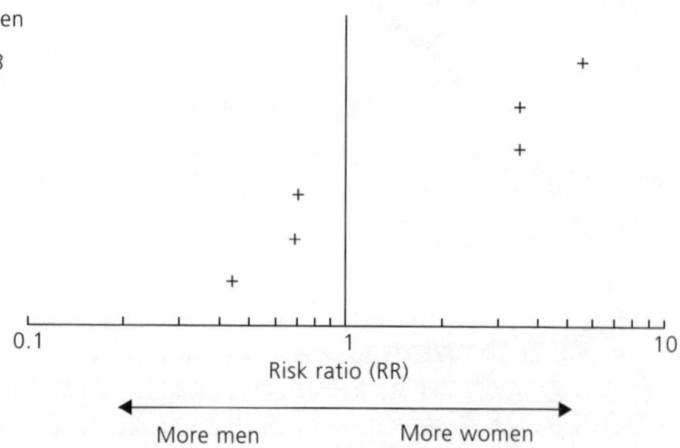

Figure 10.12 Forest plot showing relative risks of drug treatment incidence according to gender. ATC: Anatomical Therapeutic Chemical classification; PAT/1000PYs: number of patients exposed per 1000 person years. Source: Courtesy of Desiree Loikas.

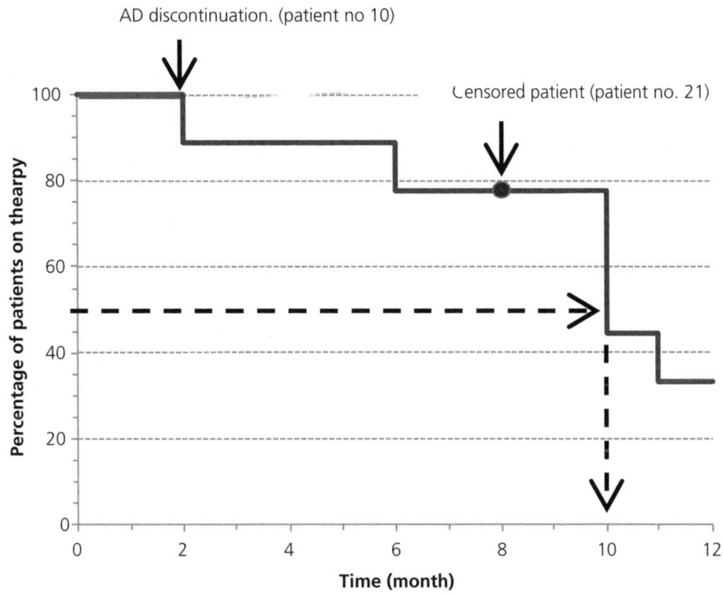

Figure 10.13 Kaplan–Meier curve for antidiabetic drug persistence. AD: antidiabetic drug (see also Table 10.2 column 12).

of the island inhabitants (Table 10.2, column 12). The event of interest here is the discontinuation of drug use (e.g. stopping treatment due to side effects). If a patient drops out for any reason during monitoring (as patient no. 21 did) or the monitoring stops before the event occurs (e.g. patient nos 4, 8 and 12), the true persistence value is replaced by a 'censored' value. One can see from the plot that in this 1-year observational study, half of the patients were on antidiabetic treatment for at least 10 months.

Further examples of Kaplan–Meier curves including more than one patient group can be found in Chapter 29.

Analysis of trends

Different chart types can visualize longitudinal drug use data. Heat maps or calendar plots and circular area charts are useful for displaying cyclical drug use patterns, while line and bar charts can effectively visualize increasing or decreasing trends.

In line charts only sequential data should be connected with lines, non-sequential ones (gap in time-series, missing data) should not. Heat maps are constructed of sequences of squares where each square represents a data value and its colour stands for the value's magnitude (see Figure 10.14, based on data in Table 10.3).

Table 10.3 Hypothetical consumption of two drugs over 2 years expressed in DDD/1000 inhabitants/day. D2 represents a drug with gradually increasing use, while D1 represents a drug with seasonal fluctuation in use.

Drug	Year	Jan	Feb	Mar	Apr	May	June	July	Aug	Sept	Oct	Nov	Dec
D1	2013	5	5.2	4.8	4.7	3.9	3	2	2.1	3	3.1	4.1	4.2
D2	2013	2.1	2.5	2.6	2.8	2.9	3.2	3.3	3.6	4.1	4.5	4.9	5.2
D1	2014	4.7	4.7	3.8	3.6	2.9	2.9	2.1	2.4	3	3.5	4.1	4.2
D2	2014	5.5	6	6.1	6.3	6.4	6.9	7.4	7.7	8	8.2	8.3	8.8

Practical hints for static graphs

Once the correct graph type has been selected for presentation of findings, the graph must still be customized to the individual use. In order to be understandable to someone who has not read the article, the graph should be accompanied by an informative title, an explanatory legend (abbreviations, statistics used, etc.) and sufficient information on sample size(s). Box 10.1 provides some general advice on customizing graphs, while Box 10.2 gives information on the use of colours.

Box 10.1 General principles of graphical displays.

- Generate the simplest graph that represents the information you want to convey.
- Increase the data-to-ink ratio (or information-to-ink ratio) by removing decorative elements and maximize contrast between your data and the background. Avoid the coin bar charts, cone bar charts, pseudo-3D and 3D bar or line charts offered by Excel and other programmes.
- Add structure and clarity to your chart by sorting by a metric of interest.
- When absolute magnitudes are important (e.g. in bar charts, histograms and boxplots), the vertical axis should begin at zero to avoid conveying false impressions. When relative magnitudes are important (e.g. scatterplots), scale limits closer to the actual values may be used (i.e. axes need not start from zero).
- Graphs should be large enough to make the information easy to perceive. The aspect ratio (the ratio of height to width) has a strong effect on the perception of graphics, especially in time series. If you want to show a gradual change, grow the horizontal axis and shrink the vertical one; if you want to show a dramatic change, do the opposite.
- To facilitate data interpretation and comparison tasks, navigational elements (tick marks, grid lines and axes) can be added. When using multipanel figures, use fixed axis scaling across panels (a common y-axis is a good alternative) to facilitate comparison.
- Figure legends are easier to understand if categories are displayed in the same order and in the same direction as in the figure itself (see Figure 10.2), especially if there are more than two categories. If possible (e.g. if trend lines can be separated easily or intersections are sparse), a useful alternative to a legend is to label the individual data series directly (see Figure 10.14a).
- For further reading, see Chen et al. [3], Kelleher & Wagener [11] and Krzywinski [36].

Box 10.2 Use of colours in graphics: the three types of colour scheme and other practical hints.

- Sequential schemes are used when ordering values from low to high (with low values in lighter shades and high values in darker shades of a specific colour). Sequential schemes should be used for quantitative data (e.g. number of drugs).
- Divergent schemes are used when the values are ordered and there is a critical midpoint (e.g. an average or zero). Diverging schemes use a light, neutral colour to represent average values and contrasting dark hues for low and high values. In drug utilization research, divergent colour schemes are used to visualize, for example, Likert scales.
- Categorical/qualitative schemes are used when data fall into distinct groups (e.g. gender or ATC groups) and therefore require contrast between adjacent colours. To display 'similar' categories (e.g. cephalosporin generations), shades of the same colour should be used. As some colours have particular associations (red = danger, improper use, contraindication; green = optimal, desirable), their use can be suggestive. It should also be borne in mind that some people are colour-blind, so green should be supplemented by blue.
- For a series of figures within an article or slideshow, colours should be used consistently: the same item should be displayed with the same colour throughout.
- When colouring bars, use solid (flat) colours to ensure that the end points are visible.
- ColorBrewer.org is a free online tool for the generation of colour scales [37,38].
- For further reading, see Kelleher & Wagener [11].

Interactive visualization – including time and geospatial visualization

The aim of this section is to raise some important considerations to keep in mind when deciding on whether to visualize data interactively in order to communicate a message to, for instance, decision-makers or prescribers. Interactive visualization is seldom used in the presentation of drug utilization study results.

The main goal of interactive visualization is to provide a deeper understanding of a dataset and to offer insight into the presented analysis, by allowing either the presenter or the audience to explore the dataset

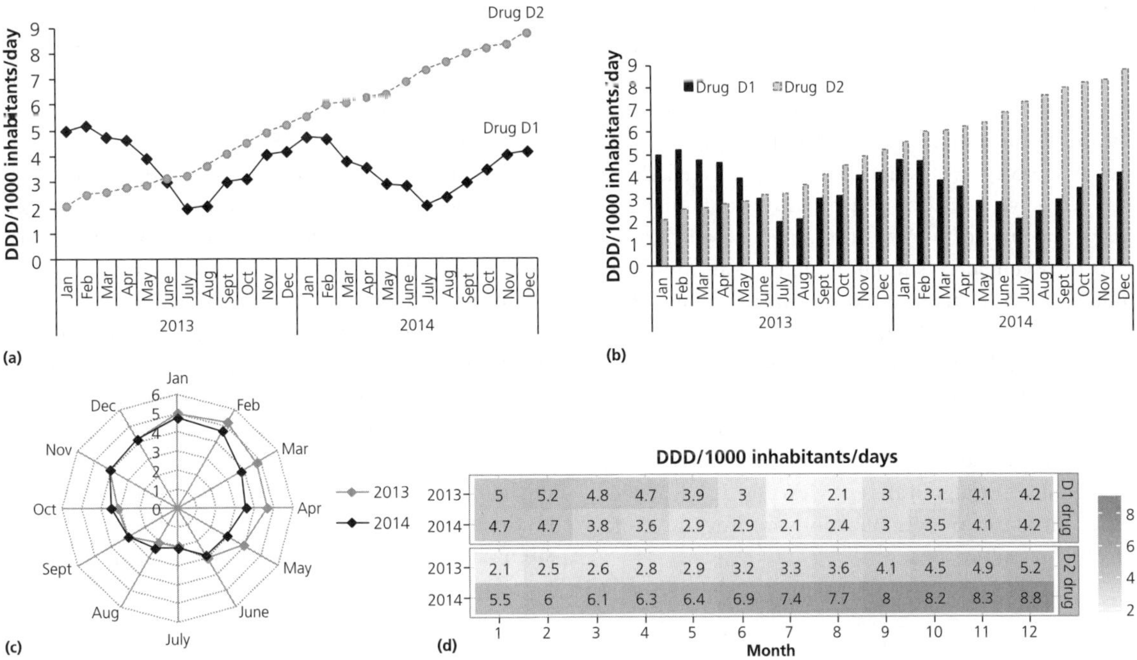

Figure 10.14 Longitudinal drug use displayed in (a) a line chart, (b) a bar chart, (c) a circular area chart and (d) a heat map. Based on data in Table 10.3.

interactively during a presentation [1,2]. A well-designed interactive visualization can empower participants to question the validity of the complete dataset, the analysis and the conclusions drawn by the presenter. It might also lead to new insights through dialogue between presenter and participants.

Interactive visualization involves several interlocking feedback loops, from selection and exploration of data to the analytical stage, and possibly to a direct problem-solving step. All loops in the different steps have their own cognitive fallacies. A deeper understanding of these processes is important to creating effective interactive visualizations [1].

More dimensions (variables) can be presented in parallel in an interactive visualization than in a basic graph or figure. Another strength is the possibility of presenting an overview and of offering the ability to zoom in and filter the dataset on demand. It is also possible to change the presentation format and variables, creating new insights into associations.

Why and when?

An interactive visualization can be used in order to reach different goals. It can simplify the understanding of a given analysis or proposal. It can help an audience to structure, analyse and remember a dataset and any conclusions drawn from it. A well thought-out interactive visualization can thus simplify the communication of the presentation's main messages.

When communicating drug utilization data, beyond the time and geospatial issues, it is often necessary to relate different dimensions to one another. For instance, the choice of a specific substance within a subgroup very often benefits from being analysed in the context of the use of the subgroup in relation to other therapeutic substitutes and/or the volume for the total subgroup. As an example, a high or low fraction of a specific statin can easily be related not only to other statins but also to the total use of statins and/or other blood lipid-lowering agents within the population studied.

When not?

The best visualization is the one that fits the dataset and can easily and quickly be understood by the audience. There is no inherent value in having either a static or an interactive visualization. The simplest way to convey a message is to be preferred. Most interactive visualizations incorporate tools and use views that part or most of the audience will not be used to. Even such 'simple' designs as an animated bubble chart (Figure 10.15) or linked graphs (Figure 10.16) can be confusing for an audience used to single graphs with the x-axis representing time. Because of this, special competence is needed in both designing and presenting a dataset through interactive visualization. In most cases, the audience has to be guided through different views by a skilled presenter of interactive visualizations in order to avoid misunderstandings.

One major caveat to consider for any visualization with several related variables is the risk of identifying associations between variables over time that are not causal associations but a consequence of confounding. Several other caveats must also be borne in mind before using interactive visualization, especially when covering longer time periods which include major changes in demography that might influence the measures used. Indiscriminate use of measures such as currency (instead of inflation-adjusted currency or purchasing power parity) or number of individuals (instead of data standardized for age and sex) may lead to misinterpretation by the audience. The same problems exist for static visualizations, but a specific problem with interactive visualization is that user interaction might lead to the creation of graphs – not previously considered by the presenter – that create a false impression of the strength of a correlation and/or of causality.

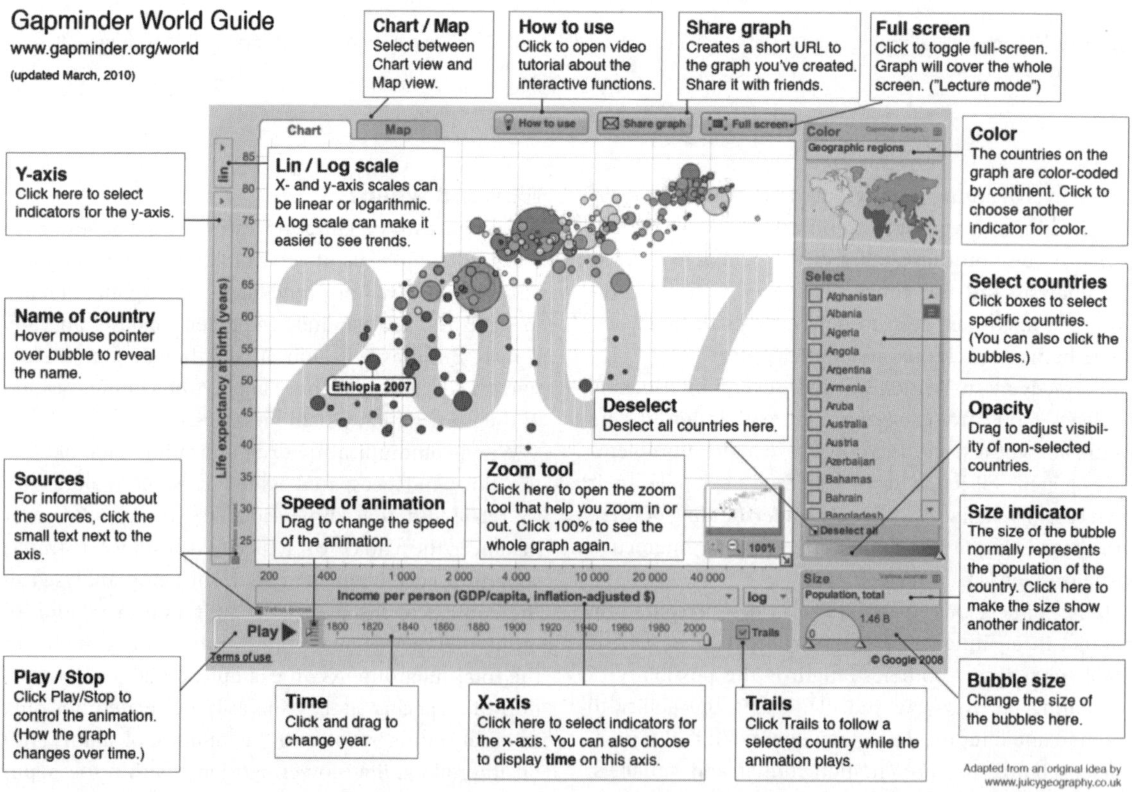

Figure 10.15 Static view of an animated bubble chart. Guide to the Gapminder World – Health and Wealth of Nations. The illustration shows the basic functions of the Motion Chart tool, originally developed by the Gapminder foundation [39,40]. For colour details, please refer to the colour plates section.

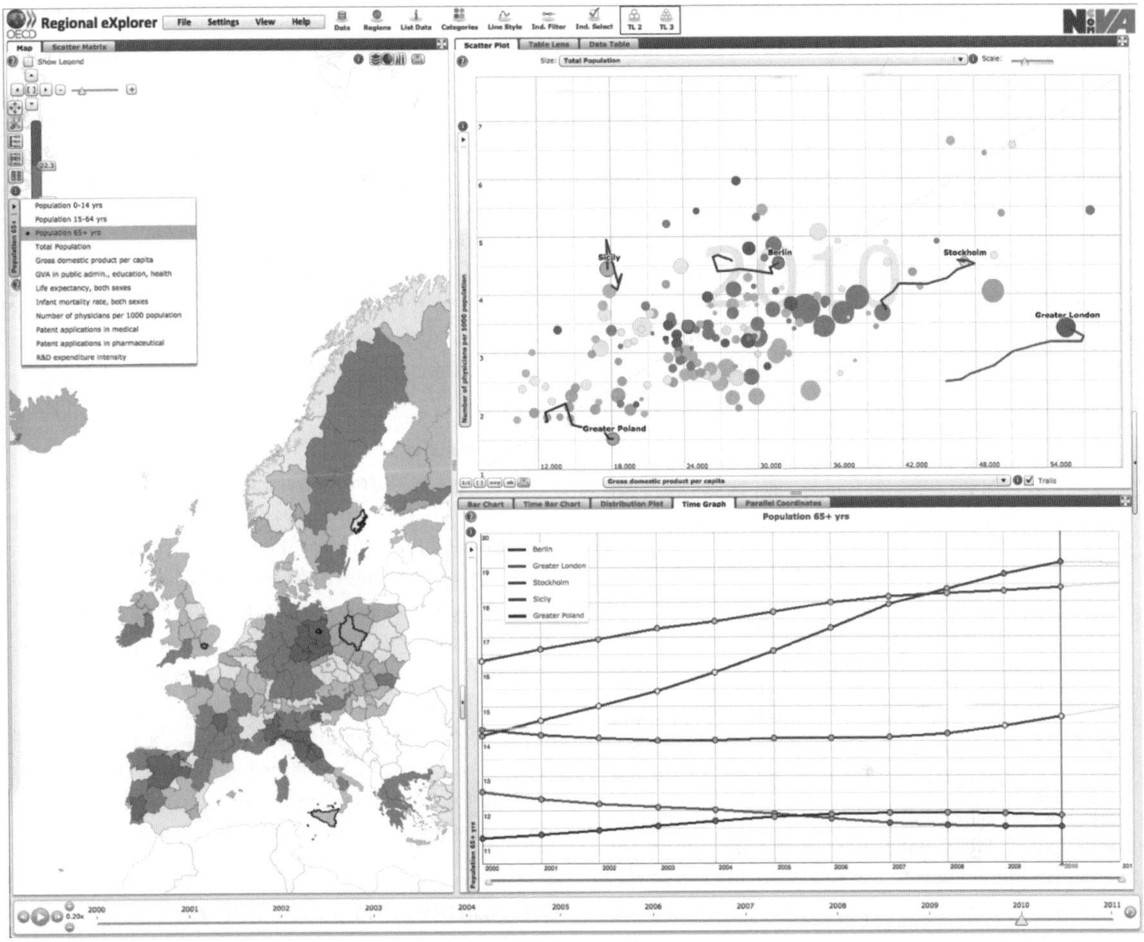

Figure 10.16 Static view from a visualization tool showing data linked between different graphs. For colour details, please refer to the colour plates section.

Source: OECD Factbook [41,42].

Practical hints and tools

Gapminder/Google Motion Charts

The Gapminder tool (or Google Motion Chart), featuring animated bubble graphs, is one of the most well known and accessible interactive tools for time and geospatial visualization [39,40]. A basic bubble graph is a scatterplot relating two variables on the x- and y-axes. Two additional variables can be visualized by the use of size and colour for each observation/bubble. Time introduces a fifth variable. The software was developed and popularized by the Gapminder foundation and later acquired by Google and introduced as a component (Motion Chart) of their cloud-based office suite, Google Drive.

The Gapminder tool is a strong method for conveying focused messages and responding to questions from an audience. In general, humans are very bad at tracking more than seven moving objects at a time, and this type of visualization is thus not suited to tracking multiple bubbles simultaneously. The success of the Gapminder tool is to a large degree a consequence of well-prepared presentations with a compelling message that is highlighted by focusing on a small subset of the data.

Linked highlighting

An often important feature of interactive visualization is the ability to combine different visual presentations and at the same time filter and highlight the same subset of data (e.g. geographical areas).

Figure 10.16 is an example from the OECD Factbook [41,42] showing a snapshot of 2010 (from an animated time series covering 2000–11). Clicking on the play button at the bottom or sliding the time ruler will animate the graph, showing change over time. Variables to include can easily be changed and datasets from other sources can be uploaded to the visualization tool. In the image in the figure, five different European regional areas have been selected by the user and thus simultaneously highlighted in three different graphs. To the left is a map with a drop-down menu with available variables unfolded. The fraction of the population aged over 65 years is used to colour-code both the map and the scatterplot in the upper right corner. The five regions highlighted in the map are also automatically highlighted in the scatterplot and selected for the time graph in the lower right corner. Different visualizations can be chosen by the tabs in each section, variables can be changed and highlighted everywhere and other types of geographical regions (countries, regions, municipalities) can be chosen. In the scatterplot, the variables selected are the gross domestic product per capita (in price parities) on the x-axis, the number of physicians per capita on the y-axis, the colour code (as on the map) and the total population (as size of bubbles). Changes over time for the selected regions are shown as tracks. All selected regions except Sicily have increasing GDP during the time period (movement to the right). Sicily and Greater Poland have the lowest GDP per capita (x-axis), but Sicily has more physicians per capita (y-axis) and a higher fraction of the elderly (colour coding) in 2010. The number of physicians per capita increases in Stockholm and Greater London (movement upwards, as shown by the tracks). The time graph in the lower right corner (time on the x-axis and fraction of the elderly on the y-axis) shows the striking increase in the fraction of the elderly in Berlin over the period. This is not matched by an increase in physicians per capita in the bubble-graph and can be further explored by changing the x-axis in the scatterplot to fraction of elderly instead of GDP per capita.

Brushing and filtering

As the dataset becomes more complex, it becomes more important to be able to focus on specific subsets of the data, perhaps by brushing or filtering the data [43]. The same basic considerations are relevant for all visualizations, whether they are interactive or not. It is important to consider the type of data – univariate, bivariate or multivariate – when deciding on how the dataset should be presented.

Brushing is a technique by which an interaction with one item (e.g. highlighting a country) changes the encoding of other, related items. This allows simple relationships to be visualized, as shown in Figure 10.16.

One commonly employed method by which to filter multivariate data interactively is the parallel coordinate plot [44]. In this graphic interface, the user can choose to filter the data according to many different variables at the same time (Figure 10.17).

Storytelling

Storytelling, or narrative visualization, is a way of packaging information into a structure that is more easily remembered than isolated data [45]. It can be described as an ordered sequence of steps, with a clearly defined path through it. This can be achieved through traditional lectures and/or sequential static graphs, but also by using specific software or functions included in visualization tools. Tools for storytelling make it possible to publish a visualization as a story on a website with discrete defined and explained steps, but still make it possible for the audience to interact with the data during these steps.

Distributing and publishing on the Internet

Links to Google Motion Chart can be distributed and the visualization itself can be published on the Internet [39]. Several other commercial solutions are available [46–48], and there are some free desktop applications or services, but these are often only for personal use. In order to distribute and/or publish an interactive visualization, a software license is generally necessary. There are also several open-source projects, such as Ggobi [49] and Orange [50]; while versatile tools, in general these have a steeper learning curve than commercial solutions. A hands-on guide to visualisation in R is available [51].

When publishing on a website, whether an open or a password-protected site, it is important to clearly state the origin of the dataset and any limitations on use and to provide basic instructions on how to use the visualization. If possible, storytelling should be used to guide the audience.

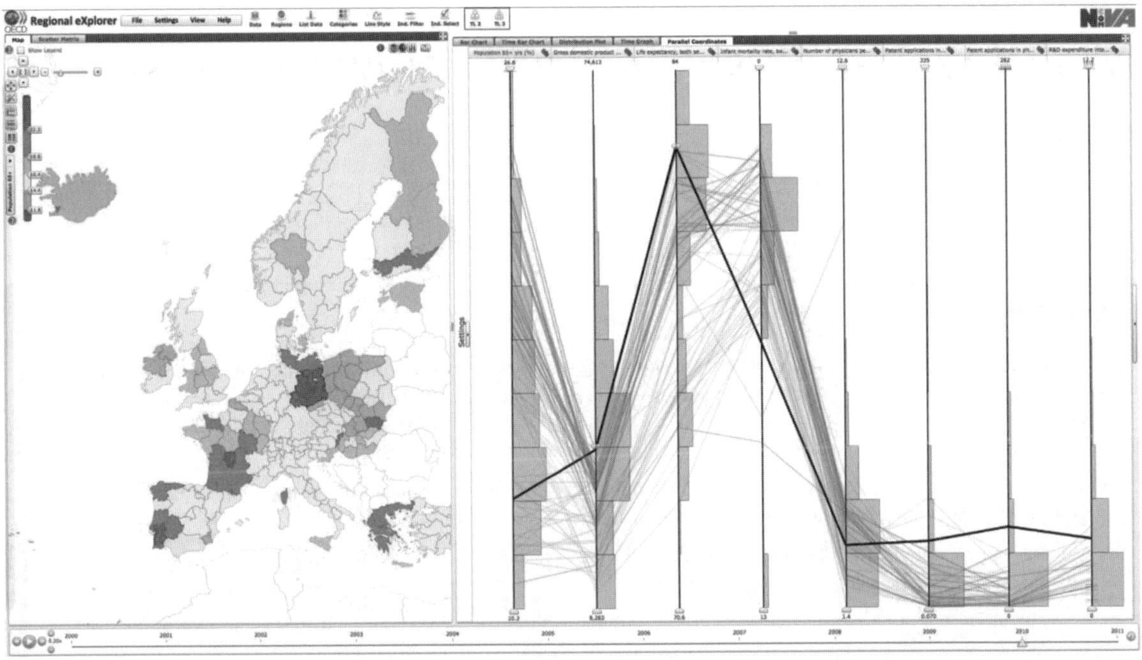

Figure 10.17 Parallel coordinate plot [44] used to filter a multivariate dataset (the same as that in Figure 10.16). By repositioning the sliders on each vertical line, the dataset is successively filtered not only in the parallel coordinate plot, but also in all associated visualizations (in this case, only the map is shown). Each remaining coloured line represents a geographically defined population that fulfils all criteria. Source: OECD Factbook [42]. For colour details, please refer to the colour plates section.

Conclusion

Static graphical display – when thought through and worked out properly – is an important tool for efficiently conveying one's message to one's audience/readers. One should be informed about the general rules and limitations of certain graphic types and consider several alternatives before choosing one that best suits the data, the objectives of the visualization and the audience/readership.

An interactive visualization can engage the audience and help them understand the dataset better. In order to achieve this, the correct tools have to be selected based not only on the dataset itself, but also on how experienced the audience is with them and with the different modes of presentation.

CHAPTER 11

Multilevel analyses in drug utilization research

Juan Merlo

Unit for Social Epidemiology, Faculty of Medicine, Lund University, Skåne University Hospital, Sweden

KEY POINTS

- As in many other fields of research, there are structures in drug utilization research that generate dependence among observations. For example, patients prescribed by the same doctor tend to use the same medications, and physicians working at the same primary health care centre tend to prescribe similar drugs. In such situations, we say that the patients' medication use is correlated within physicians or that physicians' prescribing behaviour is correlated within health care centres.
- If an outcome (e.g. medication use) is correlated in a multilevel structure (e.g. patients at the first level and physicians at the second), traditional statistical analyses such as simple logistic regression will be unsuitable.
- Multilevel regression analysis (MLRA) is a statistical technique that is appropriate for the study of correlated outcomes. MLRA provides an improved estimation of standard errors.
- In MLRA, variance is not a nuisance but a source of substantive information for understanding the influence of, for example, geographical, institutional or physician levels on individual medication use or other outcomes.
- MLRA provides an improved measurement of medical practice variation and institutional ranking (what is sometimes referred to as 'league tables').

Introduction

Multilevel regression analysis (MLRA) [1–6] is a statistical technique that is suitable for the study of correlated outcomes within multilevel structures. To be considered a 'higher level', a candidate category must condition the variance of the lower level. Examples of simple multilevel structures are patients with the same physician and physicians at the same health care centre [7]. Physicians are a higher level for the patients because doctors decide their patients' treatment. Therefore, patients with the same doctor are more likely to use the same kind of medication than are patients with different doctors. That is, patient medication use is correlated within physicians. If information is correlated in a multilevel structure, the normal statistical regression analyses will be formally inappropriate and should not be applied.

MLRA provides an improved estimation of standard errors (SEs) and an appropriate measurement of medical practice variation and institutional ranking (league tables). In MLRA, variance is a source of substantive information for understanding the influence of, for example, geographical, institutional or physician levels on individual medication use or other outcomes [1–4].

MLRA is known by a variety of names, including 'hierarchical linear models', 'nested models', 'mixed models', 'random coefficients models', 'random-effects models' and 'random parameter models'. It was developed for the study of repeated measurements within individuals [8], which are encountered relatively frequently in clinical pharmacology. It has been extensively applied to the investigation of school performance [9], as it is expected that pupils at the same school will share a common degree of learned knowledge. MLRA is being increasingly applied in the investigation of small-area variations in health [10], in the evaluation of health care performance [11,12] and in drug utilization research [13–20].

The main purpose of this chapter is to provide a short introduction to MLRA. The intention is to offer

Drug Utilization Research: Methods and Applications, First Edition. Edited by M. Elseviers et al.
Published 2016 by John Wiley & Sons, Ltd.

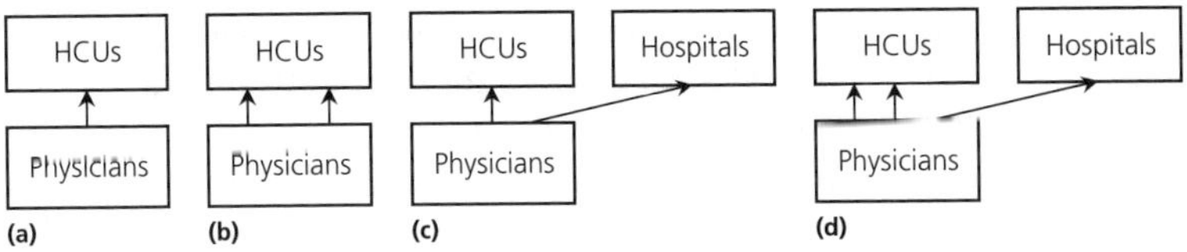

Figure 11.1 Classification diagrams for two level (a) hierarchical, (b) multiple-membership, (c) cross-classified and (d) multiple-membership cross-classified structures. HCU, health care unit.

a conceptual rather than a mathematical understanding of multilevel concepts and techniques. After reading this chapter, you will be able to recognize the presence of multilevel structures in drug utilization research and tell when MLRA is necessary. By following a didactical example and consulting the references, you will acquire the basic knowledge required to perform and interpret MLRA in drug utilization research. A more extended introduction can be found elsewhere [1–4]. It is also recommended that you look at the free online course offered by the Centre for Multilevel Modelling at the University of Bristol,[1] where you can learn both basic and advanced multilevel techniques and gain access to many resources of help in understanding MLRA, including references to appropriate software and other courses.

Multilevel structures

The term 'multilevel' refers to the existence of arrangements of information that present a hierarchical or categorical structure. Examples of multilevel structures are repeated measurements of blood pressure for the same patient, pupils within schools, patients with the same physician and physicians within health care centres. It is worth insisting that in order to be considered a 'higher level', a candidate category (e.g. the health care unit, HCU) must always ***condition the variance of the lower level*** (e.g. patients' differences in use of medication). However, multilevel structures are not always hierarchical. For instance, a patient might be treated at different HCUs (termed 'multiple membership') or at both an HCU and a hospital ('cross-classification'), or both ('multiple membership multiple classification') [21]. These structures can be represented in a ***classification diagram*** as shown in Figure 11.1. They can all be modelled using available software [22].

Why are MLRA techniques necessary?

If there are structures that generate dependence in observations (e.g. physicians' prescribing behaviour is correlated within health care centres), then we need MLRA techniques for both statistical and substantive reasons.

Statistical reasons

Correct estimation of standard errors

From a statistical perspective, MLRA allows a correct estimation of the SEs of the β-coefficients in a regression analysis. A condition for performing normal (single-level) regression analysis is that the residuals are not correlated. If residual correlation exists and is not considered then the statistical 'significance' or precision (95% CIs) of the measures of association (e.g. the odds ratios, ORs) for the variables at the higher level will be overestimated. In fact, the stronger the residual dependence, the less statistical information is available and the lower the effective sample size, and, therefore, the lower the statistical power [23]. MLRA accounts for this residual dependence and thereby provides correct estimations.

To understand this fundamental notion, we need to have a clear idea of the concepts of 'residual', 'variance', 'components of variance' and 'intraclass correlation' (ICC). We also need to be sure of the basic distinction between individual-level and ecological analyses and to distinguish these study designs from multilevel analysis. (If you want to refresh these concepts, see Appendix 11A on the companion website.)

[1] Learning Environment for Multilevel Methodology and Applications (LEMMA 1, 2, 3) (http://www.bristol.ac.uk/cmm/research/lemma/1/). The Centre for Multilevel Modelling provides numerous other resources in multilevel analysis, including information on the MLwiN software (http://www.bristol.ac.uk/cmm/software/mlwin/). The MLwiN is free to UK academics and can be run within Stata and R. The site also provides information on other software, including HLM, aML, Mplus, SAS, SPSS, Stata, BAYESX, BUGS, GeoBUGS, GLLAMM, MIX, R and R/S.

More parsimonious analyses

Let's say that we wish to quantify the differences between 24 HCUs concerning use of recommended statins (yes vs. no) among patients on treatment with statins [7]. A classical approach would be to apply a simple logistic regression analysis modelling 23 dummy variables and using one of the HCUs as a reference. In this way, we would be able to obtain an OR for each of the remaining 23 HCUs. That is, we would have a logistic regression model with an intercept β_0 (the reference) and 23 regression coefficients (β_1 to β_{23}) that quantified the difference between the reference and the value of each HCU:

$$logit\ (p_j) = \beta_0 + \beta_1 + \beta_3 \ldots \ldots \ldots \beta_{23} \tag{11.1}$$

However, when we apply MLRA, we have a model with just one intercept, β_0, and its variance, σ_u^2:

$$logit\ (p_j) = \beta_0 + u_j$$
$$u_j \sim N(0, \sigma_u^2) \tag{11.2}$$

where u_j is the intercept for each HCU. The intercept, u_j, also denominates the HCU residual that quantifies the difference between the overall mean β_0 and the mean value of the HCU (see also Appendix 11A).

In both the classical and the MRLA approach, we can include in the models individual-level variables to adjust for patient characteristics and account for patient mixes that might confound the observed differences between the HCUs. However, in the MLRA we can also include HCU characteristics and investigate HCU variance. Understanding HCU variance is fundamental to quantifying the general influence of the HCU on drug prescription. It is not possible to measure HCU variance in the classical approach, as the dummy HCU variables explain all the variance between the HCUs and prevent the inclusion of HCU characteristics in the models [24].

Another alternative could be to perform a simple ecological analysis and compare the use percentages of recommended statins between HCUs. However, this approach is not recommended because it neglects individual-level variation. Later in the chapter, and in Appendix 11B, we discuss how individual-level information is essential to interpretting HCU variance. Furthermore, aggregated ecological analysis has many other weaknesses, including ecological and sociological fallacies that are explained in detail elsewhere [10,25,26].

Better measurement and evaluation of medical practice variation and institutional ranking (league tables)

Understanding unjustified medical practice variation (e.g. variation in prescribing that is not motivated by differences in patient comorbidity between medical practices) is very relevant for the evaluation of health care quality, since it can reflect, for example, inappropriate clinical decisions that are susceptible of improvement.

In the analysis of medical practice variation, it is common to construct ranking lists (e.g. league tables) or coloured atlases that explicitly show variation and evaluate geographical areas or health care institutions on the basis of performance indicators [15,27]. However, for several reasons, MLRA provides a better methodology for ranking institutional performance than the classical approaches.

MLRA applies techniques that account for the reliability of the information in each HCU. Small units with few patients provide unreliable information that expresses itself by very high or very low values due to random chance. Therefore, in MLRA, small units are smoothed or shrunken towards the mean (see Appendix 11C). MLRA moreover provides an improved estimation of the uncertainty of the ranking of HCUs [28–34].

Notably, the ranking of institutions based only on average values is insufficient for evaluating institutional performance. We need to analyse both differences between institutional averages and the total individual variance. The analysis of variance in MLRA provides information on the share of the total individual variance at the institutional (e.g. HCU) level. Therefore, it provides information on the relevance of the HCUs to understanding individual-level variation. When investigating medical practice variation, the main aim is not to evaluate differences between institutional averages but, rather, to quantify to what degree those differences are relevant to understanding the total individual variation. More information can be found in the literature [4,10,12,15,35,36], and an overview is given in Appendix 11B.

More flexible analysis of variance

We normally assume that the higher-level (e.g. HCU or the neighbourhood) variance is the same for all individuals in a population. However, it could be that this variance is higher (or lower) for specific groups of individuals, defined by age, sex, specific diseases or any other characteristic. That is, the higher-level (e.g.

neighbourhood) variance could be a function of the lower-level (e.g. individual) variables.

For instance, in a previous World Health Organization (WHO) publication, the MONICA project [37], we allowed the associations between body mass index (BMI) and blood pressure-lowering drugs, on the one hand, and blood pressure, on the other, to be different at the second level (i.e. the MONICA population). In this way, we observed, for example, that population differences were higher for overweight women who used blood pressure-lowering drugs. This finding can be explained by differences in the effectiveness of health care systems in different countries.

In another publication [38], investigating trends in adherence to guidelines for statin prescription, we allowed the slope (β-coefficient) of the association between time (calendar month) and prescription of a recommended statin to fluctuate at the HCU level. On doing so, the variance between HCUs became a function of time (see the original publication for an extended explanation [38]). Besides the study of trends, this analytical approach can be applied to investigate the influence of HCUs on drug prescription for different types of individual (e.g. men and women, different age groups, patients with different diseases, etc.) [3,39].

For information on the concepts of 'random slope' and 'variance function', see Appendix 11E.

Substantive reasons

The advantages of MLRA are not only grounded in statistical reasons. MLRA also conveys a number of substantive benefits concerning the evaluation of health care performance and geographical and medical practice variation.

General and specific contextual effects

In MLRA, variance is not considered a nuisance that needs to be modelled in order to obtain correct estimations of SE. Rather, it is a source of substantive information of use in understanding the influence of geographical, institutional and physician levels on individual medication use and other outcomes. The existence of residual dependence is not only the *sine qua non* for performing multilevel regression analyses but might also indicate that the context (e.g. HCU) conditions the individual outcome over and above individual characteristics (see elsewhere for an extended explanation of this idea [10,15,40,41]). This conditioning has been termed ***general contextual effects*** because it does not specify any other contextual characteristic than the very definition of context (e.g. HCU). The term 'general' stresses the difference from the habitual ***specific contextual effects*** that focus on the association between specific contextual characteristics and the individual-level outcome. For instance, we could observe that the HCU level conditions the prescription of recommended statins, since the ICC[2] is 30%, which is a general contextual effect. Simultaneously, we could detect that prescription of recommended statins is three times more frequent in public than in private HCUs (OR = 3), which is a specific contextual effect.

This distinction is relevant, since similar specific contextual effects can be found alongside very different general contextual effects, so general and specific contextual effects must be interpreted together. For more information, see Appendix 11B.

Considering both averages and variation around the average in evaluation of health care performance

As we have already noted, if league tables or coloured atlases are to be used as a tool for evaluating quality in health care, it is essential that they are complemented by a measure of general contextual effects, such as the variance partition coefficient (VPC), the ICC [4] or the area under the receiver operating characteristics curve (AU-ROC) for random effects (see Appendices A and C) [36,42]. These measures allow us to estimate the extent to which differences between individuals' outcome are conditioned by the context under consideration, such as the health care facility [41]. The higher the value of these measures, the more important is the context for understanding the individual differences in the outcome under study. The median odds ratio (MOR) is another useful measure for quantifying general contextual effects, but it has a different interpretation than the ICC (see also Appendix 11C) [43].

This information has direct practical consequences. If the share of the total variance at the higher-level units is low, interventions should not be focused on specific units at this level. Therefore, league tables are not necessary [41,44]. In conclusion, observing only differences in means between contextual units (as is the norm when analysing league tables or coloured atlases) is insufficient for the purpose of evaluating quality in health care (see also Appendices A and B).

[2] See Appendix 11A for more on the concept of ICC.

Basic concepts in MLRA: a didactic example

In order to understand the fundamental concepts in MLRA, it is most appropriate to begin with an example modelling a continuous variable such as systolic blood pressure (SBP) in a multilevel *linear* regression analysis. Statistical technicalities apart, the concepts and interpretation of MLRA are similar for dichotomous variables modelled by multilevel logistic regression analysis [4]. Nevertheless, MLRA is easier to explain and understand in the case of continuous variables. The data presented in this section are fictive, but are inspired by a real empirical analysis [37]. We also recommended following a free online tutorial [1–4] and taking an online course at the Centre for Multilevel Modelling at Bristol University (http://www.bristol.ac.uk/cmm/learning/online-course/index.html).

Assume that we want to investigate the SBP of 25 000 patients treated at 39 different primary HCUs. We have, therefore, a multilevel structure with patients (level 1) nested within HCUs (level 2). For the sake of simplicity (and excepting solo practices), we do not consider the physician, even though such a level is certainly relevant, as many patients can share the same doctor and several doctors can work within the same HCU. We also have information on the age of every patient and we know whether each HCU is a private or a public practice.

The ***first goal*** of our study is to audit health care quality. From this perspective, we develop a quality indicator that is just the mean SBP of the HCU. The goal is to achieve a value equal to 120 mmHg. Using this indicator, we aim to rank the HCUs and construct a league table for use by decision-makers and the public. We plan to adjust the analysis for individual age, since SBP increases with age and there may be differences in the age distributions of patients attending the different HCUs. The league table will be complemented by the ICC value, which provides information on the general contextual effects of the various HCUs.

The ***second goal*** is to investigate whether average SBP differs between public and private practices. That is, we hypothesize that the financial management of the HCU influences treatment quality and is thus associated to individual SBP. We also think that, alongside individual age, the financial management will also explain differences in average SBP between the HCUs.

We now present a step-by-step guide to analysing the data. We see in Table 11.1 that we distinguish between ***analysis of individual variance components*** and ***analysis of averages***. This distinction is specific to MLRA, since most classical regression analyses only focus on the analysis of averages. Most of the times, the analysis of components of variance refers to the analysis of general contextual effects, while the analysis of averages includes the study of specific contextual effects.

Table 11.1 Example of a multilevel analysis of components of variance in systolic blood pressure (SBP) in a population of 25 000 patients from 39 primary health care units (HCUs). Values are mmHg if not otherwise indicated. The analysis is fictive and is given only for didactical purposes.

	Model 1 Empty components of variance	Model 2 Individual characteristics	Model 3 Contextual characteristics
Analysis of individual variance components			
• Between HCU (SE)	38.2 (9.5)	36.4 (9.0)	26.3 (6.6)
• Within HCU (SE)	433.4 (3.9)	349.2 (3.1)	349.2 (3.2)
VPC	8.1%	9.4%	7.0%
PCV			
• Between HCUs	Reference	4.7%	31.2%
• Within HCUs	Reference	19.4%	19.4%
Analysis of averages			
Population mean SBP, intercept (SE)	130.1 (1.0)	129.9 (0.85)	132.6 (1.0)
Age (1 year increasing), β-coefficient (SE)		1 08 (0.01)	1 08 (0.01)
Private vs. public HCU, β-coefficient (SE)			6.5 (1–5)

SE, standard error; VPC, variance partition coefficient; PCV, proportional change in variance.

In the first step (Table 11.1, model 1), we estimate only the mean SBP in the whole population (the intercept in the MLRA) and perform a simple analysis of components of variance.

It is intuitive that the patients treated at the same HCU may have a more similar level of SBP, and that this level may differ between HCUs because of, for instance, different practice traditions concerning treatment of high blood pressure or differences in the characteristics of the patients (e.g. age). That is, even if the individuals from the same HCU have different SBP values, they share a common level of SBP over and above their own individual level. This common SBP level is, in turn, different from that at other HCUs. In other words, a part of the total individual difference (i.e. variance) in SBP is at the HCU level. When this phenomenon exists, we say that there is intra-HCU correlation in SBP. In statistical terms, this situation is named 'residual dependence' and is a fundamental characteristic of a multilevel structure (see Appendix 11A).

In the simple analysis of components of individual variance, we do not include any individual or HCU variables (e.g. individual age, being a private HCU); we only include the individual SBP (i.e. the outcome) and the patient and HCU identification numbers. Measures of variance are based on the so-called 'residuals'. We know from basic statistics that the ***variance*** is the average of the squared differences from the mean (i.e. the average of the squared residuals; see also Appendix 11A).

The variance is not a measure of probabilistic uncertainty (as it is sometimes interpreted), but expresses a natural phenomenon that corresponds to the underlying interindividual heterogeneity [45] in the outcome variable (i.e. blood pressure, in our example). Probabilistic uncertainty is quantified by the SE of the mean and by the SE of the variance. Note that, unlike the variance, the SE of the variance will decrease as the number of individuals in the sample increases. In short, the individual heterogeneity (variance) may be large but is estimated with high precision (i.e. a low SE of the variance) [46].

The simplest MLRA of variance just models how the total individual variance (i.e. differences around the overall mean) is distributed across levels. This information is expressed by the VPC, which in the example of patients nested within an HCU is:

$$VPC = \frac{\text{Variance between HCUs}}{\text{Variance between HCUs} + \text{Variance within HCUs}} \quad (11.3)$$

The VPC informs the share of the total individual variance that is at the HCU level, and in our case corresponds with the ICC (see Appendix 11A). In Table 11.1, we can see the values of the variances between HCUs and within HCUs, which in model 1 renders VPC = 0.08. This value means that 8% of the individual differences in SBP are at the HCU. In order to understand this concept, we can actually plot the individual SBP values in every one of the HCUs and observe what 8% really means (Figure 11.2). We see that there is a rather considerable individual SBP heterogeneity around the SBP mean of each HCU. In fact, the overlap between the individual SBP distributions of the HCUs is considerable. This implies that we cannot discriminate the SBP of a specific individual just by knowing his or her HCU.

A high VPC tells us that HCUs are very relevant to understanding individual differences in SBP. When the VPC is close to 0, we do not need to apply multilevel analysis. It does not matter if the difference between the HCU averages is statistically 'significant' (see Appendix 11B). Whether to consider a VPC 'high' or 'low' is a decision for the investigator [41]. As a reference, we can keep in mind that the VPC for repeated measurements of SBP within individuals is around 80–90%, which is actually a very high value. On the other hand, a VPC close to 0 suggests that the populations at HCUs are similar to random samples taken from the whole population and thus that HCUs are not relevant to understanding SBP differences. In drug utilization research, ICCs are higher when studying behavioural outcomes (e.g. adherence to guidelines for prescription of statins) than when studying medication for medical conditions, such as use of blood pressure-lowering drugs [7,15,47]. The size of an ICC is also conditioned by the validity of the definition of context as such [41]. In other fields of research, such as the evaluation of school achievement, the ICC for schools and classrooms is normally rather high (about 20–30%).

Applying MLRA, we can obtain improved estimations of the mean SBP in every HCU. These averages correspond to the so-called *shrunken* residuals (see Appendix 11D) around the overall SBP mean. MLRA provides an improved estimation of the rank, which takes into account the reliability of the information and avoids fallacious results produced by statistical noise (see Appendix 11A). Besides, the MLRA provides 95% CIs/credible intervals around every mean, which also informs on the uncertainty of the ranking [15].

Using the concepts we have learned so far, we can evaluate the first goal of our study: to audit the performance of HCUs by constructing a league table based on their average SBPs.

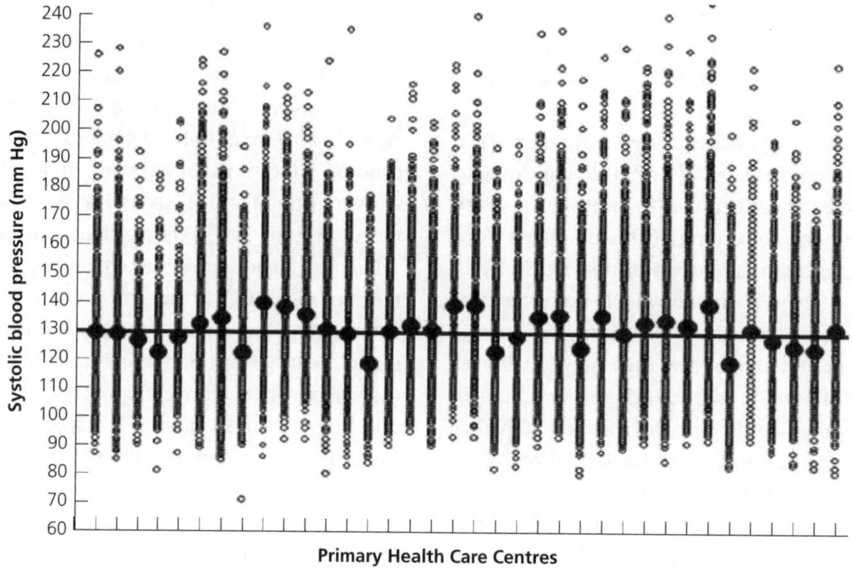

Figure 11.2 Individual distribution of systolic blood pressure (SBP) values in different health care units. The data correspond with ICC = 8%.

Source: Merlo et al. 2005 [1]. Reproduced with permission from BMJ Publishing Group Ltd.

Figure 11.3 shows the ranking of the HCUs in our fictive example. The black spots are the shrunken residuals and the white circles the raw residuals, calculated as the simple difference between the observed SBP mean in the HCU and the overall SBP mean in the county. In our example, the raw and the shrunken residuals are difficult to distinguish. They are similar because the number of patients within each HCU is large enough to produce a reliable estimation of the mean SBP of the HCUs.

A classical interpretation of Figure 11.3 would be that there is considerable HCU variation and that there are 'large' and 'significant' differences between the HCUs in terms of average SBP. However, this classical

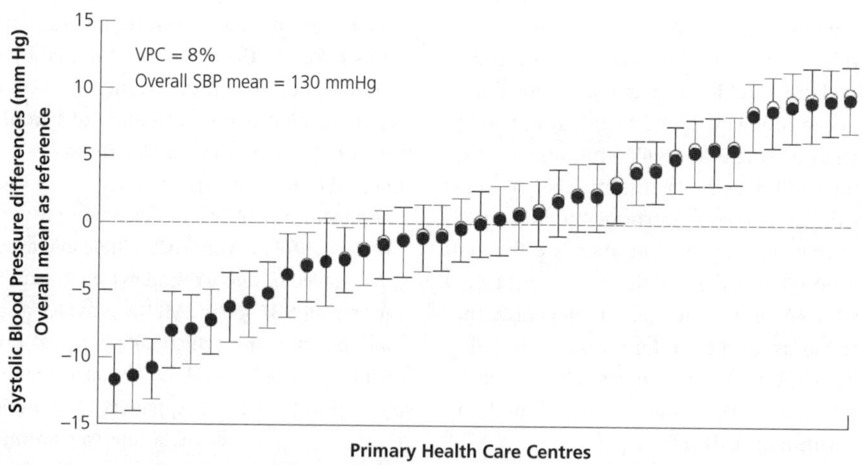

Figure 11.3 Ranking of health care units (HCUs) according to HCU residuals (i.e. the difference between the SBP mean of the HCU and the SBP mean of the whole population). The black spots are the shrunken residuals and the white circles the raw residuals.

Source: Merlo et al. 2005 [1]. Reproduced with permission from BMJ Publishing Group Ltd.

interpretation is insufficient. We must simultaneously consider that the information on HCU variation is only meaningful when it can be related to the total individual-level variance using measures such as the VPC [15,48]. In our example, the VPC is only 8%, so the information on HCU does not help much in classifying the SBPs of individuals (see Figure 11.2). In other words, focusing an intervention on the HCUs with the highest SBP average will leave untreated many individuals with high SBP who are visiting the HCU with the lowest SBP average.

The exclusive analysis of differences between averages in league tables or coloured maps is still frequent but misleading. This approach has been questioned regarding classical studies of hospital variation [11,24], studies of 'small-area variation' in mortality [10] and drug utilization research studies [15].

Once we have performed the simple analysis of components of variance, the next step (Table 11.1, model 2) is to quantify to what extent individual age explains SBP variance. It could be that HCU variance is caused by differences in the age of patients. In order to quantify how much of the individual SBP variance is explained by patient age, we compute the proportional change in variance (PCV) as:

$$PCV = \frac{\begin{matrix}\textit{Variance of the} \\ \textit{initial model}\end{matrix} - \begin{matrix}\textit{Variance of the} \\ \textit{more elaborated model}\end{matrix}}{\textit{Variance of the initial model}} \qquad (11.4)$$

Analyzing the PCV in Table 11.1, model 2, we observe that the inclusion of patient age explains 19.4% of the individual variance within HCUs and 4.7% of the between-HCU variance in SBP. The VPC, however, becomes slightly higher (i.e. 9.4%), indicating that the general influence of the HCU on individual SBP remains after adjusting for age.

Finally, in Table 11.1, model 3, we see that private HCUs have on average a 6.5 mmHg higher SBP than do public HCUs. Since this variable has the same value for all patients within an HCU, it cannot affect the within-HCU variance, but only explains the variance between HCUs.

How can we apply the results of our analysis in public health practice?

Understanding medical practice variation is very pertinent for the evaluation of health care quality, since it can reflect, for example, inappropriate therapeutic behaviours that are susceptible to improvement. This kind of analysis promotes benchmarking in health care [49] and helps to evaluate health care performance by monitoring specific quality indicators. The goal is to strive towards an ideal degree of performance and identify HCUs with relatively lower performance that can be targeted to improvement.

In our example, we observed that the overall SBP was about 10 mmHg higher than the goal of 120 mmHg, which indicates the need to improve SBP control. We also observed differences between HCUs in mean SBP. However, those differences only explained a relatively low share of the total individual differences in SBP (VPC = 8%). In other words, the individual distributions of SBP within the different HCUs overlapped each other to a considerably high degree. Therefore, it would be inefficient only to launch interventions in the HCUs with higher SBP means. Rather, any intervention should engage all HCUs. This could be done by primary prevention (e.g. promoting physical activity by adequate policies) or by secondary prevention (e.g. improving blood pressure control in patients with hypertension). It is also recommended that analyses are repeated every year.

A real empirical example

Now that we know the fundamental concepts in MLRA, we can discuss a real empirical MLRA using a dichotomous variable that is modelled by multilevel logistic regression [4]. Dichotomous variables are common in drug utilization research (e.g. use of medication: yes/no).

In a previously published study [7], we investigated the impact of a decentralized budget on physicians' adherence to guidelines for prescription of statins. The decentralized budget conveyed that the economic responsibility for tax-financed prescription drug costs was transferred from the regional administrative level to the local HCU level.

Obviously, official guidelines promoting evidence-based and cost-effective prescribing are desirable. Therefore, it is relevant to understand to what extent these guidelines are followed and the role that physicians and HCUs play in adherence to the guidelines. In our study, we expected that increased local economic responsibility would promote the prescribing of recommended, cheaper statins. Therefore, our hypothesis was that the decentralization would increase the prevalence of use of recommended statins and decrease the variance between HCUs in adherence to the guidelines.

From the Skaraborg Primary Care Database (SPCD) in the county of Skaraborg (Sweden), we obtained data on individual prescriptions for lipid-lowering drugs from all 24 public HCUs in the county before (2003) and after (2005) the budget decentralization.

We applied MLRA in order to study the distribution of the variance in the propensity of being prescribed a recommended statin. We distinguished between patient, physician and HCU levels. The outcome variable on the patient level was the prescription of the recommended statin (yes/no). In the 2003 dataset, the recommended statins were simvastatin (Zocord or generic simvastatin) and pravastatin (Pravachol). In the 2005 dataset, only simvastatin (Zocord or generic simvastatin) was recommended. The sex and age of the patients and the sex, age and occupational status of the physicians were included as explanatory variables. We could have used the ICC to measure the general effect of the HCU and of the physician on adherence to recommendations, but we chose instead to apply the MOR [4] (see Appendix 11C).

We performed analyses before (2003) and after (2005) the introduction of the decentralized budget and observed that the prevalence of adherence to guidelines for the prescription of statins increased from 77% in 2003 to 84% in 2005. The MLRA showed that in 2003 the variance was equally distributed between the HCU and physician levels ($MOR_{HCC2003}$ = 1.89 vs. $MOR_{PHYSICIAN2003}$ = 1.88). We also observed that the variance between physicians and between HCUs decreased considerably between 2003 and 2005. The inclusion of individual and physician characteristics did not explain any of the remaining variance. From these results, we concluded that both the HCUs and the individual physicians were relevant actors when it came to adherence to guidelines, so an intervention at those levels was appropriate. We also concluded that the decentralized budget increased adherence to guidelines and reduced inefficient variation in prescribing.

As an example from this study [7], we show in Figure 11.4 the (logarithmic) ORs or shrunken residuals (see Appendix 11D) of the HCUs and of the physicians

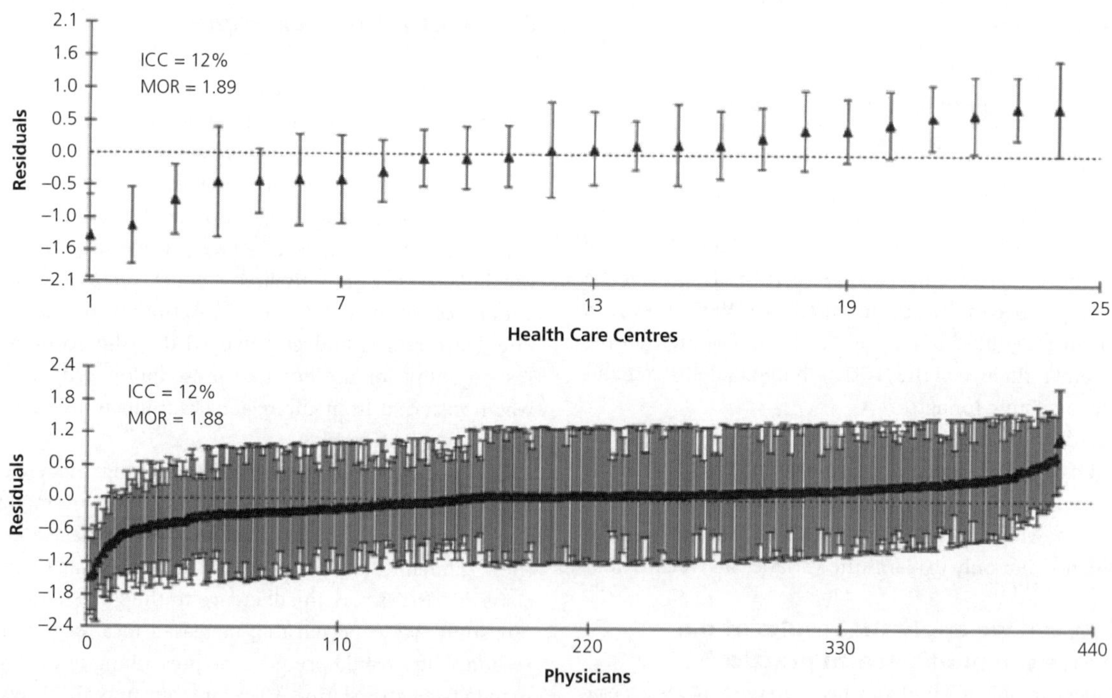

Figure 11.4 Shrunken residuals (logarithm odds ratios, ORs) from the MLRA of prescriptions of recommended statins in Skaraborg in 2003. The values of the intraclass correlation (ICC) and median odds ratio (MOR) are also indicated.

Source: Hjerpe et al. 2011 [7]. Reproduced with permission from Springer Science and Business Media.

in 2003. The differences between these higher-level residuals need to be interpreted alongside the ICC or MOR, which provides information on the relevance of these levels to understanding individual differences in the likelihood of being prescribed a recommended statin. In this study, both levels play a similar role, as expressed by the MOR value of about 1.9. Using the ICC, we see that the share of total individual variance at these levels is considerable (i.e. ICC = 12%). See elsewhere for methods of computing the MOR [4,50] and the ICC in logistic regression [4,51–53]. See also Appendices A and C.

Conclusion

Many studies in drug utilization research have an underlying multilevel structure that requires analysis by MLRA, as single-level regression analyses are inappropriate in such situations. MLRA provides an improved estimation of SEs and a better measurement of medical practice variation and institutional ranking.

In MLRA, the analysis of variance is a source of substantive information for understanding the influence of, for example, geographical, institutional or physician levels on individual medication use or other outcomes.

When evaluating medical practice variation, the main aim is not to evaluate differences between institutional averages but, rather, to quantify to what degree those differences are relevant to understanding the total individual variation.

Acknowledgements

I am grateful to the members of the Unit for Social Epidemiology at the Faculty of Medicine, Lund University for reviewing the draft of the text and providing useful comments.

CHAPTER 12

Defining and developing quality indicators for drug utilization

Stephen Campbell[1], Björn Wettermark[2] & Morten Andersen[3]
[1]Centre for Primary Care and Patient Safety Translational Research Centre, Institute of Population Health, University of Manchester, United Kingdom
[2]Clinical Pharmacology and Centre for Pharmacoepidemiology, Department of Medicine, Karolinska Institutet, Sweden
[3]Centre for Pharmacoepidemiology, Department of Medicine, Karolinska Institutet, Sweden

KEY POINTS

- Quality indicators are important tools in quality improvement initiatives such as continuous professional education, benchmarking and disease management programmes.
- A prescribing quality indicator can be defined as 'a measurable element of prescribing performance for which there is evidence or consensus that it can be used to assess quality, and hence in changing the quality of care provided'.
- Quality indicators can be classified in different dimensions, such as structure–process–outcome. In drug utilization, quality indicators can be classified as drug-oriented, disease-oriented or patient-oriented.
- Prescribing quality indicators should be developed using systematic methods such as evidence from randomized controlled trials (RCTs), high-quality observational studies or clinical guidelines, or by combining the available scientific evidence with expert opinion.
- A good indicator should fulfil several attributes. The most essential attribute is validity, which can be defined as the degree to which the measured value reflects the characteristic it is intended to measure.

Introduction

There is room for improvement in drug utilization. In some cases, inappropriate use simply results in the absence of any clinical effect. In other, more serious cases, the consequences may include increased morbidity or mortality, interactions caused by polypharmacy, adverse drug reactions, increased antimicrobial resistance or the wasting of money. All these manifestations of inappropriate drug utilization are increasingly being discussed in medical journals and in public debate [1–4].

Quality use of medicines, previously often referred to as 'rational drug use', was defined originally by the World Health Organization (WHO) as 'patients receive medication appropriate to their medical needs, in doses meeting their own individual requirements, for an adequate period of time and at the lowest costs to them and to the community' [5]. Since drug utilization research focuses on all steps in the process, from prescribing to consumption, quality of medicines use may focus upon all of these aspects. It has been suggested that rational drug prescribing involves a decision on whether to use a drug and, if so, the selection of a suitable drug and regimen, consideration of compatibility between the drug and patient and any other drugs being given, a legibly written prescription and appropriate instruction about the use of the drug and the expectations of treatment and follow-up [6]. In recent years, the importance of patient-centred communication has been increasingly emphasized, as the physician's communication skills can positively affect the patient's adherence to the prescribed medication, leading to better health outcomes [7]. The role of the pharmacist in promoting

Drug Utilization Research: Methods and Applications, First Edition. Edited by M. Elseviers et al.
Published 2016 by John Wiley & Sons, Ltd.

quality use of medicines has also been emphasized, with responsibilities going beyond rational drug dispensing to involving, for example, long-term supervision, patient education activities, consideration of patient needs and of medication-related issues (e.g. drug interactions) and optimization of medicinal treatment and adherence [8]. Other examples of pharmacy services include pharmacist-led information technology intervention for medication errors [9] and safety alerts in electronic patient medication record systems at the point of pharmacy order entry [10]. The patient perspective has been less discussed, but rational drug consumption from a patient perspective may include aspects of adherence to medication, concordance/shared decision-making and a team-based approach to promoting rational use of drugs among patients [11–14].

Assessment of the quality use of medicines requires valid and reliable indicators. A range of performance, quality and safety indicators has therefore been introduced and is increasingly being used [15–17]. The quality of prescribing has been measured for many years by other names, including 'measures of rational prescribing' [18], 'standards of prescribing performance' [19], 'indicators of appropriateness' [20], 'indicators of quality or cost minimization' [21], 'desired responses' [22] and 'quality markers' [23].

Quality indicators are important tools in improving quality of care [24]. However, they should not be used in isolation, but as part of quality improvement initiatives such as continuous professional education, benchmarking and disease management programmes [4,21,25–28]. During the last decade, quality indicators have been increasingly linked to payment, accreditation and financial incentives aimed at regulating providers of care, ensuring accountability, promoting quality improvement, stimulating cost-effectiveness and encouraging cost control [29–31]. Since drug prescribing is one of the most important processes in health care, quality indicators for medicines need to be included in these initiatives. Consequently, skills in quality indicator theory and practice are important for those involved in drug utilization research. The aim of this chapter is to describe the terminology and theories underlying the development and validation of prescribing quality indicators. The conceptual framework needed to delineate quality aspects that can be assessed using prescribing indicators, including some examples and practical applications, is described in Chapter 43. In this methodology chapter, we focus on medicines prescribed in primary care, but the theories and concepts are also applicable to medicines used in the hospital setting or as part of long-term care, as well as to over-the-counter (OTC) medications, herbals, natural health products, vitamins and minerals and nutraceuticals.

Definition of a quality indicator

The original definition of a health care quality indicator was proposed by Lawrence and Olesen in 1997 as 'a measurable element of practice performance for which there is evidence or consensus that it can be used to assess the quality, and hence change in the quality, of care provided' [32]. This was further developed in the more specific definition of a prescribing quality indicator proposed by the European Drug Utilisation Research Group (EuroDURG): 'A measurable element of prescribing performance for which there is evidence or consensus that it can be used to assess quality, and hence in changing the quality of care provided' [15,33]. Thus, a quality indicator needs to be measurable, and there should be evidence or consensus that it can be used to assess quality. Consequently, it is important to emphasize that all indicators are not quality indicators. Performance indicators, for example, can be defined as 'statistical devices for monitoring performance without any necessary inference about quality' [24]. Other terms, such as 'activity indicators', 'comparators', 'markers' and 'ratios', are also used for statistical parameters that enable comparisons between health care units but do not have any inherent association with quality. Some have argued that it is relevant to distinguish between a 'quality indicator' and a 'performance or quality measure' [24,34]. While a quality indicator specifies particular cases for which a defined process should (or should not) be performed, a performance measure translates this into a definition of a numerator and a denominator.

Dimensions and classifications

Improving a health system requires simultaneous pursuit of three different aims [35]:

- improving the population health;
- improving the experience of care;
- reducing the per capita costs of health care.

These three aims have become the goal of many health care organizations, employers and communities around the world. In the United States, the Institute for Healthcare Improvement (IHI) has developed a population health framework for the monitoring of these aims [36]. This framework focuses on the causal pathways among the determinants and outcomes of health. It includes social and physical environmental factors, individual factors such as behaviours and physiology, intermediate outcomes of disease burden and injury, outcomes of health/functional status, mortality and well-being. The experience-of-care framework is based on the six aims for health care formulated by the Institute of Medicine: health care should be safe, effective, patient-centred, timely, equitable, and efficient [37]. Indicators for measuring cost include multiple perspectives, such as supply (health care providers), intermediary (health plans and insurers) and demand (consumers, public and private payers and the overall community).

Structure, process and outcomes indicators

Quality indicators can be classified within the dimensions just mentioned or under other dimensions of quality, such as access and effectiveness (i.e. whether patients get the care they need and whether the care is effective when they get it) [38]. Within effectiveness, two key components may be defined: effectiveness of clinical care and effectiveness of interpersonal care. The latter may be described as the interaction of health care professionals and users, so it includes the social and psychological aspects of the consultation. Indicators can also be placed within the structure–process–outcome model advocated by Donabedian [39,40]. The structure comprises the organizational factors that define the health system under which care is provided (e.g. staff, competence and equipment, but also regulation and contracting), while the process is the interaction between users and the health care structure (i.e. what is done – the care provided) and the outcome is the consequences. Outcome may be influenced by both structures and processes (e.g. a patient may die if there are no physicians with appropriate skills available (structure) or if the patient was prescribed an inappropriate drug (process)). Drug prescribing is a health care process and therefore most quality indicators of prescribing are process-oriented. However, outcome indicators are important, as improvement in patient health (outcome) is the aim of drug prescribing. Some examples of dimensions of quality within the structure–process–outcome model of relevance to drug utilization studies are shown in Table 12.1. The triad of structure, process and outcome was designed as an 'approach to the acquisition of information about the presence or absence of the attributes that constitute or define quality' [39]. In essence, it facilitates the measurement of quality.

The relationship between process and outcome may not always be very clear. It has been proposed therefore that if process indicators are to be credible, it must be demonstrated that variations in the attributes they measure lead to differences in outcome [41,42]. Correspondingly, if outcome indicators are to be credible, it must be demonstrated that differences in outcome will result if the processes of care under the control of health care professionals are altered [41,42]. This may be a specific challenge when deriving indicators for rational drug therapy, given the discrepancy between the efficacy demonstrated in clinical trials and the effectiveness of drug therapy in real-life settings [43]. In practice, a combination of process and outcome indicators is required for a balanced assessment of quality. However, while process indicators may have only nominal meaning to patients unless a link to outcomes can be shown, attributing process to outcome is problematic given the many factors outside the control of the prescriber/practitioner/provider and in the context of patients in receipt of multiple interventions and with multiple morbidities. Prescribing data are based on population-level measures that provide values for 'average' rather than individual patients [21,44,45], but there is no such thing as an average patient, so unspecific indicators must be complemented by more specific prescribing indicators [46,47]. Moreover, it is important to emphasize that while prescribing quality indicators are tools for assessing quality, the preferences for specific types of indicator may differ between stakeholders [48].

Drug-, disease- and patient-oriented indicators

Quality indicators for drug utilization may also be classified based on the amount of clinical information they incorporate [15,33]. This can be illustrated by the step model presented in Figure 12.1. Higher steps indicate an increasing level of complexity in the clinical information, but may also indicate increasing credibility to health care professionals or an increasing feasibility of demonstrating that the indicator is a quality indicator and not simply a performance indicator. Indicators may complement one another. As an example, simple drug-oriented indicators can be used to screen for potential

Table 12.1 Dimensions of quality applicable to drug utilization studies.

Domain	Dimension	Areas where quality indicators could be developed
Structures		
Physical characteristics	Resources	Financial, personnel, buildings, equipment, availability of information (e.g. a drug formulary or interaction database), clinical data and registries
	Organization of resources	Provider continuity, hours of operation, organization of prescribing and supply of medicines
	Management	Administration, operational and strategic management to support rational drug prescribing (e.g. drug and therapeutics committees)
Workforce characteristics	Skill mix	Skills/knowledge of staff
	Teamwork	Team functioning: delegation, role in promoting quality of medicines use
Systems characteristics[a]	Engineering activities	Organizational or managerial interventions, such as prescribing targets and price–volume agreements
	Educational activities	Extent and nature of prescribing guidance. These may range from simple distribution of printed material to more intensive strategies such as educational outreach visits by trained facilitators
	Economic interventions	Insurance and reimbursement systems, patient copayment (including tier levels), positive and negative financial incentives and physician budgets
	Enforcement	Regulations by law, such as generic substitution at pharmacies or prescribing restrictions for physicians
Processes		
Clinical care • acute • chronic • preventive		History-taking, including medication history, relevant measures taken (e.g. lab test) when initiating drug treatment, appropriate drug prescribing, medicines reconciliation
Interpersonal aspects of care		Communication with patients: information exchange and motivational interviewing, patient adherence and persistence
Outcomes		
Health status	Freedom from disease, comfort, longevity	Functional status, symptom relief, quality-adjusted life years. May include both positive and negative effects of the drug therapy, including hospitalizations and adverse events
User evaluation	HRQOL	Satisfaction, communication, self-esteem
Systems	Efficiency, efficacy and equity	May include patient outcome at a population level, but also the outcomes of interventions to promote rational use of drugs

[a]Activities to promote quality of prescribing. These have been categorized using the four Es: education, engineering, economics and enforcement [4].

areas of improvement, which can be further studied in depth using more sophisticated disease- or patient-oriented indicators.

Aggregate data on the volume and expenditure of prescribed or dispensed drugs are useful for physicians and other health care professionals in promoting quality use of medicines. Such data could, for example, be presented as time trends or top-ten lists and used as a catalyst to stimulate discussion and cognitive dissonance around drug therapies and to raise questions around potential areas for improvement. The aggregated data could also be used to construct simple drug-oriented indicators by which to compare practices, clinics or regions. Such drug-oriented indicators are based on drug prescribing/dispensing data alone and can be used irrespective of the indication for which the drug is prescribed. Access to patient-level data enables construction of more clinically relevant drug-oriented indicators linking different drugs to one another or over time.

Disease-oriented indicators include information on drugs linked to the diagnosis or health problem. They may indicate either to what extent patients are being

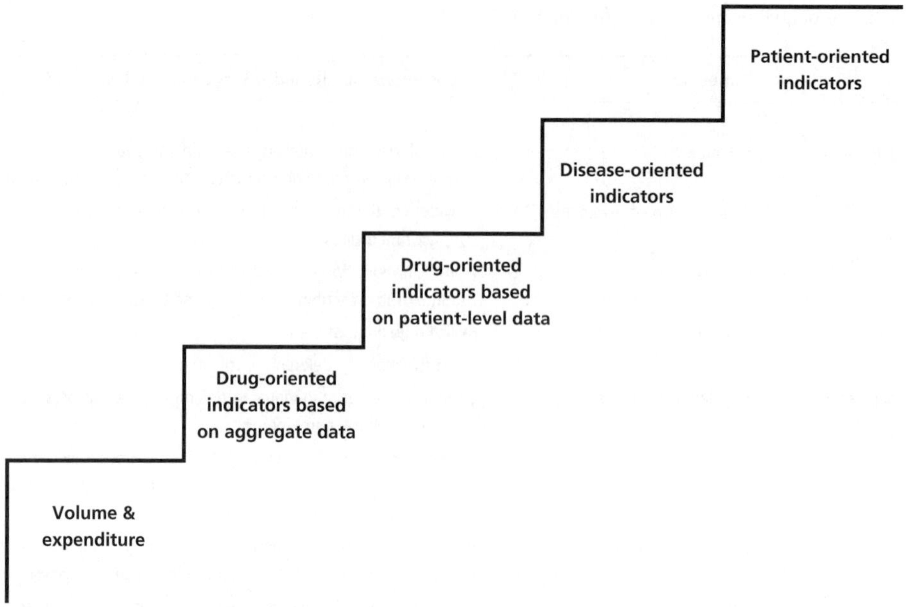

Figure 12.1 A proposal for a theoretical model to describe different types of quality assessment and quality indicators of drug prescribing.

treated with the recommended drugs for a certain condition or to what extent drugs are avoided in patients with conditions for which they should not be used.

Patient-oriented indicators include information on drugs linked to individual clinical patient characteristics, such as the severity of a disease and whether a certain treatment is suitable for a specific patient. Some examples of drug- and disease-oriented prescribing quality indicators are described in the sections that follow.

Data sources

Quality indicators should preferably be independent of subjective judgment, since it is known that this produces gross overestimations of adherence to guidelines [49]. Consequently, it is favourable if the indicators can be derived from routinely available data. A common problem, however, is that the more clinically relevant indicators are, the less they can be used with data available in routine care [15,50,51]. Data on drug prescribing are often only available in a structured form in administrative databases, designed for other purposes than the evaluation of quality or provision of feedback. These databases can seldom be used to derive valid patient- or disease-oriented indicators. However, during the last decade, the rapid development of electronic medical records and registries that provide opportunity for record-linkage, using the unique identifier of each patient, has facilitated the creation of disease-based quality indicators independent of subjective judgment. Still, it is important to emphasize the need for validation, since such readily available data may have large bias in the recording of diagnoses and may suffer from variations in quality [52].

There are specific challenges in getting access to data that allow comparison of quality across health care systems. The Organisation for Economic Co-operation and Development (OECD) and the WHO regularly publish data on different aspects of the performance of health systems in different countries [53,54]. Initiatives have also been taken from the consumer perspective to rank healthcare systems and the Euro Health Consumer Index produces an annual report with indicators grouped into five categories including pharmaceuticals. [55]. However, there are many methodological challenges inherent in these comparisons, and studies have shown that indicators cannot be transferred directly between countries without taking an intermediate step to account for variation in professional culture and clinical practice [56]. A review showed that quality indicator research conducted today varies substantially between countries and that further progress is partly hampered by data availability [57]. Issues to be addressed include the use of unique patient identifiers to facilitate linkages between separate databases, standardized measurement of the experiences of patients and others and deepening collaboration between key agencies, such as Eurostat, the WHO, the Healthcare Effectiveness Data and Information Set (HEDIS), the Agency for Healthcare Research and Quality (AHRQ) and the OECD, to facilitate the availability of internationally comparable performance information.

Drug-oriented prescribing quality indicators

Aggregate data

The simplest indicators focus on drug expenditure or volume, e.g. defined daily dose (DDD)/1000 inhabitants daily in ambulatory care and DDD/100 bed days in the hospital setting. Even though most of these indicators are not that closely related to quality, they are important in drug utilization studies as they form the basis for more in-depth analyses. In some cases, time trends in expenditure or volumes can be used to identify areas for quality improvement. For further information on aggregate measures of drug utilization, see Chapter 6.

Several drug-oriented indicators that do not require patient-level data have been developed and are commonly used (e.g. in feedback to physicians or in incentive programmes using claims or dispensing data) [43,58–62]. A common indicator is the ratio between recommended/not recommended drugs. It is easily constructed using aggregate data, placing the volume of the recommended drug (measured in DDDs or prescriptions) as the numerator and the volume of the pharmacological group it belongs to (including the not-recommended drugs) as the denominator (Figure 12.2). Such indicators have often been used to promote the use of cost-effective generic substances versus patent-protected me-too drugs. Some examples include the ratio

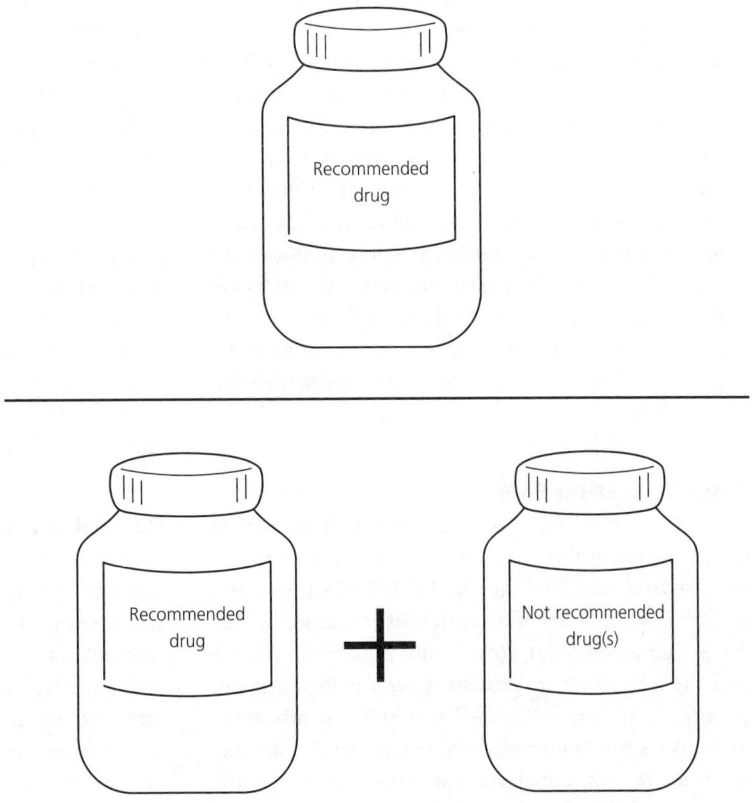

Figure 12.2 Illustration of an indicator constructed as a ratio between a recommended drug and its corresponding treatment alternatives.

Table 12.2 Drug-oriented quality indicators that do not require individual-level data.

Category	Quality indicator	Ref.
Drugs of limited clinical value	Use of peripheral vasodilators	Avorn & Soumerai 1983 [65]
Drugs to be avoided	Long-acting benzodiazepines in the elderly[a]	Beers 1997 [66]
	Off-label prescribing to children[a]	Carnovale et al. 2013 [67]
Ratios between drugs	Ratio of cox-2inhibitors to all nonsteroidal antiinflammatory drugs (NSAIDs), measured in DDDs	Muijrers et al. 2004 [61]
	Ratio of simvastatin to statins	Godman et al. 2010 [63]
	Ratio of angiotensin-converting enzyme (ACE)-inhibitors to all renin-angiotensin drugs	Fernández Urrusuno et al. 2013 [62]
Range of drugs	Range of NSAIDs prescribed	Avery et al. 1996 [68]
Global adherence[b]	Global adherence to guidelines	Kamps et al. 2000 [69]
Patient safety	Prescribing safety indicators	Avery et al. 2011 [16]
	Indicators of preventable drug-related morbidity	Mackinnon & Hepler 2002 [70]

[a]These indicators require information on the age of the patient, but can be measured with aggregate data as the number of DDDs/1000 inhabitants dispensed to a certain age group.

[b]The proportion of drugs prescribed according to guidelines, regardless of whether they are prescribed to the right patients (in contrast to specific adherence, which is the proportion of patients with a certain disease/diagnosis who receive the appropriate drugs).

of simvastatin to statins and the ratio of omeprazole to proton pump inhibitors (PPIs) [63]. It is important to note that these indicators, based on current prescribing recommendations and/or drug costs, may be highly specific to the health care setting, country and time.

Other indicators that may be constructed with aggregate drug data include the prescribed/dispensed volume of drugs of limited clinical value (inadequate evidence-based documentation or safety profiles), the range of drugs and the global adherence to guidelines (Table 12.2). Properly used, these indicators can be used as screening devices to reveal important areas for improvement, but they may also have substantial limitations [64].

Drug utilization 90%

A simple method for assessing the overall quality of drug prescribing using aggregate data is the drug utilization 90% (DU 90%) method [71–73]. DU90% is a further development of a top-ten list focusing on the drugs that account for 90% of the prescribed volume and the adherence to guidelines within this segment (Figure 12.3). The 90% level was selected arbitrarily to focus on the majority of prescribing while allowing some leeway for individual variation. The remaining 10% might include drugs used for rare conditions, to treat patients with drug intolerances/adverse events or complex comorbidity and/or therapy initiated by other physicians than those assessed.

The rationale behind using number of drugs (constituting 90%) as a quality measure is the assumption that high-quality prescribing is associated with the use of a relatively limited number of evidence-based documented drugs. Standards for comparison might be evidence-based guidelines, meta-analyses or local formularies. The DU90% method can be applied for all drugs or for drugs within a selected therapeutic area. It can be used for international comparisons of drug utilization and in feedback to prescribers, as a way of implementing guidelines [28,74–76].

Patient-level data

Access to data at the individual patient level allows for analysis of drugs that are linked to one another and of drug use over time. These indicators can focus on important quality issues such as duplication, drug–drug interactions, polypharmacy, in what order therapy is initiated and patient compliance/persistence. Some examples are presented in Table 12.3. Patient-level data may also be used to analyse coprescriptions with other drugs as

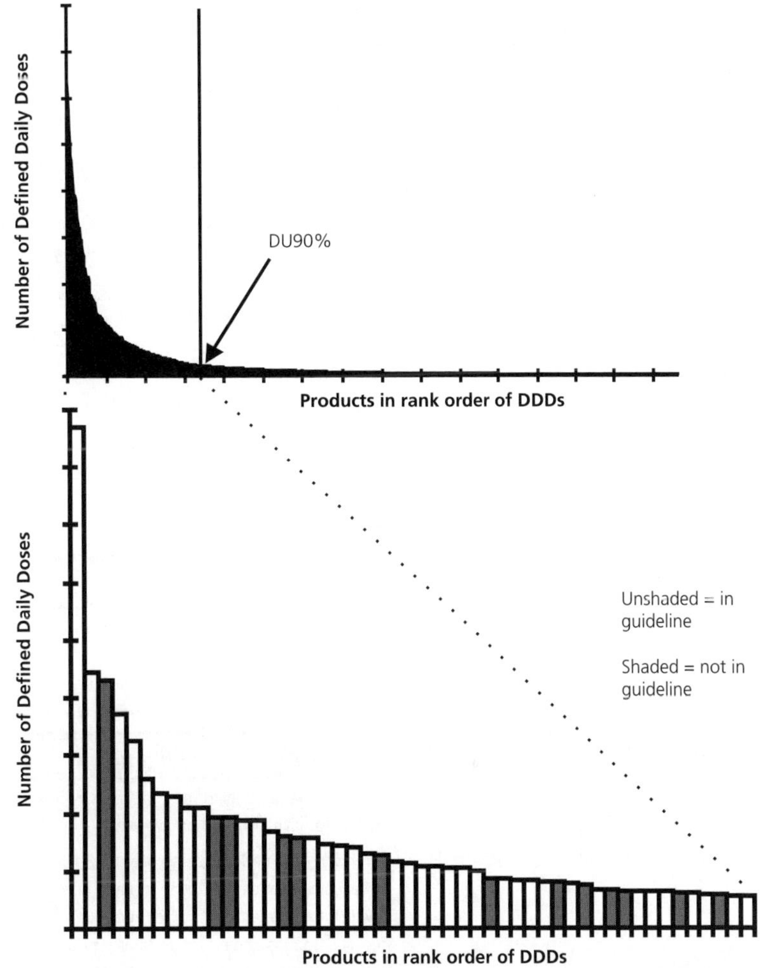

Figure 12.3 Drug utilization 90% (DU90%) method. (a) Number of drugs (products or substances) ranked by volume of DDDs. The arrow indicates the number of drugs accounting for 90% of the DDDs. (b) The DU90% segment enlarged, indicating drugs listed (unshaded) and not listed (shaded) in guidelines. For colour details, please refer to the colour plates section.

Source: Bergman et al. 1998 [71]. Reproduced with permission from Springer Science and Business Media.

markers for risk factors or diseases [77]. Furthermore, these data may be used to estimate the prevalence and incidence of drug use, in order to assess over- or underuse in relation to disease patterns. For further information on patient-level data analyses, see Chapter 7.

Disease-oriented prescribing quality indicators

Disease-oriented indicators include information on drugs linked to the diagnosis or health status of a patient. A large number of such indicators are used jointly with other indicators in assessing the quality of care for different diseases [87]. These indicators may be derived from medical-records data or through record linkage between diagnosis and drug data. There are also examples of disease-oriented indicators that utilize a prescribed drug as a proxy for the disease. Some examples of disease-oriented indicators are presented in Table 12.4.

Disease-oriented indicators may be further developed by integrating other clinical data. For example, if a patient with diabetes is also treated for hypertension and has proteinuria, an ACE inhibitor should be preferred. The prescription of an ACE inhibitor can then be further linked to a second indicator, so that a patient receiving an ACE inhibitor should have their creatinine and potassium measured within 1 month of starting treatment [94].

Disease-oriented prescribing quality indicators have been used for many years in quality-improvement

Table 12.3 Drug-oriented quality indicators that require individual-level data.

Category	Quality indicator	Ref.
Coprescribing	Use of inhaled corticosteroids in heavy users of inhaled β-adrenoceptor agonists	Gaist et al. 1996 [78]
	Coprescribing of β-adrenoreceptor antagonists and agonists	Arnlind et al. 2010 [79]
Sequential therapy	Proportion of patients initiated on angiotensin II receptor blockers (ARBs) who were previously dispensed ACE inhibitors	Frisk et al. 2008 [80]
Duplication/polypharmacy	Use of more than one drug from the same drug class	van Dijk et al. 2003 [81]
Drug interactions	Interacting drugs (questionable combinations) prescribed to individual patients	Linnarsson 1993 [82]
Prescribed daily dose	Deviations from recommended doses	Van Dijk et al. 2003 [81]
Overuse and misuse	Heavy users of sumatriptan	Gaist et al. 1998 [83]
	High annual consumption of short-acting β-agonists in asthma	Davidsen et al. 2011 [84]
Adherence/persistence	Proportion of days covered by statins	Yeaw et al. 2009 [85]
	Proportion of patients discontinuing treatment with antihypertensives	Qvarnström et al. 2013 [86]

Table 12.4 Drug-oriented quality indicators that require individual-level data.

Disease	Quality indicator	Ref.
Arthritis	Use of NSAIDs for arthritis in patients >65 years old who have not tried paracetamol	Dreischulte et al. 2012 [88]
Asthma	Proportion of patients using over 0.25 DDDs of inhaled bronchodilators per day on average without antiinflammatory treatment (inhaled corticosteroids and cromoglycates), among all patients receiving inhaled bronchodilators	Veninga et al. 2001 [87]
Atrial fibrillation	Proportion of patients with atrial fibrillation receiving anticoagulants	Cheng et al. 2007 [89]
Depression	Proportion of patients >18 years old diagnosed with a new episode of depression who are treated with antidepressant medication for at least 180 days	Hermann et al. 2004 [90]
Diabetes	Proportion of patients dispensed an oral antidiabetic agent also dispensed a statin	Strøm et al. 2008 [91]
Ischaemic heart disease	Proportion of myocardial infarction patients prescribed a statin for secondary prevention	Ashworth et al. 2002 [92]
Respiratory tract infections (RTIs)	Percentage of patients aged between 18 and 75 with acute bronchitis/bronchiolitis prescribed antibacterials for systemic use	Adriaenssens et al. 2011 [93]
Urinary tract infections (UTIs)	Percentage of female patients >18 years old with cystitis/other urinary infection prescribed antibacterials who receive the recommended drugs (ATC: J01XE or J01EA or J01XX)	Adriaenssens et al. 2011 [93]

initiatives in primary care [92,95]. The development of electronic medical records has facilitated the integration of these indicators into systematic quality-improvement initiatives [96].

Other types of indicator

Cross-sectional and sequential indicators

Studies that employ a cross-sectional approach use measures of processes and/or outcomes of care at a single point in time. These may be supplemented by successive cross-sectional measurement at several 'single' points of time (e.g. annually) and by analyses as part of a time-series design. However, the cross-sectional sample at each point will not normally contain the same participants. The value of cross-sectional indicators is that they enable assessment of data against set parameters; for example, high-risk prescribing has been found to be more common in patients prescribed long-term drugs [97], and correlations have been found between prescribing quality and pharmaceutical expenditure [98]. Sequential indicators embed the longitudinal nature of the measurement of care; for example, they are valuable in estimating the quality of risk factor management and may provide a more accurate and fair judgment than cross-sectional indicators [99].

Indicator sets and combinations of indicators

A single indicator is seldom enough to serve as a basis for decision-making. Consequently, many stakeholders develop indicator sets with a defined number of validated indicators. Such indicator sets can focus on various aspects of drug therapy (e.g. by combining drug-oriented and disease-oriented indicators), but they can also integrate drug therapy with other aspects of care. A critical first step in defining a set of indicators is to identify the target audience and the purpose of the set. Attention should also be given to the processes of indicator development, addressing the following questions:

- Who will be responsible for the final selection and publication of the indicators?
- How will the relevant stakeholders be involved?
- Will an expert panel of specialists be established to provide guidance?
- Will public consultation be undertaken?
- How will the indicators be revised and kept up to date over time?

Indicators can also be combined to provide a better degree of knowledge, such as by plotting two indicators against each other to form a paired indicator (Figure 12.4).

A composite indicator is created when individual indicators are averaged together and compiled into a single index. The individual indicators must share an underly-

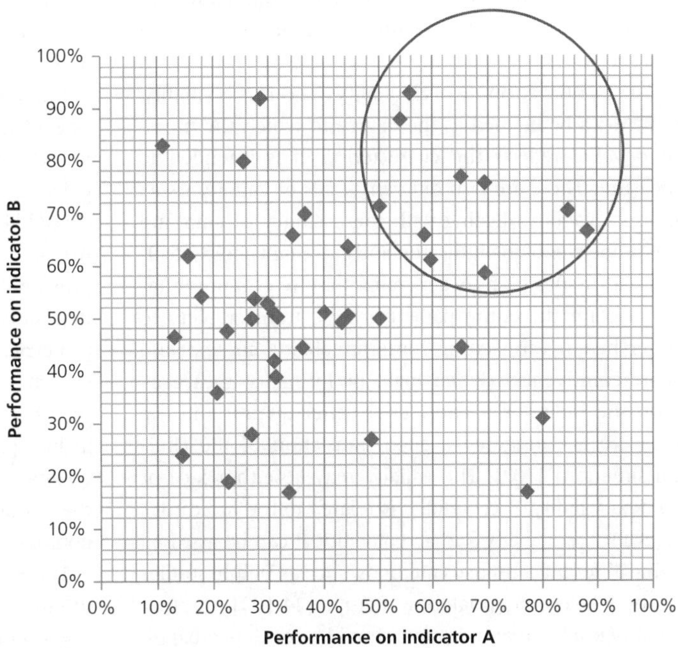

Figure 12.4 Example of paired indicators used to identify 'best practice'. The circle shows those practices scoring well on both indicators.

ing model or concept that is under measurement. The added value of a composite score depends on the *a priori* reasons for the measurement [100]. There are various ways of computing and measuring the same set of individual indicators, such as the 'all-or-none', the '70% standard', the 'overall percentage', the 'indicator average' and the 'patient average' [101]. The all-or-none and 70% standard are criterion-referenced methods that assess the degree to which a threshold for quality of care for each patient has been reached (100 or 70%). The threshold (%) can be set to any level required, but this must be *a priori* rather than following measurement. The remaining absolute methods produce scores representing the proportion of required care that has been successfully provided. Fundamentally, different methods of computing composite quality scores can lead to different outcomes concerning both relative and absolute quality among health care providers. Moreover, different methods are suited for different types of application [101].

Development and validation of prescribing quality indicators

Prescribing quality indicators should be developed using systematic methods, such as by taking evidence from randomized controlled trials (RCTs) and high-quality observational studies, following clinical guidelines or combining the available scientific evidence with expert opinion [24].

An essential attribute of all quality indicators is validity, which can be defined as the degree to which the measured value reflects the characteristic it is intended to measure. There are two different kinds of validity issue: internal validity, dealing with the accuracy of data and the properties of the indicator, and external validity, dealing with issues such as generalizability (e.g. representativeness for the entire patient group), transferability to other health care settings, interpretability, context and representativeness (when high, performance measured with the indicator is considered better quality and the measure is considered a good translation of the clinical situation) [102]. The validity may be either face or context validity. Face validity is related to the indicator's relevance, credibility and acceptability. It can be assessed using different consensus methods, such as Delphi studies or the RAND appropriateness method [24,103]. Content validity implies that indicators should be evidence-based, in accordance with updated recommendations and current guidelines, which in turn are based on the latest available results of meta-analyses, RCTs and high-quality observational studies. For some indicators, it is desirable to compare them to a gold-standard assessment of quality (concurrent validity). This should be widely accepted as the best available reference assessment, and it may be established by assessing detailed clinical data [104].

When quality is measured at the individual patient level, indicators can be evaluated using the same framework as is used for a diagnostic test, comparing the indicator's assessment of suboptimal treatment to that of the reference. An indicator of suboptimal treatment can thus be characterized by its sensitivity (the proportion of cases of suboptimal treatment found using the reference assessment, also identified by the indicator) and positive predictive value (PPV; the proportion of suboptimally treated cases identified by the indicator that are confirmed by the reference assessment). Ideally, both values should be high, but a high sensitivity is particularly important in screening and identifying individual patients with potential quality problems. For monitoring of changes, the PPV may be relatively more important than the sensitivity [15]. If a reference quality assessment is difficult to obtain, a comparison of several indicators can instead provide indirect information on their validity. To examine the concurrent validity of aggregate indicators at the practical level, correlation analysis can be used [87,105], and factor analysis may be informative concerning which indicators should be chosen among a larger candidate set [106].

Indicators that are developed using clinical guidelines or evidence from RCTs or high-quality observational studies have high face validity, while those based on rigorous evidence possess high content validity. However, these should be a minimum prerequisite for any quality measure, and subsequent developmental work is required to provide empirical evidence for a set of attributes of good indicators within a formal testing protocol [24,44]. Such a protocol should also ensure that those health care providers who will be assessed by the indicators are involved in their development. The assessment should preferably also include patients, since they play a crucial role in measuring quality. An example of a testing protocol, exemplified for the development of indicators for the managed introduction of new medicines, is presented in Box 12.1.

The purpose of using an indicator testing protocol is to ensure that valid indicators are developed. The testing protocol should also address implementation issues,

Box 12.1 Testing protocol for the development of indicators for the managed introduction of new medicines.

Necessity

- The therapeutic arena has been analysed, in terms of current challenges, existing therapeutic recommendations, unmet needs and the possibility that the new drug will address these needs.
- Current indicators and their applicability for the new drug have been assessed.
- Each indicator is underpinned by a published evidence base related to need (e.g. evidence of better efficacy, feasibility, safety or cost-effectiveness than the existing drug).
- Economic modelling has been undertaken.

Clarity

- The indicator's wording is clear and precise, with unambiguous language that reflects a specific domain of quality.
- The indicator is within the control of the prescriber/provider that will be assessed.

Content validity

- The indicator represents high-quality care. There is sufficient evidence/professional consensus to support it and it shows clear benefits to the patient receiving the care (or the benefits significantly outweigh the risks).
- Each indicator is underpinned by a published evidence base (e.g. a guideline or a well-conducted clinical trial).
- Adherence to the indicator is based on physicians/staff adhering to it providing a higher quality of care/service than those who do not.
- The indicator shows likely patient benefit.

Technical feasibility and the reliability of data extraction/data availability

- It is possible to write and integrate data extraction specifications from all relevant providers into health information systems.
- It is possible to generate reproducible test reports from all relevant providers within a reasonable time frame and budget.

Acceptability

- The testing protocol has been evaluated.
- The indicator aligns with the health care system and societal values.
- The indicator aligns with patient values.
- The indicator aligns with professional values.

Implementation

- The indicator discriminates between providers.
- The indicator's current baseline and its potential baseline at the end of a piloting period have been assessed.
- Clinical staff are able to interpret the indicator.
- Potential for gaming/manipulation is limited.
- Changes required to implement the indicator have been assessed (i.e. acquisition and/or modification of IT, changes in physical capital/staffing, changes to regulation, policies and education).
- The workload implications of implementing the indicator have been evaluated.
- Potential barriers among different stakeholders to the implementation of the indicators have been discussed.
- Unintended consequences of implementation have been considered, whether positive or negative in nature (e.g. disruption to clinical or organizational workflow, 'spillovers' such as diversion of effort (negative) or general quality improvement (positive)).

Source: Campbell et al. 2015 [107]. Reproduced with permission from John Wiley and Sons.

such as the ability of the indicators to discriminate between providers, the changes required to implement the indicators, potential barriers among stakeholders to implementation and unintended consequences of implementation [44,107].

Finally, the benefit for patients of using indicators depends on their impact on patient outcomes when implemented in actual practice [108]. Indicators that are content-valid can be used on the assumption that higher performance is likely to result in patient benefit. Evidence supporting this assumption is scarce, however [109,110].

Conclusion

Prescribing quality indicators are important tools for improving the use of medicines. A range of different types of indicators can be derived from medical records, claims databases, dispensing registries and patient-reported data. Four aspects should be considered when assessing quality of care using prescribing indicators. First, indicators should be tested for their validity, reliability, acceptability, unintended consequences, feasibility, sensitivity to change and how communicable and understandable they are. Second, indicators should not be used in isolation, but as part of more comprehensive quality improvement initiatives. Third, indicators should be flexible, in order to minimize measure fixation and ossification. Fourth, and most importantly, patients as individuals play a crucial role in measuring quality and should be involved in the assessment process.

CHAPTER 13

Qualitative methods in drug utilization research

Anna Birna Almarsdóttir[1] & Pia Bastholm Rahmner[2]

[1]Clinical Pharmacology, Department of Public Health, University of Southern Denmark, Denmark

[2]Medical Management Centre, Department of Learning, Informatics, Management and Ethics, Karolinska Institutet, Sweden

KEY POINTS

- Qualitative research methods derive from the social sciences. Their use in drug utilization research is increasingly widespread, especially in understanding patient and prescriber perspectives.
- The main focus in qualitative research is exploration of a given phenomenon in order to get a wider understanding of why and how it appears.
- Qualitative research methods build on various theoretical underpinnings/schools of thought.
- The same validity and quality criteria cannot be used for both qualitative and quantitative methods.

Reasons for using qualitative methods in drug utilization research

Most health care research is biomedical in nature, but since the 1980s there has been an increasing awareness within the field that the social sciences can fill an important gap in understanding and evaluating health systems. The use of qualitative methods came about when it was recognized that patient and prescriber behaviours and perspectives were important in improving the use of medicines.

This understanding of the utility of qualitative methods is illustrated by a series of articles published in the *BMJ* between 1993 and 2000 introducing its readership to qualitative methodology, which indicated a turn towards a less dogmatic approach to health care research [1–6]. This was also apparent in drug utilization research, which increasingly became a cross-disciplinary field involving medical, pharmaceutical and various social sciences.

The chapters in this book have so far mainly focused on research methods that can be labelled as quantitative. The definition of drug utilization research outlined in Chapter 1 provides the background for the need for various research methods. Quantitative methods can be used for describing, understanding, evaluating and intervening in medicines use. In this chapter, we turn our attention to an often less understood realm of drug utilization research methods: those labelled as qualitative. The chapter necessarily cannot cover all these methods, but seeks first to provide an insight into their role within drug utilization research and the types of research questions that it would be important to answer using qualitative methods, and second to briefly review the most common types of data collection. Finally, it contrasts sampling, analysis and validity concepts between qualitative and quantitative research methods.

The WHO's *Introduction to Drug Utilization Research* states that 'The ultimate goal of drug utilization research must be to assess whether drug therapy is rational or not' [7]. From the perspective of qualitative research, this evokes such thoughts and reflections as: What is *rational*, and in whose eyes is it rational? That is, is

Drug Utilization Research: Methods and Applications, First Edition. Edited by M. Elseviers et al.
Published 2016 by John Wiley & Sons, Ltd.

the definition of 'rational' the same for the prescriber of drugs as for the patient or the pharmacist? Would paediatricians describe rational drug therapy differently from geriatricians? Even understanding of the concept of 'drugs' or 'medicines' is far from being uniform among lay persons [8]. Further arguments can be seen in Chapter 33, where the authors state that understanding the patient perspective is a necessary challenge for drug utilization research. They argue that researching the patient perspective may necessitate employing qualitative methods and including researchers from other disciplines, who bring with them experience in studying the patient perspective and a wealth of expertise in theories and methods not often used in current drug utilization research. Similar arguments may be employed regarding the rationale of prescribers in their decisions about medicines.

The role of qualitative research methods in drug utilization research

In drug utilization research, it is often necessary to describe situations, understand peoples' rationales and design and implement interventions aimed at improving utilization. In qualitative research, this means collecting data in direct interaction with people, either on a one-to-one basis or in a group. The main methods of data collection are individual interviews, group discussions and observation.

Research using qualitative methods is aimed at answering questions that typically start with a 'why'. As an example, drug utilization researchers have a long-held interest in understanding why patients do not use their medicines according to schedule: Is it because they forget? Is their understanding or are their beliefs concerning medicines preventing adherence? Another example is why physicians sometimes make seemingly non-evidence-based prescribing decisions. Are they not keeping up to date? Do they consider other aspects than the evidence base? Or are there other, more complex answers to both these questions? Qualitative methods have gained in acceptance within drug utilization research due to their ability to address these multifaceted 'why' questions.

Although the term ***description*** (or ***describing***) is often used in reference to qualitative methods in drug utilization research, the main focus and purpose of these methods is to ***understand***. Therefore, the act of describing in these types of study is an attempt to go beyond surface knowledge about a phenomenon and delve deeper into rationales and interrelationships between explanatory factors. Qualitative methodology thus has goals more commonly seen in analytic drug utilization research, whereas descriptive methodologies within the quantitative realm focus on generating hypotheses based on patterns found in descriptive data analysis (see Chapter 2). Conversely, qualitative methodology springs from a tradition that is focused on broadly and deeply exploring, whereas analytic quantitative methodologies aim at evaluating interventions or testing very specific hypotheses.

Qualitative research data often take the form of an individual's written or spoken words, which are interpreted by the researcher either to form a theory or in relation to an established theory. Table 13.1 provides a few examples of drug utilization studies that use qualitative methods: their research questions, samples, settings and theoretical frameworks (if used). Further discussion about the role of theory is covered in other, more comprehensive works [9,10]. Drug utilization research's theoretical frameworks can originate in a number of ways: they usually stem from theories within sociology about topics such as health and illness, organizations, professions and socialization, but they can also come from other social sciences, such as medical anthropology, social psychology, education, business and political science. Examples in Table 13.1 include Noerreslet et al. [11], who used theories of consumerism in the design and analysis of their study, and Kardakis et al. [12], who employed diffusion of innovation to identify and explore determinants that supported or challenged the development and sustainability of the Pharmacotherapy Centre (established to increase rational use of medicines in Stockholm county).

Some drug utilization researchers use grounded theory [13], which is a gradual development of analytical concepts from unstructured qualitative data with the goal of formulating hypotheses. The researcher focuses on incidents (e.g. a decision to use a medicine) and how they are dealt with, instead of on the more common subject of people. Examples in Table 13.1 include Deschepper et al. [14], who sought to understand the different consumption levels of antibiotics between Flanders and the Netherlands, and Björnsdóttir et al. [15], who were interested in seeing what evidence

Table 13.1 Examples of drug utilization research studies using qualitative research designs and methods.

Reference	Research question/ objective	Data collection method(s)	Setting and sample	Theoretical framework (or other framework)
Noerreslet et al. 2009 [11]	To understand active and informed patients' perceptions of medicines and physicians, and how these perceptions fit with the wider trends of society	In-depth interviews with patients or parents of patients with atopic dermatitis	Denmark, specialist clinic in dermatology. 12 adult patients and 12 parents of juvenile patients	Consumerism in health care
Kardakis et al. 2013 [12]	To identify and explore determinants that support or challenge the development and sustainability of the Pharmacotherapy Centre (PTC) in Stockholm	Semi-structured interviews among key informants involved in the establishment of PTC	The regional Board of Health in Stockholm, Sweden. 11 informants held key positions within Stockholm County Council and had varying professional backgrounds	Diffusion of innovations
Deschepper et al. 2002 [14]	To understand how different consumption levels of antibiotics are related to cross-cultural differences in lay perspectives towards disease labelling, initial coping strategies and antibiotics utilization	Semi-structured interviews with 3-month diaries of upper respiratory tract infections	Two neighbouring cities in two adjacent countries (the Netherlands and the Dutch-speaking part of Belgium). 30 informants recruited through three community pharmacies and one child day care centre in each city	Grounded theory
Björnsdóttir & Hansen 2001 [15]	To understand the use of evidence by GPs in the diagnostic process preceding antibiotic prescribing	Observations of doctor–patient communication during consultation and in-depth interviews	Iceland, primary health care practices. Three GP observations and 10 GP interviews to reflect variation in: age, professional experience, gender, practice organization, employment, geographical area, country of specialist training	Grounded theory Observations used to improve semi-structured interview guide and as validity check
Friend-du Preez et al. 2013 [16]	To understand the role of medicines as both a predisposing and an enabling factor in the health-seeking process in urban South Africa	Mixed methods, including a survey, focus groups and semi-structured interviews	Soweto, Johannesburg, South Africa. Recruiting for the focus groups was through the Birth of Twenty (Bt20) cohort. The interviewees were representatives of Western health care and of traditional healing, as well as mothers of children	Background empirical knowledge of the South African health care environment
Chen et al. 2014 [17]	To understand the perceptions, attitudes and concerns that might influence adherence to imatinib treatment among patients with chronic myeloid leukaemia (CML)	Semi-structured interviews	CML patients (n = 42) who regularly attended oncology outpatient clinics in a medical centre in southern Taiwan	Background empirical knowledge of chronic patients' adherence patterns and rationales for nonadherence

(continued)

Table 13.1 *(continued)*

Reference	Research question/ objective	Data collection method(s)	Setting and sample	Theoretical framework (or other framework)
Holmström et al. 2014 [18]	To understand how and where adolescents acquire their knowledge and attitudes regarding over-the-counter (OTC) drugs. What perceptions do they have about the use of OTC drugs?	Focus groups (semi-structured)	10 focus groups with upper secondary school students aged 16–19 years in different parts of Sweden	A pragmatic policymaker question prompted this research. The primary question led the thematic analysis
Carter et al. 2012 [23]	To investigate factors that might motivate patients to participate in a collaborative medication management programme	Focus groups (semi-structured)	14 focus groups held throughout Australia, recruited by outpatient pharmacists or at a meeting of the New South Wales Council of the Ageing	Theory of motivated information management
Latif et al. 2013 [24]	To explore the impact and consequences of the English Medicine Use Review (MUR) service on pharmacy support staff	Ethnographic-oriented observations and interviews	Two English community pharmacies. Interviews with 5 pharmacists and 12 members of support staff	The role of pharmacy support staff within the organization of community pharmacy when introducing a new service
Hayward et al. 2013 [25]	To understand how general practitioners interact with prescribing clinical computerized decision support systems	Multichannel video recordings	United Kingdom. 112 primary care consultations in 3 general practices with 8 general practitioners	Impact of technology on interactions between a patient and their health care professional

general practitioners (GPs) in Iceland used in prescribing antibiotics.

Many drug utilization researchers build on existing (often quantitative) research that has uncovered important factors relating to the question of interest. This is exemplified by the work of Friend-du Preez et al. [16], who built on results from previous field studies in South Africa regarding health care utilization, and that of Chen et al. [17], who built on the premise that chronic myeloid leukaemia (CML) was no longer a life-threatening disease and was becoming a chronic disease due to oral treatment with the drug imatinib, which meant that adherence patterns might change.

Another inductive approach, without theoretical underpinnings, is where there is no theory with which to explain a phenomenon convincingly. One example of this type of study was carried out by Holmström et al. [18]; in this case, the authorities had to know rather quickly whether the availability of over-the-counter (OTC) pain relievers could introduce abuse problems in young people.

All these different approaches, theory-driven or not, are inductive and focus on exploring a phenomenon.

Research questions within drug utilization research that require qualitative research methods

As already mentioned, qualitative studies are strong when it comes to answering research questions starting with a 'why'. The studies in Table 13.1 provide some examples of rationales for using qualitative methods in their respective research questions.

Björnsdóttir et al. [15] needed to know why GPs in Iceland prescribed many more antibiotics than their colleagues in the other Nordic countries. Most GPs are trained in Scandinavia, and the illness burden could not account for this difference. The researchers could not construct a survey that could adequately address the issues, as they did not know what issues were of importance in the decisions made by the GPs. Instead, they carried out observations of doctor–patient consultations, and from these constructed an interview guide.

Questioning people about their knowledge cannot really be done quantitatively unless they are tested directly. This approach is not always applicable to patients, however. Using qualitative face-to-face interviews with patients with CML, Chen et al. [17] found that the patients frequently misunderstood the purpose of diagnostic tests and their main drug, imatinib. This in turn adversely influenced their adherence. This research helped tackle inappropriate dosage changes made by patients.

Although the most straightforward explanation of what constitutes qualitative research is that it does not aim to measure, but rather to describe and understand, there are grey areas where qualitative data material can form the basis for quantitative description. A good example is provided by Richard and Lussier [19], who coded audio recordings of 422 medical encounters, focusing on any mention of a drug. Conversely, quantitative description can be a prelude to qualitative research, as seen in the work of Friend-du Preez et al. [16] (Table 13.1). A survey of a cohort in Johannesburg found significant differences between mothers seeking different types of health care for their children with respect to choice of medicine or remedy for diarrhoea, cough, fever and constipation. The qualitative focus groups and interviews shed an important light on how pharmaceuticals obtained at public health clinics were viewed as inferior to medicines obtained at hospitals and private clinics, leading to overuse of these types of more expensive health care setting.

Starting a study by using qualitative methods to inform quantitative data collection is becoming more common. For example, qualitative methods can be used to identify issues of importance to patients as a first stage in questionnaire studies, in order to increase validity and willingness to participate. As an example, focus groups were advantageously used by Holmström et al. [18] (Table 13.1) at the preliminary or exploratory stages of a study when there was little knowledge about the topic (young people's beliefs about OTC pain medications). Another important role for qualitative methods is in exploring why a given intervention does not work. Bjerrum et al. [20] sought to understand the reasons for the lack of impact of sending feedback on prescribing patterns to GPs using semi-structured interviews. They found that the feedback did not motivate GPs to change and that it was only effective if the GPs knew the identities of the treated patients and were given relevant advice on how to optimize prescribing.

Common qualitative data collection methods that could benefit drug utilization research

Data collection for qualitative research usually involves either interaction with individuals on one-to-one basis, interaction with groups of individuals or observation of a specific behaviour in a group of individuals. The first two approaches involve asking the individuals questions.

The common feature of these data collection methods is that they generate a large amount of textual data. The individual interviews and group discussions should be audio-recorded and transcribed verbatim for analysis. The observational methods require that the researcher carefully collects data in structured field notes or a diary. The advantages and disadvantages of the data collection approaches described in this section are summarized in Table 13.2.

Interviews in qualitative research

Data collection through interviews is common in qualitative research. It involves a research process that is just as tight and rigorous as other forms of research. In all interview research, the methods and data analysis require diligence and loyalty to the material; they do not simply involve starting an audiotape and asking questions. The approach is nuanced, and a scientific mindset is required to collect data that will provide useful information on the subject matter. In addition, the researcher needs to have certain skills, such as open-mindedness, flexibility, responsiveness, patience, keen observation and the ability to listen well.

An interview can be structured in different ways. As mentioned in Chapter 3, interviews can range from closed answers, as in a survey, to a narrative with minimal structure, whereby the informant speaks freely about a topic.

In qualitative research, a common typology distinguishes between two types of structure – the semi-structured interview and the unstructured interview – but there is a continuum of the level of structure. The different levels of structure are linked to some extent to the depth of response sought. The choice of which interview methods to use is related to the research question, the level of knowledge already in place about the subject matter and the ability of the interviewee to speak about the topic without prompting. Whereas quantitative research

Table 13.2 Advantages and disadvantages of common qualitative data collection approaches.

Data collection approach	Advantages	Disadvantages
Semi-structured and unstructured interview	Complex, unknown and sensitive issues can be explored Probing can provide rich data Allows the possibility of investigating underlying motives	Expensive and time-consuming Requires trained interviewers, to reduce bias Requires careful preparation on behalf of the interviewer Interview must be transcribed – one 1-hour tape takes 10 hours to transcribe fully
Focus groups	Exploration of cultural values and health beliefs Provides broader understanding of why target groups behave or think in a particular way and what influences their beliefs and values Increases the amount and range of data by collecting from several people at the same time Group dynamics help focus on the most important topics People who cannot read or write are not discriminated against	Potential for group thinking not allowing for other attitudes and beliefs Requires a trained moderator to handle passive informants, resolve conflicts in the group and create a relaxed and welcoming environment Makes it difficult to explore sensitive issues
Observation – participating and nonparticipating roles of the researcher	Takes into account nonverbal behaviour The observer gets a real picture of behaviours and events as they manifest in natural settings Systematic and unbiased observation can produce an accurate representation of the individual's natural set of behaviours Certain phenomena can be accessed and properly understood only through observation	The observer has little control over the situation they are interested in observing The observer can affect the situation Many extraneous factors influence the phenomenon under observation Subjects who are observed may change their activities in the presence of the observer It is difficult to assess what causes or determines the behaviours of interest Observer bias Ethical problems Time-consuming – the researcher must wait until the event of interest takes place in a natural setting

usually uses a predefined set of methods, in qualitative research there is a flexibility of approach. Methods can therefore change during the study, but the impetus is on being transparent about what was done, why and when.

Semi-structured interviews are by far the most common approach in drug utilization research. They consist of a predetermined set of questions, or at least themes, but the order can be modified based upon the interviewer's perception of what seems most appropriate. Unlike in fully structured interviews, question wording can be changed and explanations given, questions that seem inappropriate for a particular interviewee can be omitted and additional questions can be included. This type of interview can include both the topics of interest to the researcher and additional topics raised by the interviewee. The researcher also has the freedom to probe the interviewee in response to something they have said, possibly opening up a new line of inquiry.

Table 13.1 provides some examples of research involving semi-structured interviews. Kardakis et al. [12] asked their informants the questions presented in Box 13.1, while Noerreslet et al. [11] used a more schematic method of eliciting information, shown in Figure 13.1. This simple scheme was shown to atopic dermatitis patients at the

Box 13.1 Examples of questions from a semi-structured interview (Kardakis et al. [12]).

- How would you describe the early development of this organization?
- What factors influenced your work?
- What stakeholders influenced your work?
- How did the organization proceed in relation to the original development plan?
- How have you been working with the implementation of the knowledge and decision support?

beginning of the interview in order to understand their perceptions of conventional medicines and contribute to our knowledge about patients as consumers.

Unstructured interviews are less frequently used within the realm of drug utilization research, although there has recently been a call to use the narrative approach in the related field of pharmacy practice research [9]. Narratives are stories told by the interviewee (usually a patient), with a beginning, middle and end, made up of a series of actions and centring on the illness. The interview starts with very general health questions and moves to focus on the interviewee's use of medicines, before then panning out again to reflect on the process. The argument for its increased use is that it can come closer than semi-structured interviews to the patient perspective.

Unstructured interviews tend to have a research topic but no predetermined questions, and they are generally informal. This means that the interviewer has a general

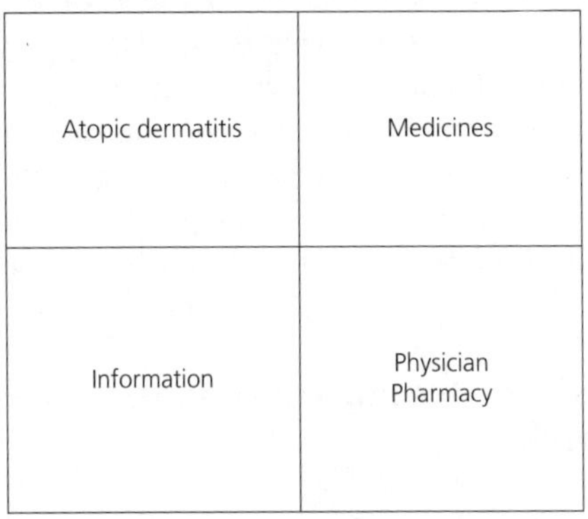

Figure 13.1 Simple schematic interview guide.

Source: Noerreslet et al. 2009 [11]. Reproduced with permission from Elsevier.

area of interest and lets the conversation develop within this area. The interviewer frames their next question based on the interviewee's previous response, which allows them to cover areas in great detail. The interviewee speaks freely about the areas of relevance, in whatever way they choose, with minimal interviewer direction.

Focus groups

As a qualitative method, focus groups aim to explore issues and problems from the perspective of groups of individuals in the context of their experiences, views, priorities and concerns.

Compared to individual interviews, which aim to obtain individual attitudes, views and experiences, focus groups are valuable in examining how people think and how ideas operate within a given cultural context [21]. Focus groups explicitly use the group interaction of about four to eight persons [21,22] as part of the method. The idea behind the focus group method is that group processes can help participants to explore and clarify their views in ways that would be less easily accessible in the face-to-face interview [21]. The group interactions help in focusing on the most important areas, and it is fairly easy to assess the extent to which there is a consistent and shared view.

Table 13.1 provides examples of the use of focus groups in drug utilization research. Carter et al. [23] investigated psychosocial factors that might motivate patients to participate in the Australian Home Medicines Review (HMR) programme using the question schedule illustrated in Box 13.2. As in face-to-face interviews, the group did not have to follow this schedule rigorously, but could flex to a question lower on the list.

Another common approach is to show a group a number of objects and ask the participants to discuss them. A research project in South Africa [16] asked a group to sort traditional and Western medicines into piles according to how they were used by mothers for their children under 6 years old. This opened up a discussion of the rationales and beliefs of mothers regarding medicines for their children.

A moderator or group facilitator is important in leading a focus group. The moderator encourages debate, helps participants feel at ease and facilitates interaction between group members, while keeping the discussion focused on the topic. However, the moderator of a focus group has less control over the data produced [21] than does the researcher in either quantitative studies or face-to-face interviewing. Group dynamics play a large

Box 13.2 Examples of questions used in focus groups (Carter et al. [23]).

1. How do you obtain your medicines?
2. What sort of medicine problems do you experience? How do you manage them? How do you cope? Do you use dose administration aids? Do you have a carer?
3. How likely are you to: get sick from your medicines; see a doctor; or need to go to hospital because of them?
4. How much do you worry about your medicines?
5. Who do you approach for advice regarding medicines and medicine problems? Where else do you go for information?
6. How did you first hear about Home Medicines Review (HMR)? Did you already know about it? What did people say about HMR? What did you expect?
7. What was it like during the interview? What did the pharmacist cover? What happened after the interview?
8. Overall, how do you feel it benefitted you? How would it benefit people, generally?
9. Would you want another HMR? Why or why not?

role in the breadth and depth of the data gathered in focus groups.

Observation methods

There are a wide range of approaches to doing observational research. The researcher may take a participating or a nonparticipating role [3]. The participating researcher becomes involved in the activities taking place, in addition to observing them, while the nonparticipating researcher merely observes.

Although it has a similar name, this type of research is not like the observational research methods used in analytical drug utilization research [3]. Here, instead, the drug utilization researcher has borrowed a well-established methodology from anthropological field research. Instead of focusing on asking questions, the researcher can watch people and events and learn about their behaviours and relationships. As mentioned later, asking people about how they act in certain situations can lead to bias.

An important reason for using this kind of method is that people or groups of people often have ways of doing things of which they are not consciously aware. They may not find certain behaviours or rules to be of any interest, and they are often unaware of how their social environment is constructed, but the naïve observer may be able to see these things. Table 13.1 includes a study in which Björnsdóttir et al. [15] observed physician–patient encounters in order to better understand how these related to the decision to prescribe antibiotics. They found that the patient's practical life situation played an important role in prescribing decisions, and they were subsequently able to add a new question to the GP interview guide. Until Björnsdóttir et al. made their observations, this important aspect had been taken for granted by the GPs, without being voiced. The observations also served to check the credibility of doctors' responses in the interviews.

The observer can be either someone who belongs to the environment under study or an outsider who enters the group. Doing an outside observation without becoming a participant is difficult unless the situation being studied is a very public space, such as a clinic waiting room. An example in Table 13.1 is Latif et al.'s [24] study of the provision of Medicine Use Reviews (MURs) in community pharmacies, in which the first author – a pharmacist – observed MURs provided in two pharmacies over 5 weeks each. In order to lower the risk of the Hawthorne effect (the influence of the observer on the environment under study [25]), video recording can be used, as was done by Hayward et al. [26], who used multichannel videos of consultations in GP surgeries to study how computerized decision support systems interact with the prescriber in the process of a consultation.

One of the challenges of participant observation is the requirement to immerse oneself in the environment and gain acceptance by the observed. Once this is achieved, another risk presents itself: the researcher may lose their novel perspective on the environment and 'go native' [3]. The most important weakness of this kind of method is that in order to learn about the environment, the researcher is required to stay there for long periods of time. Often, researchers devise a system whereby they stay in an environment at varying times until they find the best one at which to gain the most insight. Finally, there is an ethical problem around not telling those under study that they are being observed.

Sampling strategies in qualitative research

In a qualitative approach, representativeness, with randomization of informants, is not a primary concern [1]. When the aim is to gain an idea of how a certain phenomenon manifests itself in a group of people or to identify and explore unknown phenomena in society, informants are selected strategically. A 'strategic' or 'purposeful' sample selection refers to information-rich cases; that is, people who have the best possible knowledge, experience or overview with respect to the study's research topic [27]. Moreover, the informants should be willing to share this information with the researcher.

There are several different strategies for purposefully selecting information-rich cases (see Box 13.3). The logic of each strategy serves a particular purpose and, as always, the choice of strategy depends on the research question under study.

Analysis of data gathered in qualitative research

There is no single set of conventions for analysing qualitative data corresponding to that for quantitative data, but there are ways in which qualitative data can be dealt with systematically (e.g. using the United Kingdom framework approach [28] or the grounded theory approach [13]). The most important feature of qualitative data analysis is the focus on text, usually taking the form of interview transcripts or notes on observation sessions. Researchers commonly seek to describe their textual data in ways that capture the setting or the people who produced them.

The researcher's interest is often in explaining a phenomenon or constructing theories from collected data. Hence, the process of analysis in qualitative research often starts at the same time as data are collected, as the researcher searches for saturation in data [29]. Saturation in qualitative research is the point in the data collection at which no new or relevant data emerge in relation to the research question (or phenomenon under study). Consequently, the researcher decides that no more data need to be collected. When no new information comes forth and the categories or theory appear to be robust, with no unexplained phenomena, saturation has been reached. Saturation is a matter of achieving quality in qualitative studies, as inadequate sample size can undermine the credibility of research findings, but power analysis can never be used to determine sample size in qualitative research.

As qualitative research usually generates a large amount of raw data (transcripts and field notes), the researcher can use computer software programmes to organize and sort the data. Software programmes help the researcher in the development of consistent coding schemes but cannot provide explanations. It is still the researcher's task to interpret the data.

Validity concepts in qualitative research

One of the most important concerns with qualitative studies is that asking people about how they act in certain situations may lead them to report only intentions or socially desirable behaviours. Giorgi states that a relationship can be anticipated between what people say and do [30], and that one way to increase the validity between 'saying and doing' is to ask questions that reflect the interviewee's ways of acting. By letting the interviewee describe and give concrete examples from their own practice, we can gain insight into their experiences, increasing the link between 'saying and doing'. Another way of approaching this dilemma is to use observations, as already mentioned.

The problem many drug utilization researchers have with qualitative methodology is that it does not apply the same validity criteria as quantitative methodologies; at least, it does not meet the classical criteria of reliability, internal validity and generalizability. As the reader has probably noted by now, qualitative methods cannot

Box 13.3 Strategies for the systematization of sampling methods in qualitative research.

Maximum-variation sample
- Searching for heterogeneity among informants' background and experiences.

Homogeneous sample
- Searching for informants who have something in common, but who are sufficiently different to allow for contrasting views.

Snowball or chain sample
- Asking key informants to recommend useful people to talk to (this is useful where researchers don't know where they can find people who are sufficiently knowledgeable about the subject of interest).

Theoretical sample
- Beginning by interviewing one key informant and then building interpretative theories from emerging data; subsequently selecting a new sample with which to examine and elaborate on this theory (constant comparative method of analysis).

and will not seek generalization in the way quantitative methods will, simply due to the sampling methods and the number of research units. Here, the effort is instead put into seeking sensitivity to the context of the research. By the same token, the researcher is the instrument of data collection, and therefore internal validity is not an option, as each researcher will have preconceived notions and biases.

Establishing validity is still as fundamental in research using qualitative methods as in quantitative drug utilization research. Four criteria by which to create trustworthiness in qualitative studies have been developed: credibility, dependability, confirmability and transferability [31,32]. Table 13.3 briefly explains these concepts.

Triangulation and use of mixed methods is also highly recommended by many publications relating to the quality of qualitative research. The Qualitative Research Guidelines Project suggests a few publications that relate to assessing the validity and the general quality of a

Table 13.3 Validity concepts in qualitative research. Building on texts by Guba and Lincoln [31] and Hamberg et al. [32].

Concept of validity	What is it?	How is it evaluated?	Corresponding term in quantitative methods
Credibility	The researcher's ability to communicate how the research process affects the validity of the knowledge produced. It is important that the analysis is true to the collected data and encompasses critical reflection	A detailed description of the research process with: • sampling strategy; • the informant's motive for taking part in the study; • the researcher–informant relationship; and • the structure of the process from data collection to analysis.	Internal validity
Dependability/consistency	Focusing on exploring, and not testing whether the findings are repeated in the same context with the same subjects. People live in a changing environment, where nothing is constant	The researcher's task is to describe the research process so that it can be easily followed by the reader, despite this changing environment	Reliability
Confirmability/neutrality	The research should convincingly show how the results are grounded in the material. In qualitative research, the researchers themselves are seen as an instrument, whereby they are subjective in relation to informants, as they often interact with them directly	The researchers must be objective in relation to the data. This demands that they be open-minded, that they listen and that they be sensitive to the effect and influences that they might have on the informants. A researcher has to try to set aside their own beliefs, perspectives and preconceptions in order to understand people from their own frame of reference. Their awareness of and willingness to reflect on these choices is the only way of securing rigour in research	Internal validity
Transferability	Findings that are more generally applicable, for example in contexts, situations and times other than those directly studied. The onus is on the reader to evaluate the methods, setting and findings and decide whether they are transferable to their own situation	The researcher has a responsibility to provide a thorough description of the findings and context. Transferability of findings is conceptual rather than numerical	Generalizability

research study, and the reader is referred to www.qualres.org for further information. Three studies in Table 13.1 employed this approach. Friend-du Preez et al. [16] used a mix of surveys, focus groups and semi-structured interviews with various informant groups in a mixed-methods approach. Latif et al. [24] triangulated observations of MUR counselling sessions with interviews with patients and pharmacy staff, enabling them to better observe that there was scope for developing a much more effective and joined-up MUR service that transcends traditional boundaries between GPs and pharmacists. Björnsdóttir et al. [15] used observations to inform the development of the interview guide with GPs.

Conclusion

There are a range of different approaches within qualitative research, all of which involve the systematic collection, organization and interpretation of data [33,34]. Although there are some common characteristics within the qualitative research tradition, there are also some differences in terms of the history, strategy, epistemology and ontology of each approach [35]. The diversity among qualitative methodologies can be compared to that within quantitative methods, and there are guidelines for interpreting texts in qualitative analysis, just as there are for constructing and interpreting tables and figures in statistical analysis [33,36].

It is of great importance that drug utilization researchers learn to balance quantitative and qualitative methodologies and use them appropriately according to the research question at hand. It is also highly recommended that researchers not shy away from utilizing more than one method and triangulating their results or from using mixed-method designs in order to get a fuller picture of the phenomenon of interest [27,37].

PART 3

Applied drug utilization research

CHAPTER 14

Comparison of drug utilization across different geographical areas

Vera Vlahović-Palčevski[1,2], Björn Wettermark[3,4], Luisa Ibáñez[5] & Robert Vander Stichele[6]

[1]*Department of Clinical Pharmacology, University Hospital Center Rijeka, Croatia*
[2]*Department of Pharmacology, University of Rijeka Medical Faculty, Croatia*
[3]*Centre for Pharmacoepidemiology, Department of Medicine, Karolinska Institutet, Sweden*
[4]*Department of Healthcare Development, Stockholm County Council, Sweden*
[5]*Foundation of the Catalan Institute of Pharmacology*
[6]*Heymans Institute of Pharmacology, Ghent University, Belgium*

KEY POINTS

- Geographical comparisons of drug utilization can stimulate discussions areas around improvement in the quality of prescribing, dispensing and consumption of medicines.
- A common methodology is small area analysis, which includes calculations of utilization rates for a drug in each area, descriptive statistical analyses, identification of important differences between areas and attempts to seek explanations for these variations.
- Several studies have shown a large variation in drug utilization between countries or between different regions within the same country. These differences are only to a limited extent explained by differences in morbidity.
- It is difficult to compare drug utilization across countries, since there are large variations in data availability, population demography, disease prevalence and the organization and provision of health care.
- Checklists for conducting cross-national studies are helpful tools in ensuring the validity of comparisons.

Introduction to comparative studies

Comparative drug utilization studies aim to promote an efficient, effective, equitable and safe use of medicines. They may be either descriptive or analytical. Descriptive comparative studies can be valuable in identifying areas requiring more in-depth studies using other designs and in stimulating discussions around areas for improvement in the quality of prescribing, dispensing and consumption of medicines. Analytical comparative studies aim to gain a deeper understanding of the explanatory factors behind observed differences in drug utilization. These studies may also seek to determine the consequences of the observed differences or to identify ways in which one comparator (e.g. region, setting, group of patients) might benefit from the experience of another.

Consequently, comparative studies are closely related to benchmarking; that is, to the process of establishing best practices through comparison of an organization's performance with that of one or more other organizations. This is usually done to determine standing against peers and to identify improvement opportunities. Many studies have shown a widespread variation in the translation of best available evidence to clinical

Drug Utilization Research: Methods and Applications, First Edition. Edited by M. Elseviers et al.
Published 2016 by John Wiley & Sons, Ltd.

practice. There are multiple, diverse reasons behind these variations, reflecting personal, organizational and system-level characteristics. The reasons for gaps between evidence and practice are complex, and efforts to improve care are unlikely to be successful if they are one-dimensional or focus on individual health professionals. Reducing unwarranted clinical practice variation is important from a quality and safety perspective; it encompasses patient-focused care, appropriateness of care, reduced mortality and morbidity and efficiency in meeting increasing health care expenditure [1].

The development of comparative studies is closely linked to the history of drug utilization research. A strong wish to compare drug use between different countries was one of the main reasons for the development of the discipline, as well as the development of internationally acceptable drug classifications, methods and metrics [2]. Other pioneering studies focused on assessing differences in drug utilization between regions and other populations. The historical development of drug utilization research is further described in Chapter 1. This chapter focuses on geographical comparisons of drug utilization, while Chapter 16 looks at comparisons over time. The other chapters in this section present comparative studies from the perspectives of health care providers, patients, prescribers and health systems. For further reading on the explanatory factors behind variation in drug utilization, see Section E.

Practical guide to geographical comparisons of drug utilization

Geographical comparisons of drug utilization may be conducted at different hierarchical levels, from intercontinental, international (cross-national) and national studies to local studies in small regions or towns. A common methodology in local studies is small area analysis (SAA), which includes calculations of utilization rates for a drug in each area, descriptive statistical analyses, identification of important differences between areas and attempts to seek explanations for these variations [3]. There are no strict rules for defining a small area, but it is typically an area defined by physical or demographical boundaries for which data such as health care consumption are available: a particular region, city or postcode area. The general procedure for SAA is presented in Box 14.1. The same principles are also relevant when comparing geographic areas between different countries, but it is important to acknowledge the additional challenges in such comparisons (see later).

Box 14.1 How to conduct a small area analysis (SAA) of drug utilization.

1. Identify and define the geographic boundaries of the areas of interest (e.g. cities, municipalities, regions).
2. Estimate the amount of drugs prescribed or dispensed to the population of each area. This may be done either by using aggregate data on defined daily doses (DDDs), packages or prescriptions or by using patient-level data on number of individuals exposed.
3. Calculate utilization rates. This may be done on a crude basis or adjusted by age, sex and social characteristics, usually using the indirect method of standardization.
4. Analyse the results, normally through one of the following methods:
    a. Compare rates between areas of high and low utilization.
    b. Conduct correlation analyses to establish relationships between drug utilization patterns and other variables (e.g. morbidity, socioeconomy, access to health care facilities).

SAA has some important limitations that must be taken into consideration when conducting these studies:

- Small numbers of individuals can increase the risk of chance and random variation.
- It can be difficult to allocate events to a particular area (e.g. when patients living in one region purchase drugs in another).
- Geographical boundaries can change over time (leading to difficulties for longitudinal studies).
- There may be a lack of appropriate denominator data, such as population size and composition.
- Case mix in populations can make direct comparisons difficult. Standardization or adjustment may address this.

In a small area, it is also possible that only a limited number of patients will be using a particular drug. This can lead to problems around patient confidentiality.

Regional drug utilization comparisons

Several studies have shown a large variation in drug utilization between different regions within the same country, and these differences can only be explained to a limited extent by differences in disease patterns, sociodemography or reimbursement/financing systems.

As an example, a study examined geographic variation in drug expenditure among elderly people affiliated to the US Medicare insurance plan. The findings were adjusted for differences in demographic factors (age, sex and ethnicity), insurance coverage and health [4,5]. Drugs in the area with the highest cost per capita were 60% more expensive than in the area with the lowest cost. Health care costs showed an even greater variation, and there was no clear association between either prescription spending and other health care costs or prescribing costs and quality. Similar results were found in another US study of 4.7 million Medicare beneficiaries comparing prescription drug use and overall expenditure, as well as expenditure on angiotensin-converting enzyme (ACE) inhibitors, angiotensin II receptor blockers (ARBs), statins and antidepressants [6]. The authors found that regional variation in spending resulted to a large extent from differences in choice of treatment, rather than prescription volumes.

Aimed at investigating regional differences in prevalence, incidence and adherence to guidelines for drug treatment of asthma, a study using data on antiasthmatic drugs dispensed to all Swedish citizens aged 18–44 years between July 2005 and December 2008 found a large regional variation in utilization, with substantial room for improvement [7]. There was, however, no clear explanation behind the variation. No relation was found between models for allocating prescribing budgets or Drug and Therapeutics Committee recommendations and adherence to guidelines.

An Italian study assessed differences in child and adolescent drug prescription patterns at the regional and local health unit (LHU) levels [8]. A total of 3.3 million children and adolescents were included. The correlation between mean latitude (indication north–south differences), average annual income, hospitalization rate, number of paediatricians per 1000 resident children and prevalence rate was evaluated by LHU. Large differences in drug utilization were found across the regions and LHUs, with prevalence rates ranging from 43 to 70%.

There may be even greater variation in the utilization of newly introduced drugs used by specialists in secondary care. A study analysing the uptake of TNF-α inhibitors and trastuzumab in Swedish regions found annual TNF inhibitor sales increased 9-fold from 2000 to 2009, from 195 to 1779 million SEK (from 0.7 to 5.0% of total drug expenditure in the country) [9]. The regional variation was initially 6.2-fold, but decreased to 2.3-fold in 2009. For trastuzumab, a 3.2-fold variation was observed in 2009.

Substantial regional differences in drug utilization have also been demonstrated from low- and middle-income countries. A study on the diffusion of interferon beta for the treatment of patients with multiple sclerosis in Iran showed a more than 100-fold difference in utilization in DDDs/1000 inhabitants between the 28 provinces, with a rapid uptake in the capital and much lower diffusion in the poor provinces [10]. An Ethiopian study analysed the utilization of antiretroviral treatment (ART) in towns, administrative zones and regions and found a marked variation between urban and rural communities [11]. The suggested explanation was a combination of differential accessibility of ART sites, patient knowledge and health-seeking behaviour.

Large regional differences in prescribing within a country are often criticized as inequitable. In the United Kingdom, differences in access to drugs according to which treatments local health boards are willing and able to provide have been decried as 'postcode prescribing', and efforts have been taken to reduce the variations (e.g. through the instigation of national guidance) [12]. Similar activities are ongoing in other countries. Drug utilization studies have been important in this development, as they can show where large variations in prescribing exist and whether there is any rationale behind the differences. Today, many countries regularly publish comprehensive overviews of drug utilization data comparing regions and/or practices. This is done in the United Kingdom, the Nordic countries, the Baltic countries, the Netherlands, Germany, Italy, Catalonia (Spain) and Belgium, for example. However, more analytical studies on the explanations behind such differences and their consequences for patient outcomes are needed. Such studies are difficult to conduct in many countries, due to the large population case mix between geographic areas and the limited access to other relevant data that can be linked to drug utilization patterns.

Cross-national drug utilization comparisons

It is difficult to compare drug utilization across countries, as variations in data availability, population demography and disease prevalence may be much greater than within a single country. There is also a large variation between countries in how health care is organized and provided. Over the years, many attempts have been made to harmonize descriptions of data sources and their validity and comparability. After a first attempt by the European Drug Utilisation Research Group (EuroDURG) [13], the European Association of Microbiologists set out, with support by EuroDURG experts, to map the utilization of antibiotics in Europe. The European Surveillance of Antimicrobial Consumption (ESAC), granted by DG/SANCO of the EC Commission [14], was a retrospective survey of antimicrobial usage data collected from various sources across 31 European countries (ESAC I). The aim of the study was to collect publicly available comparable and reliable data on antibiotic use across Europe. The ESAC I project was followed by the ESAC II project, which collected additional data on ambulatory care, hospital care and nursing homes, performed pharmacoeconomic evaluations and aimed to deepen our knowledge of antimicrobial consumption. The ESAC III project then aimed to consolidate the continuous collection of comprehensive antimicrobial consumption data from ambulatory and hospital care across 32 countries. The ESAC project as a whole set out to provide timely information on antimicrobial consumption, to develop indicators of antimicrobial use and to create evidence-based guidelines and educational tools for managing the risk of infections and antimicrobial resistance (see Chapter 26). The ESAC project has been an important contribution to the development of cross-national comparisons (CNCs) in Europe.

Other efforts have been made throughout the years to collect and compare information on available data sources in Europe. The EURO-MED-STAT project collected information on the availability of data and suggested a number of indicators for comparisons of the availability and utilization of drugs in different countries [15]. The more recent Pharmacoepidemiological Research on Outcome of Therapeutics by a European Consortium (PROTECT) project, part of the European Innovative Medicines Initiative (IMI), compiled information on nationwide administrative databases containing drug consumption data, updating its list annually. Finnally, 27 European countries and 31 databases have been included. In addition, it provides information on sources of measurement error in these databases, in order to help interpret studies from different countries [16].

Scientific CNC studies have been conducted in a number of different therapeutic areas, with early studies conducted on antidiabetic agents, cardiovascular drugs and psychotropic agents in the first years of the 1970s [17–20]. During the 24th International Conference of Pharmacoepidemiology (ICPE) in Copenhagen, EuroDURG and the special interest group for Drug Utilization organized a structured CNC poster session with data from more than 20 countries. At the 26th ICPE in Brighton, a methodological workshop was held. EuroDURG also organizes scientific meetings with CNC as a central part of the programme. A literature review was conducted for the EuroDURG conference Better Public Health through Pharmacoepidemiology and Quality Use of Medicine (Antwerp, 2011), collecting information on 100 CNC studies published between 2000 and June 2011 that included at least one European country (for a total of 37 European countries) [21]. The country that participated most frequently in CNC was Sweden, followed by the Netherlands, Denmark, Germany and Italy; overall, these countries were included in more than half of all CNC studies. The studies were based on a range of data sources, from administrative databases on reimbursed drugs to specific disease-based registries. The Anatomical Therapeutic Chemical (ATC)/DDD methodology was applied in most studies, but some used other metrics. One-third of all studies were conducted on antibiotics. Studies on cardiovascular drugs, psychotropics, analgesics and drugs for asthma/chronic obstructive pulmonary disease (COPD) were also common. Most studies were descriptive, but some made attempts to explain the variability between countries. This work laid the basis for cooperation between EuroDURG and the PROTECT project in producing guidelines for conducting CNCs.

The development of national registers on drug consumption in many European countries has facilitated a number of recent large CNC projects, including the Arrhythmogenic Potential of Drugs (ARITMO) project, funded by the European Commission in the 7th Framework Programme [22–24]. The aim of this project was to analyse the arrhythmic potential of drugs in the following classes: antipsychotics, antiinfectives (antibacterials, antimycotics and antivirals) and H1-antihistamines. Drug utilization data were used to provide a population perspective on the arrhythmogenic potential of drugs belonging to the therapeutic classes of interest across 19 European countries. Large European CNC studies have also been conducted through the Piperska group, aimed at understanding the impact of differences in pharmaceutical policy between different European countries [25,26]. These studies are described in Chapter 18 and Section B.

The literature review created for the Antwerp meeting identified a number of non-European countries in comparison studies containing at least one European one. The most active were the United States (included in 10 studies), Australia (9), Canada (9), New Zealand (3), Japan (1) and South Africa (1)[21]. Studies have also been conducted wholly on other continents, such as one comparing lipid-lowering drug prescribing and persistence between Canada and the United States [27,28] and one comparing different drug classes between Asian countries, using different data sources [29–32]. In recent years, many Asian countries have established large claims databases covering their entire populations, similar to corresponding databases in Europe. In 2012, the Asian Pharmacoepidemiology Network (AsPEN), a special interest group of the International Society for Pharmacoepidemiology (ISPE), was established with the aim of developing and advancing multinational database research in pharmacoepidemiology in the Asia/Pacific region [33]. The situation in Latin America has been more scattered, due to the large difference between countries in terms of data availability [34]. Some CNC studies have been conducted in Africa and the Middle East, with corresponding difficulties in finding comparable data [35].

Data collection for CNCs

Regardless of the geographical hierarchical level at which a drug comparison is conducted, it can be based on either primary or secondary data sources. Most European CNC studies are conducted on databases, while most from settings other than Europe have been based on samples of medical records or physician/patient questionnaires. It is important to emphasize that field studies that include primary data collection may be more difficult to perform, not only because health care systems vary widely between countries, but also due to cultural differences in beliefs and attitudes, which influence the comparability of the data collected. Primary data collection is also time-consuming, and there may be large problems around selection bias and poor response rates. There have been some attempts at conducting CNC studies using structured surveys. For example, the ESAC project has organized a coordinated point-prevalence survey with a 1-day registration of antibiotic consumption in European hospitals [36]. In another recent CNC study, drug utilization data for pregnant women were collected across four continents via an anonymous online questionnaire [37]. For further guidance on primary data collection and surveys, see Chapter 2.

Some disease-based registries have been developed to facilitate international comparisons of medication use. For example, a study assessing the utilization of antiepileptic drugs (AEDs) between 1999 and 2005 was conducted in 4798 prospective epilepsy pregnancies from 38 countries participating in EURAP, an international AED and pregnancy registry. Exposure to second-generation AEDs varied greatly. Even wider variation was recorded in exposure to individual AEDs. Prominent differences in utilization patterns were observed across the various countries, probably reflecting a lack of evidence concerning the optimal treatment of epilepsy in women of childbearing age [38]. Disease-based registries offer the opportunity to analyse drug utilization in relation to clinical data. The development of disease-based registries for CNC is important in adaptive licensing and safety assessment of new therapies, particularly for orphan drugs and other rare conditions where data collection across countries is needed. This is further described in Chapter 29 and Section G.

Disease-based registries may also be the preferred source when comparing drug utilization in the hospital setting. While there has been a rapid growth in ambulatory care databases in many countries recently, it is important to acknowledge that it is still a challenge to find comparable data on hospital drug consumption [39,40]. More efforts are needed to monitor drug utilization patterns from different sources. One rare example of such a longitudinal effort to collect and integrate commercial and publicly available data from different sources in order to provide a comprehensive picture of consumption of over-the-counter (OTC) medication, prescription medication not reimbursed, reimbursed ambulatory care medication and hospital consumption is a Belgian study providing data from 1990 to 1999 [41].

Finally, it is important to acknowledge that some comparative studies are based on data from marketing research. IMS Health is the largest commercial drug data provider. It gathers data from multiple sources of information, namely manufacturers [42], wholesalers [43], community and hospital pharmacies, prescribers [44] and electronic medical records [45]. One of the advantages of IMS Health is that it collects nationwide data on drugs for which there is no register in many countries [46,47].

Methodological challenges in CNCs

Many CNC projects yield huge amounts of data. The ESAC project concluded that methodological rigor is needed to ensure the validity of data and the reliability of comparison [13]. In addition, corrections need to be made for bias by parallel export and OTC sales, as well as by incomplete census. As there is no European administrative drug database, the attribution of national brands to specific ATC classes and the local calculation of the number of DDDs in medicinal product packages need to be validated in national registers [13]. Similar experiences came from the EURO-MED-STAT project [15,48]. Walley and colleagues compared data on statin utilization and expenditure across Europe between routine administrative databases (reimbursement data) and a commercial source (IMS Health) [48]. Substantial differences were found, and it was concluded that standards for data collection were urgently needed for administrative databases. The importance of checking whether the ATC/DDD methodology is applied similarly in all countries has also been emphasized [49].

To combat these challenges, a checklist was developed by the ESAC group (Box 14.2) [13], suggesting that all datasets be checked for possible bias related to sampling or census procedure, methods of extrapolation to the population, drug coverage (undetected consumption of nonreimbursed medicines in data collection systems based on reimbursement), ambulatory/hospital care mix, undetected OTC consumption (in data collection systems based on prescription databases), parallel import and export and errors in the attribution of national brands to the ATC classification. According to this checklist, the quality of data collection in each country participating in the ESAC project was evaluated as valid, valid with a minor bias or not valid [13].

Another checklist was proposed by PROTECT with the aim of helping explain differences in drug use across countries in CNC projects [50]. This list was developed based on previous publications by the ESAC group and others [13,51–53]. The factors it takes into account are differences in disease patterns, adherence to national clinical guidelines on disease treatment, advertising policies, cultural differences, sociodemography and reimbursement/financing system features, as well as the characteristics/validity of the drug utilization data sources in each of the countries. Correlation analysis with the variables related to several of these factors are

Box 14.2 Checklist for evaluating the validity of data in CNC projects (ESAC).

1. Problems with population coverage:
   a. Sample bias in samples of less than 90% of the population, not or incorrectly extrapolated.
   b. Census bias in census data covering less than 90% of the population, not or incorrectly extrapolated.
   c. Census bias in census data covering at least 90% but less than 100% of the population, with significant differences in consumption between rest of population and population covered, not properly weighted.
   d. Underdetection bias in countries where the reimbursement system does not cover substantial segments of the population (in data collection systems based on reimbursement data).
   e. Under- or overdetection bias by parallel import and export (in data collection systems based on distribution data).
2. Problems with drug coverage:
   a. Underdetection bias by OTC sales (in data collection systems based on reimbursement data).
   b. Underdetection bias in countries where specific classes of antibiotics are excluded from reimbursement (in data collection systems based on reimbursement data).
   c. Measurement bias caused by problems with ATC classification/DDD assignment.
3. Problems with ambulatory care/hospital care mix:
   a. Assignment of data from nursing homes, daycare centres and dental care to one or both settings (ambulatory care or hospital care).
   b. Assignment of specialist prescribing (prescribing by specialists based in ambulatory care, prescribing by hospital-based specialists to outpatients or dispensing by hospital pharmacists to outpatients).

Source: Vander Stichele et al. 2004 [13]. Reproduced with permission from John Wiley and Sons.

commonly used to determine the degree of relationship between amount of drug use and the selected variables, as well as time-series regression analysis when sufficient points of observation along time are obtained.

Globalization has increased the need to compare the quality of drug treatment between countries. There are many methodological challenges to such comparisons, and studies have shown that quality indicators cannot simply be transferred directly between countries without an intermediate process to allow for variation in professional culture or clinical practice [54]. In 2004, an expert meeting on indicators of prescribing quality was held, bringing together 40 researchers from 19 European countries, the United States, Canada and Australia. It was organized by EuroDURG, the Belgian National Health Insurance Institute (RIZIV-INAMI) and the World Health Organization Regional Office for Europe (WHO-Euro). This meeting discussed a conceptual grid for the classification of quality indicators, listed databases available for continuous monitoring of drug utilization in Europe (including a description of their content, the richness of their data and their impact on the potential to develop quality indicators) and provided an overview of the (in)appropriate uses of indicators. It also defined the state of the art in the development and application of prescribing quality indicators in all represented countries and proposed a first draft of a database of prescribing quality indicators, already subject to validation procedures [55]. More on the challenges in constructing and validating quality indicators can be found in Chapter 12 and Section H.

National activities that can facilitate CNCs

CNCs can be facilitated when countries organize their data collection processes in such a way that the national data are suitable for international comparison.

The EURO-MED-STAT project in 2004 issued a report on recommendations for national registers of medicinal products and proposed the minimal set of data that these registers should collect, promoting the ATC/DDD methodology as a means of making validated comparisons of drug utilization and expenditure across countries [56]. It proposed that the collection of information should be consistent over time.

The Nordic countries have developed national prescription databases, using similar data collection and classification approaches, that allow longitudinal comparisons between countries, building on the tradition of a common approach to working on wholesaler data that has existed since the 1970s [57]. In recent years, all Nordic countries have established nationwide prescription registries that save the unique identifiers of all individual purchases of prescription drugs. A review analysed to what extent these prescription registries had been used for pharmacoepidemiologic research [58]. A total of 515 studies were found, published between 2005 and 2010, of which only 4 took the opportunity to use data from more than one Nordic country, demonstrating that such patient-level CNC studies require time and energy.

A comprehensive review of all drug utilization studies conducted in a given country provides an excellent overview of the possibility of establishing international collaboration and CNCs. Such a literature review using electronic databases was conducted in Mexico, focusing on original studies published between1990 and 2004 looking at access to and use of medicines. This review identified two priorities for Mexico's pharmaceutical policy and strategies: tackling the irrational use of medicines and improving access to medicines [59]. Another example is a review of 466 studies of the rational use of drugs in Iran, which showed many areas for improvement in prescribing [60]. Similar reviews may be available from other countries. It is difficult, however, to find appropriate papers in this field, due to the eclectic nature of drug utilization research. It is important to emphasize that national approaches to contributing to CNCs may be very different and hard to define. The examples presented here just point a way forward.

Conclusion

The ultimate aim of performing comparative studies is to identify factors influencing drug use and to find areas for improvement in drug utilization. There are many challenges in performing comparative drug utilization studies across different geographical regions, some of which are briefly mentioned in this chapter. Although not always successful, steps are being taken internationally to make these comparisons fully reliable, by making the methods of drug utilization studies as uniform as possible.

CHAPTER 15

Comparison of drug utilization in different health care settings

Sean MacBride-Stewart[1], Ksenia Zagorodnikova[2], Irene Langner[3] & Gisbert W. Selke[3]

[1]*NHS Greater Glasgow and Clyde, United Kingdom*

[2]*North-Western State Medical University n.a. I.I.Mechnikov, Russia*

[3]*AOK Research Institute (WIdO), Germany*

KEY POINTS

- The hospital and ambulatory care settings are the most common environments for drug utilization research.
- Hospital studies often involve reviewing the prescribing for selected patients and focus on quality measures in a small number of settings.
- In the ambulatory setting, datasets collected by insurers or funders for reimbursement purposes are often used for drug utilization studies. These can compare prescribing in terms of quality, patient safety or financial governance.
- In some countries, prescribing for ambulatory care is recorded within hospital datasets.
- Comparative drug utilization research in these settings can serve such purposes as increasing transparency, explaining variation, improving quality of care and enhancing the cost-effectiveness of prescribing.

Introduction

This chapter provides an overview of the application of comparative drug utilization research in different health care settings. The examples are drawn from published comparative studies in a variety of settings that highlight an aspect of drug utilization research that is considered particularly important or relevant; they are illustrative only. This chapter will provide information on where and when comparative drug utilization research can be of practical value. The key attributes of applied comparative drug utilization research are summarized in Table 15.1.

There are numerous settings in which comparative drug utilization research can be undertaken. Chapter 14 dealt with comparative drug utilization research between countries, regions and population groups. This chapter will focus on studies and practical applications comparing individual prescribers or organizations.

Comparative drug utilization studies have a wide range of uses. They provide insight into international organizations, national governments and nongovernmental organizations (NGOs) with a strategic responsibility for the effective utilization of health care resources. They are used to evaluate the safe, effective and efficient use of drugs by health care commissioners, insurers and other organizations with clinical and corporate governance responsibilities for prescribing; these organizations also use them as a basis for strategic decisions on resource allocations and to shape contractual frameworks (e.g. P4P). The pharmaceutical industry uses them to better understand market share development of the drugs that they and their competitors sell. Researchers use them to gain insight into medical, economical and administrative questions. They can be used to search for possible modifiable factors, points for intervention and measure intervention effectiveness in order to increase rational use of medicines. They are used by prescribers to reflect on their practice and to compare and contrast themselves with their peers. Other organizations similarly use them

Drug Utilization Research: Methods and Applications, First Edition. Edited by M. Elseviers et al.
Published 2016 by John Wiley & Sons, Ltd.

Table 15.1 Exemplary contexts of comparative drug utilization research.

Who performs or initiates it?	Prescribers (e.g. doctors (specialists or GPs), nurses, pharmacists)
	Organizations (e.g. hospitals, practices or other groups of physicians, health authorities, health care funds)
	Pharmaceutical industry
	Academic researchers
	Regions/countries
What is the aim?	To drive improvements in prescribing
	To improve quality of care
	To improve cost-effectiveness
	To provide transparency
	To provide input for other areas of research (hypothesis generation)
What is evaluated?	Variation in prescribing between individual prescribers, between regions and between groups of patients
	Changes in prescribing behaviour over time
	Adherence to guidelines
	Impact of health care delivery
	Uptake of new drugs
	Inappropriate prescribing
	Impact of population demographics on prescribing and health care

for educational purposes, such as academic detailing, and to promote rational prescribing. Drug utilization research can provide insight into the effect of demand-side measures on prescribing patterns within countries [1].

Health care settings

The main health care settings for applied drug utilization research are hospitals, ambulatory care and nursing/care homes. This chapter will focus on the first two; nursing/care homes are dealt with in Chapter 25.

Patients in hospitals may receive medicines that are not used in ambulatory settings because they have medical conditions that require intensive care or they are being prescribed newly authorized medicines. Information about these medicines, including individual variability of response, drug–drug interactions and safety profile, may be lacking. Hence, their higher use in this setting renders drug utilization research especially important for hospitals.

Inpatient hospital medication use may represent only a minor part of all medication expenditures in most countries. It is about 9% in the United States [2], 3–14% in various European countries [3] and 17% in Russia [4]. It may be influenced by the variable provision of hospitals; within Organisation for Economic Co-operation and Development (OECD) countries, the numbers of acute beds per 1000 inhabitants in 2011 ranged from 7.95 in Japan to 1.64 in Mexico [5].

Hospitals offer a varying range of acute, convalescent and terminal care using diagnostic and curative services in response to acute and chronic conditions arising from diseases, injuries and genetic anomalies [6]. Hospitals are characterized by a higher number of parenteral medicines compared to ambulatory settings, medicines that can only be given under professional observation and medicines related to intensive care or surgery, as well as generally used medicines.

The size and function of hospitals can vary. The spectra and severity of patient states, the range of departments or specializations, the number of beds and the length of stay are among the observable differences. In some hospitals, patients may only attend for daytime observation and not stay overnight. All these factors make drug utilization within the hospital setting variable.

Hospitals generally have centralized drug delivery, and different hospitals vary in sources of funding. Medicine availability is dependent on the hospital's level, financing and profile. Most common hospital departments receive medicines from hospital pharmacies. Hospitals may implement explicit restrictions for certain drugs [7].

Patient-specific data are available in hospitals where electronic health records (EHRs) are used. Prescribing may be analysed at the patient level, and in some countries outcomes after discharge may be analysed. Where EHRs are not used, the amount of medicine dispensed to select departments from hospital pharmacies may be the only hospital data available. Insurance data may also be a source of prescription information, but generally additional work is required to make such data applicable to drug utilization research. For more details on data sources for drug utilization research, see Chapters 3 and 4.

Patients in the ambulatory care setting are seen primarily by practitioners of family medicine, often termed family practice physicians, family physicians or general practitioners (GPs). These consult with and prescribe to people with acute illnesses and long-term conditions. In some countries, other nonmedical health care professionals (e.g. physician assistants, nurses, pharmacists and physiotherapists) increasingly provide family medicine care, including prescribing medicines [8]. In the ambulatory setting, specialist care may be available, too, which provides for a focused range of illnesses that do not require admission to hospital but warrant a specialized input. The provision of these differs between countries [9]. In some systems, they are provided as an outpatient service in a hospital building, while in others they are provided from clinics within the community. They are often set up to provide a single location that includes diagnostics, medical specialists and a multidisciplinary team specific to a particular illness, so that patients can have all aspects of care provided in an efficient manner. In other countries, office-based specialists form an integral part of ambulatory care. These differences between countries and the inevitable changes that occur over time as health systems develop within countries means it is important to understand the systems in which drug utilization research is undertaken [10–16]. For more on differences in health care settings, see Chapter 31.

In many countries (e.g. Canada, Germany, Sweden, the United Kingdom), most drugs consumed within the ambulatory setting are prescribed by family doctors in the primary care setting and supplied through community pharmacies [17]. In such countries, medicines dispensed in ambulatory care provide an opportunity for drug utilization research where reimbursement data are collated and made available. Repurposing such data is referred to as 'secondary data research'. Depending on the setting, additional information, such as details of the prescriber or the patient, are collected according to the requirements of the reimbursement mechanism and the extent of automation of electronic processes. In other countries (e.g. Russia), although medicines are prescribed in outpatient clinics and supplied through community pharmacies, only a limited set of medicines is reimbursed, and a great number of drugs are available over the counter (OTC). In such countries, only sales data are available for drug utilization research, without any medicines/patient/prescriber details.

In countries where there is limited access to office-based doctors and limited provision of community pharmacy services (e.g. China), the drugs consumed in the ambulatory setting are mostly prescribed within the hospital outpatient setting and dispensed within hospital dispensaries [18–20]. Therefore, drug utilization research in the ambulatory setting requires analysis of data sourced from hospitals. Applications of drug utilization studies in hospitals are in many instances similar to those in ambulatory care, but with more emphasis on routine hospital management tasks such as quality assessment.

The relevance of drug utilization research in the hospital and ambulatory care settings

Almost all hospital inpatients receive medication, often in life-threatening situations. Treatment, therefore, should be provided on the best quality level to every patient. Medication-related problems in hospitals are not uncommon – the median rate of medication errors is about 10% [21], and adverse drug reactions (ADRs) have a variably estimated occurrence from 1 to 30% in different countries and are associated with almost 20% of additional increases in health care costs and 8% of increases in average length of hospital stay [22].

Prescribing within the ambulatory care setting should also be of the highest quality. Medicine-related ADRs in ambulatory care lead to hospital admissions at a median rate of 5.3% of cases [23]. Higher rates are found in elderly patients, who are likely to be receiving multiple medicines for long-term illnesses. It is estimated that at least 50% of these admissions are avoidable [24]. In Germany, drug utilization is routinely monitored for individual practitioners. The results serve as a foundation for academic detailing and for work in quality circles aimed at improving the quality and cost-effectiveness of prescribing [25]. Recently, this has been expanded to managing medication at the patient level, decreasing undesired drug interactions and increasing appropriate prescribing [26]. In Scotland, nationally published prescribing indicators provide an analysis of ambulatory prescribing by general practices and, just as in Germany, are used to improve the quality and cost-effectiveness of prescribing [27]. Similar activities are undertaken in many other countries [28–32]; however, published evaluations of these activities are scarce.

Adherence to guidelines may be compared between hospitals, as was done in Canadian and Australian studies of acute exacerbation of chronic obstructive pulmonary disease (COPD) [33,34] (Table 15.2). These studies

Table 15.2 Comparative drug utilization studies identifying and targeting variation in prescribing behaviour and adherence to guidelines.

Country	Setting	Year	Ref.	Study summary	Main finding	Purpose of drug utilization research
Canada	Hospital	2013	[33]	A retrospective chart review of 293 patients admitted to a hospital for an acute exacerbation of COPD. 58% of patients received corticosteroids and 84% received antibiotics.	The respiratory medicine service demonstrated significantly better adherence with current treatment guidelines compared with general medicine and the hospitalist service, but even this was less than optimal. This study identified significant care gaps in the treatment of patients with acute exacerbation of COPD, both on admission and on discharge.	Comparison of hospital (inpatient and outpatient) adherence to guidelines.
Australia	Hospital	2013	[34]	A retrospective chart review of 201 acute exacerbations of COPD in two hospitals. In comparison to the respiratory specialists in one hospital, the general medical physicians in the other one performed fewer spirometry tests and blood gas analyses and treated patients less frequently with guideline-recommended medicines.	The study found differences in the management of acute exacerbations of COPD by general medical physicians and respiratory specialists, but these did not translate into different clinical outcomes between their patients. Suboptimal adherence to national COPD guidelines by both groups of clinicians was also observed.	Between-hospital comparison of adherence to guidelines.
Japan	Hospital	2005	[35]	Point-prevalence survey in 4 public-sector hospitals and 14 private hospitals. Using the tree-based model analysis, factors related to the total antipsychotic dose (chlorpromazine equivalent) were analyzed in 1674 patients.	Age of patient, presence of hallucination, age of first psychiatric hospitalization and change(s) in attending physician (while hospitalized) were all contributing factors to the chlorpromazine-equivalent dose.	Identification of factors influencing in-hospital prescribing.
Denmark	Hospital	2013	[36]	Comparison of hospital drug use in 10 hospitals representative of the country based on hospital pharmacies data for 2010. Adherence to hospital formularies within the DU90% segment and costs per DDD were analysed.	University hospitals were found to consume higher numbers of medicines and to have higher costs per DDD. Despite large variation between hospital drug formularies, adherence to them for the most common ATC groups was high.	Country-wide comparison of adherence to hospital drug formularies and costs per DDD.
Sweden	Primary care	2005	[37]	A retrospective analysis of statin prescribing using the Skaraborg Primary Care Database (SPCD). Multilevel regression analysis (MLRA) was used to disentangle the variances at different levels of data (patient, physician, health care centre).	The prevalence of adherence to guidelines for the prescription of statins increased from 77% in 2003 to 84% in 2005. The variance between physicians and between health care centres decreased considerably between 2003 and 2005.	Description of changing adherence to guidelines across a period of time.

(continued)

Table 15.2 *(continued)*

Country	Setting	Year	Ref.	Study summary	Main finding	Purpose of drug utilization research
Denmark	Primary care	2000	[38]	A retrospective study of 173 general practices (99 single-handed and 74 group practices) in the County of Funen, Denmark. The study reported the number of different drugs prescribed by each practice. Multivariate regression analysis was employed to determine practice characteristics that predict the number of different drugs prescribed.	The number of drugs prescribed ranged from 102 to 381 (median 236). Four practice characteristics were significant predictors of the number of different drugs prescribed: number of GPs, number of patients per doctor, percentage of listed patients ≥60 years and rate of consultations per day.	Comparison of prescribing patterns and identification of its predictors.

used retrospective review of patient records. The numbers of charts reviewed or medication administrations analysed are in the hundreds for each hospital and the scope of the studies is limited to a small number of hospitals; large, multicentre drug utilization reviews across many hospitals are uncommon. Prescribing behaviour may be compared between hospitals representative of a whole country, as was done in Denmark, where adherence to the hospital drug formularies within specific Anatomical Therapeutic Chemical (ATC) groups and costs per defined daily dose (DDD) were used as factors of comparison [36]. As in many other studies, hospital pharmacies were used as a universal source of data available for any hospital.

Drug utilization research within the primary care (ambulatory) setting mainly utilizes databases that hold records of the drugs dispensed to entire populations. These databases therefore contain millions (even billions) of prescription records, as well as other data for which linkage is possible. Examples include the Skaraborg Primary Care Database (SPCD) in Sweden, which contains all data on drug prescriptions, laboratory tests and current diagnoses at every consultation with everyone in the region. By means of a unique anonymized identification number, the SPCD is able to identify the health care centre, the physician and the patient [37].

These datasets are often used for retrospective analyses. Data quality is high because the primary use is for reimbursement. They generally contain all details of the medicines under investigation and do not normally require any additional data collection, but may require linkage to other information to add meaning, such as details of the organization for which the prescriber works. The Danish Odense University Pharmaco-Epidemiologic Database contains identifiable records of all prescription refunds for inhabitants in the County of Funen [38].

Comparative DU studies are used to evaluate and compare evidence-based prescriptions in hospitals with different characteristics. These hospital characteristics may be a target for further intervention as described in a Russian study evaluating evidence-based prescriptions for acute coronary syndrome patients [39]. Prospective observation may be used to investigate the effects of activity of specialist services (e.g. clinical pharmacologist service) on rationality and cost of treatment, as was demonstrated in an Israelian study on antibacterial use in different wards of one hospital [40]. Drug utilization research may be directed to identification of quality of use indicators requiring improvement in similar hospitals of different countries, which is exemplified by the study by Vlahovic-Palcevski et al [41].

Indicators are measures of processes and outcomes of health care that can be used to guide and monitor the quality and appropriateness of health care delivery with the aim of bringing about continuous healthcare improvement [46] (Table 15.3). Quality indicators in these examples include frequency of evidence-based prescribing [39], overall volume of antibiotics use, duration of antimicrobial prophylaxis and frequency of intravenous antibiotics use [41]. When identifying quality indicators, it is important to check that they are likely to drive clinical practice improvement, that there is evidence that examining practice leads to improved outcomes, that there is a need to improve the use of

Table 15.3 Comparative drug utilization studies identifying measures and targets that can drive improvements in prescribing.

Country	Setting	Year	Ref.	Study summary	Main finding	Purpose of drug utilization research
Russia	Hospital	2009	[39]	From seven districts, one municipal and one clinical hospital in the Saratov region, 1276 randomly selected case histories of acute coronary syndrome (ACS) without ST elevation were analysed. Demographic data, basic diagnosis, complications, disease duration, concomitant disorders and the medicines prescribed during the first day of inpatient treatment were manually collated.	Prescribing of drugs with proven efficacy in ACS was higher in the clinical hospital compared to the municipal or district hospitals, but was far from optimal when compared to other studies in Western Europe and the United States.	Comparison of the rationality of disease-specific drug use in different types of hospital.
Israel	Hospital	2004	[40]	Prospective comparison of two inpatient internal medicine units. Prescription-point prevalence survey twice a month from hospitalized patient charts over a 12-month period. Individual antibiotic utilization pattern and antibiotic costs were collected.	The intervention of a clinical pharmacology specialist in one of the units was effective in creating a significant statistical difference in antimicrobial volume and cost between the two units. This difference was observed using the prescription-point prevalence methodology.	Evaluation of effects (volume and cost of medicines) of a clinical pharmacology specialist intervention.
Croatia, Latvia, Estonia, Lithuania and Sweden	Hospital	2007	[41]	Benchmarking of antimicrobial drug use through a point-prevalence survey of five European university hospitals in order to identify potential problem areas in prescribing practice and to aid in establishing appropriate and attainable goals.	Frequency of antimicrobial drug use was lowest in Lithuania (14%) and highest in Sweden (34%). Rate of intravenous administration, compliance with guidelines and surgical prophylaxis were areas where problems were identified, and the authors concluded these deserved specific attention at all centres.	Identification of areas of treatment with a potential for improvement.
Sweden	Primary care	2003	[42]	The number of drugs constituting 90% of the volume (DU90%) and the adherence to local drug committee guideline ('Wise List') within this segment were presented to prescribers within 38 primary health care centres in Stockholm. All data were taken from the Swedish National Prescription Register. This register consists of dispensing data from all pharmacies. It contains information about drug use in aggregated defined populations and by primary health care centre.	The prescribers found the DU90% profiles clear and relevant. Providing DU90% profiles with guideline adherence as feedback was found to be a valuable tool for assessing the overall quality in prescribing in general practice.	Description of measure to identify quality prescribing.

(continued)

Table 15.3 *(continued)*

Country	Setting	Year	Ref.	Study summary	Main finding	Purpose of drug utilization research
France	Primary care	1999	[43]	Assessment of drug prescribing by primary care physicians in France for various types of condition, and identification of patterns and risk factors for prescribing practices. The study utilized details of prescriptions written by a random sample (stratified design) of physicians in France, collated, coded and priced by IMS-France.	Drug interactions, age problems, inappropriate frequency of administration and overdose were found in up to 40% of orders, depending on the target disease considered. Up to 8% of orders included a contraindication. Ineffective prescribing was assessed to have occurred in 30–90% of drug orders, according to the target disease. This included drug(s) classified as not proved to be effective.	Identification of the prevalence of prescribing assessed as ineffective and of poor quality.
Canada	Primary care	2012	[44]	In Quebec, 113 physicians consented to an analysis of all electronic prescriptions written between 2005 and 2009. Details of prescriptions were collected by the Medical Office of the XXI Century (MOXXI) primary care electronic health record (EHR) network research programme, where documentation of treatment indication is mandatory.	The prevalence of off-label use was 11%. Strong scientific evidence for the use of off-label medicines was lacking in 79% of cases. Off-label prescribing is common and varies by drug (most common for central nervous system (CNS) drugs), patient (sicker patients are less likely to receive off-label drugs) and physician characteristics (those with evidence-based orientation are less likely to prescribe off-label).	Identification of the prevalence of prescribing assessed as off-label and of its predictors.
Scotland	Primary care	2011	[45]	Data from 315 general practices in Scotland contributing to the Scottish Programme for Improving Clinical Effectiveness in Primary Care (SPICE-PC) were extracted from the dataset held by the Primary Care Clinical Information Unit at the University of Aberdeen. Patient details, prescribing and practice characteristics were analysed for frequency of high-risk prescribing in patients particularly vulnerable to adverse drug events and for how reliably the indicators could distinguish between practices.	Of patients defined as particularly vulnerable to adverse drug events, 13.9% were prescribed one or more high-risk drugs. A composite indicator of high-risk prescribing was able to identify practices as having above or below average high-risk prescribing rates with reasonable confidence.	Identification of the prevalence of prescribing assessed as posing a risk, particularly to vulnerable patients.

medicines and that indicators have widespread application across the system [47].

Drug utilization research is long established in primary care as a mechanism by which to measure and give feedback on quality prescribing to GPs. The DU90% method developed in Stockholm is an example of such a measure (the number of drugs accounting for 90% of drug use) that has been related to quality prescribing (adherence to the 'Wise List' of recommended drugs) [42]. The 'Wise List' mainly contains first-line drugs use to treat common diseases; in other settings, it would be known as a formulary (see Figure 15.1a). The DU90% concept has also been tested as a tool by which to relate antibiotics use and current cumulative microbial resistance levels in hospitals where overall resistance rates are significantly high (see Figure 15.1b).

Not all drug utilization research in primary care utilizes data from reimbursement datasets. In France, prescriptions from family doctors collected in a 7-day period were assessed against 17 quantitative indicators of drug prescribing quality. This information was collected expressly for drug utilization research and details of the disease being treated were recorded by the prescriber simultaneously with the drug order [43]. Most reimbursement datasets do not include this information, so while these data are only a sample for a small period of time, insightful measures of quality

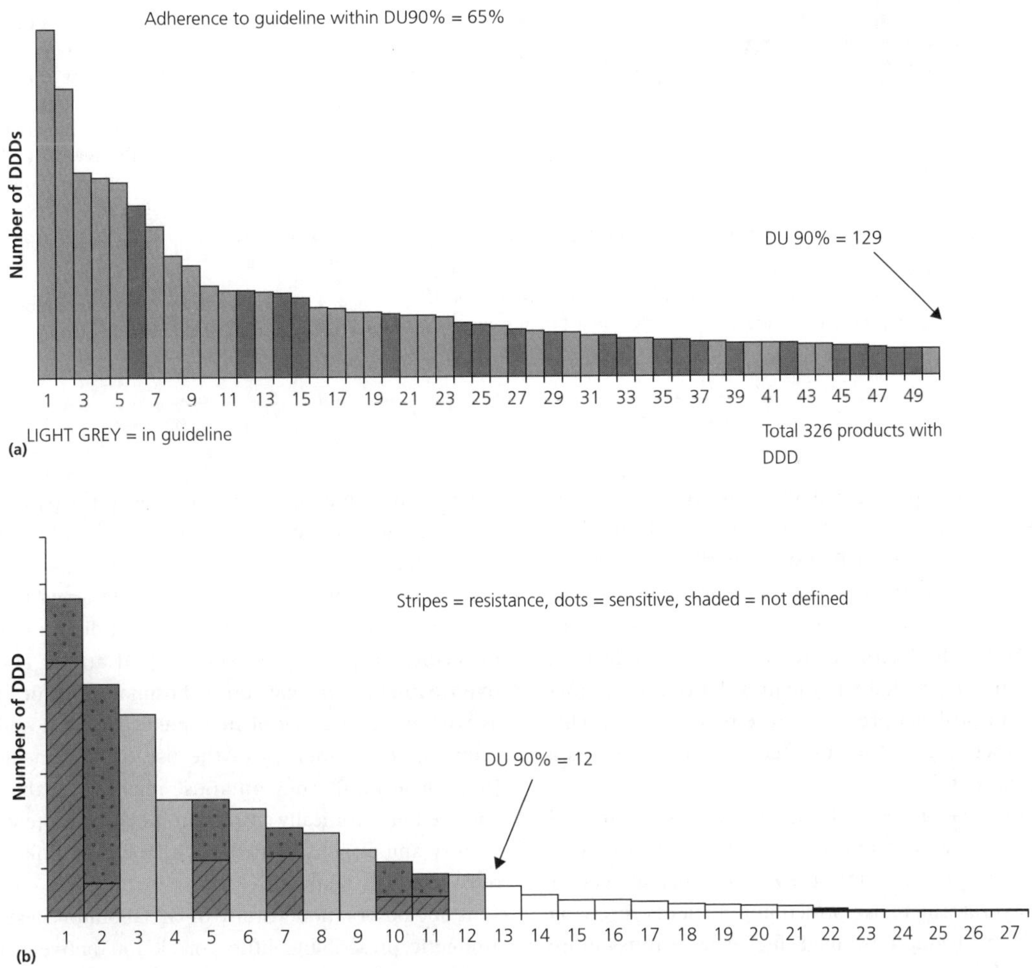

Figure 15.1 (a) Example of a prescribing profile that reports the DU90% and adherence to the 'Wise List' sorted by volume (DDDs) and cost (SEK, Swedish Crowns) for a primary health care centre in Stockholm. In this example, the DU90% is 129 of a total 329 different drugs prescribed by the center. (b) DU90% of antibiotics use and cumulative microbial resistance in a Russian hospital: a tool to alert physicians. It is generally agreed that in order to create the DU90% list, cumulative percentage of DDDs must be used, with the last medication in the list being the one that provides attainment of the full coverage of 90% of use, even though the final percentage may become slightly higher. For colour details, please refer to the colour plates section.

Sources: Figure 15.1(a) Wettermark et al. 2003 [42]. Reproduced with permission from John Wiley and Sons. Figure 15.1(b) Zagorodnikova K, Goryachkina K. 2013 [62]. Reproduced with permission from Ksenia Zagorodnikova.

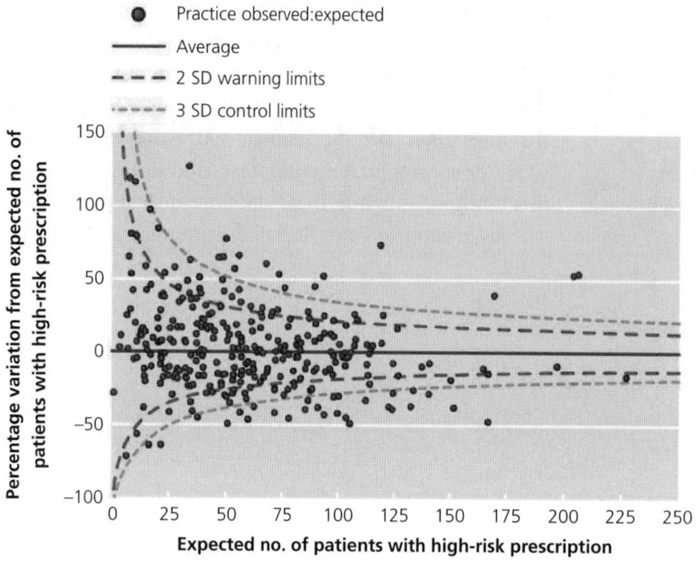

Cross-sectional control chart for observed versus expected number of patients with a high-risk prescription. Practices lying outside the 3-SD control limit are statistically significantly different from average

Figure 15.2 Results from a study of 315 general practices in Scotland contributing to the Scottish Programme for Improving Clinical Effectiveness in Primary Care (SPICE-PC). Observed numbers of patients with a high-risk prescription differ from those expected in each practice after adjustment for patient case mix. Variability between practices' prescribing of high-risk medicines is considerable even after prescribing rates are adjusted to account for patient-level variables (age, sex, number of regular drugs). Practices lying outside the three-standard-deviation control limits are statistically different from the average and vary from having half the expected rates of high-risk prescribing to having a 50–125% excess rate. For colour details, please refer to the colour plates section.

Source: Guthrie et al. 2011 [45]. Reproduced with permission from BMJ Publishing Group Ltd.

can be quantified (e.g. whether the drug prescribed was contraindicated or effective). The Medical Office of the XXI Century EHR system in Canada is a primary care EHR network research programme that also records treatment indication, but in this case, electronically. For each electronic prescription, the indication for treatment is added and the prevalence and characteristics of off-label prescribing are reported [44]. Off-label prescribing that is not effective and safe poses a risk to patients.

Drug utilization research can also use data extracted from the physician's practice IT systems. In Scotland, a composite measure was used to identify above- or below-average high-risk prescribing. Patients receiving more than 11 long-term medicines were 8 times more likely to be exposed to high-risk prescribing [45] (see Figure 15.2).

Various Italian regions have set up information systems to collect data on their inhabitants (birth year, sex, hospital care, pharmaceutical care, outpatient care, reasons for exemption from copayment) and GPs (age, gender, type of association). One study used the ability to link the databases using a unique patient identifier to create a longitudinal utilization history for patients. It assessed the influence of practice size on quality of care [49] (Table 15.4).

Drug utilization studies have been designed to evaluate, in a real-life setting, the effects of disease-specific medicines on patients' prognoses [53] and of alternative treatment strategies on in-hospital outcomes [54], as well as the efficacy of new medicines [51] and the economic consequences of the use of new medicines [55] (Table 15.5). They often use readily available data collected electronically in routine health care (e.g. laboratory and dispensary data), which can be linked and retrospectively analysed.

In one observational study of GP laboratory tests and antibiotic prescribing, little correlation between antibiotic prescribing and bacterial resistance was found [52] (see Figure 15.3).

Drug utilization studies using various sources of information can be used to identify usage patterns of new medicines. Variation in use is invariably observed, and the characteristics of both the prescriber and the population associated with the utilization of new drugs have been reported [56–59] (Table 15.6).

Table 15.4 Comparative drug utilization studies measuring variation in health care delivery.

Country	Setting	Year	Ref.	Study summary	Main finding	Purpose of drug utilization research
Saudi Arabia	Hospital	2014	[48]	A prospective study in three Saudi private hospitals of randomly selected prescriptions for patients with chronic diseases between October 2011 and January 2012.	A total of 363 patients' prescriptions were analysed, 75% for insured and 25% for uninsured patients. Insured patients in each hospital had a higher number of brand medicines, more items and a higher total price than uninsured patients.	Description of differences in prescribing, depending on patients' health care insurance.
Italy	Primary care	2013	[49]	A retrospective longitudinal analysis of utilization history for all patients in 21 health districts across 6 regions in Italy. Patients with diabetes, ischaemic heart disease and heart failure at 1 January 2008 were detected on the basis of health care service utilization in previous years. Prescribing by 2082 GPs for 164 267 people with one or more of the selected chronic conditions was analysed.	Quality indicators (% of patients receiving appropriate care) were selected (four for diabetes, four for congestive heart failure, three for ischaemic heart disease) and a total score was computed for each patient. No significant difference was found between team and solo practice for diabetes and heart failure. For ischaemic heart disease, a marginally significant impact was observed (0.040; 95% CI: 0.015, 0.065).	Assessment of quality of chronic disease management (in part measured by prescribing) in relation to GP practice size.

Table 15.5 Comparative drug utilization studies measuring the outcomes of real-life drug use patterns.

Country	Setting	Year	Ref.	Study summary	Main finding	Purpose of drug utilization research
England and Saudi Arabia	Hospital	2012	[50]	Observational study in two large teaching hospitals in England and Saudi Arabia. An intensive chart review was undertaken to identify medication errors for all children aged 0–18 years admitted to the medical ward, paediatric intensive care unit and neonatal intensive care unit for 1–3 months.	A total of 737 patients were included, of whom 333 suffered from 478 drug-related problems (DRPs). Overall DRP incidence was 45.2%, and the incidence was highest in the paediatric intensive care unit. Dosing problems were the most frequently reported DRPs. Overall, 80.3% of DRP cases were assessed as preventable, 72.2% as minor and 27% as moderate.	Search for risk factors for DRPs based on prescription and laboratory data.
France	Hospital and primary care	2014	[51]	A prospective, multicenter, observational study with a 2-year follow-up of patients with type 2 diabetes treated with vildagliptin. GPs and specialists in endocrinology, diabetology and metabolic diseases recruited patients they were treating into the study.	Of the 1700 patients recruited, 82% completed the 2-year follow-up. Glycosylated hemoglobin (HbA1c) decreased from a mean baseline of 7.8 ± 1.2% to 7.0 ± 1.1% at 6 months once vildagliptin was started and remained stable thereafter over the 2 years. It was concluded that vildagliptin efficacy was in line with existing data from randomized clinical trials.	Evaluation of real-life consequences of certain medicines use.

(continued)

Table 15.5 *(continued)*

Country	Setting	Year	Ref.	Study summary	Main finding	Purpose of drug utilization research
England	Primary care	2001	[52]	The correlation between antibacterial prescribing and resistance to urinary coliforms and streptococcus pneumonia was measured in 405 GP practices in England using routine data collected from Public Health Laboratory Service laboratories and the Department of Health Prescribing Support Unit.	Antibacterial resistance in urinary coliform isolates was found to be common, but the correlation with prescribing rates was relatively low for individual practices. Resistance of streptococcus pneumonia to both penicillin and erythromycin remained uncommon and no clear relation with the rate of prescribing was found.	Evaluation of real-life consequences of certain medicines use.

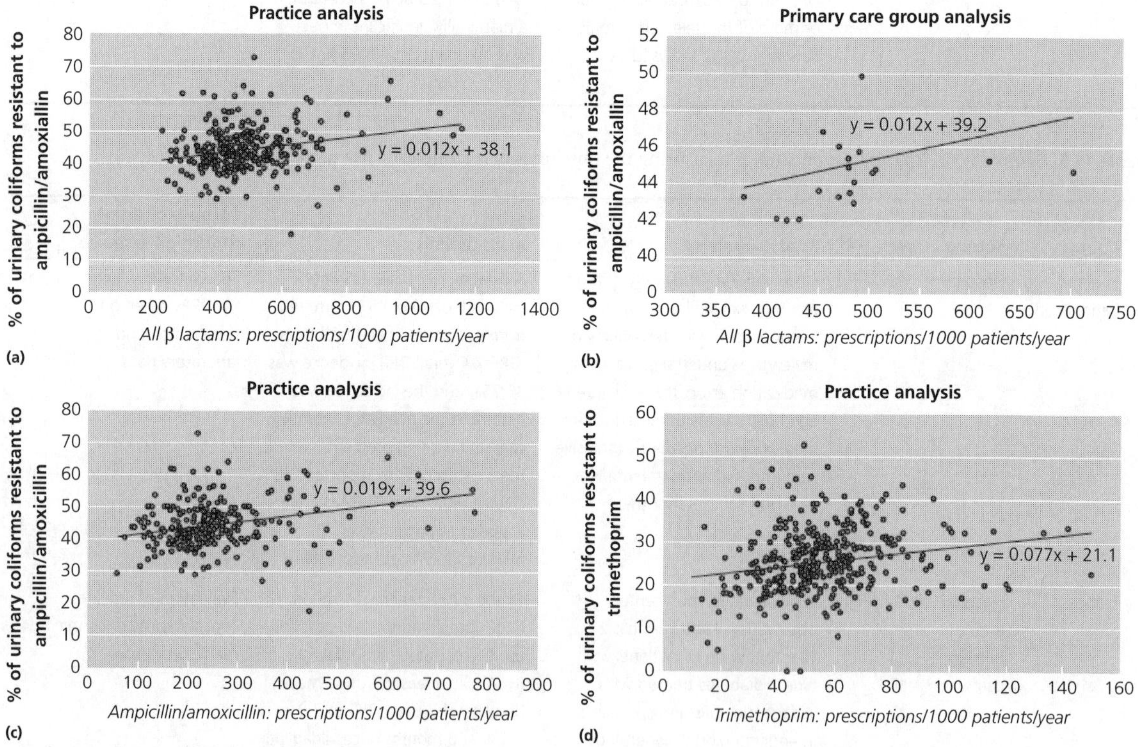

Relation between prescribing rate of antibacterial drugs and proportion of resistant urinary coliform isolates by individual general practice and (for all β lactams only) primary care group

Figure 15.3 Observed relationships between resistance to an antibacterial drug among routine urinary coliform isolates and ambulatory care prescribing of that drug.

Source: Priest et al. 2001 [52]. Reproduced with permission from BMJ Publishing Group Ltd.

Table 15.6 Comparative drug utilization studies measuring the uptake of new drugs.

Country	Setting	Year	Ref.	Study summary	Main finding	Purpose of drug utilization research
Canada	Primary care	2003	[56]	Analysis of the universal health insurance programme for persons aged 65 years and older, which covers the costs of prescription drugs. New drug utilization rates were assessed in 20 drugs that entered use between 1989 and 1994, in a stratified random sample of 1842 physicians.	The 20 new drugs were prescribed by 1.3–22.3% of physicians, and there was an 8–17-fold difference in new drug utilization rates. Characteristics associated with higher rates of utilization differed for GPs and specialists. Physician sex, specialty, medical school, years since graduation, practice location, volume and relative proportion of elderly patients influenced the utilization of new drugs.	Evaluation of prescriber and population characteristics that influence the utilization of new medicines.
Denmark	Primary care	2005	[57]	Analysis of the association between GPs' adoption of new drugs and previous prescribing of drugs belonging to the same therapeutic class. Information on all prescriptions redeemed at pharmacies in the County of Funen for esomeprazole, selective cyclo-oxygenase-2 inhibitors, new triptans and angiotensin-II receptor blockers was included in the study.	For esomeprazole and the new triptans, there was a higher preference for new drugs among 'high prescribers'. For the remaining two drug classes, the associations were weak. There is no consistent association between GPs' level of drug prescribing and their adoption of new drugs of the same therapeutic group.	Evaluation of the characteristics of prescribers that influence utilization of new medicines.
Sweden	Primary care	2009	[58]	Investigation of the role that patient characteristics and factors related to outpatient health care practice played in physicians' propensity to prescribe rosuvastatin following its introduction. Used the Swedish Prescribed Drug Register (SPDR) and a dataset from the Skåne region.	Prescribing of rosuvastatin was observed to be greater in younger patients (compared to older) and in patients with higher socioeconomic status (compared to lower). It was concluded that there was an inequity in health care, as the socioeconomic status of the patients appeared to influence the prescribing behaviour of the physicians irrespective of medical need.	Evaluation of prescriber and population characteristics that influence utilization of new medicines.
France	Primary care	2013	[59]	Statin prescribing habits from 341 GPs included in the IMS-Health Permanent Survey on Medical Prescription in France, which was conducted between 2009 and 2010 and involved 14 360 patients.	There was significant variability in the prescribing of different statins depending on patient and physician profiles, where young patients were prescribed patented statins more often if they suffered from heart disease. Also, older male physicians and GPs in solo practices were more likely to prescribe patented statins.	Evaluation of prescriber and population characteristics that influence utilization of new medicines.

Comparative drug utilization studies provide transparency and input for other areas of research

In Germany, analyses of all prescriptions reimbursed by the statutory health care system using World Health Organization (WHO) methodology (ATC and DDD), reporting drug utilization status and trends, are published annually as a book containing detailed volume information for the 3000 top sellers in the drugs market. This is used by researchers in fields as diverse as policy and public health [60].

In many countries, such as the Netherlands [28] and Wales [61], information and solutions for the proper, safe, affordable and effective use of medicine are available in primary care. These include comparative drug utilization analysis of GP prescribing behaviour and reports on individual GPs or GP practice groupings.

Conclusion

Comparative drug utilization research has many applications across acute and ambulatory care settings and is an effective tool for investigating and influencing prescribing. This chapter provided examples of where comparative drug utilization research studies have investigated adherence to guidelines, variation in prescribing, the uptake of new medicines and the influence of prescribed medicines on the health of patients and the wider community. In hospitals, these studies tend to require dedicated data collection and involve a relatively small number of patients compared to studies in the ambulatory care setting, where details of prescriptions dispensed by community pharmacies are collected when they are reimbursed by insurers (government or private). The ambulatory data are comprehensive for the population covered by the insurance programme but often do not include key pieces of information (e.g. diagnosis, dose), and therefore are often linked to other datasets in order to fill in the gaps. Collecting data expressly for the purposes of drug utilization research can be time-consuming and is therefore often done only for a sample of the population or for a short period of time (e.g. point-prevalence surveys), but it can provide an in-depth understanding of prescribing variation, quality and safety that is not possible with data collected for other purposes.

Future improvements in comparative drug utilization research will come from an increasing use of integrated electronic medical records in the hospital setting and the linking of these records with those that already exist in ambulatory care to create a comprehensive record of prescribed medicines. This will allow for improved techniques to account for variation in prescribing (e.g. the difference in case mix between prescribers, practices and hospitals). Integrating this with reimbursement data will provide an opportunity for increasingly in-depth and comprehensive comparative drug utilization research.

CHAPTER 16

Time-dependent and seasonal variations in drug utilization

Eric Van Ganse[1], Laurent Laforest[1] & Niels Adriaenssens[2]

[1]*PharmacoEpidemiology Lyon (PEL), HESPER Unit, Claude-Bernard University-Lyon1, and CHU-Lyon*

[2]*Centre for General Practice, Department of Primary and Interdisciplinary Care (ELIZA) and Laboratory of Medical Microbiology, Vaccine & Infectious Disease Institute (VAXINFECTIO), University of Antwerp, Belgium*

KEY POINTS

- Drug use varies over time for a number of reasons, including normal life cycle changes, emerging safety concerns and interventions from health authorities.
- There are a number of stages in the life cycle of a drug: launch, uptake and growth, plateau and decline.
- Decline can occur due either to safety issues or to the emergence of new (safer and/or more effective) therapeutic interventions.
- The season can influence drug use, but seasonal variation transcends calendar dates.
- Evaluation of time-dependent or seasonal variations in drug use may be a useful tool in public health surveillance.

Introduction

This chapter provides an overview of variations in drug use over time. While this aspect of drug use is often overlooked, it is nonetheless of major interest in terms of public health surveillance and health policy. The chapter starts with a general discussion of the life cycle of a drug, then presents a nonexhaustive list of factors potentially explaining drug variations over time, with examples of these variations in different domains of public health. It also provides illustrative examples of seasonal variations in drug utilization. Time variations in drug use related to patient adherence are addressed in Section F.

Life cycle of a drug

Even in the absence of external events (safety issues, regulatory interventions), drug utilization patterns change over time.

Once a drug is marketed, variable rates of uptake are observed during the initial post-launch period, with more marked trends if the new drug provides new benefits compared to pre-existing therapy. Figure 16.1 illustrates the uptake of tiotropium after its launch in France in 2006. Tiotropium was the first drug of a new chronic obstructive pulmonary disease (COPD) therapy class – long-acting antimuscarinic agents – considered to be the cornerstone of COPD management [1].

Progression of drug use tends to slow over time, suggesting that a peak number of users will eventually be reached (see Figure 16.1). Interestingly, treated patients do not necessarily correspond to the population actually targeted by the drug ('target population'). Such slowdown does not mean that a plateau will always be reached after launch, as patterns of use over subsequent years depend on many factors. First, the prevalence of the targeted disease may change over the years, as might the quality of the diagnosis (e.g. screening or identification of new phenotypes that respond to treatment), the characteristics of the populations of interest or the population's access to medical care. Likewise, changes in disease management may occur following a release of new guidelines, when new medications or drug safety

Drug Utilization Research: Methods and Applications, First Edition. Edited by M. Elseviers et al.
Published 2016 by John Wiley & Sons, Ltd.

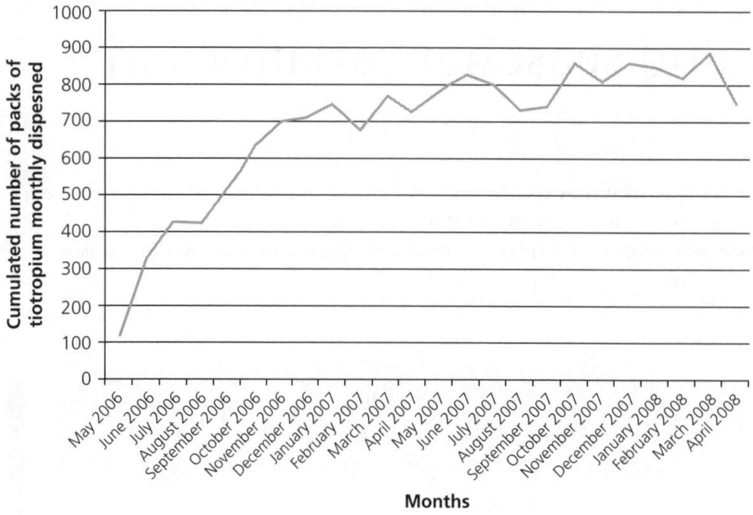

Figure 16.1 Tiotropium uptake in the French Rhone-Alpes region.

Source: Regional claims data (URCAM Rhone-Alpes).

concerns appear, or in case of extensions of the target population or of drug indications. For instance, a steady upward trend has been observed over recent years for statin users (Figure 16.2) [2], given the ageing of the population [3], improved screening and management of cardiovascular risk factors [3] and other potential benefits (pleiotropic effects). Incidentally, the prevalent use of statins has resulted in corrective actions by health authorities in some countries, in order to foster the use of generics or cheaper statins.

Acute interruptions or alterations in the process of the natural life cycle of a drug are possible. For example, the withdrawal of cerivastatin in Italy in 2001 resulted in a temporary slowing down of the upward trend of global statin use (Figure 16.3) [4]. Interestingly, the withdrawal of a medicine may temporarily impact the overall use of the corresponding drug class.

Although the precise timing of such occurrences is unpredictable, the use of some drugs may decline progressively over time due to the introduction of safer or more efficacious ones. This decline can lead to a limited level of use or to commercial withdrawal. In asthma, for example, cromones have been almost totally overshadowed by inhaled corticosteroids, which are more effective [5]. A similar decline has been observed for xanthines in Western countries [5,6]. Finally, changes in reimbursement rules or in conditions of dispensation (from prescription-only medication (POM) to over-the-counter (OTC) drugs), the emergence of generic drugs and transitory episodes of drug shortages should not be overlooked as potential modifying factors during a medication's life cycle.

However, not all older drugs disappear when more effective and/or better tolerated new drugs are introduced into the market. Some may eventually get a second life with the discovery of a new pharmacological effect of interests. As an example, aspirin was once one of the most commonly used pain relievers. Today, it has been widely replaced for this indication by safer and/or more effective new molecules, but it still remains a pivotal therapy for its platelet-aggregation-preventing properties at low dose. Another reason for drug revival might be the discovery of therapeutic problems with the replacement drugs.

Examples of factors influencing the natural life cycles of drugs

Improved knowledge about drugs

The improved knowledge of pharmacotherapy provided by medical research (randomized controlled trials (RCTs), pharmacovigilance and pharmacoepidemiology studies) contributes to changes in drug utilization through its impact on medical guidelines, physicians' drug prescribing habits and patients' drug use. Drug research studies can highlight the points of interest in new drugs, by comparing their properties with those of the existing therapy. Observational studies may also reveal beneficial/adverse properties of an existing drug

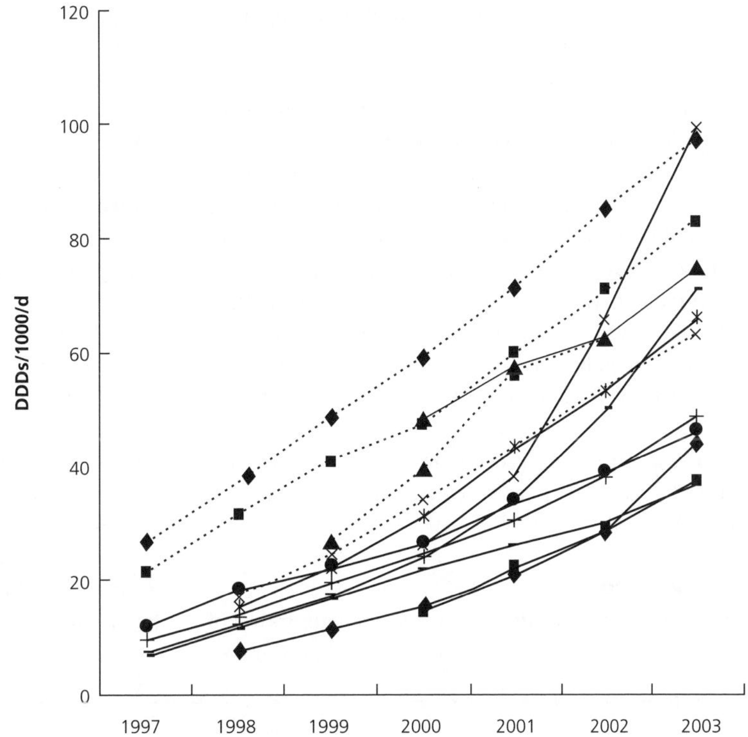

Increase in stain utilization. Norway (··◆··), Netherlands (··■··), Belgium (··▲··), Sweden (··×··), Finland (—✳—), Germany (—●—), Spain (—+—), UK (—▬—), Austria (—▬—), Denmark (—◆—),Italy (—■—), France (—▲—), Ireland (—×—)

Figure 16.2 Statin utilization from 1997 to 2003: annual defined daily doses (DDDs)/1000 inhabitants/day of statins.

Source: Walley et al. [2]. Reproduced by permission of John Wiley and Sons.

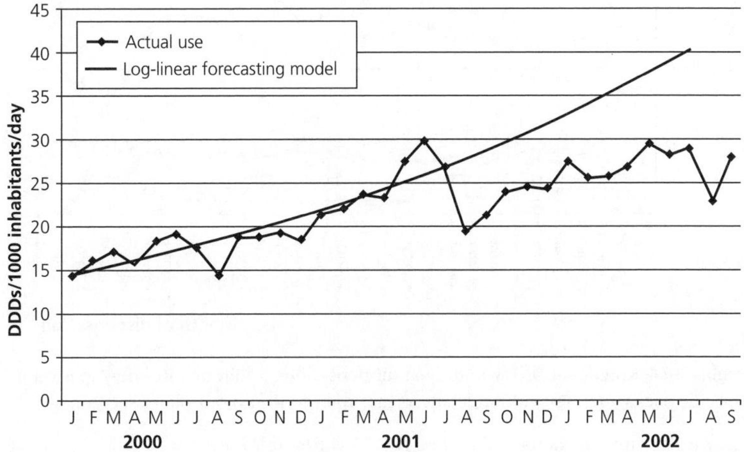

Figure 16.3 Monthly trend in statin use in Italy in the period January 2000–September 2002. Italian National Drug Utilisation Monitoring Centre (OsMed) data.

Source: Maggini et al. 2004 [4]. Reprinted with permission from Elsevier.

that were either unsuspected or difficult to highlight using short-term RCTs. Additionally, they can detect potential drug misuse and safety concerns, allowing corrective actions by the health authorities, care-givers or public health managers. More particularly, key landmark studies reporting pivotal findings of interest for medical practice have a marked influence on drug use after publication. For instance, the Scandinavian Simvastatin Survival Study highlighted a prolonged survival when patients with a history of coronary heart disease (CHD) received long-term treatment with simvastatin [7]. This key publication, and similar ones, contributed to the sizeable development of statin use at the population level during the following decades, notably for cardiovascular secondary prevention. The role of the marketing activities of pharmaceutical companies should not be ignored.

Safety issues

Rather than a gradual decline over years, withdrawal of a drug over safety issues entails its abrupt disappearance at the population level. Yet, this disappearance may occur stepwise if the initial safety concerns are not immediately followed by the withdrawal decision. Such was the case for dextropropoxyphene (DXP). In June 2009, the European Medicines Agency (EMA) [8] recommended the removal of DXP from the European market as the risk of potentially fatal overdose was felt to outweigh the drug's benefits. The recommendation to withdraw the molecule was announced almost 2 years in advance of the actual withdrawal, to allow time for the safe transfer of patients to appropriate alternative therapies. In France, DXP was withdrawn in March 2011 by the national health authority. The withdrawal pattern was investigated in the French Rhone-Alpes region using local claims data, and it was found that withdrawal occurred stepwise: the decline of dispensations was closely related to the successive decisions issued by the different health authorities (Figure 16.4). A two-stage downward trend was identified, with an initial drop during the summer of 2009 after the EMA recommendation, followed by a 16-month plateau and

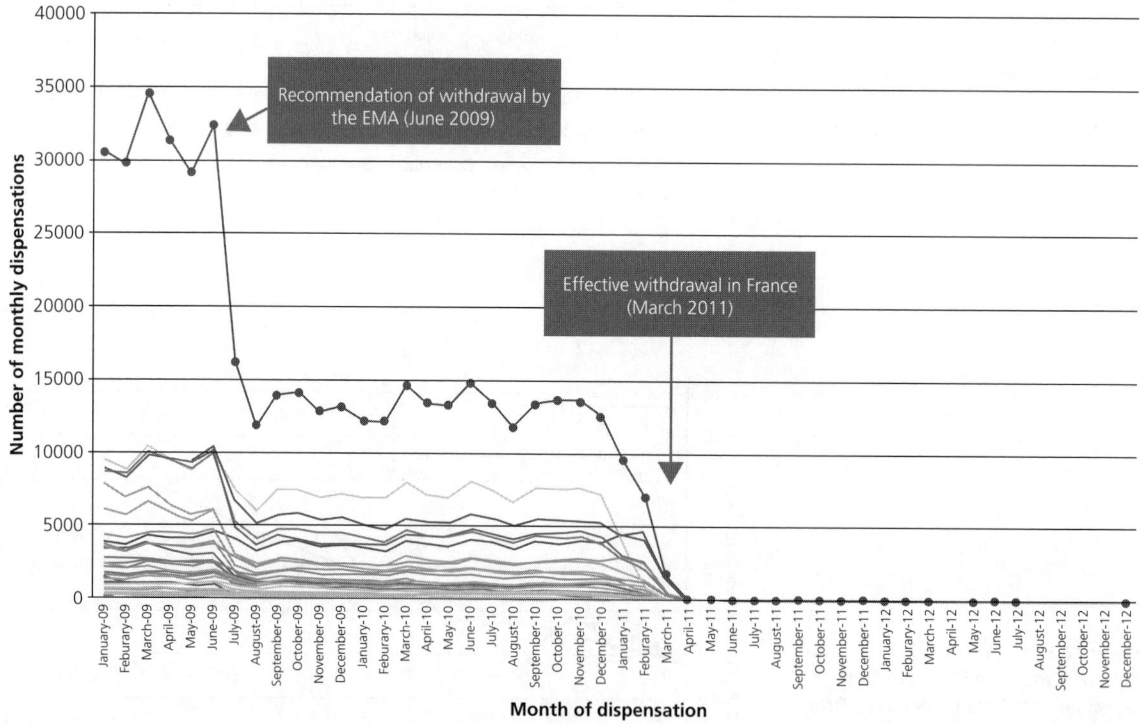

Figure 16.4 Kinetics of DXP withdrawal (dispensations) in French Rhone-Alpes claims data, 2009–2012. Different curves show specific packagings. For colour details, please refer to the colour plates section.

Source: Data from Regional claims data (URCAM Rhone-Alpes).

then full dispensing cessation in spring 2011. If the actual consumption of DXP (rather than dispensing data) had been studied, a tail distribution throughout 2011 and possibly 2012 might have been observed, due to storage of the drug by patients.

When a drug is withdrawn or its use is in natural decline, it is of interest to investigate by which drugs it is replaced, and particularly by which drug class. An increasing use of substitutive drugs might entail other specific public health issues. Rofecoxib was used chronically in rheumatoid arthritis and in osteoarthritis before its withdrawal due to cardiovascular concerns. Several surveys suggested that this withdrawal was accompanied by a concomitant decline of the other COX-2 molecules, such as celecoxib [9]. In turn, a higher use of more basic therapies, such as nonselective nonsteroidal antiinflammatory drugs (NSAIDs), was observed, raising concerns about gastroprotection in the management of these diseases [10]. These episodes suggest that a drug that is supposed to be replaced by a more effective and/or safer molecule may unexpectedly regain interest if safety concerns occur with the replacement therapy [10].

Another example is the common use of antidepressants, which may be problematic during pregnancy, given the potential increased risks of neonatal adverse outcomes [11]. These risks prompted the release of public health advisories in the United States and Canada in 2004, the impact of which was assessed using an interrupted time-series design (see Chapter 11) in Medicaid-insured pregnant women [12]. It was found that antidepressant prescribing levels decreased by 1.48 prescriptions per 1000 women per month during the post-warning period (October 2004–June 2005), while they had increased at a rate of 0.46 prescriptions per 1000 women per month during the pre-warning period).

Reimbursement restriction and incentives

Public health interventions based on reimbursement restrictions may impact acute or chronic drug exposure over time by encouraging a more rational use and/or correcting potential misuses, which may facilitate rational use of health care resources and optimize costs. For instance, a steady increase in statin consumption in Italy triggered an intervention from the national health authorities in 2004 to improve the appropriateness of prescribing. The revision of the reimbursement criteria was associated with a significant slowdown of the upward trend observed for statin dispensing levels over the 2004–07 period: the average monthly increase declined from +1.7% before intervention to +0.5% afterwards [13].

Although an increase in patient copayments may be efficient in limiting drug misuse, it can also negatively impact quality of care. For instance, an increase in copayments in Australia in 2005 expectedly reduced the overall dispensing volume of drugs in subsequent months (January 2005–September 2007) compared to the initial reference period (January 2000–December 2004). However, this measure also affected the use of preventive therapy for chronic and/or serious diseases, such as asthma, diabetes, epilepsy and glaucoma (from −3.2 to −10.9%, according to the different drug classes) [14]. Such decreased use of preventive therapy may have detrimental consequences for quality of care. Indeed, inadequate therapeutic prevention is a well-known source of disease-related severe adverse events in preventable chronic diseases.

More generally, changes in the organization of health care and in access through local subsidy schemes can entail large variations of drug consumption over time.

Educational campaigns/academic detailing

In chronic diseases, long-term community-based educational programmes can be useful in rationalizing management and limiting induced costs, by modifying patients' inappropriate drug use. Rational management in asthma, for example, primarily necessitates a regular use of maintenance therapy (controllers) to prevent exacerbations. Controllers are often inadequately used by patients, at the expense of symptomatic drugs (relievers).

For instance, a pharmacy-based educational campaign conducted in asthma patients in Australia [15] showed that patients provided with asthma education significantly improved adherence to controllers (OR = 1.9, 95%CI = [1.1–3.3], $p = 0.03$) compared to control group, while the average reliever consumption declined (−149 µg, $p = 0.03$). No significant changes appeared in the control group with no education. Although changes in drug habits induced by education can result in higher medication-related costs, these are widely compensated by the savings caused by fewer exacerbations. This was the conclusion of another educative programme campaign conducted in pharmacies across North Carolina [16]. Indeed, after educational activities, asthma patients had better adherence to controller therapy, which resulted in reduced exacerbations and less unscheduled medical care (notably, hospital contacts). Total asthma-related costs were significantly lower after education than the projections based on the study population's historical trends. Direct cost savings averaged US $725/patient/year, and indirect cost savings were estimated to be US $1230/patient/year. Indirect costs due to missed/nonproductive workdays decreased from 10.8 to 2.6 days/year.

Educational campaigns can also efficiently improve the use of acute drugs by limiting potential abuses. The high use of antibiotics in France remains an issue compared to other European countries [17]. A national campaign ('Antibiotics are not Systematic') was launched in 2002 to limit unnecessary prescriptions in ambulatory care. Compared to a baseline period (2000–2002), a 26.5% decrease was observed in antibiotic prescription rates over the following 5 years, after adjustment for flulike syndromes during the winter seasons [18].

Environmental factors

The environment can be a source of variation for drug consumption over time, with temporary or cyclic occurrence of exposure to allergens (e.g. pollens), infections or pollution. At a longer time scale, long-term evolution of climate can induce environmental modifications. Such changes may entail the emergence of new diseases or modify the prevalence and/or severity of existing ones [19].

Economic context

Changes in economic context, such as the occurrence of financial crises, may affect access to medications due to the development of social difficulties [20]. A receding economy can cause a general decrease in drug consumption at the population level, as less priority is given to health, which is overshadowed by more immediate issues and/or the development of financial barriers for some patients [21]. In parallel, induced social difficulties lead to more frequent major depressions [22], which can impact the use of antidepressants and benzodiazepines at the population level.

Societal factors

At the societal level, the traditional media or the Internet can influence the time variation of a given therapy by encouraging its use or its avoidance (whether justified or not). In France, the emergence of several cases of demyelinating diseases after antihepatitis B vaccination resulted in a lack of confidence regarding this vaccine among both the general population and health care providers. In addition to the initial precautionary measures taken by the authorities to limit the vaccination programme for hepatitis B, fears among the population were magnified by the lay press [23]. A marked and prolonged decline of the vaccination rate was observed [24].

Societal lobbies and patient associations can also influence drug use over time.

The main factors influencing variations in drug use over time are summarized in Table 16.1.

Table 16.1 Potential factors influencing variations in drug utilization over time.

Knowledge about drugs, health authorities and pharmaceutical firms	
Changes induced by drug research and improved knowledge about therapy	New drug discovery, identification of unknown (beneficial/adverse) properties in existing drugs, identification of misuse at the population level
	Trigger changes in guidelines, prescribing habits and patient use
Changes induced by health authorities	Safety issues, optimization of use, economic context
	Modify patient access to the drug via corrective actions (reimbursement/ withdrawal) and/or educative campaigns
Marketing activities by pharmaceutical firms	Research, commercial communication and marketing of new drugs
Changes at societal level	
Traditional media, the Internet, consumer associations	Provision of information on therapy, amplification of news and beliefs about drugs
	Modify prescriber and/or patient perceptions and use
Changes due to external factors	
Environmental climatic factors	Temporary changes (allergens, pollutions, infections)
	Long-term changes in disease prevalence, emergence of new illnesses
	Cause increased/decreased use of the corresponding therapies
Worsening economic context	Decreased access to therapy (financial conditions make access difficult), increased psychological distress (higher use of psychotropic drugs)

Utility of variation in drug utilization over time in the surveillance of health care issues

Drug surveillance over time can be a valuable tool in monitoring health problems and quality of care in a population. Indeed, measuring changes in the use of a given drug over time can provide useful signals for public health. For instance, the detection of an increased need for acute symptomatic drugs may reveal the occurrence of health problems. Drug surveillance also provides the opportunity to appraise the magnitude of an identified problem and to follow its evolution over time (including the impact of potential corrective actions). Drug surveillance presents specific interest for chronic therapy, such as maintenance therapy for chronic disease, in terms of quality of care. Monitoring a treated population over time enables the detection of changes, either in disease prevalence, prescriber management or patient access and/or adherence to therapy [25,26].

Surveillance of diseases/health-related environmental issues

Over-the-counter medication

As patients commonly seek OTC medication to alleviate mild symptoms, drug-based systems tracking temporal trends in drug use have been implemented in some countries (e.g. Slovenia) in order to survey the incidence of common flu, using a 'basket' of medications related to flu symptoms, including antitussives, mucolytics and analgesics [27]. The authors underlined the reactivity of OTC drug monitoring in the context of mild diseases; such monitoring efficiently complements traditional family physician-oriented surveillance systems.

Prescribed therapy/refill data

Changes in the prescription and/or dispensation levels of a given drug over time may also constitute useful signals for public health. For instance, pharmacy refill data can provide timely information of help in characterizing local influenza activity, as exemplified by the rise of antiviral oseltamivir and zanamivir dispensing levels in Ontario pharmacies during the pandemic H1N1 influenza A in 2009 [28]. Interestingly, pharmacy-based surveillance appears to be more reactive than traditional clinical and laboratory surveillance, even when restricted to reimbursed therapy. Furthermore, physicians tend to anticipate their prescriptions before receiving laboratory confirmation, which took 12 days on average for H1N1. In this case, virtually no lag time was observed between case onset and antiviral prescription trend lines, as shown in Figure 16.5 [28].

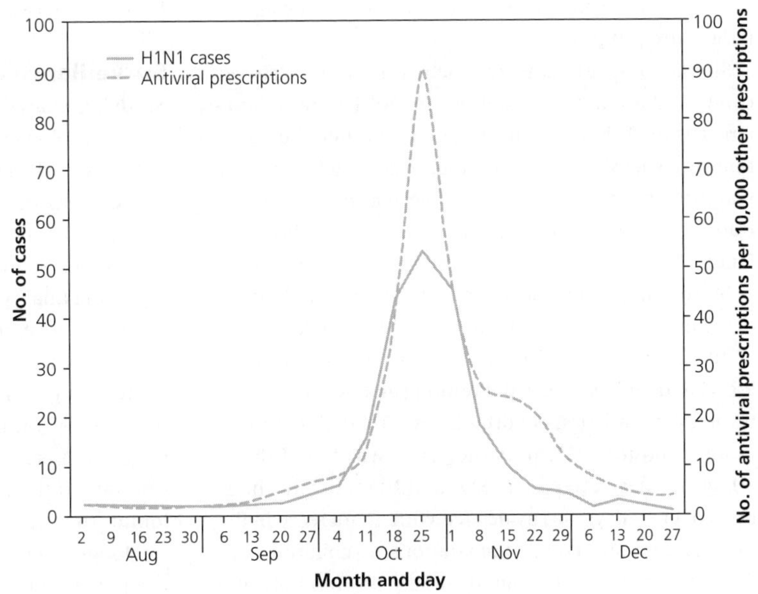

Figure 16.5 Average weekly number of influenza A (H1N1) cases and number of antiviral prescriptions per 10 000 other prescriptions reported at the local health authority level. Ontario, Canada, August–December 2009.

Source: Centers for Disease Control and Prevention. *MMWR* 2013;62:400–404 [28]. Reprinted from Value of Pharmacy-Based Influenza Surveillance – Ontario, Canada, 2009 with permission from the authors.

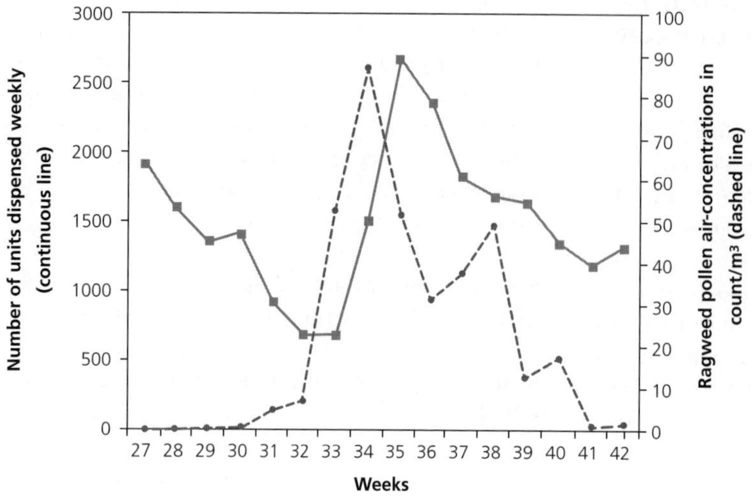

Figure 16.6 Ragweed pollen concentrations (dashed line) and antiallergic medication dispensing levels (continuous line) in community pharmacies located near a pollen collector in the Lyon-Bron area during the 2001 ragweed pollinic period (weeks 27–42).

Although mild conditions are often treated by symptomatic OTC therapy, sales of prescribed therapy can also constitute useful signals in this context.

In a study based on local claims data in Clermont-Ferrand, France, dispensations of antiallergic drugs (2000–2004) were found to vary over time with changing airborne pollen concentrations. These findings suggest that time-series analyses based on refills of reimbursed antiallergic drugs are useful in detecting and supervizing pollen-related diseases requiring ambulatory care [29].

Similar conclusions were reached in another survey conducted around Lyon during the 2001 ragweed pollen season. This study investigated whether the variation in dispensing levels of antiallergic drugs over time was influenced by changes in ragweed airborne concentrations obtained from a pollen collector, as shown in Figure 16.6 [30].

Monitoring drug use over time may also help in detecting air pollution-related health problems. An identified increase in respiratory drug use has been associated with airborne pollution peaks. A review confirmed that variations in drug use are related to air pollution exposure [31]. In particular, it was found that a 10 μg/m^3 mean increase in SO_2 and NO_2 air concentrations over 10 days was associated with an increase in the sales of cold and cough preparations in children aged 15 and younger [31]. Nonindustrial pollution may also result in increased use of asthma quick-relief medication, as exemplified by a study originating from natural, geologic sources in Alaska [32].

Interestingly, detection of health consequences of pollution peaks with variation in drug use over time, instead of collecting data on traditional outcomes such as mortality or asthma-related hospital contacts, could be an alternative when investigating pollution in small geographic areas or middle-sized cities, where counts of deaths and hospital admissions can be expected to be low [33].

Surveillance of drug abuse/misuse

Studying changes in drug use at the population level over a prolonged period may be helpful in detecting progressive deviation from recommendations, whether at the prescriber or at the patient level. Potential abuses might reflect unidentified physical or mental suffering, notably for relief medications, and could raise concerns regarding quality of care, safety and economic issues.

For instance, a steady upward trend in the prescribing of psychiatric medications has been observed in the United Kingdom over recent decades (1998–2010), particularly for antidepressants [34]. Conversely, no evidence supports a concomitant increase in the depression rate in the United Kingdom. Parallel investigations found that treated patients received antidepressants for longer periods, suggesting potential difficulties in stopping therapy or a lack of regular review of patients' prescriptions by their physicians. An extension of the prescription of antidepressants to other indications was also identified, notably for anxiety. Such identification of the suboptimal use of a drug can lead to corrective interventions from health authorities.

Examples of seasonal drug use variability

While some drug use remains continuous throughout the year, other use will increase or decrease with changes in the season or other specific repetitive and predictable events throughout the year. The description of seasonal drug use variability can help us better understand drug utilization, but it can also lead to misinterpretation. Statistical methods can be implemented to eliminate the impact of seasonality. The examples in this section will illustrate these concepts.

Antibiotics

Antibiotics are usually used to treat respiratory tract infections (RTIs). The incidence of most respiratory pathogens and the consumption of antibiotics follow a clear seasonal distribution, with a noticeable rise during the winter months [35,36].

In a longitudinal data analysis (1997–2009) of outpatient antibiotic use in Europe, a mixed-effects model was applied, taking into account (shifts in) seasonality (Figure 16.7) [37]. The results showed that the timing of the upward winter peaks and downward summer troughs in outpatient antibiotic consumption shift significantly

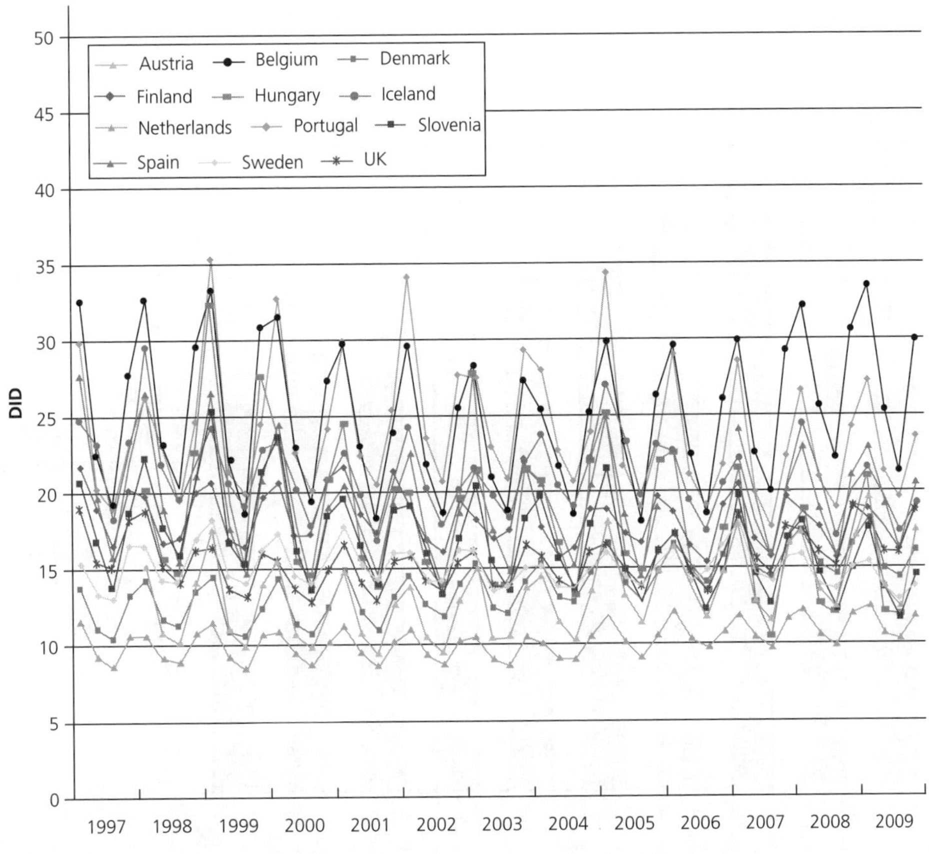

Figure 16.7 Seasonal variation in outpatient antibiotic use in 12 European countries, expressed in DDD/1000 inhabitants/day (DID). For colour details, please refer to the colour plates section.

Source: Adriaenssens et al. 2011 [37]. Reproduced by permission of Oxford University Press.

from one year to the next (phase shift) and that there is a significant positive correlation between volume of use and seasonal variation. This means that, in terms of absolute amounts, countries with high antibiotic use (suggesting use for nonbacterial RTIs, such as influenza) tend to have greater seasonal variation [36]. Therefore, time-dependent variation of antibiotics can also be used as a quality indicator of care [38] (see Chapters 13, 43 and 44).

Although seasonal variation is a constant factor in the interpretation of antibiotic consumption data, variations in the peak incidence of influenza and other RTIs can influence the interpretation of antibiotic consumption. In 1998, Belgium had the second highest rate of community antibiotic consumption in Europe. Nationwide campaigns promoting rational use of antibiotics in the community, organized by the Belgian Antibiotic Policy Coordination Committee, were launched in November 2000. Three successive winter campaigns (November to February) targeted both the public and prescribers [39]. Reimbursement data on antibiotic use in the period 1997–2005, expressed in antibiotic packs (as a surrogate for treatments), indicated that community antibiotic usage steadily decreased in the period 2000–03, with a larger decrease in 2004 and then a rise in 2005. To assess the effect of the campaigns on antibiotic sales, Bauraind et al. [40] suggested applying a statistical time-series analysis, controlling for the influence of the seasonal variation of influenza-like illnesses (ILIs). Weekly indices of ILIs were collected by the Belgian Scientific Institute of Public Health and revealed a peak in December 2003 (2003–04 winter season) and January 2005 (2004–05 winter season). Hence, in the 2004 calendar year (from January to December), the incidence of pathogens causing respiratory infections was lower compared to that in other years. Annual assessment of epidemiological seasons of RTIs (from July to June), rather than of calendar years, seems to reflect observed trends more accurately (Figure 16.8).

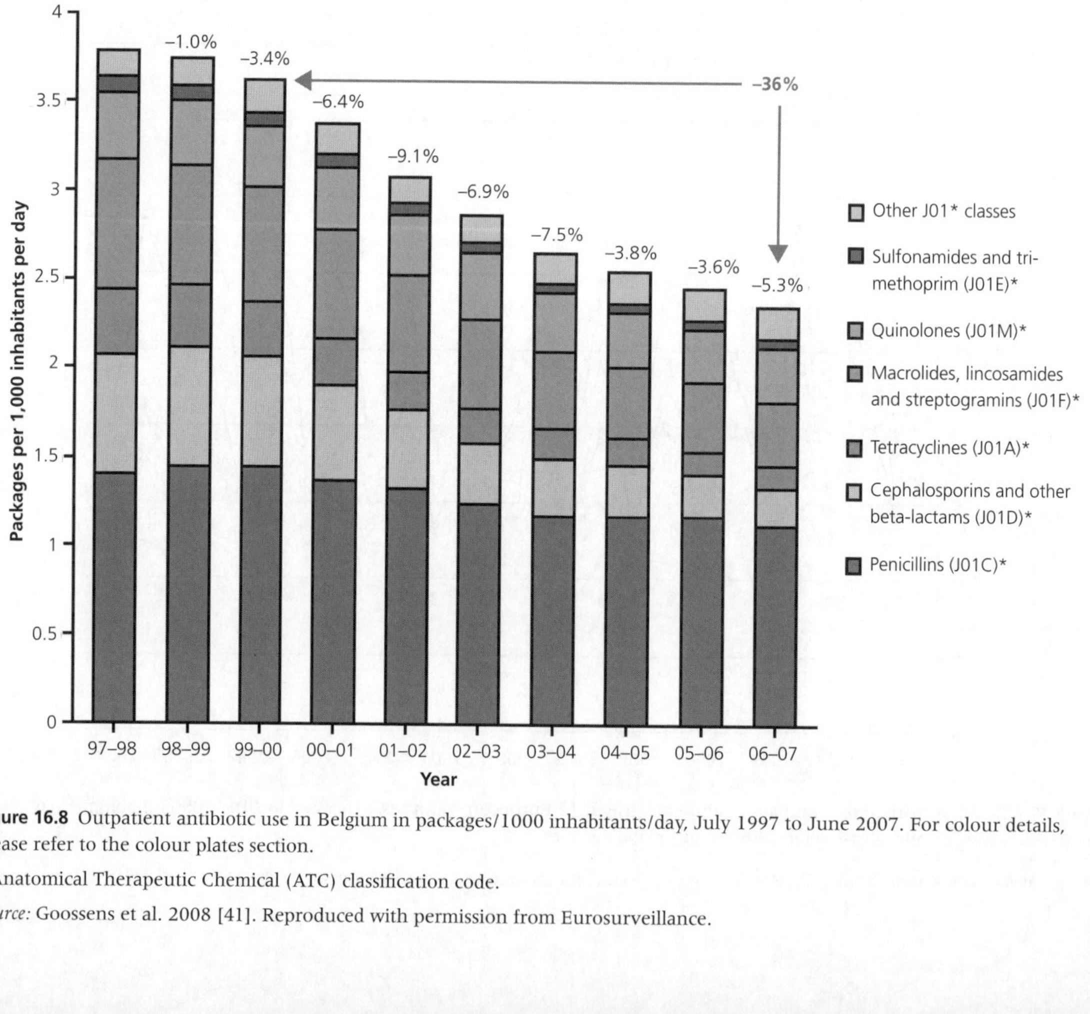

Figure 16.8 Outpatient antibiotic use in Belgium in packages/1000 inhabitants/day, July 1997 to June 2007. For colour details, please refer to the colour plates section.

* Anatomical Therapeutic Chemical (ATC) classification code.

Source: Goossens et al. 2008 [41]. Reproduced with permission from Eurosurveillance.

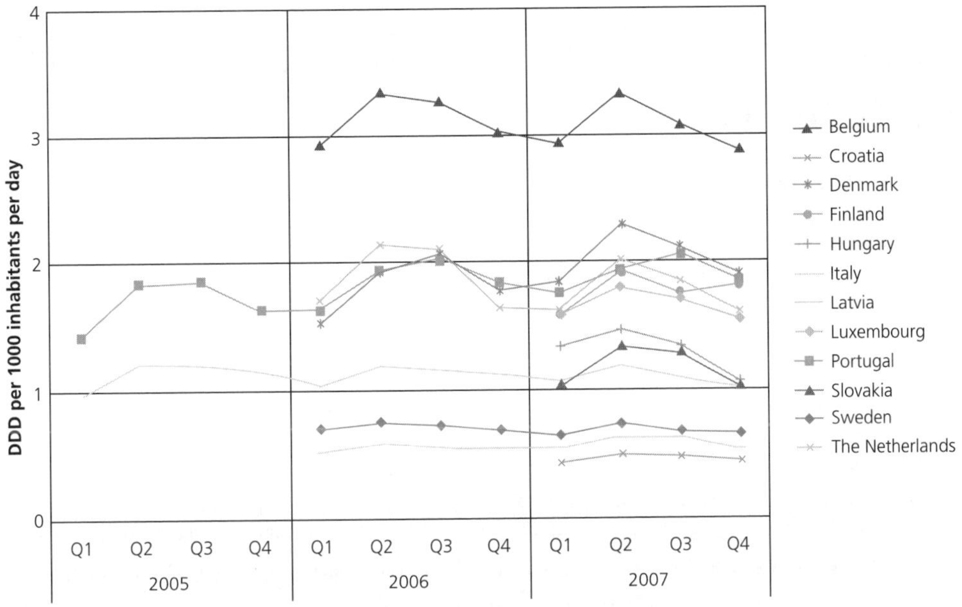

Figure 16.9 Seasonal variation in outpatient systemic antimycotic and antifungal use in 12 European countries. Data by quarter (Q) for 2005, 2006 and 2007. For colour details, please refer to the colour plates section.

Source: Adriaenssens et al. 2010 [42] Reproduced by permission of Oxford University Press.

Antifungi

For other types of antimicrobials, such as antifungal agents, a reversed seasonal variation can be observed; that is, lower use in winter and higher use in summer (Figure 16.9). However, it has not been established that this seasonal variation is due only to the incidence of dermato- and onychomycoses [42]; it has been hypothesized that, for aesthetic reasons, people who wear skin-revealing clothes and shoes may be more likely to consider seeking treatment for fungal infection, thereby contributing to the increased use of antifungal agents.

As already described, the use of antiallergic drugs is of interest for the surveillance of pollens and induced allergic diseases. Hence, prescribing patterns of antiallergic drugs can act as an indicator of variations in airborne pollen concentrations over time (see Chapter 5).

Conclusion

The examples presented in this chapter highlight the diversity of factors contributing to variations in drug use over time. Monitoring of drug utilization patterns over time can help detect infectious and/or environmental risk factors and thus lead to interventions by which to modify the consequences of these factors. Studying changes in drug exposure at the population level over an extended time period may be helpful in detecting progressive deviations from recommendations, whether at the prescriber or the patient level, thus providing information on the changes needed to improve quality of care. Evaluation of drug utilization over time is deserving of more attention by clinicians and researchers in pharmacoepidemiology.

CHAPTER 17

Comparative studies of patient and prescriber characteristics

Irene Eriksson[1], Ulf Bergman[2], Vera Vlahović-Palčevski[3] & Mia von Euler[4]
[1]*Centre for Pharmacoepidemiology, Department of Medicine, Karolinska Institutet, Sweden*
[2]*Department of Clinical Pharmacology, Karolinska Institutet, Karolinska University Hospital, Sweden*
[3]*Department of Clinical Pharmacology, University Hospital Center Rijeka, Croatia*
[4]*Department of Clinical Science and Education, Karolinska Institutet, Södersjukhuset, Sweden*

KEY POINTS

- Age, sex and socioeconomic factors, such as education and income, as well as the interaction between these factors, can influence patient health and well-being and have an impact on the utilization of both prescription and over-the-counter drugs.
- Prescribing preferences may vary between physicians and can be influenced by physician age, sex and specialty.
- Research exploring the impact of patient–physician concordance on drug utilization is scarce and has so far been limited to the assessment of single-measure concordance (e.g. language concordance). When studying patient–physician concordance, it is recommended that the cumulative impact of the concordance of patient and physician characteristics (social concordance) be assessed.

Introduction

Age, sex and socioeconomic factors, such as education and income, can influence patient health and well-being and have an impact on the utilization of both prescription and over-the-counter (OTC) drugs. Moreover, prescribing preferences can vary between physicians according to physician age, sex and specialty. The interaction of patient and prescriber characteristics can also impact the decision on whether or not the patient should receive a prescription and, if so, what drug to prescribe. Comparisons of drug utilization across patient and prescriber subgroups can help address a variety of questions, ranging from the appropriateness of drug use to the identification of subgroups to be targeted in academic detailing. In this chapter, we provide examples of drug utilization studies that illustrate how patient and prescriber characteristics, as well as the concordance of these characteristics, can influence drug use.

Patient characteristics and drug use

Age

As a consequence of age-related differences in the incidence, prevalence, presentation and prognosis of disease, medical needs can vary markedly between age groups. Assessment of drug utilization across ***age groups*** can give insight into the disease panorama by providing an overview of epidemiology, current treatment patterns and pharmacotherapeutic approaches to the prevention and treatment of diseases and related complications.

Age-associated changes in body composition and organ function, particularly in children [1] and the elderly [2], warrant close follow-up to ensure the safe and effective use of medicines in these populations. The very young and the very old have historically been underrepresented in clinical trials, resulting in limited information on drug safety and efficacy in these populations. Such limited inclusion in

Drug Utilization Research: Methods and Applications, First Edition. Edited by M. Elseviers et al. © 2016 John Wiley & Sons, Ltd.
Published 2016 by John Wiley & Sons, Ltd.

clinical trials may be explained by concerns over susceptibility to adverse drug reactions (particularly in children), multiple comorbidities and comedications (in the elderly) and inability to grant informed consent [3]. As medical needs are high in these age groups, particularly the elderly, so too is the demand for effective medical treatment. Assessment of drug use across age groups can provide information on over- or underuse of certain medications and inform prescribers, payers and regulators whether off-label use (outside licensed indications) is prevalent.

Given the growing pressures on health care systems and emerging unmet medical needs due to ageing populations, studies comparing age groups provide information that can help us understand and plan health care resource utilization. Table 17.1 provides some examples of studies comparing drug use among different age groups. For more examples of drug utilization studies in children and the elderly, as well as in pregnant women, see Section C.

Table 17.1 Examples of studies comparing drug utilization in different age groups.

Study	Country	Study summary	Main findings
Morbidity and medical care utilization of old and very old persons [4]	United States	The morbidity, health care, drug utilization and health status of random samples of HMO-enrolled Medicare beneficiaries (study period 1980–82) aged 65–79 and ≥80 years were compared	The health care needs of old and very old persons did not differ in terms of the type and extent of health care services and drug treatment required. The findings support the idea that noninstitutionalized very old persons are the healthy survivors of their cohort
Financial disparities in prescription drug use between elderly and nonelderly Americans [5]	United States	Out-of-pocket spending for prescriptions, copayment rates and the proportion of family income spent on prescription drugs were examined in elderly and nonelderly adult populations based on data from the 1998 Medical Expenditure Panel Survey	Elderly consumers overall were financially disadvantaged in out-of pocket spending for prescription drugs, out-of-pocket proportion and income proportion compared with working-age adults
Utilisation of medications recommended for chronic heart failure and the relationship with annual hospitalisation duration in patients over 75 years of age [6]	France	Patient characteristics, medications at discharge, outpatient medications and hospitalization frequency and duration were compared in all adult patients admitted to a teaching hospital with a main diagnosis of chronic heart failure over the course of a year (2000) using reimbursement claims data	At discharge, diuretic use was similar in the younger groups, but fewer older patients were prescribed angiotensin-converting enzyme (ACE) inhibitors or β-blockers. Thus, medications recommended for chronic heart failure patients were underused in the elderly
Treatment with statins after acute myocardial infarction in patients ≥80 years: underuse despite general acceptance of drug therapy for secondary prevention [7]	Norway	Information on demographic variables and drug therapy for acute myocardial infarction patients was obtained from hospital records and by direct patient contact or questionnaire in 1999/2000. The main indications for prescribing were recorded	Cardiovascular drugs were prescribed to about the same extent for very old and younger patients. The exception was lipid-lowering drugs, which were prescribed to a limited extent in the older patients
Drug use in centenarians compared with nonagenarians and octogenarians in Sweden: a nationwide register-based study [8]	Sweden	Drug utilization among elderly patients (July–September 2008) was compared using data from the Swedish Prescribed Drug Register. Age was categorized into three groups: 80–89, 90–99 and >100 years	On average, centenarians used a similar number of drugs compared to octogenarians. Institutionalization increased markedly with age
Effect of age on the profile of psychotropic users: results from the 2010 National Ambulatory Medical Care Survey [9]	United States	Psychotropic coprescribing, psychiatric diagnoses and other clinical characteristics of adult patients were compared based on data from the 2010 National Ambulatory Medical Care Survey	Psychotropic use in the absence of a psychiatric diagnosis was higher in every drug class for adults aged 65 and older

Sex and gender

Comparing drug use in ***men and women*** may yield important information on over- or underuse of medications. It has been observed that women in general are dispensed more prescribed drugs compared to men, even if hormonal contraceptives are excluded [10–12]. To what extent this reflects a higher medical need, overuse in women or underuse in men is unclear. Differences in drug use between men and women might be influenced by sex, gender or a combination of both [13]. Sex differences are due to biological differences between women and men, such as hormones, sex-specific gene expression from autosomes and body composition. Gender differences concern behavioural differences that arise as a result of a sociocultural process.

While it has been noted that life expectancy is lower in men [14], the perception of health and well-being has been shown nonetheless to be higher in men than in women [15]. It is possible that attitudes towards health and health-seeking behaviour vary between the sexes [10,16–18]. Studies have found that women seek health care more frequently and participate in preventive health care measures more readily than men [10,19,20], which results in women having a higher chance of being diagnosed and treated. Reproductive health and screening programmes for breast and cervical cancers lead to an increased number of health care consultations for women during a large part of their lives [19]. Screening for prostate cancer and urological disorders should do the same for men, but it starts later in life and is less well established. Furthermore, research shows that men may be less prone to seek preventive health care [20] or visit primary care physicians [21]. This may apply to adults only, as it has been found that there is no difference in health care-seeking behaviour between the sexes in the very young (which may, however, reflect the health care-seeking behaviour of parents) and the very old [22].

Reproduction-related differences between men and women (pregnancy, lactation, menopause) may explain some variations in the choice of prescribed drugs (see also Chapter 23). In studies of antiepileptic drug use, for example, men have been shown to use more valproic acid [23], which can be explained by its increased teratogenic risk compared to other antiepileptic drugs. Prescribers may, therefore, avoid using this drug in women of childbearing age [24].

Some sex differences in drug utilization can also be explained by differences in disease risk profiles, presentation of disease and overall morbidity, which can vary, as has been described for conditions as different as acute myocardial infarction and attention deficit disorders [25–27]. While observed differences in the use of antidepressants may reflect a higher prevalence of depression, anxiety and related disorders among women, they could also indicate that diagnostic criteria are better suited to detect depression in women or that men are more reluctant to seek medical care for mental problems [28]. Studies on differences between men and women in antihypertensive treatment show greater differences in the choice of drug than in the presence or absence of treatment [12,29].

Differences in adverse drug reactions (e.g. the higher risk of bradycardia associated with amiodarone treatment in women [30] or the higher risk of moderate to severe muscle pain on simvastatin or atorvastatin treatment in men [31]) may lead to variances in drug utilization. Physiological differences between men and women, such as the fact that women in general have a longer QT interval and are thus at higher risk of drug-induced ventricular tachycardia-type torsades de pointes, may explain susceptibility to adverse drug reactions [32].

Women have also been shown to use more diuretics and less angiotensin-converting enzyme (ACE) inhibitors than men, which may be explained by the more frequent presence of ankle oedema and the higher risk of coughing associated with ACE inhibitor use in women [12,29,33]. For angiotensin receptor blockers (ARBs), however, no differences in adverse drug reactions have been shown. As both ACE inhibitors and ARBs affect the same mechanism in the renin–angiotensin–aldosterone system, a correspondingly higher drug utilization of ARBs in women might be expected. However, studies in Sweden have shown this not to be the case, indicating a potential underuse of this drug class in women [4,33].

Interaction between age and sex needs to be considered when comparing drug utilization in men and women, as age at onset of disease can vary [34]. For example, age at first onset of cardiovascular diseases (CVDs) is, in general, 5 years earlier in men [16,35]. It is therefore important to either adjust for age or stratify analyses by age group when studying differences between drug use for conditions with differences in age of onset, as these may affect findings. This can be illustrated by a study which showed that β-blocking agents and cardiac glycosides were more commonly used in women in unadjusted analyses; after age adjustment, the observed association was reversed [12]. By contrast, in studies of anticoagulant utilization in patients with atrial fibrillation, women have been shown to use less anticoagulant drugs than men, despite women with atrial fibrillation being at a higher risk of embolic stroke [36]. After age adjustment, the difference becomes less pronounced, although it remains significant, suggesting a possible underutilization. The lower utilization of anticoagulants in women is often explained by women being older at the time of ischaemic stroke or transient ischaemic attack. Such underuse is, however, of concern, as the risk of an embolic event as the result of an untreated atrial fibrillation increases with age and is higher in women [36].

Analyses of the influence of age and sex can be performed either by stratifying the population by sex and/or age or by including these characteristics as adjustment variables in analyses. Examples of drug utilization studies comparing men and women are provided in Table 17.2.

Other sociodemographic factors

In addition to age and sex, sociodemographic factors such as ethnicity, education, occupation, income and civil status are frequently used in drug utilization studies as explanatory variables. Patterns in associations between sociodemographic factors and drug utilization are not homogeneous and may differ according to the type of health care system, therapeutic area and drug class studied.

If information on ***educational level and income*** can be collected and linked to drug utilization data, researchers can study associations between an individual's socioeconomic status and drug use. For example, a Norwegian longitudinal survey examined the relationship between socioeconomic status and antidepressant use among young adults [41]. Apart from education level of parents, all indicators of low socioeconomic status were related to higher rates of antidepressant prescription, which could be due to the association of low socioeconomic status with higher levels of anxiety and depression. Similar utilization patterns have been reported in Sweden, where the use of codeine and tranquilizers was reported to be higher in socioeconomically poorer areas [42,43].

An analysis of drugs dispensed during 2006 in Sweden showed that people with low education were generally prescribed more drugs [44]. Most differences appeared to correspond to those found in studies of the relationship between education and disease prevalence. However, some drugs, such as antibiotics, sildenafil, hormone replacement drugs, antimigraine drugs and angiotensin receptor blockers, were used in people with higher education to a greater extent than was expected from incidence and prevalence data. It should be acknowledged that these patterns may not be completely similar in other countries; this was illustrated when Danish and Swedish counties were compared and an opposite relationship between antibiotic utilization in children and the educational level of their parents was found [45]. Another drug utilization study of elderly persons in Sweden indicated that low educational attainment was associated with a greater likelihood of polypharmacy and potential inappropriate drug use [46]. This association persisted even after controlling for age, sex, place of residence and comorbidity. Moreover, the *type* of education may have an impact on prescribing patterns, as was shown in a Taiwanese study of diabetic patients with and without medical training. Patients with medical training were more likely to receive brand-name oral antidiabetic drug prescriptions than other diabetic patients [47].

Differences in health care service use among individuals with different ***ethnic and cultural backgrounds*** have been well established but are not fully understood [48–53]. Some of these disparities may be explained by socioeconomic status, attitudes towards health, adherence to physician advice, patient–physician communication, physician practice style and prescribing habits [54]. For example, a study on ethnic differences in access to prescription medication in New Zealand showed that ethnicity played a critical role in facilitating access to health care: the odds of postponing buying a prescription drug were approximately three times higher in the Maori and Pacific population compared to the New Zealand European population [55]. Beliefs and culture may also impact perceptions of health and health-seeking behaviours, as suggested in a study of insomnia and the use of hypnotics in the Sámi people of Norway [56].

Finally, a patient's ***social environment*** may have an impact on drug utilization. Thus, factors such as marital status and living arrangements (e.g. living alone, with a partner and/or with children) have been compared in drug utilization research, particularly in studies of psychotropic drug use [57,58]. Table 17.3 provides some selected examples of studies comparing drug use across various sociodemographic factors, including ethnicity, education, income and civil status.

Table 17.2 Examples of studies comparing drug utilization in men and in women.

Study	Country	Study summary	Main findings
Factors associated with the consumption of psychotropic drugs in a cohort of men and women aged 50 and over [18]	France	Sociodemographic, clinical and drug utilization data collected using self-administered questionnaire as part of the SUVIMAX (inclusion year 1994) prevention trial were compared in men and women	Socio-occupational factors in men and medical factors in women influenced the extent of use of psychotropic drugs
Gender and the use of neuroleptics in schizophrenia [37]	Finland	Prescribed daily doses of neuroleptics were recorded for schizophrenia patients, who were discharged from hospital (1982, 1986, 1990, 1994 cohorts) and followed up for 3 years. Daily doses of neuroleptics were compared	Men were prescribed higher daily doses of neuroleptics than women in practically all age groups, especially when the effect of age at first admission was controlled. There was no consistent increase in daily doses of neuroleptics in women after menopausal age
Gender differences in hypertension treatment, drug utilization patterns, and blood pressure control among US adults with hypertension: data from the National Health and Nutrition Examination Survey 1999–2004 [38]	United States	Drug utilization, medical history and blood pressure data for hypertensive male and female participants in NHANES 1999–2004 were compared	Hypertensive women were significantly more likely to be treated than men, but were less likely to have achieved blood pressure control. Additional efforts may be needed to achieve therapeutic goals for the hypertensive population, especially in women
Sex differences in risk factor control of treated hypertensives: a national primary healthcare-based study in Sweden [33]	Sweden	Sociodemographic, clinical, drug utilization (treatment with antihypertensive and lipid-lowering drugs) and smoking data were collected from primary care patients' medical records	Women were more often treated with diuretics and β-receptor blockers and men with ACE inhibitors, calcium channel blockers and lipid-lowering drugs. Both men and women were prescribed an equal number of antihypertensive drugs
A comparison of the frequencies of medical therapies for overactive bladder in men and women: analysis of more than 7.2 million aging patients [39]	United States	Frequencies of overactive bladder diagnoses and medical therapies by age and sex were compared using administrative claims data	Despite overactive bladder prevalence, many patients received no medical treatment. Men were significantly less likely than women to be treated with overactive bladder medications
Treatment utilization by gender in patients with borderline personality disorder [40]	United States	Parents of children diagnosed with borderline personality disorder (BPD) completed a 100-question anonymous Internet survey. The survey assessed aspects of treatment that included provider, setting, type, frequency, duration and cost	Male patients received significantly less lifetime psychotherapy and pharmacotherapy than female patients, although the duration of medication and psychotherapy treatment did not differ by sex
Differences in drug utilisation between men and women: a cross-sectional analysis of all dispensed drugs in Sweden [12]	Sweden	Drug dispensation data were used to compare drug utilization. All pharmacological groups with ambulatory care prescribing accounting for >75% of the total volume in defined daily doses (DDDs) and with a prevalence of >1% were included in the analysis	Women were dispensed more drugs in all age groups except <10 years. Substantial differences in the prevalence and incidence of dispensed drugs were found between men and women

Table 17.3 Examples of studies comparing drug utilization across various socioeconomic categories.

Study	Country	Study summary	Main findings
Ethnicity			
Ethnicity and prescription patterns for haloperidol, risperidone, and olanzapine [62]	United States	Administrative claims data were analysed for people with a diagnosis of schizophrenia or schizoaffective disorder who started treatment with olanzapine, risperidone or haloperidol	African Americans were significantly less likely to receive the newer antipsychotics. Among those who received the newer antipsychotics, ethnicity did not affect medication choice
Equality in the care and treatment of immigrants and native Swedes – a comparative study of patients hospitalised for heart failure [63]	Sweden	Medical records of immigrant and Swedish patients hospitalized for heart failure or chronic heart failure during 1994–2003 were analysed	The Swedish health care system had achieved its aim of equality in the care and treatment across patient groups
Ethnic differences in access to prescription medication because of cost in New Zealand [55]	New Zealand	Sociodemographic, health and health-behaviour data collected in a survey were analysed	Ethnicity independently predicted deferred prescription medication due to cost, with Maori and Pacific people having higher odds of deferring medication purchase than New Zealand Europeans
Use of hypnotics in Sámi and non-Sámi populations in northern Norway [56]	Norway	Sociodemographic, drug utilization, medical and other data were collected using a questionnaire and compared in the Sámi and non-Sámi populations	The stronger the Sámi affiliation, the lower the prevalence of use of hypnotics. In general, insomnia was less frequently stated in the Sámi than in the non-Sámi study population. This may reflect a different attitude to sleep as a phenomenon among the Sámi
Education			
Education and drug use in Sweden – a nationwide register-based study [44]	Sweden	Prescription drugs dispensed in Sweden in 2006 were analysed. Data on educational level were obtained from the National Education Register	Large differences were found in drug utilization between groups with different educational levels. Some disparities reflected differences in need, but there were also inequalities in drug use
Patterns of psychotropic medicine use and related diseases across educational groups: national cross-sectional survey [59]	Denmark	The prevalence of psychotropic drug use and related diseases in educational groups were studied using data from the Danish Health and Morbidity Survey 2000 (face-to-face interviews)	Psychotropic drug use was congruent with the distribution of related health problems, which means that the least-educated groups most in need of treatment had the most frequent drug use
Brand name or generic? What are the health professionals prescribed for treating diabetes? A longitudinal analysis of the National Health Insurance reimbursement database [47]	Taiwan	Drug utilization data, as well as data on medical training background, were obtained from the NHI Research Database. Drug prescribing patterns (brand versus generic) for patients with and without medical training background were compared	Patients' medical training background, in addition to the characteristics of patients, prescribers and medical settings and market competition, may influence physicians' prescribing choice of brand-name versus generic oral hypoglycaemic agents. Health professionals suffering from diabetes were more likely to be prescribed brand-name drugs

(continued)

Table 17.3 *(continued)*

Study	Country	Study summary	Main findings
Income			
Statin prescribing in Australia: socioeconomic and sex differences. A cross-sectional study [60]	Australia	Sociodemographic and drug utilization data were obtained from administrative data. The Socioeconomic Indexes for Areas was used to assign the quintile of Index of Relative Socio-Economic Disadvantage	Among men, there was either overprescribing of statins in the highest socioeconomic quintile or underprescribing in the lowest
Cardiovascular drug utilisation and socio-economic inequalities in 20 districts of the Czech Republic [64]	Czech Republic	Aggregate district-level drug utilization data from the General Health Insurance Company for the period 1997–2000 were analysed. Socioeconomic status was assigned at a district level	There was a significant gradient in the utilization of mainly newer CVD drug groups within districts, which might be explained by their socioeconomic characteristics
Patterns of benzodiazepine and antidepressant use among middle-aged adults. The Brazilian longitudinal study of adult health (ELSA-Brasil) [61]	Brazil	Sociodemographic, clinical and drug utilization data were collected for participants in the Brazilian Health Longitudinal Study. Antidepressant and benzodiazepine use were compared among sociodemographic groups	Higher educational level (>15 years of schooling) and having private health insurance were associated with antidepressant use. In Brazil, the higher antidepressant use among the higher socioeconomic strata may reflect difficulties in accessing public mental health care for most of the population; those from the higher socioeconomic strata can afford private mental health services
Civil status			
Socioeconomic determinants of psychotropic drug utilisation among elderly: a national population-based cross-sectional study [57]	Sweden	Psychotropic drug utilization data from the Prescribed Drug Register were linked to socioeconomic data. The associations between psychotropic utilization and marital status and income were assessed	There was an association between socioeconomic determinants and psychotropic drug utilization. The probability of using potentially inappropriate psychotropics was higher among individuals with low income and among the nonmarried
Living alone and antidepressant medication use: a prospective study in a working-age population [58]	Finland	Data on living arrangements (living alone versus not), psychosocial factors, sociodemographic factors and health behaviours were collected in a baseline survey in 2000. Antidepressant medication use was followed up from 2000 to 2008 through linkage to national prescription registers	People who live alone were more likely to have material and psychosocial problems, which might have contributed to excess mental health problems in this population group

Prescriber characteristics and drug use

While patient sociodemographic characteristics can influence which drugs are prescribed and how they are taken, decisions regarding whether or not to prescribe a drug and which drug to prescribe are reserved to the prescriber. Researchers compare prescribing patterns to determine whether certain characteristics may influence drug utilization patterns (e.g. uptake, prescriber adherence to guidelines, patient adherence to the prescribed regimen and appropriate use). In determining prescriber characteristics associated with drug utilization, age, professional experience (including number of years in practice) and specialty have been more extensively studied (see selected examples in Table 17.4). Such comparative studies are typically performed to help guide education programmes and interventions targeting prescribers in order to improve care and patient outcomes.

Table 17.4 Examples of studies comparing drug utilization across prescriber characteristics.

Study	Country	Study summary	Main findings
Age and time since graduation/certification			
Medical decision making in antipsychotic drug choice for schizophrenia [65]	Germany	Semistructured interviews with 100 psychiatrists on drug choice for 200 patients suffering from schizophrenia were conducted and data were analysed using multiple logistic regression	Older physicians were up to five times more likely to prescribe first-generation antipsychotics. Patient variables did not significantly influence treatment decisions
Quality of cardiovascular disease preventive care and physician/practice characteristics [66]	United States	A standardized online survey and experimental case studies were administered. Multivariable regression models tested physician age, sex, specialty and practice type as independent predictors of guideline awareness/adherence	Although guideline awareness was high, efforts to promote their utilization were needed to improve quality outcomes
Effect of board certification on antihypertensive treatment intensification in patients with diabetes mellitus [67]	United States	Demographic, laboratory data, billing codes and physician notes were obtained for hypertensive patients. Year of physician board certification was obtained from the American Board of Internal Medicine	Physician intensification of pharmacological therapy for blood pressure levels above the recommended treatment goals decreased with time since last board certification
Sex			
Association of physician's sex with risk factor control in treated hypertensive patients from Swedish primary healthcare [68]	Sweden	Physician age and sex, as well as sociodemographic, clinical and drug utilization (treatment with antihypertensive and lipid-lowering drugs) data, were collected from primary care patients' medical records	Female physicians appeared to reach the treatment goal for blood pressure in female patients and cholesterol level in all patients more often than did male physicians
Physician and patient gender concordance and the delivery of comprehensive clinical preventive services [74]	United States	Consecutive adult patient visits to family physicians were observed by research nurses. Delivery of sex-neutral preventive services was assessed by direct observation and medical record review	The interaction effect of physician and patient sex was not significantly associated with delivery of screening, counselling or immunizations
Is physician gender associated with the quality of diabetes care? [69]	United States	Patient data were obtained through survey, medical record review and health plan administrative records. Physician data were obtained from health plan administrative records	Patients of female physicians received similar quality of care to patients of male physicians
Physician gender and changes in drug prescribing after the implementation of reference pricing in British Columbia [70]	Canada	Administrative claims data on female and male physicians treating elderly Pharmacare enrolees who were prescribed a high-priced ACE inhibitor before the implementation of reference pricing were analysed	Physician sex was associated with slightly different patient management strategies regarding physician-requested exemptions after the start of a new drug cost-sharing policy
Physician gender, patient gender, and primary care [73]	United States	Data from the US National Ambulatory Medical Care Surveys 1985–92 concerning encounters between adult patients and primary care physicians (internists, family physicians and obstetricians/gynaecologists) were analysed	Female physicians were more likely to deliver prevention procedures to women, but few other physician sex differences in primary care were observed. Physician–patient sex concordance was a key determinant of encounters

(continued)

Table 17.4 *(continued)*

Study	Country	Study summary	Main findings
Specialty			
Knowledge and practices of generalist and specialist physicians regarding drug therapy for acute myocardial infarction [72]	United States	Cardiologists, internists and family practitioners were surveyed in order to assess their knowledge about and practices regarding drug therapy for myocardial infarction	Internists and family practitioners were less aware of or less certain about key advances in the treatment of myocardial infarction than were cardiologists
Differences in generalist and specialist physicians' knowledge and use of angiotensin-converting enzyme inhibitors for congestive heart failure [71]	United States	A national systematic sample of family practitioners, general internists and cardiologists was surveyed concerning knowledge of ACE inhibitors	Compared with cardiologists, family practitioners and general internists probably underutilized ACE inhibitors, particularly among patients with decreased ejection fraction who were either asymptomatic or post-myocardial infarction
Variations in management of common inpatient pediatric illnesses: hospitalists and community pediatricians [75]	United States	Hospitalists and community paediatricians were surveyed in order to collect data on the frequency of use of diagnostic tests and therapies for common inpatient paediatric illnesses	Overall, in comparison with community paediatricians, hospitalists reported greater adherence to evidence-based therapies and tests in the care of hospitalized patients and less use of therapies and tests of unproven benefit

While physicians with more experience accumulate knowledge and skills, their drive to adopt newer health technologies and incorporate the most recent advances in knowledge may be lower [76]. This can result in poor adherence to clinical guidelines and inappropriate prescribing, which may negatively affect patient outcomes [76]. On the other hand, rapid adoption of new drugs may lead to poor patient outcomes if knowledge about the safety profiles of new treatments and technology is lacking. Thus, physicians who prefer prescribing well-established drugs that are both effective and safe to rapidly adopting emerging technologies may in fact deliver better patient care.

Specialists tend to be more knowledgeable than general practitioners when it comes to clinical guidelines in their specific field and are more likely to follow these guidelines when prescribing [72]. This observed relationship does not always hold, however [77]. Furthermore, primary care physicians often need to consider comorbidities and make allowances for them when interpreting and implementing guidelines, and such considerations may affect prescribing. According to recent reviews, there is limited evidence on how comorbidity should best affect guideline recommendations [78,79]. Given ongoing initiatives to shift some health care services towards general practice, comparative research can be used to identify differences in prescribing among specialists and general practitioners and help guide interventions to improve prescribing.

When comparing drug utilization in subgroups of prescribers, researchers should bear in mind that certain patients (e.g. sicker patients or patients with higher expectations) may cluster with certain prescribers, so the population treated should be taken into account (e.g. adjustment for patient case mix can be done [80]) when analysing the data. Given that not all relevant information can be captured in data, it may be that observed associations between characteristics and prescribing patterns are just that – associations – and other factors explain the patient or prescriber behaviour. For example, among benzodiazepine users, long-acting benzodiazepine use was found to be more common among male patients and patients of earlier-graduating prescribers and specialist prescribers [81]. However, the effects of the latter two factors were modified by patient self-reported anxiety. This study demonstrated that consideration of patient factors may be necessary in order to obtain an accurate estimate of the association between at least some physician factors and the use of long-acting benzodiazepines. Furthermore, the complex interplay between patient and prescriber characteristics discussed in the next section may also play a role.

Concordance of patient and prescriber characteristics

Concordance can be defined as the degree of similarity or agreement across a given dimension [82]. Research suggests that among providers of care, concordance may result in less biased interpretations of viewpoints and symptoms, potentially improving communication and decision-making. Similarly, among patients, concordance has been shown to encourage more active participation in care, thus potentially improving communication with providers and optimizing health behaviours [83].

Language discordance (differences in proficiency in a given language) is an obvious barrier to communication between patient and health care provider. If given the choice, some patients might prefer to receive care from a physician able to communicate in their primary language. A US study examining the association between patient–physician ***language concordance*** and medication adherence rates found that language concordance was positively associated with adherence in Spanish-speaking patients [84]. American researchers also noted the preference for a ***race/ethnicity concordance*** among some groups of patients and suggested that people with limited English proficiency might be more likely to have same-race/ethnicity physicians as they feel more comfortable with a health care provider from the same cultural background [85]. Furthermore, ***gender concordance*** can also play a role in the delivery of health care services [73]. For certain interventions (e.g. cervical cancer screening) [86] and questions (e.g. questions about sexual health) [87], there may be some discomfort if the patient and physician are of opposite sex. In general, however, the evidence supporting improved outcomes in gender-concordant compared to gender-discordant dyads is limited [74,88].

Research exploring the impact of patient–physician concordance on drug utilization is scarce. A study in Medicaid enrolees found that while in the white population race concordance between patient and physician did not affect prescription use, it was however a significant predictor of drug utilization among the black population – black people with black physicians had lower rates of prescription use compared to those with white physicians. The study investigator postulated that this might be due to there being a better relationship between patient and physician, which helps them consider and implement lifestyle changes as a substitute to medicines [89].

Findings from studies examining the association between race concordance and medication adherence are inconsistent [84,90–93]. It is possible that a single-factor explanation may be an oversimplification of a complex interplay between patient and provider characteristics [82]. It has also been observed that increased patient trust is associated with significantly better adherence in all patients, irrespective of their being in race-concordant or -discordant pairs [93]. Race concordance has, however, been found to be associated with perceived similarity, and patients' perception of similarity to their physicians was identified as a strong predictor of their satisfaction with their care, trust in their physician and intent to adhere to treatment recommendations [94]. The same study also highlighted that in single-factor concordant dyads (e.g. race or sex), some patients rated themselves as very different from their physicians, and within discordant dyads, some patients saw themselves as very similar to their physicians.

The importance of understanding the cumulative impact of patient–physician concordance was highlighted by Thornton et al. [82], who established a framework for a multidimensional measure of shared social characteristics, called ***social concordance***, and recommended that researchers move beyond one-dimensional measures of patient–physician concordance to understand how multiple social characteristics influence health care quality.

Conclusion

Drug utilization results from a complex chain of events, beginning with the patient's decision to seek health care and continuing with the physician's interpretation of symptoms, diagnostic findings and medical history. A subsequent diagnosis may then be followed by the prescriber recommending a certain drug, which the patient may, or may not, agree to use. Once a drug is prescribed, it is finally up to the patient to decide whether or not to fill the prescription and take it as recommended. Patient and prescriber characteristics, such as age, sex and socioeconomic status, as well as the interaction between these factors, need to be considered when studying drug utilization.

CHAPTER 18

Comparative studies of health systems

Tatiana Chama Borges Luz[1], Claudia Garcia Serpa Osorio-de-Castro[2] & Björn Wettermark[3]

[1]*René Rachou Research Center, Oswaldo Cruz Foundation, Brazil*

[2]*Department of Pharmaceutical Policies and Pharmaceutical Services, Sergio Arouca National School of Public Health, Oswaldo Cruz Foundation, Brazil*

[3]*Clinical Pharmacology and Centre for Pharmacoepidemiology, Department of Medicine, Karolinska Institutet, Sweden*

KEY POINTS

- Countries across the world have organized their health care systems in different ways in terms of funding, structure and mode of operation. Comparative studies on drug utilization are valuable tools to promote development of health systems.
- Drug utilization studies may compare health system factors related to legislation for drug approval, prescribing regulations, drug supply structures, financing models and strategies by which to promote access to essential medicines and the quality use of medicines.
- A variety of methodological approaches have been used to compare drug utilization between health care systems. Further research is needed to develop good indicators for comparison purposes.
- There are currently few comparative studies of self-medication and drugs sold directly to the consumer without a prescription, but they have been gaining increasing attention recently due to quality and safety concerns.

Introduction

The huge disparities in health that exist between countries have been considered one of the greatest moral and intellectual problems of our time [1]. Comparative studies on health systems are valuable tools to identify these disparities and to find good examples of successful reforms and solutions. Many such studies focus on medicines, since these play an important role in all health care systems, promoting health and preventing and managing diseases.

Health care systems can be defined as a combination of all the resources, organizations and institutions that are dedicated to improving personal health through preventive, promotive, curative and rehabilitative health actions and interventions provided by both state and non-state actors [2,3]. Countries organize their health care systems in different ways in terms of funding, structure and mode of operation. The legislation and central coordination of the systems also differ, especially regarding the role of the state [2–5]. In the field of health systems research, many different typologies are used to categorize existing health care systems [6,7]. According to such aspects as funding and degree of state intervention, these systems can broadly be divided into four models: free market, social security, national health service and socialist health system [8] (Table 18.1).

In the ***free market*** model, health care is considered a commodity to be bought on the market and the state conducts a policy of noninterventionism. This model is adopted by countries such as the United States, South Africa and Switzerland. In the ***social security*** model, adopted by Belgium, France, Germany, Japan and the Netherlands, health care is guaranteed through mandatory insurance and the state's role is considered intermediate; that is, it has a strong influence of health care providers and (social) insurers. The ***national health service*** model, present in countries such as Australia, Canada, Denmark, Finland, Italy, New Zealand, Norway, Spain, Sweden and the United Kingdom, is a tax-based model, in which health care is seen as a guaranteed, state-supported consumer service. Within this

Drug Utilization Research: Methods and Applications, First Edition. Edited by M. Elseviers et al. © 2016 John Wiley & Sons, Ltd.
Published 2016 by John Wiley & Sons, Ltd.

Table 18.1 Health care system models and drug utilization research interface.

Source: Adapted from WHO Public–Private Roles in the Pharmaceutical Sector: Implications for Equitable Access and Rational Drug Use, 1997.

	Free market	Social security	National health service	Socialist health system
Countries	United States, South Africa and Switzerland[a]	Germany, The Netherlands, France, Belgium and Japan[b]	United Kingdom, Australia, New Zealand, Canada, Sweden, Denmark, Norway, Finland, Spain and Italy	Cuba, Belarus and China[c]
Advantages	Probably accounts for the majority of over-the counter (OTC) sales May be technically efficient: the profit incentive may enable private drug suppliers to deliver drugs to patients at low cost	May capture some of the benefits of the supposedly superior distribution efficiency of the private sector	Dedicated to providing the best possible care to each individual at the best cost for the system Comprehensive care is valued	Fully public systems can potentially be very equitable ones and monopsony (single-buyer) power in purchasing helps procure drugs at low cost
Disadvantages	In some countries, there are substantial problems with the provision of low-quality drugs, inappropriate drugs and incomplete treatment courses Cost may be high for the health benefit gained. A fully private system is also likely to impede access for those with lower incomes who are unable to pay for drugs	The cost of administrative expenditures is probably higher and there may be limited financing Potential adverse implications for equity. A special concern is rational drug use, when providers have a direct financial incentive to prescribe more drugs or more expensive drugs	Gratuity is not necessarily involved in universal care Pressures from the pharmaceutical industry for drug incorporation may make balance between universal provision of essential medicines and pharmacotherapeutic innovation difficult to achieve	May offer insufficient incentives for efficient behaviour by the distributor Total amount spent on drugs is constrained by the government budget
Characteristics of drug procurement and distribution	Patients or private insurers pay the entire cost of drugs, purchasing from private retail pharmacies and drug sellers	Pharmacies or patients are reimbursed for drugs provided through private pharmacies Drugs are supplied by government medical stores or state-owned wholesalers and dispensed by government health facilities, but paid for (in whole or in part) by patient fees	Usually, nominal universal access to health care Social agreements are sealed to make policy decisions as to medicines selection, procurement and distribution	Drugs are financed, procured and distributed by a centralized government unit
Drug market regulation	Often low	Varied	Varied	Strong
Drug information availability	Fragmented; industry harnesses considerable quantities of drug information	Drug information is less fragmented but availability is limited	Drug information is theoretically centred in the health system; patient-level information may be available for health care and research Health information systems may or not be linkable	Drug information systems are not freely accessible

[a] Most countries worldwide present this model at some level of the health care system

[b] Several countries in South America, Asia and Africa also present this model.

[c] Other former communist countries share this model.

model, the state has a strong role in controlling and financing health facilities. Finally, in the ***socialist health system***, the most centralized type of health care system, the state owns facilities and pays providers directly. Cuba, China, Russia, Belarus and other former communist countries in Central and Eastern Europe operate this type of health care system [8].

It is important to note that health care systems around the world are continuously changing [5], and these four 'pure' models can be seen in many combinations and varieties. In practice, a mixture of public and private strategies, in varying proportions, frequently exists to deliver health care in most countries [9].

All health care systems face the challenge of improving population health and improving patients' experience of care, while at the same time reducing per capita spending for health care [10]. Various measures are undertaken to improve health status, protect society against health-related financial risk and meet the needs and expectations of the population [11]. Six core components have been identified as contributors to the strengthening of health care systems: service delivery, health workforce, health information systems, access to essential medicines, financing and governance [2,12].

Medicines are integrated into these strategies, as they play a crucial role in health care, promoting health and preventing and managing diseases. They also account for an increasing proportion of health care spending, with a growth of more than 50% in the Organisation for Economic Co-operation and Development (OECD) countries during the 2000s [13]. Medicines can account for up to 60% of total health care expenditure in some countries [14]. Overall, in low- and middle-income countries, health care expenditure accounts for between 13 and 32% of household expenditures, and between 41 and 56% of households in these countries spend all their health care expenditure on medicines [15]. Medicines can also be harmful, and their inappropriate use has serious medical, social and financial implications. Inadequate supply of medicines may lead to treatment failure and loss of confidence in the health care system. Consequently, the World Health Organization (WHO) advocates that access to essential medicines constitutes the most cost-effective element of any health care system. A well-functioning health care system must, then, ensure equitable access to medicines of proven quality, safety and efficacy [2,16].

Given that misuse, overuse and underuse of medicines can result in poor health outcomes and a waste of resources, various pharmaceutical policies and interventions are implemented by governments and other third-party payers to control expenditures and facilitate rational drug use [17–22]. Globalization has facilitated countries to learn from one another and to implement strategies that have been successful elsewhere. Consequently, comparative studies on drug utilization are valuable tools to promote the development of health systems. Such drug utilization studies may compare issues related to legislation for drug approval, prescribing regulations, drug supply structures, financing models and strategies to promote access to essential medicines and the quality use of medicines, in order to serve as a basis for formulating and implementing health programmes and pharmaceutical policies.

The main purpose of this chapter is to provide an overview of studies comparing drug utilization across different health systems. It also describes drug utilization studies for over-the-counter (OTC), complementary and alternative medicines.

The role of medicines in health care systems

All health systems are heavily dependent on access to medicines of assured quality that are used in a scientifically sound and cost-effective way [23]. This is particularly important because medicines constitute the second largest component of most health budgets (after salaries) and the largest component of private health expenditure in low- and middle-income countries. Key components of a functioning system ensuring quality use of medicines include [23]:

- A regulatory system for marketing authorization and safety monitoring.
- National lists of essential medicines and national diagnostic and treatment protocols.
- Standardized equipment that can guide procurement, reimbursement and training.
- A supply and distribution system that can ensure universal access to essential medicines through public and private channels, with focus on the poor and disadvantaged.
- A national medical products-availability and price-monitoring system.
- A national programme for the promotion of rational prescribing.

Considerable efforts have been made during the last 30 years to promote access to essential medicines [24,25]. Essential medicines policies are established in almost all countries across the world. These policies have increased the availability of key drugs and limited the power of the pharmaceutical industry. Although few new drugs have been developed for high-burden diseases in poor countries, there are exceptions, including the development of malaria drugs and vaccines. There are also examples of agreements that have improved access to medicines, such as the recent agreement for new hepatitis C virus (HCV) medicines in Egypt [26].

There are several future challenges to be met. The WHO Report on Priority Medicines has identified the key challenges in drug therapy for all health systems [27]. In the report, 'pharmaceutical gaps for a number of diseases and risk factors based on the following criteria: pharmaceutical treatments for a given condition will soon become ineffective (e.g. due to resistance); the delivery mechanism or formulation is not appropriate for the target patient group; an effective medicine either does not exist or is not sufficiently effective (e.g. lack of basic scientific knowledge or lack of financial incentive due to market failure). The authors recommend that pharmaceutical innovation should be encouraged by a shorter medicine development process, a reviewed reimbursement procedure and a more attractive research environment [27]. Drug utilization studies could contribute to better treatment, particularly in addressing obstacles where effective medicines could be better delivered to the patient. The report also highlights the special needs of three population groups (the elderly, women and children), which should be addressed.

Drug utilization studies and health care systems

Health care systems are organic, complex and in constant change. All are organized in a particular way and deliver care according to their specific financing mechanisms [28]. Comparisons between different health care systems can help identify both commonalities and differences regarding drug utilization patterns and their determinants. Such studies can also provide other useful information for policy recommendations towards sustainable health care systems development.

When conducting comparative studies on health care systems, it is important to strike a good balance between avoiding blueprints that do not allow for country contexts and specificities and encouraging a degree of standardization that enables comparisons within and between countries, as well as over time. Standardized indicators allow comparisons between countries and can create the basis for mutual learning. However, caution is needed when interpreting such indicators, and it is important to emphasize that they cannot be used as definitive assessments of a health system's success or failure. A fundamental theoretical orientation that takes into account the level of complexity of the care is required, and it is important to consider the large differences that exist between countries. Even economically advanced countries are not homogeneous in respect to national gross and net wealth, population size, judicial system, human rights status, economic organization and social expectations regarding health care [29].

Given the importance of medicines in promoting health and curing disease, as well as their associated costs, drug utilization research may be understood as a critical tool by which to measure health care system performance and outcomes. Drug utilization studies can be performed to quantify and identify inappropriate drug use, to find explanations for changes in utilization patterns and to evaluate the impact of interventions. These three main objectives can all be placed in the context of the research domains recognized by Remme at al. [30] in their classification of studies aiming at improving health systems: ***operational research*** is predominantly targeted at local health care providers; ***implementation research*** is predominantly targeted at programme managers engaged in scaling up an intervention; and ***research on the health system as a whole*** (or one of its building blocks) is predominantly targeted at those who manage or make policy for the whole system [30].

Measuring drug utilization in health care systems depends not only on the way the system is organized, but also on the type of data available. It is important to consider, for comparison purposes, the source of the data (wholesalers, pharmacies, prescribers), their coverage (the whole country or particular regions) and their content (e.g. only medicines subject to prescription or both prescription and OTC medications). For further guidance on some important considerations when comparing drug utilization across countries, see Chapter 14.

Comparative drug utilization studies of health care systems

There are many studies comparing drug utilization between different health care systems. For didactic purposes, we present a typology of common focuses for this type of research and examples of research questions illustrating the types of problem that can be addressed in Table 18.2, adapted from the 'Tool to Assess the Pharmaceutical Sector in a Given Country' proposed by Seiter [31]. The table also provides some examples of selected references within each dimension. However, it is important to emphasize that these dimensions are closely linked and that some of the selected studies involve more than one of them.

Pharmaceutical market

The pharmaceutical market, as a dimension of comparison, allows mapping and analysis of market factors related to drug utilization within health care systems,

Table 18.2 Drug utilization research within different health systems: dimensions, research questions and selected references.

Dimension	Examples Questions	Study title	Reference
Pharmaceutical market	Total health care spending and categories of health care expenditure	Healthcare reform in the United States and China: pharmaceutical market implications	[32]
	Price comparison among countries	Generic drug prices and policy in Australia: room for improvement?	[33]
		Does the market share of generic medicines influence the price level?	[34]
		Prices paid for adult and paediatric antiretroviral treatment by low- and middle-income countries in 2012: high, low or just right?	[35]
	Drug shortages	Drug shortages in European countries: a trade-off between market attractiveness and cost containment?	[36]
Pharmaceutical policy and regulation	Implementation of WHO essential medicines policies	WHO essential medicines policies and use in developing and transitional countries: an analysis of reported policy implementation and medicines use surveys	[25]
	Regulatory process for approval of therapeutic agents	Regulatory review of novel therapeutics – comparison of three regulatory agencies	[37]
	Health system factors influencing the uptake of new medicines	International diffusion of new health technologies: a ten-country analysis of six health technologies	[38]
	Uptake of centrally authorized drugs	No difference in between-country variability in use of newly approved orphan and non-orphan medicinal products – a pilot study	[39]
	Access to biologic drugs	Inequities in access to biologic and synthetic DMARDs across 46 European countries	[40]
Public reimbursement and procurement	Comparison between medicine reimbursement systems	Same drugs, valued differently? Comparing comparators and methods used in reimbursement recommendations in Australia, Canada, and Korea	[41]
	Analysis of government purchasing power	Analysis of prices paid by low-income countries – how price sensitive is government demand for medicines?	[42]
Service delivery and logistics	Comparison of estimates of medicine availability at health facilities	Pharmaceutical availability across levels of care: evidence from facility surveys in Ghana, Kenya, and Uganda	[43]
	Adoption of e-prescriptions	Electronic prescriptions are slowly spreading in the European Union	[44]

Dimension	Examples Questions	Study title	Reference
Out-of-pocket spending on drugs	Variation in out-of-pocket prescription drug spending across regions	Pharmaceutical out-of-pocket spending on prescription drugs	[45]
	Impact of the cost of medicines	Quantifying the impoverishing effects of purchasing medicines: a cross-country comparison of the affordability of medicines in the developing world	[46]
Rational use of drugs	Comparing adherence to guidelines and formularies	Adherence to WHO's essential medicines list in two European countries	[47]
	GPs' attitudes to following clinical guidelines	Guidelines; from foe to friend? Comparative interviews with GPs in Norway and Denmark	[48]
	Variations in health care and clinical decision-making	Between-country variation in the utilization of antihypertensive agents: guidelines and clinical practice	[49]
		How do doctors in different countries manage the same patient? Results of a factorial experiment	[50]

serving to guide policymakers' decisions. The considerable variation around pricing structures and the number of pharmaceutical manufacturers, for instance, are factors that influence the availability of medicines. Hence, evaluation of market trends, price comparisons and studies analysing drug shortages hold significant implications for health care systems. An example of such a study would be the one conducted on market projections by Daemmrich & Mohanty [32] in order to evaluate the sustainability of free-market pricing for drugs in the United States and China, which showed that spending on prescription drugs will continue to grow, reinforcing tensions concerning drug prices and universal access to medicines.

As to the introduction of generic drugs into the market, Mansfield [33] found that it does not necessarily translate into lower overall drug prices, since both the regulation of such medications and their exposure to market forces vary substantially between different health care systems. Dylst & Simoens [34] also found that the extent to which price competition from generic medicines leads to price reductions varies according to the market share of generic medicines, with countries with high generic market shares seeing a larger decrease in medicine prices over time than low-market-share countries.

Regarding drug shortages, Pauwels et al. [36] compared data from seven European countries and reported that over 50% of such events affected medicines included in one of the five major Anatomical Therapeutic Chemical (ATC) classes (the cardiovascular system, antiinfectives for systemic use, antineoplastic agents, immune-modulating agents and the nervous system). Causes for drug shortages were largely underreported, but production problems dominated among the known factors.

Pharmaceutical policy and regulation

This is another relevant dimension for comparison purposes, with implications for health care performance and outcome. Issues around the national implementation of essential medicines policies, regulatory processes for the approval of new therapeutic agents and variations in drug uptake across health care systems, for instance, are valuable tools by which to identify whether a policy is effective. As an example, Holloway & Henry [25] aimed to determine whether public-sector medicine use is better in low- and middle-income countries that have implemented essential medicines policies than in those that have not, and found a positive correlation between the number of medicine policies countries reported implementing and the quality of their medicine use.

When appraising new drug applications, health care systems differ highly in the complexity of the processes they follow. Downing et al. [37] compared the time to completion of the first review and the total review time for all applications involving novel therapeutic agents approved by the US Food and Drug Administration (FDA), the European Medicines Agency (EMA) and Health Canada from 2001 through 2010 and showed that the FDA reviewed applications more quickly, on average, than did the EMA and Health Canada, with the vast majority of novel therapeutics being approved for use in the United States before either Europe or Canada.

Another question relates to the variation in uptake of new medicines in different health care systems. Packer et al. [38] compared the uptake of four new drugs and two other health technologies between 10 countries and related the differences to health technology assessment (HTA) in the different countries. Above-average health spending and the presence of HTA or other guidance reports were associated with increased diffusion. Early-warning activity and national coverage decisions were more likely to be associated with a reduced diffusion. Stolk et al. [39] determined for six European countries that there was a large difference in access to medicines between health care systems. However, there seemed to be no systematic difference between 'orphan drugs' (drugs used for the treatment of rare diseases) and other expensive medicines without an orphan medicine status, despite the joint EU efforts to promote rapid access to orphan drugs. Putrik et al. [40], on the other hand, found appreciable differences in the utilization of biological and synthetic disease-modifying antirheumatic drugs (DMARDs) for patients with rheumatoid arthritis across Europe. Differences resulted from financial factors (including high patient copayment levels, especially in lower-income European countries) and administrative factors (e.g. prescribing restrictions, relegating such medicines to second–line use).

Public reimbursement systems and procurement

It is well known that medicines account for an appreciable proportion of costs within health care systems, and it is always difficult to find a balance between the needs of the patient and the optimal allocation of resources. A considerable number of studies comparing aspects of public reimbursement systems or procurement have been conducted, contributing to our understanding of variation in drug access. Bae et al. [41], for example, investigated reimbursement decision data from Australia, Canada and Korea and found that, in spite of marginal differences regarding the methods used by each country for reimbursement recommendations, the same drug was evaluated differently across jurisdictions. Srivastava et al. [42] investigated the pattern of medicine prices across 16 low-income countries and found significant cross-country variation both between and within therapeutic drug classes, demonstrating that access to medicines is still a complex public health issue.

Service delivery and logistics

Another pertinent way to compare different health care systems regarding the performance of pharmaceutical services is through aspects of service delivery and logistics. A wide variety of relevant questions can be addressed. Masters et al. [43], for instance, compared the availability of medicines in health facilities in Ghana, Kenya and Uganda and showed poor availability of essential medicines across all three countries. They also showed that rates of pharmaceutical stock and stock-out varied by country and supplier (hospital, health centre, private clinic, pharmacy).

Another example would be how the introduction of new technologies is changing the way health care is delivered. Electronic prescriptions, for instance, have been considered to improve the quality and safety of patient care and to be important in facilitating administrative tasks such as reimbursement. Mäkinen et al. [44] investigated whether the adoption of electronic prescriptions had increased in the 27 member countries of the European Union in the beginning of the second decade of the 21st century, and found that nationwide use of electronic prescriptions is still scarce in everyday practice and that several countries are still piloting projects on this technology.

Out-of-pocket spending on drugs

Access to medicines varies from country to country and largely depends on the characteristics of each country's health care system. For example, in systems that are nominally more restricted in regard to access to health, access to medicines is also restricted, and medicine expenses will mostly be out-of-pocket. On the other hand, health systems that promote universal access will tend to project and extend this outlook to access to medicines, and to health technologies in general. Thus, comparisons of out-of-pocket spending on drugs can shed light on possible disparities in access to and availability of health care services. A Canadian report analysed whether Canadian spending on prescription medicines had increased over time and if there was any variation due to household income, age and region [45]. Such comparisons could also be made between different countries. Niëns et al. [46] analysed the purchasing of medicines by individuals in 16 developing countries and showed that such purchases could lead to the impoverishment of large numbers of people. They also suggested that in many countries, the affordability of such treatments is low.

Studies of out-of-pocket spending may also include OTC drugs, herbal products and complementary medicines; these products are described later in this chapter.

Rational use of medicines

The last dimension shown in Table 18.2 is rational use of medicines. Support for the rational use of medicines through adoption of guidelines and other strategies to maximize patient safety can greatly contribute to a well-functioning health system. Studies on adherence to guidelines and professional practices abound, underlying particular characteristics of different health care systems. In a Croatian-Swedish comparison, the total consumption of prescription medicines in each country was compared with the WHO essential medicines list in order to identify areas for improvement [47]. In another example, Carlsen & Kjellberg [48] interviewed a sample of general practitioners (GPs) in Norway and Denmark about their attitudes to guidelines, showing that the Norwegian GPs were sceptical about guidelines that incorporated economic evaluation, while the Danish GPs regarded these guidelines as important and legitimate. Stolk et al. [49] assessed guideline preference in relation to the use of antihypertensive agents in Denmark, Finland, Germany, Norway, Sweden and the Netherlands. These authors found that none of the guidelines discussed current utilization and that in some countries they seemed disconnected from drug use in clinical practice. McKinlay et al. [50] conducted factorial experiments to compare physicians from the United States and the United Kingdom with regard to management of coronary heart disease (CHD) and depression, looking at the influence of patients, providers and the health care system. The authors detected significant differences between the two health care systems regarding patient management.

Drug utilization studies of self-medication and nonprescription drugs

An important area of inquiry relates to self-medication and OTC drugs, sold directly to the consumer without a prescription. Grigoryan et al. [51] compared public attitudes, beliefs and knowledge concerning antibiotic use and self-medication between 11 European countries. The most pronounced differences they found were in awareness about resistance, followed by attitudes towards situational use of antibiotics. Awareness about antibiotic resistance was lowest in countries with a higher prevalence of resistance. In another study, the same authors looked at the impact of predisposing patient- and health system-related factors on self-medication with antibiotics [52]. Some health system factors associated with a lower likelihood of self-medication were higher gross domestic product (wealth) and exact dispensation of prescribed tablet quantities by pharmacies. Other studies have shown that the problem of self-medication with prescription drugs may be greater in low- and middle-income countries [53].

There are fewer comparative studies of OTC medicine use, despite the increasing attention this area is receiving due to quality and safety concerns. In many countries, OTC drugs are selected by a regulatory agency to ensure that they contain only substances that are safe and effective when used without physician oversight. As a general rule, OTC drugs have to be used primarily to treat conditions that do not require direct supervision by a qualified prescriber, and they must be proven reasonably safe and well tolerated. OTC drugs are usually required to have little or no abuse potential. As many medicines are available both over the counter and on prescription, it is important to take OTC availability into consideration if performing drug utilization studies of therapeutic areas where drugs are available over the counter. A drug's status – OTC or prescription – may differ between countries, and this should be borne in mind when performing cross-national comparisons of drug use.

It is difficult to use the same methodological tools for nonprescription drugs as are used for prescription drugs, as the use of OTC drugs is not as closely monitored. OTC drug utilization can be estimated by subtracting sales on prescription and to hospitals from total drug sales utilizing aggregate drug data [54]. This does not allow OTC use at the individual patient level to be studied, however, so information on OTC use has often been obtained through primary data collection. The extent of OTC drug use is largely unknown, but some prevalence studies have been published in different settings. In a cross-sectional population survey of 2816 randomly selected Swedish residents conducted between

2001 and 2005, 71% of respondents used some kind of a drug, 52% used one or more prescription drugs, 38% used OTC drugs and 8% used one or more herbal preparations [55]. A US study evaluated the use of prescription and OTC medications among more than 3000 older adults and found that 81% used at least one prescription medication and 42% used OTC drugs [56].

There are some published studies on the impact of switching a drug from prescription to OTC status [57–61]. For example, the switch to OTC status of chloramphenicol eye drops and ointments in the UK increased the total usage of ophthalmic chloramphenicol [57]. Similarly, the availability of OTC triptans in Sweden did not affect prescription volumes [58]. On the other hand, decreasing prescription volumes were observed for H_2 receptor antagonists, loratadine and low-dose simvastatin when they became prescription-free [59–61]. It is likely that the impact of switches differs considerably between therapeutic areas and between countries/health care systems, due to differences in pricing and reimbursement regulations and to variations in marketing activities by the pharmaceutical industry. In a cross-national comparative study, Gauld et al. [62] compared the impact of OTC switches between the United States, the United Kingdom, Australia, Japan, the Netherlands and New Zealand and found that New Zealand was the most active in progressive switches, while the United States, Australia and the Netherlands were the least active. Few medicines for long-term conditions were switched, and the switch of certain medicines took considerably longer time in some countries than in others.

A systematic review of complementary and alternative medicines showed considerable uncertainties about the true prevalence of their use. The costs of complementary and alternative medicines can be considerable, yet their popularity seems to be increasing [63]. An estimated 29% of US adults used at least one complementary and alternative medicine therapy in the past year, with nearly 10% of this consisting of herbal medicines [64]. In an evaluation of demographics and beliefs regarding the safety and efficacy of herbal medicines in nearly 800 randomly selected adult patients, 42% reported herbal medication use. Women with higher education were more likely both to use herbal medicines and prescription drugs [65]. Studies of complementary and alternative medicine use may also assess physician attitudes. A cross-sectional survey assessing the attitudes of German outpatient care physicians showed that half were in favour of complementary and alternative medicine use, with primary care physicians being significantly more inclined to use them than specialists [66].

Overall, comparative data on OTC drugs and complementary and alternative medicines are very limited.

Conclusion

Most drug utilization studies comparing health systems have cross-sectional study designs that compare drug utilization patterns and policies at a certain point in time. Also, many studies are ecological. Such studies may give misleading estimates of the influence of system characteristics, due to the large number of other factors that can affect drug utilization, such as marketing, mass media and various changes in health care organization and delivery, insurance/reimbursement and demography. There may be limited evidence and availability to do in-depth research with existing registries. Consequently, there is a need for primary data collection and for qualitative studies, combined with a growing need for well-designed intervention studies that can generate evidence on the performance and outcomes of different health care systems. It is also important to develop reliable, valid, understandable and evidence-based quality indicators that can be applied in comparative research.

CHAPTER 19
Drug utilization and health policy

Brian Godman[1], Hye Young Kwon[2], Marion Bennie[3] & Anna Birna Almarsdóttir[4]

[1]*Division of Clinical Pharmacology, Karolinska Institute, Karolinska University Hospital Huddinge, Sweden*

[2]*Institute of Health and Environment, Seoul National University, South Korea*

[3]*Strathclye Institute of Pharmacy and Biomedical Sciences, University of Strathclyde, Glasgow, UK*

[4]*Clinical Pharmacology, Institute of Public Health, University of Southern Denmark, Denmark*

KEY POINTS

- Pharmaceutical policy is a complex arena that works at various levels (cross-national, national, regional and local) and through various actors. It can be defined as the conscious attempt by public officials to achieve certain objectives through a set of laws, rules, procedures and incentives.
- The chosen policy options will depend on the income level of the country implementing them, the method of financing health care and the agreed objectives.
- The costs of pharmaceuticals can be controlled in a number of ways, including formal pricing and reimbursement systems, profit controls, patient copayments, devolution of budgets to physician groups and generic substitution.
- Health care organizations, including governments, can potentially instigate multiple measures to enhance the rational use of medicines. These can be collated under the 4Es: education, engineering, economics and enforcement.
- Rational guidance within pharmaceutical policymaking can only be achieved when policymakers and researchers come together and learn from one another or when initiatives exert their influence in other countries (cross-country learning).

Introduction

Medicines have made an appreciable contribution to improving health outcomes [1,2]. However, pharmaceutical expenditure is coming under increasing scrutiny [3,4], having risen by more than 50% in real terms during the past decade among Organisation for Economic Co-operation and Development (OECD) countries [5]. This growth has resulted in pharmaceutical expenditure becoming the largest, or equalling the largest, cost component in ambulatory care, in some countries forming up to 60% of total health care expenditure [4,6]. The scrutiny over pharmaceutical expenditure will continue in the future, driven by multiple factors, including ageing populations, rising patient expectations and the continued launch of new premium medicines [3,7–11]. This combination of factors has resulted in even high-income countries struggling to fund medicine purchasing with their available resources [12–14]. The observed consequence is the adoption of multiple policies within and across countries in an attempt to maximize the use of medicines and achieve or maintain comprehensive, equitable health care [14–17].

This chapter will describe what is meant by 'pharmaceutical policy' and how this is developed and influenced through key drivers, and will provide an introduction to the issues and types of measures surrounding the rational use of medicines. These subjects will be further explored in Chapters 20 and 21.

Drug Utilization Research: Methods and Applications, First Edition. Edited by M. Elseviers et al.
Published 2016 by John Wiley & Sons, Ltd.

Defining pharmaceutical policy

Health care policy has been defined by the World Bank as the conscious attempt by public officials or executives entrusted with public funds, including those working in health authorities, health insurance agencies and managed care organizations, to achieve agreed objectives through a set of laws, rules, procedures and incentives [17].

Pharmaceutical policy is a subset of this, designed to improve the safe and effective use of medicines. Pharmaceutical policy debates incorporate a number of areas, including (i) issues of unmet need, (ii) access to medicines, (iii) pricing and cost containment, (iv) rational use of medicines and (v) innovation and service provision [18,19]. All policymaking is naturally prone to debate and potential disagreement, and is impacted upon by differences in ideology, politics and variable evidence [17]. However, good policy analysis, through the application of drug utilization studies of past policies and their evidentiary impact, will help inform and predict the impact of future pharmaceutical policy initiatives.

Forming pharmaceutical policy across the globe

Political traditions and national income are key drivers in shaping pharmaceutical policy objectives. Figure 19.1 lists these objectives for high-, middle- and low-income countries.

In low-income countries, the principal policy goal is to improve access to essential medicines in order to reduce maternal and child mortality, as well as mortality from acquired immunodeficiency syndrome (AIDS), malaria and tuberculosis [17]. Overall, in low- and middle-income countries, health care expenditure typically accounts for between 13 and 32% of household expenditures, with one in four poor households in low-income countries incurring potentially catastrophic health care expenses when family members become ill [20]. Between 41 and 56% of households in these countries spend 100% of their health care expenditures on medicines [20–23]. The goal in these countries is to move towards universal access to health care, including medicines.

In contrast in high income countries, the main goal is to sustain universal coverage in the face of a rapidly growing elderly population and an increasing prevalence of chronic diseases, as well as to fund new, high-priced drugs [11,14,24,25]. This has generated significant activity in pharmaceutical policy development, aimed at managing the introduction of new medicines and maximizing the use of existing ones [12,14,16,26,27]. Table 19.1 presents some illustrative examples of pharmaceutical policies in high-income countries.

Some countries have very explicit national pharmaceutical polices, such as the recently approved national medicines plan in Malaysia [28] and the national plans in Australia (Table 19.1), while others do not [17]. Where such policies exist, they define the overall objectives for the country.

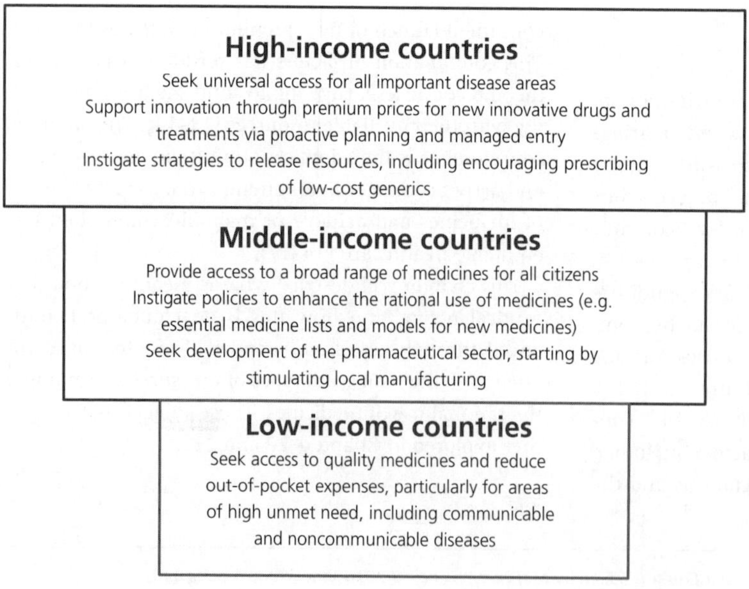

Figure 19.1 Core pharmaceutical policy objectives by country income level.

Source: Data from [14,16,17].

Table 19.1 Ongoing initiatives to improve the quality and efficiency of prescribing for both new and established medicines in select countries worldwide.

Country	Policies
Australia [67–71]	The National Medicines Policy (NMP) aims to optimize the use of medicines in order to improve health outcomes for all Australians. It proposes to meet medication and related service needs through four central objectives: • Timely access to medicines that Australians need at a cost individuals and the community can afford. • Provision of medicines meeting appropriate standards of quality, safety and efficacy. • Quality use of medicines. • Maintenance of a responsible and viable medicines industry. Potential ways of achieving optimum use of medicines include: • Providing timely access to accurate information and education about medicines and their use to consumers and health practitioners. • Establishing public health and health education programmes and other programmes relating to the quality use of medicines. This includes NPS MedicineWise, as well as drug and therapeutic committees (DTCs), which have existed in hospitals in Australia for a number of years and aim to promote best practice in therapeutics. • Involving industry and health practitioners through the contribution of appropriate information, education and promotion activities. • Demanding accurate and responsible reporting of issues relating to the use of medicines by the media.
Canada [45,46,72–74]	The CADTH Common Drug Review (CDR) conducts objective, rigorous reviews of the clinical effectiveness and cost-effectiveness of new medicines for Canada's publicly funded drug plans, excluding Quebec (Quebec requires manufacturers to guarantee the best available prices for private and public plans). Increasingly, this includes confidential discounts/product listing agreements (PLAs) to enhance the potential for reimbursement of new premium-priced medicines. However, there are concerns, which have led to suggestions for greater collaboration among the provinces. The potential for drug utilization studies in Canada is enhanced by drug policy research networks and the National Prescription Drug Utilization Information System (NPDUIS) (http://www.cihi.ca/CIHI-ext-portal/internet/en/document/types+of+care/pharmaceutical/npduis_metadata, last accessed 18 November 2015), which contains data on prescription claims from publicly financed drug benefit programmes in Canada
Korea [4,75,76]	Recent reforms aimed at improving access to medicines and care delivery include (i) abolishing patient copayments for drugs that treat cardiovascular and cerebrovascular diseases, rare diseases and cancers, (ii) increasing the incremental cost-effectiveness threshold (ICER) in these four disease areas. These reforms are intended to protect citizens against financial catastrophes associated with poor health and prohibitive increases in health insurance premiums.
New Zealand [14,77–80]	The reimbursement body of New Zealand (PHARMAC) operates within a fixed budget, prioritizing funding for new medicines based on strict criteria, and has the ability to fund their use in defined subpopulations where their value is greatest. Cross-company deals exist, with PHARMAC agreeing to fund a new medicine at an agreed price in a defined patient population in exchange for the manufacturer lowering the cost of their other listed medicines. A recent comparative analysis of the approval and funding of new drugs showed only 59 (43%) of the 136 medicines listed in the Australian PBS between 2000 and 2009 were listed in the New Zealand reimbursement I schedule, with listings first appearing on average just under 3 years after they appeared Australia. This may be at least in part due to the reimbursement body in New Zealand operating within a fixed budget and so prioritizing new medicines both against one another and against all existing medicines.
Scotland [41,51,56,81,82]	The Scottish Medicines Consortium (SMC) assesses the value of new medicines and new indications for potential funding. Overall, approximately one-third of new medicines are approved for funding at licensed indications, one-third are restricted and one–third are rejected. This is changing with greater involvement of patients and clinicians in decision making (PACE Patient and clinician engagement). The Scottish model for the rational use of medicines, including the SMC, emphasizes the involvement of both ambulatory and secondary care physicians in DTCs and in developing joint prescribing guidance and guidelines. Local prescribing guidance and guidelines are based primarily on evidence of effectiveness and safety, and adherence to agreed prescribing guidance is monitored by health board pharmaceutical advisers.

Legal and institutional framework

The legal and institutional hierarchy that governs the medicine market within a country shapes pharmaceutical policy at the international and national levels. The typical hierarchy is illustrated in Figure 19.2.

The Ministry of Health or its equivalent will normally define the technical standards and provide the legal framework for regulatory agencies, as well as agencies involved in the pricing, reimbursement and marketing of pharmaceuticals [17].

Overall, the pharmaceutical market is highly dynamic, with a hierarchy of laws, regulations and implementing agencies at national, regional and local levels (Figure 19.2). For example, in Sweden, reimbursement decisions for new and established ambulatory care medicines, including potential prescribing restrictions, are under the jurisdiction of the national agency (TLV), but budgetary responsibility for medicines lies with the 21 counties (regions) [29,30]. This can lead to further prescribing restrictions at the county council (regional) level, aimed at improving the quality and efficiency of prescribing of both new and established medicines within available budgets [12,29,31].

Influencing pharmaceutical expenditure

Countries typically instigate multiple initiatives to influence pharmaceutical expenditure. These can be considered under the collective headings of supply-side measures, which are principally concerned with the pricing of medicines and associated regulations, and demand-side measures, which are principally concerned with interventions/activities designed to influence the utilization of medicines. Often, these are combined to make the most effective use of available resources, including compulsory price cuts and measures to increase the prescribing of low-cost generics [4,27,32–34].

Pricing and reimbursement of medicines

Potential supply-side measures include [27,29,32,35–46]:

- **Price and profit controls at all stages of the pharmaceutical distribution chain:** These are commonly applied to manufacturers, wholesalers, importers and pharmacies. At the manufacturer level, controls can include profit ceilings, comparative pricing systems and price negotiations. At the wholesale and pharmacy levels, interventions are typically aimed at limiting the additional handling costs that organizations apply as medicines move through the supply chain, often termed the 'marginal cost'.
- **Changes in the medicine reimbursement system:** Countries often make incremental changes in their pharmaceutical reimbursement systems in order to maintain financial budgets. Typical changes include: (i) increasing patient copayments; (ii) reclassifying prescription medicines as over-the-counter (OTC) medicines; (iii) instigating reference pricing,

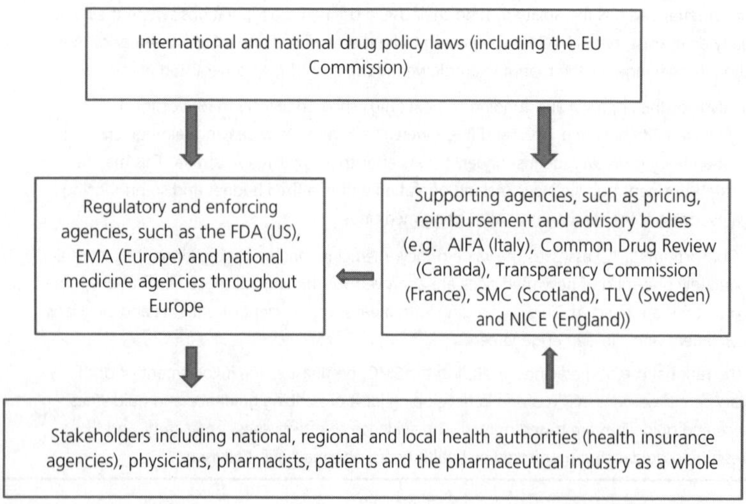

Figure 19.2 Hierarchy of laws, regulations, implementing agencies and other stakeholders involved with developing and implementing pharmaceutical policy.

Source: Data from [17].

with reimbursement based on the lowest reference price drug at Anatomical Therapeutic Chemical (ATC) class level 3, 4 or 5, with patients covering the additional costs themselves for a more expensive product; and (iv) implementing managed-entry agreements/risk-sharing arrangements (see Chapter 20).

In Europe and elsewhere, two principal approaches are used to inform decisions on the pricing and reimbursement of new medicines:

1 The reimbursed price is calculated based on an assessment of the clinical gain of the new medicine compared to the current treatment standards in the country, with graded pricing scales applied based on the assessed level of health benefit (e.g. Austria, France and Germany) (Table 19.2) [38,47–49]. Typically, there are robust processes and guidelines in place to assess the level of innovation, based on health technology assessment principles [38].
2 Pricing and reimbursement decisions are based on the evaluation of economic criteria, such as the incremental cost/quality-adjusted life year (QALY) metric applied through health technology appraisal (HTA) systems for new medicine versus current standards [38] (e.g. Australia, Canada, New Zealand, Norway, Sweden, Korea and the United Kingdom) [14,38,50–53].

Studies have shown that countries that use economic evaluations in their decision-making are typically more sensitive to uncertainties attached to health outcomes or costs, or both. This hypothesis is endorsed by the fact that they reject funding applications for new drugs on the grounds of uncertainty more often than do countries that do not use economic evaluations in decision-making [38].

There has also been a growth in risk-sharing schemes and managed-entry agreements (MEAs), certainly across Europe, as health authorities increasingly challenge the perceived level of innovation and associated requested prices [36]. These schemes include price–volume arrangements [36,37] and are a means

Table 19.2 Linking the health gain of new ambulatory care medicines in Austria, France and Germany to reimbursed prices.

Source: Data from [38,83].

Country	Subdivisions	Potential prices
Austria (3 subdivisions)	Substantially added benefit	Average of prices among selected European countries combined with a pharmacoeconomic study to justify the requested price
	Added benefit	Maximum of 10% above current standards, depending on population size
	Marginal or similar benefit	Minimum of 10% below current standards in Austria
France (5 subdivisions)	ASMR I: Major improvement (new therapeutic area, reduction in mortality) ASMR II: Significant improvement in efficacy and/or reduction of side effects ASMR III: Modest improvement in efficacy and/or reduction of side effects	Based on prices of the new drug in selected European countries (Germany, Spain, Italy and the United Kingdom)
	ASMRIV: Minor improvement	Typically, similar prices to current standards in France
	ASMR V: No or inadequate improvement	Lower prices than current standards in France
Germany (6 subdivisions)	Substantial additional benefit Considerable additional benefit Small additional benefit Unquantifiable additional benefit No additional benefit Less benefit than current therapies	Either assigned to a preexisting reference price group (typically limited or no added benefit) or put forth for price negotiation between individual sickness funds and the manufacturer, based on the level of health gain and prices in 15 European countries, including any current discounts

ASMR, Amelioration du service medical rendu.

Table 19.3 Areas of concern around the rational use of medicines and their potential causes.

Source: Data from [17,40,58,84–90].

Parameter	Possible prescriber factors	Possible patient factors
Overprescribing	Safety, where there are concerns with diagnosis Meeting patient expectations Financial incentives, through procurement	Perception that more medicines are better than one Limited opportunity for follow-up to assess the effectiveness of current treatments
Overuse of antibiotics	Difficulty with identification of causal agent(s) Pressure from patients/parents	Expectation of quick relief, even for viral infections
Over use of injectable drugs	Better control of potential over dosing Higher remuneration for hospitals and/or physicians for using injectable versus oral medicines	Believing injections have a greater effect than oral tablets
Use of premium-priced newer drugs	Pharmaceutical industry and patient pressures (via the media)	Believing newer agents are more effective
Use of more expensive originators than generics	Believing the quality of originators is superior to that of generics	Perceiving generics to be of lower quality than originators
Underuse of treatments for patients with chronic diseases	Access barriers, including income Incomplete knowledge of prescribing in chronic diseases, including optimal doses Lack of quality targets (e.g. blood pressure and lipid goals for patients with cardiovascular diseases) Lack of systems for the routine monitoring of patients with chronic diseases	Stopping treatment upon feeling well/absence of symptoms Experiencing side effects or affordability issues with current regimens

Table 19.4 Definitions and explanations of the 4Es.

Source: Data from [16,42,54,91].

Measure	Explanation and initiatives aimed at improving the quality and efficiency of prescribing
Education	Activities range from simple distribution of printed material to more intensive strategies, including academic detailing and monitoring of prescribing habits against agreed criteria and colleagues (benchmarking)
Engineering	Organizational or managerial interventions, such as prescribing and quality targets for physicians
Economics	Financial incentives for physicians, patients and pharmacists including co-payments for patients
Enforcement	Regulations enforced by law, such as prescribing restrictions for certain medicines, compulsory generic substitution and compulsory international nonproprietary name (INN) prescribing

by which pharmaceutical companies can enhance the value of their new medicines without altering the list price; alternatively, they can be a means by which health authorities control pharmaceutical expenditure. They also increasingly involve drug utilization studies (see Chapter 20).

We are likely to see health authorities becoming more stringent when assessing the value of new medicines as resource pressures grow. However, this must be balanced against the need to support the development and introduction of new medicines aimed at addressing continued areas of unmet need. Health organizations will have to improve their planning around the introduction of new premium-priced medicines, and drug utilization studies will play a major role in this, starting pre- and continuing post-launch (see Chapter 20) [9,14].

Demand-side measures to enhance the rational use of medicines

Table 19.3 provides a list of broad parameters and their potential influencing factors, generated from a review of various drug utilization studies, that could be the focus of demand-side measures to improve the rational use of medicines. These parameters tend to focus either on overuse of medicines generally or on overuse of medicines specific to a therapeutic area, and they apply to the use of premium-priced rather than generic medicines, where pertinent.

Interventions designed to target the underlying drivers of prescriber and/or patient behaviour are discussed in Chapter 21 and can be collated under four headings (the 4Es): education, engineering, economics and enforcement (Table 19.4) [54]. The 4E methodology has been used in a number of countries and drug classes in order to assess the influence and impact of different health policy interventions on utilization patterns and so inform future policy [8,13,55–57]. Examples are given in Chapters 20 and 21.

An alternative way of looking at potential methods of enhancing the rational use of medicines was developed in the Canadian National Pharmaceuticals Strategy Report, which highlighted six challenges [58]:

1 improper drug selection;
2 overcoming inappropriate dosing;
3 reducing adverse drug reactions (ADRs);
4 reducing drug–drug interactions;
5 reducing therapeutic duplication;
6 improving patient noncompliance.

Whether health authorities choose to concentrate on new or established medicines, or both, for future interventions will depend on the current and projected dynamics in their country and on their policy goals. What is important is that health authorities fully assess the impact of their current policies in order to improve future planning. Drug utilization tools and research can support this endeavour, and researchers should be encouraged to work alongside health organizations (public and private) and health practitioners. Studies have shown that such engagement is welcomed by policymakers as they strive to ensure the financial sustainability of their health care systems [59]. Shared learning across countries is key; while this is already evident in some places, increasing resource pressures will require it to continue and expand in the future if countries are to meet their objectives [12,42,60].

Criteria for undertaking good quality drug utilization and policy cross-country comparative studies include: (i) the appropriate use of theory; (ii) explicit selection of comparator countries (i.e. the rationale for selecting them, including differences in epidemiology, financing and policies); (iii) the rigour of the comparative design, including the research approach; (iv) the complexity of cross-national comparisons; and (v) the contribution to current knowledge [61].

Conclusion

Pharmaceutical policy analysis is highly complex and requires a solid evidence base. This need will only increase in the future, as resource pressures grow. This will be achieved through greater collaboration between decision-makers and researchers, linking drug utilization and health policy at the regional, national and cross-national levels. Consequently, the importance of the involvement of drug utilization researchers in pharmaceutical policy analysis and the policy consultative process cannot be overemphasized. To achieve this, drug utilization researchers need a good overview and understanding of the available design and methodological options for drug utilization and policy studies, coupled with knowledge of existing health care systems. In addition, they will need access to comprehensive information regarding ongoing reforms and initiatives, as well as database sources [62–66].

CHAPTER 20

Managed introduction of new drugs

Brian Godman[1], Roberta Joppi[2], Marion Bennie[3], Saira Jan[4] & Björn Wettermark[5]

[1]*Department of Laboratory Medicine, Division of Clinical Pharmacology, Karolinska Institutet, Karolinska University Hospital Huddinge, Sweden*

[2]*Pharmaceutical Drug Department, Azienda Sanitaria Locale of Verona, Italy*

[3]*Strathclyde Institute of Pharmacy and Biomedical Sciences, University of Strathclyde, Glasgow, UK*

[4]*Clinical Professor, Rutgers State University of New Jersey, Piscataway, New Jersey, United States*

[5]*Centre for Pharmacoepidemiology, Karolinska Institutet, Karolinska University Hospital Solna, Sweden*

KEY POINTS

- New medicines are required to address continuing unmet need.
- New medicines are often costly, and it is critical to understand their health benefit (safety and effectiveness) in clinical practice (outwith the clinical trial setting) in order to support robust decision-making regarding their access and funding.
- Improved planning is needed to optimize the funding and utilization of new medicines. This can be focused around three pillars: pre- (including horizon-scanning and forecasting), peri- (including reimbursement decisions) and post-launch activities (including registry and database studies).
- Drug utilization studies will take an increasing role in generating the evidence base for the use of new medicines in clinical practice, as electronic patient records make it more feasible to access data.
- There has been a rapid development in methods to handle missing data and confounding factors to facilitate such research. This will continue.

Introduction

Expenditure on medicines accounts for an increasing proportion of health care budgets, with a growth of more than 50% in real terms among Organisation for Economic Co-operation and Development (OECD) countries during the 2000s [1]. This growing expenditure causes pressures on public resources, resulting in an increasing number of countries being unable to fund premium-priced medicines [2–4]. The drivers behind this growth include ageing populations, in part due to advances in medical research, and the launch of new premium-priced medicines [3]. Pharmaceutical companies typically seek a premium price for their new medicines to help recoup research and development costs [5], with some new biological medicines costing USD100 000–400 000 per patient per course or per year, or even more [2,3,5–9]. The challenge is in the evaluation of these new medicines and the extent to which they offer significant therapeutic advantage over existing therapies.

A number of independent reviews have examined the additional health benefit of new medicines and concluded that approximately 85–90% of all new medicines provide few or no clinical advantages for patients versus existing standards [3,10,11]. In France, in 2011, only 2% of new medicines or new indications for existing medicines were assessed as innovative and/or offering a real therapeutic advantage over existing treatments [12]. In Australia, of the 217 approvals by the Australian Therapeutic Goods Administration between 2005 and 2007, only 7 were rated as important therapeutic innovations [13]. In the United States, the Food and Drug Administration (FDA) approved 12 new medicines for various cancers in 2012 [14], of which only 3 prolonged overall survival – and in 2, this was by less than 2 months.

Drug Utilization Research: Methods and Applications, First Edition. Edited M. Elseviers et al. © 2016 John Wiley & Sons, Ltd.
Published 2016 by John Wiley & Sons, Ltd.

A second challenge is that new medicines come to the market having been exposed to relatively small defined populations in their clinical trials. Consequently, there is a lack of information on the risk–benefit ratio of these medicines in wider populations with multiple morbidities. This can result in medicines having to be withdrawn from the market post-launch following their prescribing. One example is natalizumab in patients with relapsing multiple sclerosis, which was withdrawn soon after its launch due to the development of progressive multifocal leukoencephalopathy [15,16]. Natalizumab was relaunched some 2 years later in Europe under strict regulations and with research programmes aimed at clarifying the benefit–risk ratios [15,16]. There have also been concerns with the prescribing of Dabigatran, a new anticoagulant, in more elderly and comorbid populations than those recruited into phase III clinical trials [2,17,18]. These concerns resulted in a number of professional bodies and health authorities initiating extensive pre- and perilaunch programmes [17]. Discussions have included the potential benefits of monitoring anticoagulant activity and adjusting doses in order to reduce possible major bleeds post-launch [3,19–21]. Other examples of medicines withdrawn from the market include cerivastatin, rimonabant, rofecoxib and rosiglitazone [22–25].

A third challenge is the variation in the uptake of new medicines globally. Cross-national comparisons have showed a large variation between countries in the uptake of new medicines. For instance, studies have shown physicians in the United Kingdom are less likely to prescribe new medicines compared with those in Italy, Spain or the United States [9,26–28]. Other studies have demonstrated there may be large variations in the uptake of new medicines across therapeutic areas [27,28]. Critical factors in the uptake of new medicines in either hospital or ambulatory care are listed in Table 20.1 [9,29–35].

Understanding and addressing these challenges to the introduction of new medicines is critical to supporting the advancement of clinical care through potentially more effective treatments, reduced numbers of adverse drug events, as well as improved formulations and administration regimes aimed at improving compliance [2,36,37].

New medicines will continue to challenge the European ideals of equitable and comprehensive health care for all [32]. Strategies will continue to be deployed by health authorities and others in an attempt to support the safe and cost-effective introduction of new medicines, including risk-sharing schemes/managed-entry agreements (MEAs), out-of-pocket payments and

Table 20.1 Key influencers and drivers in the uptake of new medicines in hospital and ambulatory care.

Sector	Influencers
Hospital (inpatient) care [33–35]	• Involvement of physicians in clinical trials • Role of physicians in decision-making bodies such as drug and therapeutic committees (DTCs) • Level of innovation of the new medicine • Marketing activities of pharmaceutical companies The cost of a new medicine is less of an issue, as this may well be influenced by the extent of hospital discounting among pharmaceutical companies The level of discounting in hospitals has become a driver for the creation of joint ambulatory–hospital drug formularies and other measures to improve 'interface management' at local, regional and national levels
Ambulatory care [9,29–31]	• Level of health gain/patient benefit (innovation) versus current treatments • Hospital physicians • Physician age – younger physicians have a greater propensity to prescribe newer medicines • Participation in clinical trials • Level of academic detailing and other inputs from pharmacists and physicians employed by health authorities • Marketing activities of pharmaceutical companies • Patients The cost of a new medicine is of less importance when assessing key drivers influencing uptake in ambulatory care

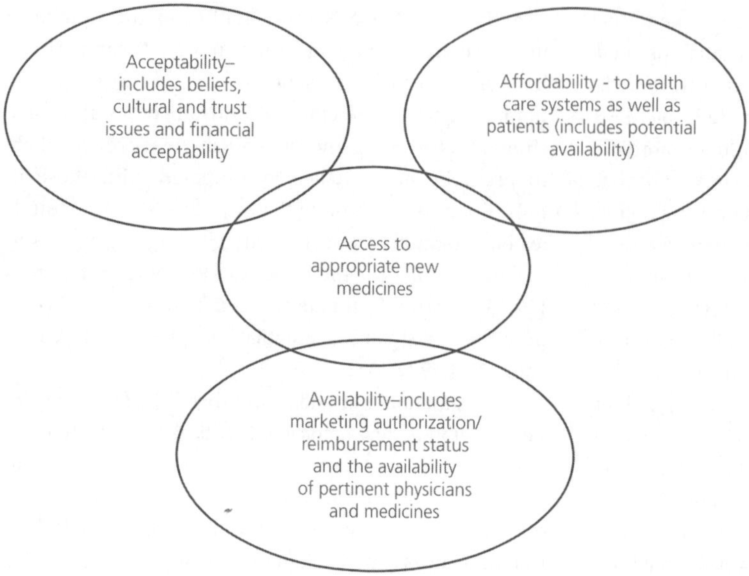

Figure 20.1 Key components regarding provision of new medicines.

Source: Adapted from Putrik et al. [50].

post-launch safety programmes [38–44]. New medicine developments will also challenge low- and middle-income countries as they struggle to increase access to medicines for their citizens, with the ultimate aim of providing universal coverage [3,45–49].

Given these multiple issues, there is a recognized need to improve planning for the introduction, utilization and monitoring of new medicines as they become available post-launch. Figure 20.1 provides a construct of four key components impacting on provision of new medicines: acceptability, affordability, access and availability [50].

This chapter will examine approaches being deployed across countries, principally by health authorities, to support the planned introduction of new medicines and how drug utilization studies can be applied to assist key stakeholders and decision-making groups in meeting the challenges associated with introducing new medicines.

New models to improve the rational use of new medicines

One helpful approach to describing the multiple activities involved in the successful implementation and monitoring of new medicines is to group activities around predictive timelines associated with market launch. Figure 20.2 presents such a model, consisting of three pillars – prelaunch, perilaunch and post-launch – and highlights where drug utilization activities can add intelligence to the process [2,3,51]. However, it must be noted that any drug utilization study undertaken with new medicines will depend on the availability of and access to data, ranging from aggregated drug sales data and more sophisticated patient-level data [52].

Prelaunch activities

Horizon-scanning can be defined as 'identifying new medicines or new uses of existing medicines that are expected to receive marketing authorisation from the Regulatory Authority in the near future and estimating their potential impact on patient care' [53–56]. There are numerous examples of different countries instigating horizon-scanning approaches [53,57,58]. Since 1999, a number of countries in Europe, North America and the Asia-Pacific region have been collaborating under the EuroScan project (International Information Network on New and Emerging health Technologies) [56,57,59]. Each member agency is unique in its approach, but they all have a common goal of informing health authorities and hospital managers, in particular, about new and emerging technologies that could have a significant impact on their health system [59–61].

Typically, activities consist of five sequenced components (Figure 20.3).

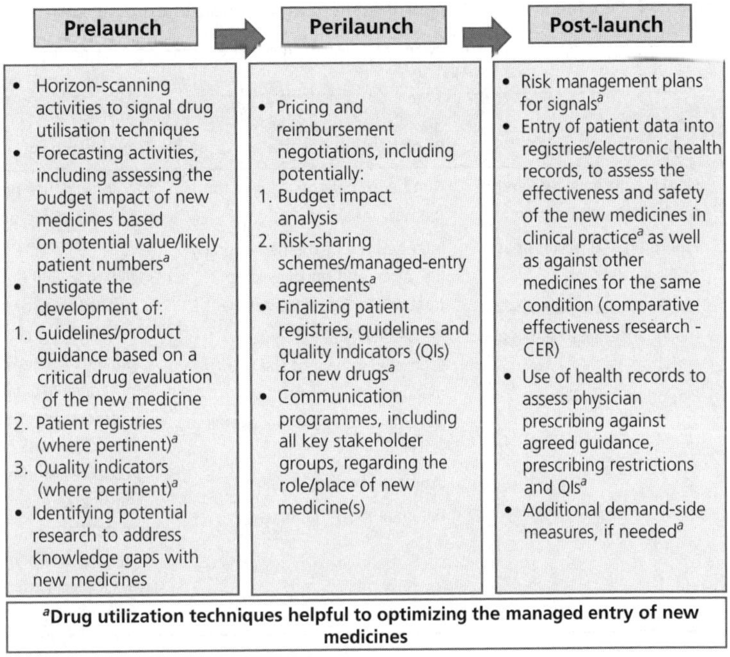

Figure 20.2 Proposed model to optimize the managed introduction of new medicines.

Source: Data from [2,3,51,53].

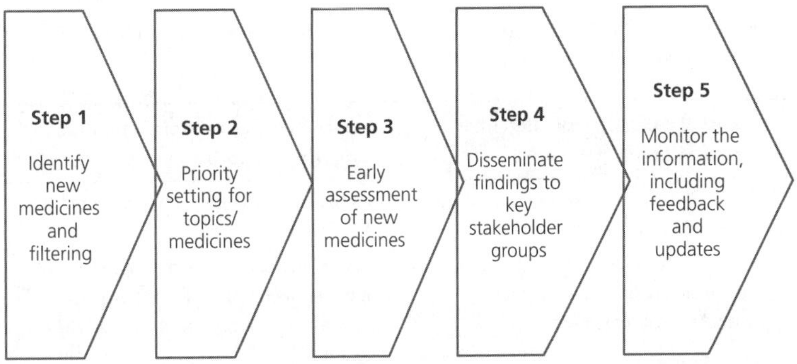

Figure 20.3 Horizon-scanning sequencing activities.

Source: Adapted from [53,59].

Information sources for the identification of potential new medicines (Step 1) include the medical scientific literature, pharmaceutical companies, regulatory agencies, conference presentations, newspaper articles and online information portals/providers such as DIA and Medscape [53,57,59,62,63]. Filtering and prioritization of topics for evaluation (Steps 1 and 2) must include the potential health benefits and budget impact of new medicines, which can include potential savings [2,53,57,64]. Table 20.2 illustrates two examples of these processes, as applied in Austria for new cancer drugs and in England for all new technologies.

Prelaunch (early) assessments of new medicines (Step 3) are typically undertaken up to 3 years before their likely launch date [2,53,57].

One example of a well-developed horizon-scanning system is the Italian Horizon Scanning Project (IHSP) [57]. This project critically reports on emerging medicines in order to assess in a timely fashion their potential impact on the Italian National Health System (NHS). IHSP issues several reports following its filtering and prioritization process (Steps 3–5) to aid in decision-making (Table 20.3).

The forecasting of drug utilization and expenditure is essential to improving planning and resource allocation for new medicines as part of their rational introduction. The planning may include: (i) the development and/or adaptation of guidelines based on a critical evaluation of available evidence; (ii) the instigation of educational activities around the therapy; (iii) budget-setting, including potentially the development of quality

Table 20.2 Filtering process and prioritization of new anticancer drugs in Austria [59] and of new technologies in England [64].

Austria		England	
Criteria for filtration	**Prioritization criteria**	**Topic selection**	**Information needs for prioritization**
New (i.e. recently received) marketing authorization Emerging (e.g. still in phase II or III) clinical trials Use in adults, including solid malignancies, leukaemia and lymphomas Extended indications	Number of patients eligible for the new medicine Intended use of the new therapy (i.e. as an add-on to existing treatments or as a replacement to existing treatments) Estimated impact of the new medicine on the health of patients (e.g. additional overall survival) Estimated budget impact Potential for off-label use	Would guidance promote the best possible improvement in patient care? That is, does the proposed guidance: • Relate to one of the NHS clinical priority areas or health-related priorities; significantly improve patients'/carers' quality of life and/ or reduce avoidable morbidity; or, if used extensively, either appreciably impact on NHS or other societal resources or free up resources? Alternatively, will it be detrimental to patient care? • Address a condition that is associated with significant disability, morbidity or mortality?	Estimated usage in England and Wales Estimated size of the patient group Burden of disease Potential cost per patient Cost of current diagnostic or therapy options Potential for savings Service requirements, including training Level and extent of evidence of benefit or harm

Table 20.3 Process and reports of the Italian Horizon Scanning Project (IHSP) prior to potential marketing authorization from the European Medicines Agency (EMA) [57].

Report 36 months before potential marketing authorization	Report 18 months before potential marketing authorization	Report 12 months before potential marketing authorization
Provides data from phase II trials and indications of ongoing phase III trials Helps identify research areas of interest to the Italian NHS not being met by pharmaceutical companies	Assesses available results of completed phase III trials Enables identification and prioritization of emerging medicines likely to have a clinical and economic impact on the Italian NHS Essentially for internal purposes	Critically reports on the efficacy and safety of selected drugs Assesses the possible level of innovation, place in therapy (target population) and social and economic impact of these drugs Seen as particularly useful for policymakers, including those involved in subsequent reimbursement decisions

indicators; (iv) potentially, developing registries to monitor the effectiveness and safety of new medicines in routine clinical practice; and (v) instigate additional research to address key information gaps [3,17,65].

Factors that drive increased expenditure on new medicines (including premium-priced medicines for the treatment of diseases that are difficult to treat with existing medicines) can be divided into those that govern prices and those that affect volumes [9,66,67]. There are well-established methods by which to predict changes related to these factors [58]. However, the traditional models had difficulties in forecasting the uptake and expenditures of new biological drugs, given their high acquisition costs compared to current therapies. This led to the development of new models. One example, combining a number of factors, is a forecasting model developed in Sweden [58]. Regression analyses are conducted on aggregate sales data and the predicted trends are adjusted for likely changes in the market, including patent expiries, new guidelines, reimbursement decisions and the introduction of new medicines. The underlying assumption is that new medicines are introduced and utilized based on the theory of the diffusion of innovations developed

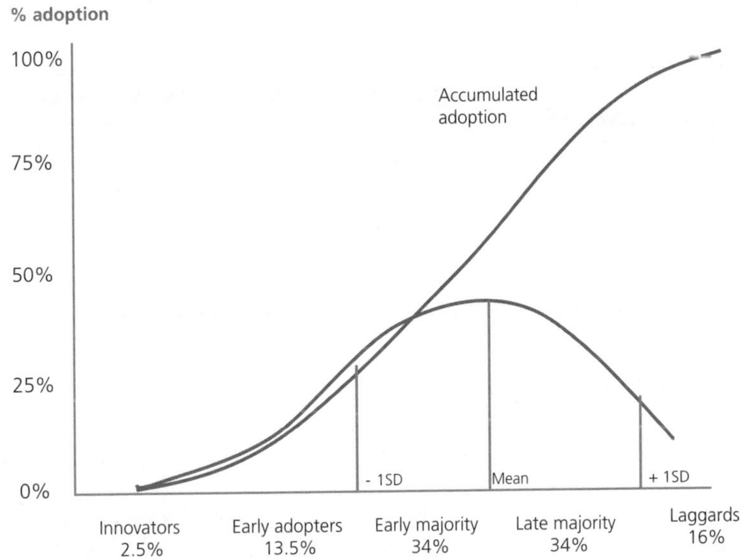

Figure 20.4 Typical adoption curves over time for new technologies [Adapted from Ref [68]; SD = Standard Deviation.

by Rogers [68] (Figure 20.4). Figure 20.5 plots drug expenditure against current predictions in Stockholm County Council, Sweden. This includes the sales patterns in 2011–14 and the predicted growth in the different therapeutic areas (Anatomical Therapeutic Chemical (ATC) classification 1st level) in 2015–16. An internal assessment showed that predictions had been adequate overall, giving good guidance. However, there have been miscalculations in some therapeutic areas, due to uncertainties surrounding, for instance, the timing of patent expiries and the instigation of unexpected reimbursement restrictions by the national reimbursement agency. The figure shows that pharmaceutical expenditure has levelled off in therapeutic groups where generics are now available as standard treatment (e.g. cardiovascular, nervous system and respiratory diseases) but has increased rapidly in areas where many new medicines are being introduced (e.g. diabetes, anticoagulants, hepatitis C and oncology).

Authors in Australia recently used the Bass diffusion model to retrospectively assess patterns of adoption, distinguishing between adoption patterns driven primarily by external factors, such as regulations, and those driven by internal forces, such as social contagion [31]. The Bass diffusion model is the most common mathematical representation of diffusive adoption, describing the number of new adopters per unit time by the additive effects of external and internal forces [31].

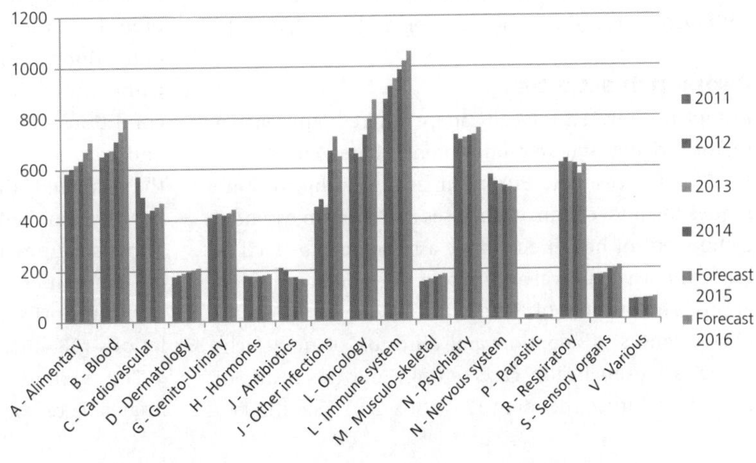

Figure 20.5 Actual and forecasted expenditure on medicines in Stockholm County Council, broken down by ATC class. For colour details, please refer to the colour plates section.

Table 20.4 Differences in the age and sex of patients discharged from hospital with nonvalvular atrial fibrillation (NVAF) and patients enrolled into phase III trials with new oral anticoagulants (NOACs) [70].

Cohort of Italian patients	RE-LY study (dabigatran) Published 2009	ROCKET AF (rivaroxaban) Published 2011	ARISTOTLE (apixaban) Published 2011
Mean age 76.3 years (SD 10.7) Median age 79 years (interquartile range 71–84) 64.6% ≥75 years of age Proportion of men: 49.8%	Mean age 71.5 ± 8.7 years 40% ≥75 years of age Proportion of women: 38%	Median age 73 years (interquartile range 65–78) 38% ≥75 years of age Proportion of women: 40%	Median age 70 years (interquartile range 63–76) Approximately 32% ≥75 years of age Proportion of women: 32%

Drug utilization data are valuable for both horizon-scanning and forecasting activities. These data can assist with: (i) estimating likely patient numbers for a new medicine; (ii) estimating the potential rate of uptake, based on historic data in similar drug classes or disease areas; (iii) estimating the level of unmet need, based on the proportion of patients currently not fully treated with available medicines; and (iv) identifying potential factors influencing uptake in particular countries [31,57,58,69]. For example in Italy, IHSP has run transferability analyses using its administrative (health authority) databases. This allows comparisons between population-based cohorts in clinical practice and those included in phase III clinical trials, as well as identification of the possible target population for emerging and/or new medicines. An illustration of this is the analysis of 13 360 Italian patients discharged from hospital with a diagnosis of nonvalvular atrial fibrillation (NVAF) and the subsequent comparison with patients included in the three key phase III studies of new oral anticoagulants (NOACs) in stroke prevention (i.e. the RE-LY, ROCKET AF and ARISTOTLE studies) [70] (Table 20.4). In this analysis, the findings highlighted the potential for increased adverse drug events with NOACs with increasing age, as renal function declines [2,19,71].

Perilaunch activities

European countries typically adopt different approaches to the pricing and reimbursement of new medicines [72,73]. Increasingly, European health authorities are requesting budget impact analyses (BIAs) as an essential component of health economic assessments, as well as for formulary approval and/or reimbursement considerations. The purpose of BIAs is to estimate the financial consequences of adoption and diffusion of new technologies within health care settings and the resultant impact on future spending [74]. Box 20.1 lists the key components of a BIA [75]. Again, drug utilization studies are crucial to enhancing the robustness of forecasted budgets by reducing uncertainties.

Box 20.1 Components of budget impact analyses (BIAs) [75].

The budget holders' perspective.

- A defined time horizon (up to 3 years).
- A clearly specified setting.
- Results expressed as undiscounted cost differences between the new scenario (including the new technology) and the current one.
- Potential trade-offs in health care resources, taking into account the variable effectiveness of the new technology.
- Sensitivity analyses responsive to the uncertainty surrounding future market developments.

Risk-sharing schemes, or managed entry schemes (MEAs) [38,40], can be defined as 'agreements concluded by payers and pharmaceutical companies to diminish the impact on the payer's budget of new and existing medicines brought about by either the uncertainty of the value of the medicine and/or the need to work within finite budgets'. In practice, the agreement lies in setting the scope and realizing the mutual obligations amongst both payers and pharmaceutical companies depending on the occurrence of an agreed condition – the "risk". The 'risk' varies by situation, and can include pharmaceutical expenditure higher than agreed thresholds or a lower-than-expected health gain, reducing the new product's value [40]. These schemes are one means by which pharmaceutical companies can gain reimbursement for their new premium-priced drugs in all or some patient populations [38–40].

The various schemes can be classified as either financial or outcome-based (Table 20.5). Financial

Table 20.5 Types of risk-sharing scheme/managed-entry agreement (MEA) [12,17,38,40,42,43,85,86].

Risk-sharing scheme/MEA	Definition and examples	Role of drug utilization data
Financial schemes		
Price–volume agreements (PVAs)	These typically involve health authorities (payers) agreeing expenditure and volume targets for single products or a range of medicines each year. Under these agreements, pharmaceutical companies typically pay monies back to the authorities if agreed expenditures are exceeded They are the most common type of MEA among European countries (39% of all MEAs) They are widely used by health authorities to control pharmaceutical expenditure, especially where there are few demand-side measures in place to counteract pharmaceutical industry marketing activities	Collection of aggregated drug utilization and expenditure data and comparison with the agreements The findings are used as a basis upon which to calculate the extent of any payback of monies from pharmaceutical companies to health authorities
Discount schemes	These can involve giving confidential discounts to a health service to better match the requested price with the product's perceived value, and hence enhance its potential for reimbursement Discounts are increasingly confidential, with European countries referencing one another regarding medicine prices. However, countries may choose not to accept such schemes due to the lack of transparency, especially with only a limited number of new medicines seen as truly innovative (Table 20.1)	Limited role
Price-capping schemes	Under these arrangements, companies cover the additional costs per patient over and above agreed limits. Examples include: • The Ranibizumab Reimbursement Scheme (United Kingdom). The first 14 injections for wet age-related macular degeneration are paid by the NHS and the drug costs of any subsequent injections are reimbursed by the company • Lenalidomide for patients with multiple myeloma (United Kingdom). The manufacturer pays the cost of the drug if more than 26 cycles are needed for any one patient	Tracking the use of products in identified patients Triggering payments from the pharmaceutical companies when dosage limits are exceeded
Outcome-based schemes		
Outcome guarantee schemes	Examples include: • Bortezomib for the treatment of the first relapse of multiple myeloma in the United Kingdom, based on a 50% reduction in serum paraprotein levels (M-protein) by the fourth cycle. The NHS continues funding treatment in responders, with the manufacturer refunding the cost of the drug if a 50% reduction is not achieved • Atorvastatin for the prevention of coronary heart disease (CHD) in the United Kingdom. The pharmaceutical company agrees to fund the health authority for wasted resources if atorvastatin fails to reduce LDL-C levels to agreed targets when a patient has been properly titrated	Tracking usage and outcomes via patient registries and other mechanisms Instigating payments, as well as (potentially) price reductions, when agreed outcomes are not reached

(continued)

Table 20.5 *(continued)*

Risk-sharing scheme/MEA	Definition and examples	Role of drug utilization data
Schemes to limit the utilization of new medicines		
Limiting the utilization of medicines to defined patient populations	Increasingly, health authorities are limiting the funding of new medicines to defined subpopulations where they believe their value is greatest. These are additional restrictions to the labelled indication, and health authorities encourage/enforce them through a number of measures, including education and financial incentives for both physicians and patients. Examples include: • Limiting the prescribing of dabigatran to prevent strokes in patients with atrial fibrillation to defined subpopulations (e.g. Austria and Slovenia) • Limiting the prescribing of duloxetine in Sweden to patients refractory to first- and second-line antidepressants, with associated price reductions for overuse • Funding only approved indications in Italy to limit the off-label use of medicines, especially those intended for patients with cancer	Tracking physician prescribing habits via patient registries. Using findings for future health authority activities, including physician penalties, price reductions and rebates for non-approved indications

NB: MEA = managed entry agreement

schemes include (i) price–volume agreements (PVAs), (ii) discount schemes and (iii) price-capping schemes. Outcome-based schemes include payment-by-result schemes [38–40,43]. There are also schemes that limit the utilization of new medicines to defined populations, with financial and other penalties for excessive prescribing. There are a growing number of MEAs for new orphan drugs, due to the high requested prices [76]. This is likely to continue.

The introduction of risk–sharing schemes/MEAs has raised concerns among health authority and health insurance company personnel regarding the level of administration necessary to implement them, given currently limited routine electronic clinical systems in place to enable ease of data monitoring. However, these concerns have to be weighed against the potential benefits of MEAs, which include [38,40]:

- Enhancing the opportunities for reimbursement and for 'payers' to work within defined budgets.
- Limiting off-label usage/indication creep in clinical practice.
- Potentially funding only treatments that produce desired health gain and/or helping target prescribing to those patients where health gain is greatest (e.g. through biomarkers).
- Enhancing the ability to monitor the safety and effectiveness of new treatments in practice.

Other aspects surrounding perilaunch activities incorporated into Figure 20.2 include finalizing the content of any planned patient registries and developing quality indicators for new medicines, as well as creating communication programmes (involving key stakeholder groups) to better manage the introduction of new medicines.

Post-launch activities

Post-launch activities include: (i) risk management plans; (ii) monitoring the effectiveness and safety of new medicines in routine clinical practice using data contained in either patient registries or electronic health records (EHRs); and (iii) monitoring the prescribing of medicines against agreed guidance based on available data sources (Figure 20.2). Risk management plans, which include risk evaluation and mitigation strategies, are normally required by the European Medicines Agency (EMA) and FDA as part of the medicine approval process, to help ensure that the benefits of a particular medicine outweigh its risks [77,78].

Drug utilization studies can contribute significantly in the post-launch phase, as data are generated through the use of new medicines in clinical practice. The type of drug utilization study undertaken will depend on the availability of and access to data [52]. Simple studies assessing time trends in the uptake of new medicines

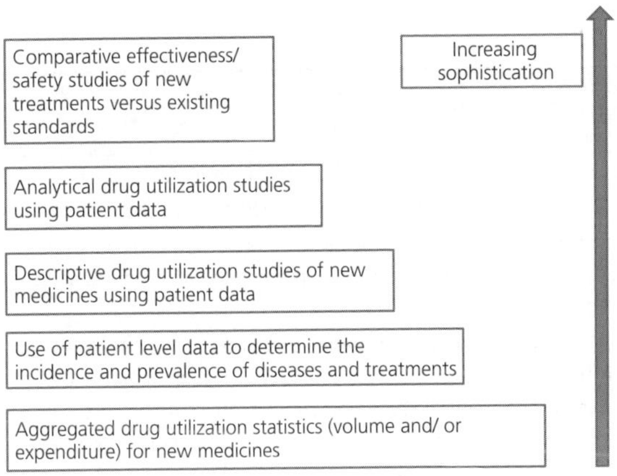

Figure 20.6 Types of pharmacoepidemiological and drug utilization study used to monitor the effectiveness, safety or utilization of new drugs.

Source: Adapted from [52].

can be conducted with aggregated drug utilization data. More analytical studies regarding the safety/effectiveness/appropriateness of the prescribing of new medicines in clinical practice require patient-level data linked to clinical information [52] (Figure 20.6, Table 20.6).

Studies can also be used to assess the impact of interventions designed to influence prescribing patterns. Typically, health authorities use a mixture of demand-side measures and initiatives (i.e. interventions) to influence the utilization of new medicines. These measures can be helpfully categorized under the 4Es (education, engineering, economics and enforcement – see Table 19.4). Examples regarding new medicines are given in Table 20.7 [79].

In the context of the United States, drug utilization studies are being increasingly undertaken in the post-launch phase (see Figure 20.2) to assess the effectiveness and cost-effectiveness of new medicines in clinical practice, in order to inform institutional organizations' (managed care organizations') formulary decisions [3]. The introduction of health care reforms, and a significant focus on specialty pipeline drugs and their increased identification [36], is reinforcing the focus on the appropriate management of patients. Models are being created by managed care organizations (MCOs) that examine comparator products in therapeutic classes, combined with their health costs, including pharmacy and medical costs, in order to identify differences in the clinical outcomes of different therapies and their associated costs. This includes comparing new medicines with older therapies and determining the most appropriate clinical end points. The models developed by MCOs typically focus on overall cost and event reduction, including reductions in hospitalizations, readmissions and emergency room visits, as well as the per-member per-month (PMPM) costs of different therapy options for the same indication. These approaches also help validate the clinical end points used in clinical trials and provide insight into potential future management tools for pertinent member populations, allowing improvement of the quality and efficiency of future care. Additionally, MCOs Pharmacy Benefit Managers (PBMs) are increasingly focusing on pragmatic clinical trials in view of their diverse patient populations (compared with the more homogeneous populations typical seen in randomized controlled trials, RCTs) and are increasingly using an active comparator arm (i.e. not a placebo [80]) in order to identify populations that will benefit optimally from given treatments. Drug utilization information is also being used in risk-based contracting, including rebates and discounts between MCOs and pharmaceutical companies.

More broadly, integration of medical data from the various US databases provides insight into the clinical effectiveness of the different therapeutic options that support MCOs in selecting the most appropriate medicine. Key initiatives are the Comparative Effectiveness Research (CER) and Drug Effectiveness Review Projects (DERP) instigated at a national level or across States [81].

Other initiatives are the collaborations under the Patient Centred Medical Homes (PCMH) initiative and Accountable Care Organizations, which provide EHR data to help better understand current management approaches and to plan for the future [82–84]. These include data on medicine use, patient monitoring and outcomes aimed at enhancing insurers' claims data, and they provide an opportunity for MCOs to conduct real-time analyses on response rates, outcomes of switches between treatment options (including new and established treatments) and disease progression. New treatments with reduced toxicities, better cure rates and shorter treatment durations will increasingly be utilized at acceptable prices, and will increasingly be accompanied by patient support programmes aimed at enhancing adherence to prescribed to achieve desired outcomes. This is because the cost of medicines in the US has increased appreciably in recent years with MCOs now typically instigating price

Table 20.6 Examples of drug utilisation studies with new medicines.

Country/region and medicine	Summary of studies undertaken
Belgium (University Hospital), dabigatran [18]	The appropriateness of prescribing of either rivaroxaban or dabigatran in patients with nonvalvular atrial fibrillation (NVAF) was evaluated using 9 of the 10 criteria of the Medication Appropriateness Index. The primary outcome measure was the prevalence of inappropriate prescribing. Secondary outcome measures included (i) categories of inappropriateness, (ii) prevalence of adverse drug events, and (iii) interventions made by a clinical pharmacist to optimize prescribing. A total of 69 patients were evaluated: 16 (23%) had 1 inappropriate criterion, and an additional 18 (26%) had more than 1 inappropriate criterion. The most frequent inappropriate criteria were inappropriate choice (28% of patients), wrong dosage (26%) and impractical modalities of administration (26%). An adverse event was found in 51% of patients (including 8 patients with transient ischaemic attack/stroke). The clinical pharmacists performed 48 interventions and 94% were accepted by the physician. Inappropriate use of dabigatran and rivaroxaban in patients with NVAF is frequent and may lead to adverse events. Reinforcing education is needed for both health care professionals and patients. Collaboration with clinical pharmacists can contribute to better use of these medicines.
Catalonia (Spain), dabigatran [87]	One-third of patients prescribed dabigatran were over 80 years old. Of these 631 patients, 103 were not receiving the recommended dose. 17% of patients had previous ischaemic heart disease and 2% had severe renal impairment, both of which are contraindications to dabigatran. Renal function was not recorded the previous year in 30% of patients, which is a concern as dabigatran is principally excreted through the kidneys and there is currently no reversal agent. Further educational initiatives are planned to address this.
Ongoing cross-national study with dabigatran [88]	As a result of continuing concerns with the prescribing of novel oral anticoagulants (NOACs) for patients with atrial fibrillation, the Global Registry on Long-Term Oral Antithrombotic Treatment in Patients with Atrial Fibrillation (GLORIA-AF) has been designed and initiated in order to investigate patient characteristics influencing choice of antithrombotic treatment in patients with NVAF and to collect data on outcomes of antithrombotic therapy in clinical practice. The GLORIA-AF is a large, international, observational registry involving patients with newly diagnosed NVAF at risk for stroke. It involves up to 56 000 patients in nearly 50 countries, and its findings will provide considerable insight for the future.
Italy and Sweden, dronedarone [89]	The study evaluated how the marketing authorization and reimbursement of dronedarone impacted on the prescribing of other antiarrhythmic drugs. In Sweden, dronedarone generated an increase in the prescription trend of antiarrhythmics, without a variation in amiodarone use. In Emilia Romagna, dronedarone marketing did not influence the prescription pattern of either overall antiarrhythmics or amiodarone. The authors concluded that while clinical guidelines place dronedarone among first-choice treatments for atrial fibrillation, amiodarone prescribing was not affected in either country by the entry of dronedarone. The authors also believed this was probably due to a cautious approach among clinicians, in line with regulatory recommendations and safety warnings.
Sweden, ARTIS (Anti Rheumatic Therapies in Sweden) [90,91]	This study involved all rheumatology clinics in Sweden with high patient involvement in data catchment. It showed that: • rheumatoid arthritis patients treated with biological drugs are not at increased risk of invasive melanoma; • rheumatoid arthritis patients selected for TNF-α inhibitor treatment are not at increased overall risk for cancer but have a 50% increased relative risk of invasive melanoma. Given the small increase in absolute risk, the authors concluded these findings do not shift the overall risk–benefit balance of anti-TNF-α medicines in clinical practice, but that they might do so in patients at high risk of melanoma for other reasons.

Country/region and medicine	Summary of studies undertaken
Sweden, antiobesity medicines [92]	Patient-level data assessing the characteristics and utilization of patients prescribed various weight-loss drugs showed: • limited persistence in routine clinical practice – 77% of patients continued treatment for less than 1 year; • 28% of rimonabant patients and 32% of sibutramine patients had a history of depression or antidepressant treatment, which is a specific contraindication for rimonabant; • 41% of sibutramine patients had a history of hypertension and/or cardiovascular disease (CVD), which is a contraindication with sibutramine; • 36% of patients had no documented weight change after treatment.

Table 20.7 Examples of the 4Es in action [2,17,93–96].

Measure	Examples
Education	Physician guidance for the prescribing of dabigatran in Ireland, Sweden and New Zealand
Engineering	Instigation of comprehensive models to optimize the managed entry of new medicines Prescribing targets for physicians with regard to new medicines (e.g. Catalonia, Spain)
Economics	Financial incentives for physicians, patients and pharmacists, including copayments for patients (e.g. TNF-α inhibitors for rheumatoid arthritis and medicines for glaucoma in Finland)
Enforcement	Prescribing restrictions for dabigatran in Slovenia: • Dabigatran is only reimbursed if it is initiated by an internist or neurologist and prescribed according to agreed indications (e.g. it is only reimbursed in patients already on warfarin if they are unstable with TTR < 65) • Patients must be followed in a tertiary or secondary anticoagulation centre; they can be followed in primary care, but only if authorized by a tertiary or secondary centre • Every patient has to be registered in a database and followed by the IT anticoagulation programme • Anticoagulation centres have to report once yearly to the tertiary centre regarding the number of patients experiencing minor and major bleeding or thromboembolic events, as well as any deaths from bleeding or thromboembolism • Failure to undertake these steps will mean patients have to pay the cost of dabigatran themselves (i.e. 100% copayment)

protection contracts. In the long term, the introduction of value based reimbursement models in the US will further promote the utilization of medicines that offer value. The increased cost share by members in premiums and copays will also affect utilization patterns. These initiatives will be enhanced by contracts with pharmaceutical companies that are outcome based, similar to the situation in some European countries, with all these initiatives leading to changes in the way new medicines are approved and used in the US. Different registries and data base are also being established to monitor the use of new medicines in select populations as soon as they become available. The involvement of CMS (Center for Medicare and Medicaid services) and individual health exchanges is also contributing to improved outcome management in US medicines.

Conclusion

Health authorities will by necessity improve their planning around the managed entry of new medicines in the future. This will be driven by increasing pressures from limited finances, ageing populations, new medicine pipelines (focusing on unmet clinical needs) and new premium-priced medicines. These challenges will result in the increasing use of drug utilization studies from pre- through peri- to post-launch, including, importantly, the analysis of associated demand-side measures, in order to optimize the use and impact of medicines. In part, such studies will be enabled through the increasing use of EHRs in clinical practice, which will make it more feasible to monitor the safety and effectiveness of new medicines.

CHAPTER 21

Management of drugs in a health care system

Brian Godman[1], Marion Bennie[2], Claudia Garcia Serpa Osorio-de-Castro[3], Vu Thi Thu Huong[4] & Saira Jan[5]

[1]*Department of Laboratory Medicine, Division of Clinical Pharmacology, Karolinska Institutet, Karolinska University Hospital Huddinge, Sweden*

[2]*Strathclyde Institute of Pharmacy and Biomedical Sciences, University of Strathclyde, Glasgow, UK*

[3]*Department of Pharmaceutical Policies and Pharmaceutical Services, Sergio Arouca National School of Public Health, Oswaldo Cruz Foundation, Brazil*

[4]*Administration Medical Services, Ministry of Health, Hanoi, Vietnam*

[5]*Clinical Professor, Rutgers State University of New Jersey, Piscataway, New Jersey, United States*

KEY POINTS

- It is necessary for health organizations to regularly review utilization and expenditure patterns for all medicines and to understand the impact of measures/interventions currently in place in their goal to promote the best use of medicines.
- Measures can be divided into supply-side measures, which are concerned with the prices of medicines and the associated regulations, and demand-side measures, collated under the 4Es (education, engineering, economics and enforcement).
- Drug utilization study design will depend on the available data and the time period over which single or multiple interventions are initiated, ranging from observational uncontrolled retrospective studies to segmented regression analysis of an interrupted time-series design.
- Increasing the utilization of generic products is a key strategy if health organizations are to achieve more equitable access to health care.
- There are certain therapeutic areas (e.g. mental health) where it is difficult for health organizations to instigate multiple measures to influence prescribing, given different mechanisms of action and appreciable interpatient variability in effectiveness and side effects of different treatments. This is accepted by health authorities.

Introduction

Pharmaceutical expenditure has grown by more than 50% in real terms during the past decade [1]. This is set to continue as a result of a number of recognized factors, including: (i) launch of new premium-priced medicines; (ii) ageing populations with greater prevalence of chronic diseases; (iii) an increase in noncommunicable diseases (NCDs) such as obesity and diabetes; (iv) rising patient expectations coupled with more demanding patient therapeutic management targets; and (v) judicial reviews of access to medicines, in some countries [2–5].

The challenge for health policymakers is balancing the desire to continue to incentivize the development of new medicines in order to address unmet clinical need [6] against the need to achieve or maintain universal health coverage within available resources [7,8]. This is particularly important in countries where health care expenditure makes up an appreciable proportion of a household's monthly expenditure. In low- and middle-income countries, health care expenditure is reported to typically account for between 13 and 22% of household expenditure, with pharmaceuticals accounting for the totality of this expenditure in 41–56% of households [9]. For example, in Vietnam, out-of-pocket payments have remained at 50–70% of total health care expenditure in recent years [10], with low-income households typically spending approximately 22% of their total income on health care [11]. Health policy focused on the attainment of universal health coverage will reduce out-of-pocket expenditures and the cost of ill-health among the most vulnerable populations [10,12,13].

Efforts to maximize the rational use of medicines within a health system are a central focus in the drive

Drug Utilization Research: Methods and Applications, First Edition. Edited by M. Elseviers et al.
Published 2016 by John Wiley & Sons, Ltd.

to secure the best use of limited resources. The World Health Organization (WHO) states that 'Rational drug use requires that patients receive medications appropriate to their clinical needs, in doses that meet their own requirements, for an adequate period of time and at the lowest cost to them and their community' [14]. There are a wide and varied number of potential measures and initiatives that health authorities can deploy to improve the rational use of medicines. These can helpfully be categorized into (i) supply-side measures, which are principally concerned with the pricing of medicines, and (ii) demand-side measures, which are principally concerned with interventions/activities to influence subsequent prescribing and utilization of medicines. For the purposes of this chapter, health authorities can include governments, ministries of health, national, regional or local health authorities and health insurance funds.

It is important to recognize that most complex health care systems now require the integration of both supply-side and demand-side measures in order to secure the best use of available resources, particularly with resource pressures growing.

This chapter will illustrate the different types of measures that can be used to support the rational use of medicines, and how drug utilization studies can be applied to inform the development of future measures and initiatives and/or assess their subsequent impact on patient care and health care resources.

Supply-side measures

Supply-side measures are principally instigated to enable health authorities to adhere to their predetermined financial budgets (see Chapter 19). This can occur at different geographical levels – international, national, regional or local. For example, as part of the response to the financial crisis in Europe, price cuts were generally implemented among health authorities to enable them to stay within allocated budgets [15]. However, pharmaceutical pricing policies typically differ between countries, as well as within countries (the latter depending on whether the medicine is the originator, a patented medicine or a multisourced medicine, i.e. a generic). For the purposes of this chapter, the originator is the original branded product, which is generally still available on the market even when generics become available, patented medicines are those that still retain their patent and generics include both branded generics and nonpatented medicines prescribed by their international nonproprietary name (INN).

The pricing of new medicines is discussed in Chapter 20. This can include both external reference pricing, based on prices in other countries, and internal reference pricing, based on Anatomical Therapeutic Chemical (ATC) class (i.e. either the therapy area (ATC level III) or class (ATC level IV)) [16–18]. There are likewise many approaches to the pricing of generics across Europe, but these can typically be categorized into three groups: (i) prescriptive pricing approaches, whereby countries define the discount expected from the manufacturer in order for their generics to be reimbursed (e.g. France and Norway); (ii) instigation of market forces to lower the prices of generics, including compulsory generic substitution with the lowest-priced product and high INN prescribing, where the pharmacist is reimbursed the price of the low-cost generic (e.g. Sweden and the United Kingdom); and (iii) a mixture of both approaches (e.g. Austria) [18–20]. There is also tendering of pharmaceuticals, including discounts and rebates, especially when generics are available at lower prices [21,22]. As a result of these various initiatives, the prices of high volume generics in some European countries can be as low as 2–10% of pre-patent-loss prices [23–25].

Demand-side measures

There are multiple demand-side measures that health authorities can potentially instigate to enhance the rational use of medicines. These can usefully be collated under the 4Es: education, engineering, economics and enforcement (see Table 19.4). This recognizes that new approaches are needed to influence physician prescribing, which can be considered under the general term 'soft regulations' [26]. This generation of the 4Es follows a literature review showing that different stakeholders across countries use a variety of different approaches to influence physician and patient behaviour, which can be categorized using this system [26]. This categorization has been shown in published studies to successfully collate and compare the influences of different demand-side measures on future prescribing in both cross-national and single-country studies [19,27–33]. Examples of the 4Es are given in Table 21.1.

Table 21.1 Examples of the 4Es [25–28,33,63,66,68,73,76,77,81–88].

Measure	Examples
Education	Educating all key stakeholder groups to allay fears and concerns regarding generics once their quality has been assured (e.g. France)
	Monitoring and benchmarking physician prescribing habits from electronic data sources; academic detailing
	Encouraging INN prescribing – starting in medical school and continuing into ambulatory care – through decision support systems and monitoring (e.g. the United Kingdom)
	Involving physicians in drug selection in regional formularies, alongside promotion, education and feedback, to enhance compliance with recommended medicines for the management of patients in ambulatory care (e.g. the 'Wise List' of Stockholm County Council, Sweden, alongside continuous medical education)
	Examining prescribing patterns among general practitioners (GPs) or both GPs and pharmacists in so-called quality circles as a basis for discussing potential improvements
Engineering	Prescribing targets for generic proton pump inhibitors (PPIs) and statins versus patented medicines in the same class
	Incentivizing physicians to achieve agreed quality standards for patient care (e.g. quality and outcome framework in the United Kingdom)
	Therapeutic switching programmes to lower cost alternatives without compromising care (e.g. the United Kingdom and the United States)
Economics	Providing financial incentives to pharmacists to achieve target substitution rates for originators to generics (e.g. France)
	Providing financial incentives to physicians for achieving prescribing targets (e.g. percentage of PPI utilization as generics or percentage adherence to the recommended medicines in the 'Wise List' of Stockholm County Council, Sweden)
	Introducing cheaper copayments per prescription for generic medicines, as opposed to appreciably higher copayments for patented medicines or originators to encourage their use (reduced copayments also appreciably enhanced compliance, especially in the elderly)
Enforcement	Compulsory generic substitution (e.g. Sweden)
	Prescribing restrictions for angiotensin II receptor blockers (ARBs) and patented statins (e.g. Austria, Croatia, Norway and Sweden)
	Removing patented medicines from the reimbursement list, i.e. 100% copayment, unless medically justified (e.g. patented ARBs in Denmark)

In many countries, a common organizational structure used to develop and coordinate such diversity of activities is the drug and therapeutic committee (DTC). These committees typically bring together key clinical and managerial stakeholders in an organization, often covering hospital or ambulatory care, and sometimes both, as the accountable authority for enhancing the rational use of medicines within established frameworks [14,34–36]. See Chapter 31 for further information on the ideal attributes of DTCs.

Drug utilization studies linked with associated health policies are a recognized methodology by which health authorities can evaluate the impact of their interventions and so improve planning for future measures. The nature of any drug utilization study will depend on the availability of and access to data (whether aggregated drug utilization or patient-level data) [37]. Simple studies assessing time trends in medicine utilization may be conducted with aggregated utilization data, while more sophisticated studies on different treatments (their safety and effectiveness) requires patient-level data linked to clinical information [37] (see Figure 20.6).

Drug utilization studies range from observational uncontrolled retrospective studies to segmented regression analyses of an interrupted time-series design [38,39]. The type of study undertaken and the analysis methodology will depend on the nature and number of initiatives undertaken in a defined time period (e.g. it will be difficult to perform segmented regression analyses if multiple supply- and demand-side measures have been instigated within a short period of time, and it is difficult to separate out individual effects). Simple statistical methods such as the chi-square test can be used to assess the level of significance of any changes in utilization patterns before and after multiple interventions [40].

Drug utilization studies can be undertaken at multiple levels both within and across countries. Within-country studies are often conducted at different levels of the health care system (i.e. at (i) a regional or local level or (ii) in ambulatory care, hospital inpatient care or nursing homes). Cross-national comparative studies (CNCs) are often undertaken where there is access to similar levels of data and/or health policy activities are focused on particular medicines of interest (e.g. atypical antipsychotic medicines, proton pump inhibitors (PPIs), renin-angiotensin inhibitors, including angiotensin-converting enzyme inhibitors (ACEIs) and angiotensin II receptor blockers (ARBs), or statins [5,27,28,30,31]). When undertaking CNCs, researchers should pay attention to a number of key issues in order to enhance the robustness of their studies. These include: (i) appropriate use of theory; (ii) selection of comparator countries, including countries with differences in health care financing, epidemiology and the extent/nature of demand-side measures; (iii) the complexity of such studies, including data sources, utilization and expenditure units; and (iv) the likely contribution of the findings to the knowledge base [41].

Irrespective of the type and scope of drug utilization studies undertaken, it is recommended that researchers work closely with health authority personnel to ensure the details of all pertinent reforms and initiatives are fully captured. This is especially important if such information is not readily available (e.g. information on laws and reforms contained in local language health authority websites or internal documents) [25,42,43]. Additionally, actively engaging with health authority personnel will better enable informed discussions on the development of possible measures to further improve the effective use of resources. Helpfully, data from research groups working in drug utilization across Europe have recently been collated [44].

Policy case histories

Supply-side measures: South Korea

Kwon et al. [45] analysed the effects of price cuts on the total expenditure on antihyperlipidemic drugs in South Korea. The authors showed that despite three consecutive rounds of price cuts, drug expenditure continued to rise for this drug class. Increasing number of patients, greater use of the newly launched generic atorvastatin and increased use of expensive statins were the major factors behind the increase [45]. The authors concluded that it is essential for health authorities to consider demand-side measures when reviewing pharmaceutical expenditure, as supply-side measures alone will be insufficient to meet medium- and long-term objectives in the face of ageing populations and other factors.

Demand-side measures

Improving the rational use of antibiotics

A number of activities have been instigated across countries to enhance the rational use of antibiotics, since inappropriate use can lead to the development of resistance and additional costs, with a clear link between antimicrobial resistance and the consumption of antibiotics [46–51]. Increasing antibiotic resistance is a growing concern, affecting physicians' ability to treat infections due to the lack of therapeutic options.

Various demand-side measures have been instigated across countries to enhance the rational use of antibiotic. Their details and impact are given in Table 21.2.

Improving the rational use of medicines in hospitals in Vietnam

The authorities in Vietnam have instigated a number of reforms in recent years to improve patient coverage and reduce out-of-pocket expenditure, as this will worsen with ageing populations [10,11]. Medicines are a key area, currently accounting for over 40% of total health care expenditure in Vietnam. Necessary steps will involve improving medicine selection in hospitals in order to reduce costs and improve patient outcomes, as most medicines in Vietnam are prescribed in hospitals. The intention will be to enhance the role of DTCs, as in Scotland, Spain (Catalonia) and Sweden [34]. The Vietnamese Ministry of Health has issued circulars stating that all public hospitals should have DTCs. However, there are still concerns about the quality of prescribing.

Studies with hospital personnel from one of the leading hospitals in Hanoi showed improvements with developing hospital formularies, including key criteria for drug selection and processes for adding new drugs [52]. There were also opportunities to enhance the rational use of medicines [52,53], with previous drug utilization studies demonstrating inadequate prescribing of antibiotics, gastrointestinal medicines and medicines for emergency use – these medicines accounted for 70% of total costs and 13% of volume in 2009 [52], with just 24 antibiotics accounting for 30% of the utilization quantity and expenditure, including cefuroxime, ceftriaxone,

Table 21.2 Demand-side measures to improve the utilization of antibiotics in a selection of European countries.

Country/countries	Intervention (typically education) and outcome
Six European countries [89]	The objective was to assess whether Internet-based training methods could alter the prescribing of antibiotics for acute respiratory tract infections (RTIs) After a baseline audit in 2010, primary care practices in 6 EU countries were randomized in clusters to usual care, training in the use of a C-reactive protein (CRP) test at point of care, training in enhanced communication skills or both CRP and enhanced communication (education) Antibiotic prescribing rates were lower with CRP training than without (33 vs 48%) and with enhanced communication training than without (36 vs 45%) The combined intervention was associated with the greatest reduction in antibiotic prescribing rates Similar findings were obtained in individual country studies (e.g. the Netherlands [90])
Belgium [91]	The Belgian Antibiotic Policy Coordination Committee (BAPCOC) was established in 1999 by royal decree with the overall objective of promoting the judicious use of antibiotics Interventions (principally education) included: • multimedia campaigns to promote the prudent use of antibiotics in the community • national campaigns to promote hand hygiene in hospitals • publication of clinical practice guidelines • staffing and technical support for the establishment of antibiotic management teams in all Belgian hospitals • surveillance programmes on antibiotic use and the promotion of research These multiple activities resulted in a 36% reduction in antibiotic prescriptions between 1999–2000 and 2006–07
France [47]	The multifaceted national programme Keep Antibiotics Working, targeting all key stakeholders, launched in 2001, coupled with the public service campaign Les antibiotiques c'est pas automatique (Antibiotics Are Not Automatic), was run each winter since 2002 (education) Compared to the preintervention period (2000–02), the total number of antibiotic prescriptions per 100 inhabitants, adjusted for the frequency of flulike symptoms during the winter season, decreased by 26.5% from 2003 to 2007 The greatest reduction in antibiotic use (36%) was seen among children aged 6–15 years
Italy (Emilia Romagna Region) [92]	Antibiotic prescribing among GPs and paediatricians was reduced by 4.3% in the Modena and Parma localities of the Emilia Romagna region compared with controls following a multifaceted, local public campaign between November 2011 and February 2012 (education) Campaigns (education) included materials (mainly posters, brochures), advertisements on local media and a newsletter on local antibiotic resistance targeted at doctors and pharmacists
Slovenia [93]	Multifaceted interventions were instigated at the end of the 1990s following a 24% increase in antibiotic consumption in recent years. These interventions were undertaken by all key stakeholder groups, including the Ministry of Health, health insurance personnel and physician groups Interventions included education, engineering, economics and enforcement, with enforcement incorporating prescribing restrictions for a number of antibiotics and classes, including co-amoxiclav, third-generation cephalosporins, quinolones and macrolides From 1999 to 2012, antibiotic consumption decreased by 2–9% per year, with an overall decrease of 31%; this was greater for restricted than for nonrestricted antibiotics Expenditures on antibiotics decreased by 53% during the study period

cefoperazone and ceftazidime. Alongside this, there was also considerable expenditure on vitamins and herbal medicines. As a result, additional activities are being planned between hospitals and the Ministry of Health to enhance the rational use of drugs. The outcomes are being used to provide examples to other hospitals [52,53].

Enhancing the utilization of generics

Generic medicines are defined by the WHO as 'a pharmaceutical product, usually intended to be interchangeable with an innovator product that is manufactured without a licence from the innovator company and marketed after the expiry date of the patent or other exclusive rights' [54,55]. Generic medicines are required to have the same active substance, strength, route of administration, identity, quality and efficacy (i.e. bioequivalence requirements) and the same intended use as the single-source (patented) medicine [18,54,55]. Published studies have shown no difference in outcomes between generics and originators across a range of products and classes [56–59].

In Europe, the increased use of low-cost generic medicines is seen as essential in the face of growing resource pressures, the need to improve adherence where copayments are a concern and the need to improve access to medicines generally to support continued comprehensive and equitable health care [7,60–64].

In the US, Managed Care Organisations (MCOs) also encourage the prescribing of generics through co-payments and other mechanisms [12,63]. However this is changing with some generics where their prices are rapidly increasing, resulting in greater scrutiny over their prices. This is leading to either no coverage or increased co-payments (higher Tier levels). There are also concerns that generics are being combined with patented medicines in a single tablet, increasing rather than decreasing overall costs. This is resulting in prior authorisation and other mechanisms to reduce future costs without compromising care.

Kaplan et al. [65] reviewed policies among low- and middle-income countries to promote the use of generic medicines. The highlighted policies focused on (i) pricing, including reference pricing and tendering, and (ii) prescribing/dispensing incentives for all key stakeholder groups [65]. Barriers to the successful implementation of generic medicine policies included: (i) legal issues (e.g. competition and intellectual property barriers); (ii) management barriers; (iii) perception/knowledge barriers, with mixed views among prescribers; and (iv) financial barriers (e.g. the financial gains to physician from prescribing higher-priced patented medicines instead of lower-cost generics) [55,65].

Potential ways of enhancing the prescribing and dispensing of generics versus originators include pharmacy substitution targets (e.g. France), compulsory generic substitution with the lowest-cost generic (e.g. Sweden) and encouraging high INN prescribing, starting with physician education in medical schools and continuing with monitoring and prescribing support tools in ambulatory care (e.g. the United Kingdom) [66–68]. The initiatives in the United Kingdom have resulted in INN prescribing in over 80% of all prescriptions, rising to 98% or above with high-volume generics [68,69].

In Sweden, Andersson et al. [67,70] undertook a study to investigate how sales patterns for substitutable and nonsubstitutable pharmaceuticals developed following the introduction of mandatory generic substitution in Sweden in 2002 and to see how sales patterns differed in different groups of the population. They ascertained that in most therapeutic groups, there was an increase in the volume of substitutable pharmaceuticals following the reform. There were few gender differences in the sales patterns of substitutable and nonsubstitutable drugs. The authors concluded that there had been a proportionally larger increase in sales of substitutable pharmaceuticals compared with nonsubstitutable pharmaceuticals since the reform. They believed this indicated that the reform may well have contributed to growing sales of less expensive pharmaceuticals [70].

There have been multiple initiatives across countries to increase the prescribing of low-cost generics versus patented products in classes or related classes where all products are seen as therapeutically similar at appropriate does. The classes include PPIs, rennin-angiotensin inhibitors (including ACEIs and ARBs) and statins [28,30, 71–74]. Some of these classes will be used to illustrate a number of points that provide health authorities with future direction; however, these points apply to all classes.

Retrospective observational cross-national studies with the statins have shown the following:

- Multiple demand-side measures, including guidelines, academic detailing, benchmarking, prescribing targets and financial incentives (Table 21.3), increased the prescribing of low-cost generic simvastatin versus patented statins between 2001 and 2007 once generics became available. The reverse was seen in Ireland, with low use of generic simvastatin and few demand-side measures [24,27].

Table 21.3 Differences in utilization and expenditure for the statins among selected Western European countries between 2001 and 2007 [24,25,27,82,86]. Utilization measured in defined daily doses (DDDs).

Country	Demand-side measures	Change in utilization[a]	Change in expenditure[a]
France	Principally education: health insurance companies benchmarking GPs; government and health insurance company campaigns to enhance the acceptance of generics, including INN prescribing	↑ 2.1-fold	↑ 38%
	Economics and engineering: pay-for-performance targets instigated after the end of the study		
Scotland	Education: physicians trained in medical school to prescribe by INN name, with follow-up in the community, treatment guidelines, health board formularies, benchmarking and academic detailing	↑ 2.4-fold	↓ 52%
	Engineering: 'Better Care Better Value' indicators to enhance the prescribing of low-cost statins, therapeutic switch programmes and decision support software		
	Economics: physician financial incentives to encourage prescribing of generics in a class		
Ireland	No incentives or sanctions encouraging GPs to prescribe generic drugs versus originators or patented products during the study period	↑ 2.4-fold	↑ 2.6-fold
	Education: published guidelines – but these were not enforced		
Portugal	Mainly education: guidelines, encouraging INN prescribing and informing physicians every quarter of available generics	↑ 3.1-fold	↑ 1.9-fold
	No incentives or sanctions encouraging physicians to prescribe generic drugs versus originators or patented products during the study period		
Sweden	Education: regional and national guidance and guidelines, e.g. the 'Wise List' of Stockholm County Council; benchmarking of prescribing, coupled with continuous feedback; computerized decision support tools; mandating at least one DTC in each region to enhance the rational use of medicines	↑ 42%	↓ 48%
	Engineering: prescribing targets (e.g. percentage of statins prescribed as generic statins)		
	Economics: physician financial incentives to achieve agreed prescribing targets, devolved drug budgets, patient copayments for more expensive brand than the reference-priced molecule		
	Enforcement: compulsory substitution with the cheapest available product for the molecule		

[a] Changes refer to 2007 vs. 2001. Reimbursed expenditure as health authority perspective.

- The multiple measures in Scotland and Sweden (Table 21.3) appreciably enhanced prescribing efficiency in these countries compared with Ireland and Portugal, with few demand-side measures at the time without compromising care. All statins were seen as therapeutically equivalent at appropriate doses in meta-analyses and observational studies, including therapeutic switching programmes [71,73,75,76].
- As a result, total statin expenditure in Sweden in 2007, when adjusted for population size, was less than one-tenth of that seen in Ireland, with its few demand-side measures. However, there was greater comorbidity among the database population in Ireland [5,27].
- Multiple demand-side measures persisted in Scotland (Table 21.3) beyond 2007. Without these, expenditure on the statins for the same overall utilization would have been GBP290 million greater in 2010 for the 5.2 million population [24].

A similar situation was seen with the PPIs and ACEIs versus ARBs across Europe [5,27,28,68].

Multiple demand-side measures in Scotland (education, engineering and economics; similar to the situation for statins shown in Table 21.3) between 2001 and 2007 limited the prescribing of premium-priced singe-source ARBs over low-cost generic ACEIs (Table 21.4) [28]. ARB utilization was appreciably higher in Portugal, again with few demand-side measures to encourage the preferential prescribing of generic ACE inhibitors first-line [28,68].

From a health policy perspective, it is encouraging to see that the multiple demand-side measures in Scotland had a similar influence on limiting the prescribing of ARBs between 2001 and 2007 as in Austria and Croatia,

Table 21.4 ARBs as percentage of total renin angiotensin inhibitor drug utilization (DDD basis) 2001–07 [28].

	2001	2002	2003	2004	2005	2006	2007	% change
Austria	15	18	19	21	22	24	25	9
Scotland	12	13	15	16	17	18	19	7
Croatia	2	3	6	9	12	14	13	11
Portugal	20	25	29	33	36	40	44	25

The differences in ARB utilization rates between Austria and Croatia may be due to more intensive follow-up of prescribing restrictions in Croatia.

where ARBs; were restricted to second-line treatment [28]. In these two countries, ARBs were only reimbursed if patients were experiencing unacceptable side effects with ACEIs otherwise, 100% copayment was required [28]. This has important implications for countries that are unable to introduce prescribing restrictions. The multiple demand-side measures in Scotland resulted in stable expenditure on renin-angiotensin inhibitor drugs between 2001 and 2007. This compares with a >40% increase in expenditure in Portugal in 2007 versus 2001, despite a greater increase in total utilization in Scotland between 2001 and 2007 [28,68]. This would seem to endorse the multiple approaches used in Scotland.

Similar findings to those with PPIs, statins and renin angiotensin inhibitor medicines were seen following the introduction of generic losartan as the first generic ARB in Western Europe. Health authority initiatives ranged from (i) delisting all patented ARBs from the reimbursement list in Denmark (i.e. just reimbursing generic ARBs) to (ii) multiple interventions, including education, financial incentives, prescribing targets and therapeutic switching, in Sweden to (iii) removing prescribing restrictions for losartan but not single-sourced ARBs in Austria and Belgium to (iv) few activities in Ireland, Scotland and Spain (Catalonia) (Table 21.5) [30]. The findings included:

- The greatest change in losartan utilization among the countries taking part in this CNC study was seen in Denmark [30]. The combination of supply-side measures reducing the price of generic losartan and the delisting of patented ARBs in Denmark (Table 21.5) resulted in a 77% reduction in ARB expenditure post generic losartan by the end of the study, despite a 16% increase in utilization [77].
- Multiple demand-side measures in Sweden (Table 21.5) resulted in total single ARB expenditure falling by 26% post generic losartan by the end of the study, despite a 16% increase in utilization [78].
- A consistent limited change in losartan utilization was seen post generics in the three countries with few, if any, specific demand-side measures encouraging its prescribing (i.e. Ireland, Scotland and Spain; Table 21.5). The findings in Scotland suggest no spillover of learnings from one class to another to favourably influence physician prescribing of generics even if they are closely related (i.e. the multiple demand-side measures that successfully encouraged the preferential prescribing of generic ACEIs versus patented ARBs [28,68] were not carried through into the preferential prescribing of generic losartan versus patented ARBs [79]). There was a similar finding in one primary care organization (PCO) in England [33]. There was no change in losartan utilization post generic losartan where there were no specific initiatives encouraging its preferential prescribing. However, there was a significant increase in losartan utilization following multiple demand-side measures, including (i) education – academic detailing, prescribing guidance, issuing information to patients and community pharmacists; (ii) engineering – prescribing targets and therapeutic switching programmes, with patients followed up; and (iii) economics – financial incentive schemes [33]. Annual net savings from this multiple programme were estimated at over eight times the cost of implementation, endorsing this approach [33].

It may not always be possible for health authorities to take full advantage of the availability of generics in a class. This is the case with atypical antipsychotic drugs in patients with schizophrenia and bipolar disease, where health authorities recognize that pharmacologic treatment should be tailored to individual patients [80]. As a result, there were generally few demand-side measures among European countries to encourage the preferential prescribing of risperidone following the availability of generics [31]. A CNC study using an interrupted time-series design showed there was no significant change in risperidone utilization as a percentage of

Table 21.5 Summary of policies initiated among European countries following the introduction of generic losartan.

Source: Adapted from [30].

Country	Activities
Austria	Economics and enforcement: Prescribing restrictions were removed for losartan but not for patented ARBs, with ambulatory care physicians still required to document the rationale for prescribing a patented ARB versus an ACE inhibitor. Potential sanctions for abuse included physicians having to pay back to the Austrian Health Insurers an estimate of the increased drug expenditure.
Belgium	Economics and enforcement: Losartan changed from a chapter IV to a chapter I medicine, while patented ARBs remained chapter IV (i.e. second-line in patients experiencing side effects with ACE inhibitors). A chapter IV medicine can only be prescribed subject to prior approval – otherwise, a 100% copayment is required. A chapter I medicine can be prescribed without restrictions.
Denmark	Economics and enforcement: All patented ARBs were removed from the reimbursement list. Patients can still be prescribed a patented ARB and have this reimbursed. However, the prescribing physician has to justify the rationale to the authorities and have the explanation accepted before patented ARBs are reimbursed. Otherwise, 100% patient copayment is required.
Ireland	No specific activities were undertaken to influence the prescribing of losartan versus patented ARBs.
Scotland	No specific activities were undertaken to encourage the preferential prescribing of losartan versus patented ARBs in view of other identified priorities by NHS Scotland and the imminent launch of a number of generics of currently patented ARBs.
Spain (Catalonia)	No specific activities were undertaken to encourage the preferential prescribing of losartan, apart from highlighting standard costs/DDDs for ACE inhibitors and ARBs in physician contracts.
Sweden	Education: county (regional) DTCs encouraging the prescribing of generic losartan; academic detailing endorsing losartan as the ARB of choice; monitoring and feedback.
	Engineering: prescribing targets (e.g. losartan as a percentage of all ARBs); therapeutic switching programmes initiated by some counties (regions).
	Economics: budget devolution; revision of physician- or practice-based financial incentives to include the prescribing of losartan versus patented ARBs.
	Enforcement: from May 2011, prescribing restrictions were lifted for losartan but not the other ARBs. In addition, originator losartan was removed from the reimbursement list.

all selected atypical antipsychotics (DDD basis) following generic availability, with good consistency of results among the countries included in the analysis [31].

Conclusion

Health authorities worldwide are introducing multiple reforms and initiatives to enhance the rational use of medicines, including promoting the prescribing of generics versus originators and patented products. This is a key strategy if the goal is to achieve or sustain universal health care and ensure the best use of limited health care resources.

There are a plethora of measures that can be initiated by health authorities to achieve a more rational use of medicines. These measures can be categorized as either supply-side, focused principally on pricing, or demand-side, which can be collated under the 4Es [26]. Drug utilization studies play an important role in both describing medicine use over time and measuring the impact of the different measures instigated by authorities in their quest to promote the best use of medicines in their populations. They have shown, for instance, that multiple demand-side measures are typically needed to influence future physician prescribing, and they highlight that there may be a limited spillover effect between drugs classes affecting changes in physician prescribing habits.

The design of drug utilization studies is dependent on the availability of and access to data, as well as the time period over which the reforms are initiated [37]. Studies assessing time trends in drug utilization are typically conducted using aggregated data, while more sophisticated studies analysing indications and the effectiveness and safety of different treatment approaches require patient-level data linked to clinical information [37].

CHAPTER 22

The pharmaceutical industry and health policy

Richard Torbett[1,2], Donald Han[3] & Indranil Bagchi[3]

[1]*European Federation of Pharmaceutical Industries and Associations (EFPIA), Belgium*

[2]*IMT Institute of Advanced Studies, Italy*

[3]*Pfizer, United States*

KEY POINTS

- Medicines have made a major contribution to population health over many decades.
- An ageing population in much of the developed world means that, despite the challenge for publicly funded health systems, maintaining provision of care in a dynamically efficient and effective way is important to avoiding great economic and societal costs.
- Medicines expenditure is kept efficient by ensuring rational use of cheaper generic medicines on the one hand and scrutinizing value for money of new medicines on the other.
- A variety of tools exist to help assess the value of medicines, increasingly involving the use of real-world data in various forms.
- There needs to be continuous improvement in assessment methods – through a multistakeholder effort – in order to keep pace with new science and to correct for any unintended biases.

Introduction

Medicines are an intrinsic part of any health system. Spending on pharmaceuticals was approximately 17% of all health care expenditure among Organisation for Economic Co-operation and Development (OECD) countries in 2011 [1], making medicines the third largest cost component after inpatient and ambulatory care. However, expenditure on medicines has fallen relative to other areas of health care expenditure in recent years, as the efficiencies generated by the loss of market exclusivity of major products have to a large degree offset the costs associated with the introduction of new medicines.

At the same time, the overall demand for health care continues to grow. This trend is likely to continue in the coming decades, as an ageing demographic in much of the developed world is likely to be associated with an increase in the prevalence of several – especially chronic – diseases [2]. As a result, policymakers everywhere are looking to ensure health systems are as efficient as possible, so that health care provision can continue in a financially sustainable way. In this context, the management of the use of medicines – ensuring an appropriate balance between the rational use of cheaper generic medicines and allowing access to innovations, especially those that address unmet need or which can help improve the quality and efficiency of care – has become an important priority.

There are broadly two categories of policy that drive health system efforts to ensure the appropriate management of medicines. First are policies that encourage the greater use of low-cost generics instead of brand-name medicines, including originators and patented medicines. Such policies can include therapeutic protocols, prescribing targets, financial incentives and prescribing restrictions [3] (see Chapters 20 and 21). Second, there is an increasingly sophisticated set of measures aimed at ensuring that when new medicines come to market, they are not only safe but effective in the real world and offer value for money. Such policies include health technology assessment, framework agreements,

Drug Utilization Research: Methods and Applications, First Edition. Edited by M. Elseviers et al.
Published 2016 by John Wiley & Sons, Ltd.

managed entry agreements and a variety of arrangements whereby use – and sometimes pricing or reimbursement – is tied to assessment of real-world data. Drug utilization research has been, and will continue to be, an important field in informing health care systems whether both sets of policies are working well and in monitoring the balance between access to innovation and rational use of older medicines [4–6].

For the research-based pharmaceutical industry, it has become increasingly important to engage with policymakers on the design of policies for how new medicines will be assessed and valued [7,8]. Indeed, failure to achieve a constructive dialogue on these issues typically leads to instability for all sides. Medicines innovation is undergoing significant transformation, as the pharmaceutical industry is producing relatively more hospital-based specialty products and targeted therapies [9] and, alongside regulators, is exploring 'adaptive models of development and licensing' [10–13]. In the future, this will mean greater emphasis on the collection of evidence throughout a product's life cycle [14,15]. Such changes also create challenges for health systems, which can struggle to reallocate budgets to areas of innovation at the same time as developing new approaches to valuation of new medicines, especially where evidence may be limited or not fully captured during initial assessments (see Chapter 20).

This chapter presents some of the current and future challenges in this area and outlines how drug utilization research can support medicines development and assessment throughout the life cycle.

Ensuring value for money when financing future health needs

Medicines have made an appreciable contribution to improving the health of patients [16–18] through reducing morbidity and mortality [11]. However, despite the progress that has been made, inequalities in health outcomes persist within and across countries. For example, in Europe, there is an approximate 10 year variance in life expectancy at birth between the healthiest and least healthy nations [19,20]. Such inequality is often associated with wealth, lifestyle and, critically, access to health care services, including medicines.

Chronic diseases, especially noncommunicable diseases (NCDs), are a particular concern, with approximately 75% of Europe's health care expenditure spent on managing patients with chronic diseases, amounting to €700 billion annually [21]. Studies have shown that medicines can reduce disease burden, with the availability of generics further helping to prevent or reduce future morbidity and mortality. The example of the statins (cholesterol-lowering medicines: HMG CoA-reductase inhibitors) is illustrated in Box 22.1. However, compliance can be a concern with statins, necessitating follow-up drug

Box 22.1 Statins and reduced morbidity and mortality.

- Pharmaceutical company-funded outcome studies such as the Scandinavian Simvastatin Survival Study (4S) have demonstrated a significant reduction in cardiac events with simvastatin in patients with coronary heart disease (CHD) [25].
- Subsequent drug utilization studies have further contributed to the knowledge base and have found statins to be effective, cost-effective and safe for a broad range of patients. However, there have been concerns over their use in combination with fibrates, especially cerivastatin. These concerns led to the withdrawal of cerivastatin in 2001 [26–35].
- National survey data from the US National Health and Nutritional Examination Study (NHANES) demonstrated that statin therapy reduced low-density lipoprotein levels by 18.8%, which translated into roughly 40000 fewer deaths, 60000 fewer hospitalizations for heart attacks and 22 000 fewer hospitalizations for strokes in 2008 [36].
- Statin therapy was associated with a 27% reduction in cardiovascular health care costs per patient, including coronary artery bypass grafts and electrocardiograms (ECGs), versus placebo [37]. From 1987 to 2008, the aggregate social value of statins was estimated at USD1.252 trillion, with the patient surplus associated with statins estimated at USD947.4 billion [37].
- The availability of generic statins in recent years has reduced concerns over access and affordability. This is exemplified by a lowering of threshold levels for the prevention of coronary vascular disease (CVD).

utilization studies to assess and help optimize treatment patterns [22–24].

The burden on chronic disease is likely to grow, given ageing populations and rising rates of obesity, hypertension, diabetes and other NCDs globally [16]. If not adequately addressed by all key stakeholder groups, this will lead to increases in lost productivity, morbidity and mortality [38]. Cost-of-illness studies have shown that the current cost of chronic diseases and their risk factors already have a sizeable impact on a country's gross domestic product (GDP), ranging from 0.02 to 6.77% [39]. In addition, poor health contributes to early labour market exit, whether directly due to ill health or in order to care for relatives [40]. It has also been shown that the share of disability life years within total life expectancy has risen; that is, although people are living longer, they are spending a greater proportion of their lives in some form of disability or illness [41].

The increasing health burden, coupled with a decline in the number of working people [42], means that society faces a dual challenge in the coming decades. On the one hand, financing increased health care demand will be difficult, especially for state-funded universal health systems. On the other, failure to provide adequate health care would lead to enormous economic cost, which would make matters even worse. Policy that considers both of these two challenges in a coherent and connected way is important. As long as systems are delivering care in an efficient and high-quality manner, they should be seen as an investment on which economic growth can be built. On the other hand, if, in the name of 'sustainability', policymakers are tempted to cut back the provision of health services – at a time when we need it most – they should be aware of the economic as well as obvious societal consequences [43].

Policymakers, health authorities, researchers, pharmaceutical companies and the public all need to work together to secure the sustainability of global public health, including providing a climate for fostering innovation [2]. Health systems need to pursue reforms that result in genuine efficiency, while concurrently ensuring enough budgetary space for new medicines that address unmet need and/or improve the quality or efficiency of care.

There are four key areas of current discussion that are worth noting here:

1 health technology assessment of the value of medicines;
2 framework agreements;
3 priority medicines development;
4 outcomes-focused health system reform.

Health technology assessment of the value of medicines

All advanced health systems have some way of assessing the value for money of new medicines. Although the exact methods, processes and data used vary from country to country, the clear trend is to try and ensure that the best available evidence on the value of medicines is used to inform decisions about their future use. There is a need for continuous improvement in such health technology assessment processes, for example to address issues related to new scientific developments or to address biases in the way in which some outcome measures, including current quality-of-life scales, are more meaningful in some disease areas than in others.

Another major point of debate is around the scope of costs and benefits used in the final decision on the funding and reimbursement of a particular new medicine. Some systems, for instance, only consider costs and benefits that accrue to the health system itself, whereas others make an attempt to consider wider societal costs and benefits, such as in terms of productivity or social care burden [8]. The debate is particularly current in Europe, where a number of health care systems are considering how to measure the wider societal impact of new treatments – especially those for chronic conditions such as arthritis, cardiovascular diseases (CVDs), diabetes and neurological conditions such as dementia, Parkinson's disease and stroke.

The question of whether or not to try and incorporate wider societal impact into assessments is, however, sometimes easier than the question of how to do so in practice. For instance, the UK National Institute for Health and Care Excellence (NICE) recently rejected a government proposal that its assessment of new medicines should include wider societal impact, following an inconclusive public consultation [44]. However, the debate is still ongoing.

The Scottish Medicines Consortium (SMC) has also recently introduced a Patient and Clinician Engagement (PACE) group in recognition of some of these concerns. PACE gives patient groups and clinicians a stronger voice in funding decisions by giving them the opportunity to better describe the added benefits of new medicines, which may not be fully captured within the conventional clinical and economic assessment process [45].

Increasing knowledge about wider societal impact through patient-specific drug utilization and other studies will help inform future debates on how to assess the value of medicines.

Framework agreements

Industry-level agreements with governments or health systems on the management of medicines usage can be an important mechanism by which to achieve stability and predictability in the medicines market. Several countries have a long tradition of establishing such agreements, such as the Pharmaceutical Pricing and Regulation Scheme (PPRS) in the United Kingdom [46] and the Accord Cadre in France [8,47]. These schemes use a variety of methods to, on the one hand, provide a framework for assessing value for money, and on the other, seek assurance that the ongoing development of valuable new medicines remains a priority. Recently, an agreement was signed in Lithuania with the similar aim of improving rational use and mix in medicine markets in order to both control cost and release resources for use on new products [48]. Drug utilization research will have an increasingly important role to play in improving the sophistication of such agreements, helping to monitor delivery against commitments for all parties and ensuring that objectives of financial management and access to innovation are met.

Priority medicines development

The World Health Organization (WHO), in collaboration with the European Commission, undertook to prepare a report on Priority Medicines for Europe and the World 2013. This report identified priority disease areas for research based on four criteria: (i) global burden of disease; (ii) risk factors amenable to pharmacological intervention; (iii) prediction of disease burden trends based on epidemiological and demographical changes; and (iv) social solidarity (where there is no market incentive to develop new treatments) [17]. This is critical in informing the priorities for pharmaceutical research and for establishing associated research funding strategies by which to create and sustain innovation in medicines. Within this report, the development of real-life data utilizing electronic health records (EHRs) is highlighted as a key route by which to better understand and inform the safety, effectiveness and affordability of medicines [2]. Others have also highlighted the increased use of EHRs in improving knowledge of future care delivery options [49,50].

Outcomes-focused health system reform

Finally, the notion of outcomes-focused health system reform is becoming an increasingly important part of the discussion about how all inputs to health care, including medicines, can be used optimally to ensure both maximum quality of care for the patient and efficient use of resources [51]. At the core of the outcomes-focused health system concept is the idea that we need to measure health outcomes more effectively than we have done in the past, make data transparent, analyse outcomes data in order to understand practice variation within each disease area and put the resulting insights to use in designing more appropriate care pathways [52]. Those responsible for care pathways should be given more flexibility to manage budgets in a holistic way, in order to configure the best care model for each disease area. By taking down previous budget silos and rewarding the mix of resources that results in the best patient outcome, more appropriate care delivery models can be developed [53]. Those inputs – medicines, other technologies and services – that add the most value for money will be naturally used more; those adding less value for money will be used less.

Application of drug utilization methods throughout the product life cycle

There is an increasing need for all key stakeholders to work together to successfully address areas of unmet need alongside issues of access and affordability. Pharmaceutical companies are increasingly undertaking and making use of drug utilization studies throughout the product life cycle to support internal decision-making and enhance the potential for future revenues through robust demonstrations of the value of their medicines (Figure 22.1).

Disease and population characteristics shaping medicine development

Pharmaceutical companies increasingly characterize disease states in terms of their current/predicted level of unmet need, which can be based on published reports, such as the recent WHO Priority Disease Report [2]. For

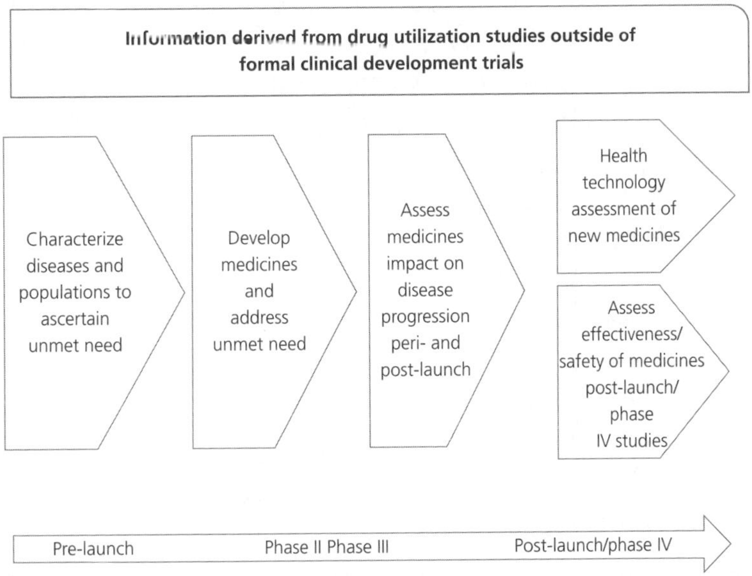

Figure 22.1 Product life cycle for new medicines: drug utilization activities supporting formal clinical trial processes.

given diseases, pharmaceutical companies will typically document current and predicted treatment patterns using pharmacoepidemiological techniques, bridging the gap between epidemiology and clinical pharmacology [4]. Pertinent issues include effectiveness, adverse drug reactions (ADRs) and adherence issues with current treatments, as these affect patient experiences' and ultimately the clinical outcome. Effectiveness rates include the number of patients needed to treat (NNT) to gain an effect, balanced against the numbers needed to harm (NNH) attributable to ADRs [12]. Increased knowledge of pharmacogenomics is leading to an increase in targeted treatments and should reduce NNTs and increase NNHs for new medicines [12].

Published studies have shown that ADRs add to the costs of health care by increasing hospital admissions and other costs [54–56]. For example, the average treatment costs for a single ADR in Germany have been estimated at approximately €2250, equating to €434 million per year [57], while the cost of drug-related morbidity and mortality exceeded USD177.4 billion in the United States in 2000 [58]. The study in Germany found that the digestive system was affected by ADRs, followed by endocrine, nutritional and metabolic diseases. The majority of ADRs were dose-dependent and predictable, with only a minority idiosyncratic.

The ability to target new treatments to patient populations where the health gain is greatest (e.g. where NNTs can be reduced and NNHs increased) should be attractive to health authorities. Currently, approximately 10% of new medicines approved by the US Food and Drug Administration (FDA) carry pharmacogenomic biomarker information in their labels [59], and this trend is expected to grow beyond the areas of oncology and specialty medicines to increasingly include chronic diseases managed in ambulatory care.

Restricting prescribing to identified subpopulations is also increasingly possible, with the growing use of sophisticated IT systems, including e-prescribing and EHRs [50,60–62].

Figures 22.2 and 22.3 illustrate how pharmaceutical companies are already concentrating new product development in areas of unmet need. In 2011, there were over 16 000 compounds in various stages of development, with over 80% of medicines focused on degenerative diseases, NCDs and cancer [11,63].

As shown in Figure 22.3, pipelines are broadly aligned with those disease areas that are estimated to yield most societal benefit in terms of disability-adjusted life years (DALYs).

There is increasing recognition of the importance of evidence that goes beyond the information required by regulatory authorities for marketing approval, collected in randomized controlled trials (RCTs) during clinical development. It is also widely acknowledged that it is increasingly difficult for pharmaceutical companies to

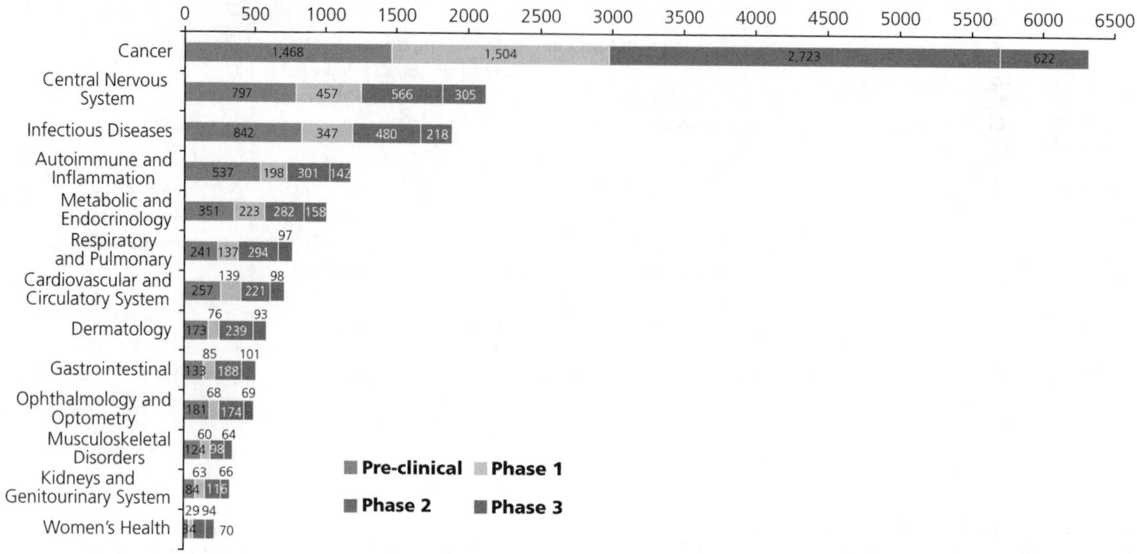

Figure 22.2 Pharmaceutical medicines in development in 2011. For colour details, please refer to the colour plates section.

Source: EFPIA. HEALTH & GROWTH – Working together for a healthy Europe. A vision towards a life sciences strategy for Europe [63].

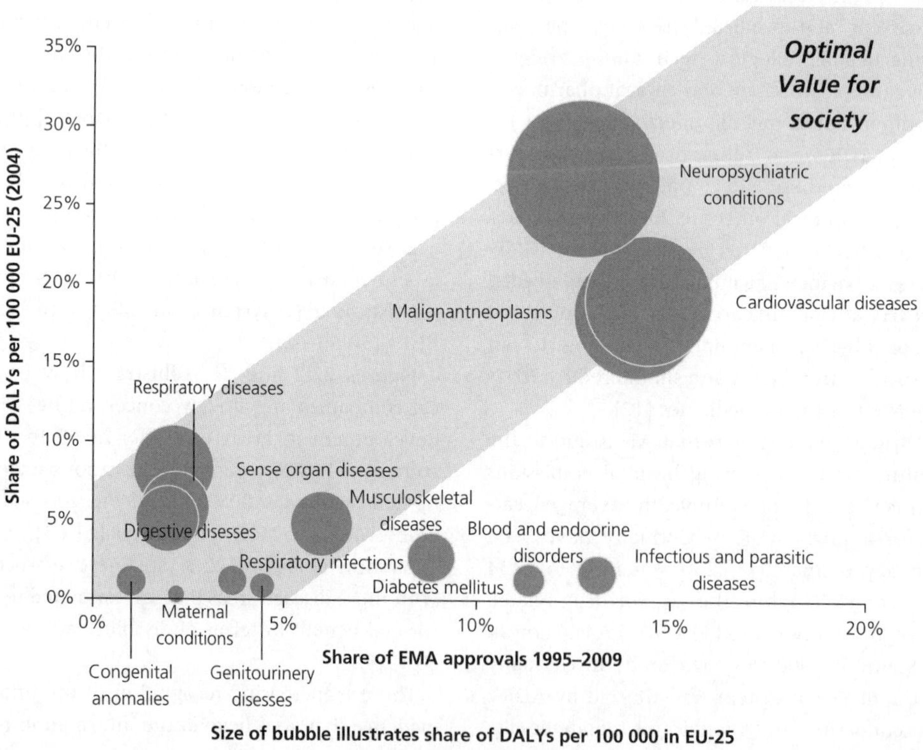

Figure 22.3 Share of EMA approvals 1995–2009 and share of DALYs per 100 000 in EU-25. Size of bubble illustrates share of DALYs per 100 000 in EU-25.

Source: EFPIA. HEALTH & GROWTH – Evidence Compendium. October 30th, 2013 [11].

achieve premium prices for their new medicines without demonstrating improvements in the effectiveness and/or safety of their new medicine versus current standards. This is a challenge for innovators, and it is exacerbated by the increasing number of effective medicines becoming available as safe low-cost generics and biosimilars [64–68].

Knowledge of current treatment patterns, outcomes and concerns/unmet needs in given disease areas can be used to design a method of data collection that is more relevant to key health authority decision-makers [7,69]. This knowledge can also be used to design predictive models of virtual trials, which can be used to aid internal decision-making within pharmaceutical companies. It allows the key characteristics of patients who should be included in phase II and III clinical trials to be identified, as well as potential indications for inclusion in future phase IV trials.

Assessment of medicines peri- and post-launch

These activities can be divided into three components, all involving drug utilization studies:

- Health technology assessments of new medicines, to support pricing and reimbursement applications.
- Managed-entry agreements (MEAs)/risk-sharing arrangements, to support reimbursement.
- Patient registry studies, to assess the effectiveness and safety of new medicines in routine clinical care to aid in future decision-making.

Health technology assessments

Health authorities are increasingly seeking information on the potential value of new medicines, to allow them to make informed judgements concerning value for money. They require different datasets for different value assessments [8]. Some authorities request cost per quality-adjusted life year (QALY) (e.g. Norway, Poland, Sweden and the United Kingdom), potentially alongside budget impact data [8,70], while others want pharmaceutical companies to provide them with comprehensive clinical datasets, to enable them to assess the level of health gain of new treatments versus current standards and so discuss potential prices for the new medicines (e.g. Austria, France and Germany) [8,71]. A recent report from the OECD provides a comprehensive summary of the data requirements for the major European markets and other countries [8].

We are also increasingly likely to see pharmaceutical companies and health authorities working together to develop robust models of the likely budget impact of new medicines in all or targeted populations [70]. These will be based on improved knowledge of the incidence and prevalence of given diseases and of current treatment approaches, helped by comprehensive drug utilization data.

Managed-entry agreements

MEAs are used to facilitate the reimbursement of new medicines and improve health authority budgeting in times of uncertainty. They have been used increasingly often in recent years, with 116 implemented in 2011 alone [72]. Despite this, however, there appears to be a lack of peer-reviewed publications assessing their impact in practice [73]. It is hoped this will be addressed through drug utilization and other studies, since MEAs can potentially help pharmaceutical companies, pricing and reimbursement agencies and physicians develop a more complete understanding of the real-world value, safety, effectiveness and optimal use of new medicines, including orphan drugs [74].

Properly used, MEAs can increase access to new treatments and give stakeholders confidence that new medicines are being used efficiently. However, they must be supported by sufficient data and technical capacity and they are not appropriate for every new medicine or for every health care system. Ideally, MEAs should address genuine uncertainties, be straightforward to implement, be aligned with regulatory post-approval commitments, be rigorously evaluated and be time-bound. However, it is accepted that the latter may be difficult given the limitations in data availability with some agreements – especially access to patient identity data.

Patient registry studies

The number of patient registry studies is increasing. They are usually used in two ways:

- Reimbursement purposes: Registries can be part of MEAs, price consideration agreements or other studies informing authorities of the value of new medicines (Box 22.2).

Box 22.2 Examples of patient registry studies informing reimbursement decisions.

- Follow-on registry studies in France under the guidance of the French authorities have demonstrated the value of omalizumab in the management of patients with severe asthma. Hospitalization and emergency room visits were significantly decreased in patients with uncontrolled severe asthma, helping with continued reimbursement [75]. These studies were conducted following concerns over the effectiveness and cost-effectiveness of omalizumab, based on clinical trials conducted by some authorities [76].
- Evidence generated by registries in Sweden has informed product reassessments and improved access. Using data from its rheumatoid arthritis registry, the National Board of Health and Welfare determined that early treatment with tumour necrosis factor (TNF) inhibitors was cost-effective. As a result, national rheumatoid arthritis guidelines prioritized early treatment with TNF inhibitors [77].
- CVS Caremark in the United States plans to conduct comparative effectiveness research using its own anonymized claims data to inform guidelines, improve patient adherence and lower costs [78].

Box 22.3 Examples of patient registry studies assessing the effectiveness and safety of medicines in routine clinical care.

- Natalizumab became available across Europe for the management of patients with multiple sclerosis in 2006 under strict prescribing regulations [80,81]. Patient registry studies are ongoing to investigate whether seropositivity for JCV antibodies will help accurately predict the development of leukoencephalopathy (PML), as well as improve understanding of the risks of patients developing PML if they remain seronegative to JCV while still taking natalizumab or of the risks of developing PML if they convert from seronegativity to seropositivity. This continual reevaluation is important in avoiding unpredictable events [80].
- The ARTIS register involved all rheumatological clinics in Sweden. Its objective was to investigate the effectiveness and safety of tumour necrosis factors (TNFs) in treating patients with rheumatoid arthritis [82]. It showed that:
  - Rheumatoid arthritis patients treated with biological drugs are not at increased risk of invasive melanoma.
  - Rheumatoid arthritis patients selected for TNF-α inhibitor treatment are not at increased overall risk for cancer, but have a 50% increased relative risk of invasive melanoma.
  - Given the small increase in absolute risk, these findings do not shift the overall risk–benefit balance of the use of TNF inhibitors in clinical practice, but may do so in patients at high risk of melanoma for other reasons.

- Effectiveness, safety and dosage of medicines: Registries can assess effectiveness, safety and dosage in routine clinical care, to inform future treatment practices (Box 22.3).

In addition, in the United States, Humana has entered into a partnership with Pfizer with the aim of using drug utilization review study results to improve health care for the elderly [79]. It is likely that such agreements will become more common in the future.

Communication of drug utilization studies

Drug utilization tools are the basis for all registry analyses and are likely to increase in use with the advent of EHRs [2] and with future developments such as adaptive licensing approaches for new medicines [10,14]. This increasing use of drug utilization studies has resulted in scientific societies concerned with the use of drug utilization data evaluating health outcomes publishing practice guidance and regulatory standards [83,84]. Care may be needed with the interpretation and communication of drug utilization studies.

Table 22.1 presents a case study in which multiple studies generated different findings. In part, this may be attributable to the differing methodological approaches applied. Consequently, caution should be exercised as new studies are published. A greater understanding of the methodologies involved and of the underlying messages is critical to making sound interpretation of the implications.

Table 22.1 Oral bisphosphonate case study.

Key characteristics	Findings
Overview	Oral bisphosphonates are used to treat osteoporosis; common side effects include trouble swallowing and inflammation of the oesophagus [85] From 1998 to 2008, the FDA received reports of 54 patients from the United States, Europe and Japan who developed oesophageal cancer after taking oral bisphosphonates [86]
Response	In 2010, two teams of independent researchers used the UK General Practice Research Database to investigate the potential link between oral bisphosphonates and oesophageal (and other) cancers: • In August, one team published a study in JAMA showing that individuals who had taken oral bisphosphonates did not have a higher incidence of oesophageal cancer [87] • In September, another team published a study in the BMJ showing that individuals taking oral bisphosphonates had a significantly higher risk of developing oesophageal cancer [88]
Outcome	The 2013 National Osteoporosis Foundation guidelines still recommended prescribing oral bisphosphonates (and other FDA-approved drugs) to treat osteoporosis and reduce fractures [85] The FDA initiated a review of the evidence to determine whether oral bisphosphonates increased the risk of developing oesophageal cancer; the review started in 2011 [89] and is ongoing [90]
Key conclusion	The oral bisphosphonates case study illustrates the need for clear standards when using real-world data-generated findings, particularly as different methodologies – even when applied to the same database – can lead to conflicting outcomes

Conclusion

Universal health care is a particularly important objective for governments over the coming decades as they attempt to meet the challenge of an ageing demographic. Failure to invest in health care will result in serious economic and societal consequences. At the same time, given the scale of demand, it is essential that health care expenditure is as efficient and effective as possible; this includes the need to provide sufficient incentive for ongoing innovation – dynamic, not static efficiency. Indeed, it has been shown that even if governments successfully implement 'cost containment', they will still face a challenge in affording health care based on current technology [91]. There is, then, no choice but to innovate.

In this context, medicines policy must ensure the rational use of older generic medicines where they are suitable for patients, as well as the appropriate use of newer innovations. An increasingly sophisticated array of tools is now available to policymakers to assist in the assessment of a given medicine's value for money. The use of real-world data, in various forms, lies at the heart of many of these tools, and drug utilization research has an important role to play in ensuring available data are appropriately interpreted. Assessment tools and methods need to be improved continually to keep pace with scientific developments and to address inherent methodological biases – such as the difficulties seen with current techniques in fully assessing the value of new medicines for orphan diseases and cancer. Improved planning, in order to optimize the managed entry of new drugs well before launch dates, is also necessary. As well as maximizing the resources released from the improved management of established drugs, such improved planning will relieve pressure on health systems that struggle to cope with the introduction of new technologies. In adopting this approach, the pharmaceutical industry will also receive clearer signals about which treatments are most valued by health systems – information vital to the direction of future innovation.

Such continuous improvement in medicines value assessments requires a multistakeholder effort. The pharmaceutical industry constitutes one of the building blocks of an effective and well-functioning health care system. The development and implementation of policies that can make an innovative and sustainable pharmaceutical market a reality will bring substantial benefits to all stakeholders within the health care ecosystem: patients, prescribers, policy makers, companies and payers.

CHAPTER 23

Drug utilization in pregnant women

Hedvig Nordeng
Pharmaco-Epidemiology and Drug Safety Research Group, School of Pharmacy, University of Oslo, Norway

KEY POINTS

- The prevalence of drug use in pregnancy ranges from 27 to 99%, with analgesics, antiinfectives, antacids and respiratory drugs being most frequently used. By far, paracetamol (acetaminophen) is the most commonly used drug during pregnancy, being used by almost half of all pregnant women.
- Ideally, information on the timing (trimester), dose and duration of medicine use in pregnancy should be recorded in drug utilization studies, as these factors impact on foetal safety.
- Studies have consistently reported the use of potentially hazardous drugs during pregnancy. The US Food and Drug Administration (FDA) and the European Union have adopted a new approach to labelling: a narrative description of the evidence available for the use of a given drug in pregnancy, rather than the risk categories previously used.
- Some medication groups have received special focus in time-trend drug utilization studies, due to new drugs being introduced on to the market, special concerns about prescription policy and debate about safety in pregnancy. This particularly affects antidepressants and antiinfectives.
- Relatively few drug utilisation studies have reported the prevalence of herbal drug use in pregnancy. Those that do show a wide range of use, from 1 to as high as 87%.

Background

Because drugs may cause injury to unborn children, we need to know which are used in pregnancy, by whom, during which trimester and for what reason. This lesson was learned in the 1960s and 1970s, when almost 10 000 children were born with malformed extremities after exposure to thalidomide during gestation (see Box 23.1) [1].

Avoiding all drugs in pregnancy is unrealistic, and may even be dangerous. Untreated diabetes, epilepsy, severe mental illnesses and infections may all be harmful to the foetus, and thus require treatment. On the other hand, superfluous use of drugs can have potential negative consequences for the health of the woman and the unborn child. The fact that over-the-counter (OTC) and herbal drugs are available without the involvement of health care professionals underlines the importance of generating information about the use of drugs during pregnancy. Therefore, drug utilization studies with the objective of generating knowledge about the use of drugs during pregnancy are important. Substantial health benefits could be obtained by preventing incorrect use of drugs and by improving the prescription of drugs to pregnant women. ***This chapter will give an overview of drug utilization studies in pregnancy and***

Box 23.1 Thalidomide advertisement from the pharmaceutical company Chemie Grunenthal, 1958.

'In pregnancy and during the lactation period the female organism is under great strain. Sleeplessness, unrest and tension are constant complaints. The administration of a sedative and hypnotic that will hurt neither the mother nor child is often necessary.'

Drug Utilization Research: Methods and Applications, First Edition. Edited by M. Elseviers et al.
Published 2016 by John Wiley & Sons, Ltd.

discuss the special challenges related to studying medication use among pregnant women.

A description of pharmacoepidemiological studies on drug safety in pregnancy is outside the scope of this book, but such studies are worth mentioning as they are often performed using the same data sources on medication exposure as are used for drug utilization studies. Typically, these studies aim to investigate associations between specific medications on pregnancy outcomes, such as malformations, stillbirth, birth weight or sometimes even long-term development in children. In fact, in practice, formal pharmacoepidemiological studies provide the best way of evaluating whether exposure during pregnancy has adverse effects on the developing foetus [2]. On the other hand, history has shown us that several drugs, such as the antiemetic Bendectin (pyridoxine/doxylamine) [3] and the antihistamine loratadine [4], have falsely been labelled as teratogens

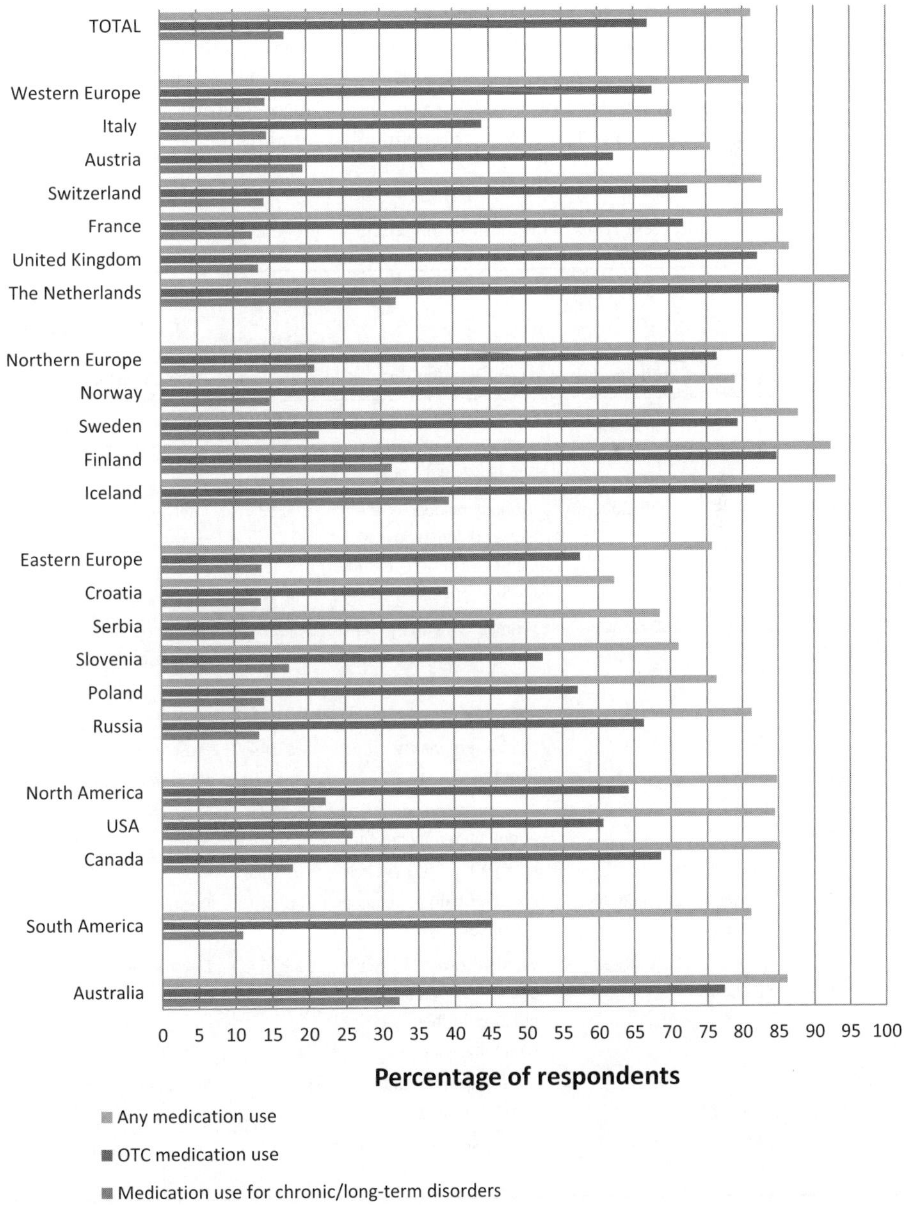

Figure 23.1 Drug utilization in pregnancy by region and country of residence. Estimates do not include vitamins, mineral supplements, iron or herbal and alternative medicinal products.

Source: Lupattelli et al. 2014 [6]. Reproduced with permission from BMJ Publishing Group Ltd.

due to signals in pharmacoepidemiological studies [5]. A major challenge in observational drug safety studies is interpretation of causal inference; often, confounding by indication and other socioeconomic and lifestyle risk factors cannot be ruled out.

Drug utilization studies in pregnancy, on the other hand, aim to describe patterns of medication use and to identify possible drug-related problems among pregnant women. The reported prevalence of drug use in pregnancy ranges from 27 to 99%. For example, 81% of women reported using drugs in pregnancy in the Multinational Medication Use in Pregnancy study in 2011 (ranging from 62% in Croatia to 95% in the Netherlands) (Figure 23.1) [6]. Another often-cited example is the Collaborative Group on Drug Use in Pregnancy (CGDUP) study, whcih documented wide variations among 22 countries in the use of psychotropics during pregnancy, ranging from 0% (Finland) to 23% (former Yugoslavia) [7]. A literature review including 17 studies from 1989 to 2010 reported that rates of prescribed medications have been found to be lowest in the Nordic countries (44–47%) and highest in France (93%) [8]. Overall, the most frequently used drugs in pregnancy are analgesics, antiinfectives, antacids and respiratory drugs [8]. By far, paracetamol (acetaminophen) is the most commonly used drug during pregnancy, being used by almost half of all pregnant women [6].

Table 23.1 shows a selection of drug utilization studies in pregnancy. For a more complete overview, see Daw et al. [8].

Table 23.1 Examples of different types of drug utilization studies in pregnancy.

Reference	Country	Study period	Study population	Study size	Data collection	Percentage of women using drugs in pregnancy	Mean number of drugs taken
Lupattelli 2014 [6]	18 countries	2011–2012	Pregnant women and new mothers with an infant aged less than 1 year	9459	Web questionnaire	81	–
Mitchell 2011 [9]	United States	1976–2008	Women included in the Slone Epidemiology Center Birth Defect Study (BDS)	25 313	Interview after delivery	94 in 2006–08	4.2 in 2006–08
Lacroix 2009 [10]	France	2004–2005	Women covered by French Health Insurance Service in the region of Haute-Garonne	10 008	Insurance claims database	93	11.0
Kulaga 2009 [11]	Canada	1998–2002	Quebec Pregnancy Registry	109 344	Prescription database	56	–
Clearly 2010 [12]	Ireland	2000–2007	Women in early pregnancy at one maternity hospital in Dublin	61 252	Hospital charts	39	–
Engeland 2008 [13]	Norway	2004–2006	Entire birthing population in Norway	106 329	Prescription database	57	3.3
Hardy 2006 [14]	United Kingdom	1991–1999	Women covered by the one of 650 primary care practices in the United Kingdom	81 975	Electronic medical records	65	–
Marchetti 1993 [7]	22 countries	1987	Women at maternity units in 148 hospitals	14 778	Interview after delivery	86	2.9
Piper 1991 [15]	United States	1983–1988	Tennessee Medicaid recipients	107 804	Insurance claims database	–	3.1

Risk factors for medication use in pregnancy

Several sociodemographic and lifestyle factors have been associated with drug use in pregnancy. These include age [16–18], maternal smoking habits [16,18,19], ethnicity [16,20], educational level [16,20,21], marital status [16,20], occupation [6,22], geographic region of residence [6], country of residence [22–24], parity [6,18], body weight [18] and social class [18], as well as personality characteristics such as risk-taking behaviour [25]. The results are inconsistent, and no homogeneous characteristics have been identified as being predictive of drug use in pregnancy.

Prescription patterns in relation to national guidelines

Results from studies on drug utilization in pregnancy have to be interpreted in a clinical context. Many drug utilization studies will be able to give important information on whether clinical guidelines are being followed; that is, whether unsafe medications are discontinued in pregnancy and replaced with safer alternatives. Bear in mind that drug utilization studies in pregnancy cannot say anything about the appropriateness of treatment on an individual level, as they normally lack or do not assess information about a woman's medical history and severity of disease. Even risky drugs may in some cases of severe illness be the best alternative for mother and child after a thorough individual risk–benefit evaluation [26].

Ideally, information on the timing (trimester), dose and duration of medicine use in pregnancy should be recorded, as these all have bearing on the potential for medications to affect the developing foetus. Appropriate timing (taking a drug at the right time in development to affect the target organ) is essential when interpreting results from studies on drug safety in pregnancy. For example, an antiepileptic can only increase the risk of neural tube defects if used in the first trimester, before closure of the neural tube; tetracyclines can only cause discoloration of the infant's teeth if used after gestational week 15, when enamel formation occurs; and nonsteroidal antiinflammatory drugs (NSAIDs) can only cause premature closure of *ductus arteriosus* if used close to term. Consequently, NSAID use in the second trimester and tetracycline use in the first are not strictly against recommendations [26].

Two examples are given here of studies comparing prescription in pregnancy with clinical guidelines; the first concerns hypertensive drugs in pregnancy and the second isotretinoin – a highly teratogenic drug that should always be prescribed together with a contraceptive in women of reproductive age.

- **Example 1.** By using UK electronic medical records, researchers found that contraindicated drugs such as angiotensin-converting enzyme (ACE) inhibitors and angiotensin II receptor blockers (ARBs) were discontinued in pregnancy by 25 and 70%, respectively [27]. Women who switched therapy normally received the safer alternatives methyldopa or an alpha/beta-blocker. The researchers concluded that prescriptions patterns were to a large extent compliant with national guidelines [27].
- **Example 2.** A Dutch drug utilization study showed that among 651 women who were prescribed isotretinoin, only 52–54% filled a prescription on contraception, in strict accordance to the Pregnancy Prevention Plan (PPP), before, during and after discontinuation of the drug [28]. A more liberal approach of a minimum of one prescription per contraception method showed 61–64% use of contraceptives among isotretinoin users [28].

Patterns of harmful drug use in pregnancy

Studies have consistently reported the use of potentially hazardous drugs during pregnancy [12,29–32]. In the examples just mentioned, specific classes of drug were studied. Other studies use risk classification systems and report use according to risk category in pregnancy. The US Food and Drug Administration (FDA) Pregnancy Risk Categories (five categories, from A to D and X) [33] are most commonly used in such studies, but other pregnancy risk classification systems also exist, such as the Swedish and the Australian Risk Classification Systems [34]. Relatively low rates of FDA category D (*'fetal risk, but benefits may be acceptable'*) (2.5%) were reported in early pregnancy at a maternity hospital in Dublin, Ireland [12], compared to 59% in a French study of 1000 prescription claims [30]. Rates of category X drugs (*'strictly contraindicated'*) were 3.2% [12] and 1.6% [30] in these two studies. Moreover, in the French study, 79% of pregnant women had used drugs that had no FDA risk category (several herbals whose safety in pregnancy was unknown) [30]. Olesen et al. [35] reported that 18% of pregnant women in Denmark used drugs classified as having harmful foetal effects according to the Swedish classification system. The relatively poor overlap between the classifications systems makes it difficult to compare studies using different systems [34].

The FDA and the European Union have adopted a new approach to labelling, as the aim of risk categories was often misunderstood; rather than assigning drugs to risk categories, they now provide a narrative description of the evidence for use of the drug in pregnancy [2,36].

For more examples of studies measuring rates of potential harmful drugs in pregnancy, see Daw et al. [8].

Secular trends in drug use in pregnancy

Several studies have focused on time trends in drug use in pregnancy, and they consistently report an increase over the last 30 years. For example, the Slone Epidemiology Center Birth Defects Study (BDS) has since 1976 used telephone interviews to collect information about 40 000 US women's medical histories, sociodemographic and lifestyle characteristics and medication use in pregnancy [9]. Overall medication use increased by 68% from 1976–78 to 2006–08, while the mean number of medications increased from 2.5 to 4.2. The proportion of women using four or more medications in the first trimester almost tripled, from 10 to 28% between these time periods.

Some medication groups have received special focus in time-trend drug utilization studies, due to new drugs being introduced on to the marked, special concerns about prescription policy and debate about safety in pregnancy. The best example of this is studies of antidepressant use in pregnancy. Throughout the 1990s, the new selective serotonin reuptake inhibitor (SSRI) antidepressants were extensively promoted, leading to increased awareness and diagnosis of depression and increased use of antidepressants in pregnancy. Although both European and American studies show a marked increase in the use of antidepressants over the last 10 years, the rates are considerably higher in North America (8.3% among pregnant Medicaid recipients in 2000–07) [37] than in Europe (2.9% in the Netherlands in 2003–04) [38] and Australia (3.6% in 1998) [39], possibly reflecting differences in pharmaceutical companies' marketing resources, therapeutic guidelines and attitudes towards these drugs among prescribers and pregnant women alike. A recent study based on six prescription databases in four European countries (the United Kingdom, Italy, the Netherlands and Denmark) found the highest prescription rates in the United Kingdom (Wales: 9.6% 1 year before, 4.5% during and 15.0% up to 1 year after delivery) and the lowest in Italy (Emilia Romagna region: 3.3% 1 year before, 1.2% during and 2.5% up to 1 year after delivery) [40]. Paroxetine was more commonly prescribed in Italy and the Netherlands than in Denmark and the United Kingdom [40].

Another group of drugs much studied in pregnancy is the antiinfectives [41,42]. Studies of this group commonly aim to evaluate antibiotic use according to therapeutic guidelines; they report that one in four [43] to one in five [42] women use at least one prescribed antibiotic during pregnancy, mostly penicillins. Conflicting results concerning the safety of erythromycin during the first trimester [44,45] have raised demand for studies on the use, effect and safety of macrolides in pregnancy.

Patterns of medication adherence and discontinuation in pregnancy

Another challenge that has recently started to receive attention is medication adherence in pregnancy. Fear of teratogenic drug effects may result in low adherence to prescribed medications. Research is underway to discover the determinants of nonadherence in pregnancy, motivated by the hope that identification and understanding of these factors might evoke strategies for the prevention of nonadherence. Generally, 30–50% of all patients are expected to be non-adherent, regardless of disease, prognosis or setting [46]. Information about the factors associated with noncompliance with guidelines is generally inconsistent [47]. Unfortunately, most factors have been analysed one at a time, and few conceptual models that take into account a combination of factors and their interrelationships have been proposed [47]. In a recent multinational study, nonadherence to prescribed medication varied by diagnosis, with high self-reported nonadherence among women with rheumatic illness (56%), anxiety (51%) and depression (47%) [48].

Herbal drug utilization in pregnancy

Most studies have shown that women use alternative medicines to a greater extent than men, and there has been an overall increase in herbal drug use over the last two decades [49]. Herbal drugs are often promoted as natural and safe alternatives to conventional drugs. Such claims may have a special appeal to pregnant women, who are often concerned about the well-being of their unborn child. Relatively few Western studies have reported the prevalence of herbal drug use in pregnancy. Those that do show a wide range of use, from 1 to as high as 87% [50]. Several of these were not specifically designed to study herbal drug use, however, so it is reasonable to believe that they underestimate the proportion of women who take herbal drugs during pregnancy. In a recent multinational study including over 9000 women from Europe, North and South America and Australia, marked differences in herbal drug use in pregnancy were reported with women from Eastern Europe (51.8%) and Australia (43.8%) twice as likely to use a herbal medicine as those from other regions. The highest reported use was in Russia (69.0%, versus an overall worldwide prevalence of 28.9%). Ginger, cranberry, valerian and raspberry were the most commonly used herbs in pregnancy [51].

For a more complete overview of herbal drug utilization studies in pregnancy, see Hall et al. [50].

Paternal medication use

A few studies have focused on patterns of ***paternal*** medication use in relation to pregnancy. In one Dutch database study of almost 26 000 fathers-to-be, 1.0–1.5% had used medication that could affect fertility or semen quality (e.g. cytotoxic drugs). In total, 35% had used medications at least once in the 3 months before conception, most commonly NSAIDs (6.0%) and antibiotics (5.8%) [52].

Sources used in drug utilization studies in pregnancy

Various sources of information on drug use in pregnancy are available. Today, studies of drug use in pregnancy are usually conducted by analysing large databases, such as prescription databases [10,35,42,53,54], reimbursement claims databases [55–58] or medical records databases [59], or by interviewing individual women [9,16,17,22,23]. Pregnancy registries [60] and teratology information services [61,62] collect valuable data on the safety of medications in pregnancy, but they are not often used in descriptive drug utilization studies.

Patient interviews

One large, successful, multicentre interview study was the Collaborative Perinatal Project, in which 50 000 women were interviewed by trained interviewers between 1959 and 1965 using standardized questionnaires. This landmark study generated information about the most frequently prescribed drugs at that time, and served as a model for later studies on drug use in pregnancy [63,64]. Another example is the CGDUP study, initiated in 1987. This was an international study including over 14 000 women in 22 countries [23]. Data on drug use in pregnancy were collected through interviews in hospital at delivery. The overall frequencies of drug use ranged from approximately 60 to 100% [23].

The main disadvantages of interview-based studies are that they are time-consuming and often costly. The subjects' recall of drug use depends on how specifically the questions are designed. Mitchell et al. [65] reported that 6–40% of the women they interviewed only affirmed use of 11 different drugs in pregnancy when they were specifically named. The EuroMap Group compared self-reported drug intake with medically notified intake for specific diseases in the Hungarian Case-Control Surveillance System of Congenital Abnormalities and found that recall bias was present, especially for drugs used for a short period of time [66]. Both Feldman et al. [33] and Mackenzie & Lippmann [67] reported better recall of prescription drugs for chronic illnesses than of other drugs used during pregnancy. Also, pregnant women may be reluctant to answer questions on sensitive topics in personal interviews, such as smoking and alcohol consumption in pregnancy.

Drug registries and administrative health care databases

Increasing attention has been paid in recent years to prescription databases produced for administrative purposes by health authorities or medical reimbursement organizations. Such registries are based upon pharmacy prescriptions or drug refund claims. Their main strengths are their size and the fact that they do not depend on individual recall of drug use. Furthermore, after initial establishment, they cost relatively little to run. In Europe, prescription registries are found in the Netherlands, the United Kingdom, France, Italy and the Nordic countries [40,68]. All such registries have been used to study drug use in pregnancy [10,13,14,31,40,42,68,69].

Prescription registries do not include a number of drugs, including OTC, nonrefundable prescription drugs and herbal drugs. However, Stephansson et al. [69] were able to link registry data with other databases in order to include OTC medication. Registries also usually lack information about the indication for use, and thus are limited by 'confounding by indication' (see next section).

An example of a reimbursement drug registry is the Medicaid health insurance system in the United States, created in 1965 to provide access to medical care for the disadvantaged. Due to its individual requirements, the Medicaid population differs significantly from the general US population.

Comparison between countries requires uniform data collection. It is difficult to compare results between studies from different countries due to the different methods used to ascertain and categorize drug use. Methodological limitations in drug utilization studies in pregnancy are usually caused by the use of a retrospective design (recall bias), poor response rates (selection bias), absence of nonprescription drugs in prescription-based studies (underestimation of drug use) and lack of information about both the indication for use and important sociodemographic and lifestyle variables. Many studies provide information on a selected group of pregnant women, such as hospitalized patients or Medicaid enrolees (see Table 23.1). Consequently, it is difficult to know whether differences in rates are a result of differences in actual use or merely differences in materials and methods. Ideally, national or cultural differences in drug use in pregnancy should be explored though multicentre studies, such as international pregnancy registries or networks. As an example, the European and International Registry of Antiepileptic Drugs in Pregnancy (EURAP) contains prospective data on over 4000 women with epilepsy in pregnancy across 38 countries. Recently, it reported large differences in the use of antiepileptic drugs (AEDs) in pregnancy. For example, use of the newer, more expensive but safer second-generation AEDs ranged from 3.5% in India to 75.0% in Denmark [24]. As another example, EUROmediCAT is a recently formed network under the European Surveillance of Congenital Anomalies (EUROCAT) network that may become a valuable source of information about drug use and safety in Europe in the future [70].

Moreover, newly emerging Web-based multinational studies may be of use in populations with high Internet use, such as women of childbearing age [71]. An example is the Multinational Study on Medication Use in Pregnancy [6], which collected data through a Web-based questionnaire in 18 countries in Europe (Western, Northern and Eastern), North and South America and Australia from October 2011 to February 2012. Both pregnant women and new mothers with a child less than 12 months old could participate. The study population included 9459 women, of whom 81% reported use of at least one medication during pregnancy and 29% reported use of herbal remedies. There was a substantial inter-region variability in the extent of medication use during pregnancy. Specific guidelines for Web-based studies have recently been proposed, aimed at promoting high data quality [72].

Methodological considerations in drug utilization studies in pregnancy

Issues that are particularly relevant to drug utilization studies in pregnancy are sample size (e.g. power), errors in measurement of medication use and bias, in the form of selection bias, information bias and confounding.

It is important to determine ***sample size*** in order to ensure that prevalence estimates are obtained with the required precision. Too-small studies may lead to inaccurate results, while samples that are too large can waste time, resources and money. For example, a prevalence of 10% in a sample of 20 subjects would have a 95% confidence interval of 1–31%, which is not very precise or informative [73]. On the other hand, a prevalence of 10% in a sample of 400 subjects would have a 95% confidence interval of 7–13%, which can be considered sufficiently accurate.

Risk of misclassification exists in all data; however, in pregnancy, ***errors in measurement of medication use*** are especially critical as they may lead to erroneous conclusions about drug safety. A specific problem in this field of research is the lack of information on gestational age at birth in several administrative health care databases. Exposure dates are important, as susceptible periods for specific malformations may be less than 1 week. For example, subtracting 280 days (= 40 weeks) from the date of birth in order to calculate the beginning of pregnancy may lead to overestimation of medication use in shorter pregnancies if use occurred prior to conception and to overestimation in longer pregnancies if use occurred post partum. Similarly, medication exposure may be erroneously classified in the wrong gestational week or trimester.

In a study based on electronic health records (EHRs) of over 200 000 mother–child pairs in British Columbia, Canada, conducted between 1998 and 2007, subtracting 35 weeks (= 245 days) from the date of birth in deliveries with diagnosis codes for preterm birth and 39 weeks (= 273 days) in those without them provided an acceptable estimate of the beginning of pregnancy [74].

Studies based upon prescription databases will make several assumptions about time of medication use in pregnancy. Prescribed or dispensed medications will be assumed to be started on the date of prescription/dispensing, for example, but for drugs that are not used daily, such as triptans (acute migraine drugs), sleeping pills and analgesics, this assumption may be severely erroneous. Moreover, some prescription database studies will classify any drugs dispensed within 3 months prior to conception as 'use in pregnancy'. This assumption is based on the fact that most patients are dispensed a 3-month supply of medications each time a prescription is filled. However, many women will discontinue use of these drugs once they become aware they are pregnant. Skurtveit et al. [75] illustrated this problem by comparing prescription data within 3 months prior to pregnancy with self-reported antidepressant use in pregnancy. They found that expansion of the time window to include intervals 3 months before pregnancy led to lower specificity and to underestimation of the risk of persistent pulmonary hypertension in the newborn.

Knowledge of drug and therapeutic guidelines will help guide the researcher in discussing misclassification. For antidepressants, discontinuation rates are high [76]; discontinuation should thus be more of a concern in such cases than in studies on, for example, the use of thyroxin among women with hypothyroidism.

Several types of ***bias*** can occur in pharmacoepidemiological studies:

Selection bias is related to the recruitment of study subjects or to losses upon follow-up. It is present when study participants differ from the target population in essential characteristics and so the prevalence of drug use and estimates of association in the study group differ from those in the target population. This may occur if the reasons for referral to the study are related to drug use (***referral bias***). For example, physicians who enrol pregnant patients may be more attentive about which drugs they prescribe to such women. Selection bias may also occur when women decide to participate themselves, or decide to leave the study, as such a decision may itself be related to drug use and health behaviour (***self-selection***).

Information bias is related to the way in which information about drug use and other study variables is collected. The specificity of questions about drug use in pregnancy has implications for recall (e.g. open-ended questions versus naming specific indications and specific drug names) [65,77]. Also, a woman's ability to remember accurately declines as the time since a drug was taken increases. Medications that are taken daily in pregnancy, such as insulin and antiasthmatics, are more accurately reported than short-term therapies, such as dermatological corticosteroids, antibiotic eye drops and decongestant nose sprays.

In descriptive drug utilization studies, bias can cause an over- or underestimation of the prevalence of drug use in pregnancy. In studies on drug safety, ***confounding*** can cause an over- or underestimation of the association between drug exposure and the outcome of pregnancy. All drug registries and administrative health care databases should validate their drug records and evaluate the appropriateness of studying drug utilization or safety in pregnancy. Sources of error or bias should be acknowledged and discussed, and should preferably be quantified, by performing sensitivity analysis of estimates under a range of assumptions about the direction and magnitude of bias.

Conclusion

There is a need for systematic studies of drug utilization in pregnancy, providing information on OTC drugs, maternal illness and sociodemographic characteristics, in both developed and developing countries. Given the widespread use of drugs, it is especially important to develop standards for calculating and reporting rates of drug use in pregnancy, in order to improve the value of future research in this area of research. Comparing drug utilization patterns in pregnancy to clinical guidelines is essential in detecting hazardous trends in drug use and ensuring safe medication use for the mother and child.

CHAPTER 24
Drug utilization in the paediatric population

Antje Neubert[1], Katja Taxis[2] & Ian C.K. Wong[3]
[1]*Department of Paediatric and Adolescent Medicine, University Hospital Erlangen, Germany*
[2]*University of Groningen, Department of Pharmacy, Unit Pharmacotherapy & Pharmaceutical Care, The Netherlands*
[3]*Research Department of Practice and Policy, UCL School of Pharmacy, London, UK*

KEY POINTS

- The paediatric population is heterogeneous, and therefore sample size is often an issue when trying to obtain valid drug utilization data, especially in rare diseases and small patient groups, such as neonatal intensive care patients. Greater cooperation among researchers in performing large (international) studies is needed.
- Off-label and unlicensed medication use is very common in children, but prevalence varies across age groups, settings and countries.
- In ambulatory care, for all paediatric age categories, antiinfective, dermatological and respiratory drugs are the most commonly used drug classes. In inpatients, systemic antibacterials, analgesic drugs, drugs for obstructive airway diseases and antiinflammatory and antirheumatic products are frequently used.
- Drug utilization research in children is particularly useful in assessing quality of prescribing (national and international studies) and in determining research needs for long-term safety, efficacy and effectiveness studies.

Introduction

The paediatric population runs from birth to the end of the 18th year. With respect to the use of medicines, this is not a homogenous population. Growth and development during the first years of life affect many physiological processes in different ways, resulting in different responses to drugs from a pharmacokinetic and a pharmacodynamic perspective [1]. To accommodate these differences, the paediatric population has been subclassified by the International Conference on Harmonisation (ICH) into different age groups (Table 24.1) [2].

Preterm neonates are particularly immature neonates, and survival is their main focus. Drug therapy concentrates on the dysfunctions of the cardiovascular system. In contrast, ***full-term neonates*** (born after 37 weeks of gestation) are more mature, and drug therapy is mainly indicated to treat problems with adoption to the extramaternal circulation, such as infections, seizures and blood glucose disturbances. Preterm and full-term neonates have the largest variability in pharmacokinetic processes, affecting all phases from absorption, distribution and metabolism to elimination. Children in their ***first 2 years of life*** are characterized by rapid growth – particularly proliferation of the liver, kidney and nervous systems. Simple infections are typical in this period of life and are important for the maturation and conditioning of the immune system. Total clearance of drugs is often increased compared to adulthood. Children from about ***3 to 11 years*** of age grow less rapidly than in the first 2 years. Nevertheless, a high prevalence of simple infections remains, particularly during the first half of this period (before school commences). Furthermore, because of the large extent of activity and increasing independency, injuries caused by accidents are more frequent in this age group. ***Adolescents*** are individuals who are changing from children into adults. Reproductive capacity is gained and full body height is reached. Emotional and psychological problems are most frequent in this period of life and require special attention.

Morbidity and mortality patterns in the paediatric population vary widely across the world, with the

Drug Utilization Research: Methods and Applications, First Edition. Edited by M. Elseviers et al.
Published 2016 by John Wiley & Sons, Ltd.

Table 24.1 Paediatric age groups according to International Conference on Harmonisation (ICH) and European Medicines Agency (EMA) guidelines.

Source: Data from [2].

Age group	Class	Focus of development
<37 weeks	Preterm neonates	Survival
<28 days	Newborn and neonates	Adoption
1 month–2 years	Infants	Growth and proliferation
>2 to <11 years	Children	Training, differentiation
>11 years	Adolescents	Gaining reproductive capacity

highest rates of childhood mortality due to infectious diseases and preterm birth complications occurring in the least developed countries [3].

The need for paediatric drug utilization studies

Drug utilization research in children is different from that in adults, due to the heterogeneous nature of the population. Furthermore, drug use in paediatrics has unique characteristics, such as the effect of drugs on maturation and adverse drug reactions (ADRs) that only occur in children. Children and adolescents are disadvantaged when it comes to drug therapy, as there is a lack of evidence guiding prescribing compared to the adult population, as well as a lack of paediatric drug formulations. In the late 1960s, children were described as 'therapeutic orphans', and this remained true until recent years [4,5]. The need for safe and effective paediatric medicines was realized in the late 1990s. Following initiatives from the United States, the European Paediatric Regulation came into force in 2007 [6]. Paediatric investigation plans (PIPs) are now part of each new licensing application and are the basis for a Paediatric Use Marketing Authorisation for older off-patent drugs. In the United States, the most recent regulation is the Food and Drug Administration (FDA) Safety and Innovations Act [7]. As a result of the Paediatric Regulation, pharmacoepidemiological studies are important, as it will always be a challenge to obtain experimental data from the paediatric population for all areas of drug use. There is thus a need to build pharmacoepidemiological research capacity and support in the areas of drug utilization, safety and effectiveness.

Drug utilization research in children is particularly useful in assessing the quality of prescribing (national and international studies) and determining research needs and priorities for long-term safety, efficacy and effectiveness studies. Furthermore, drug utilization studies can facilitate the rational use of drugs in different paediatric populations and settings. There is a need for more interventional studies, in order to enhance the quality of prescribing in the paediatric population. Drug utilization research is very important in guiding the development and evaluation of such interventions. However, this last aspect is outside the scope of the present chapter. More information on quality improvement and evaluation of interventions can be found in Chapters 45–47.

We will start the chapter by addressing some methodological issues concerning paediatric drug utilization research, including sample size, data sources, issues around measurement units and definitions (such as off-label/unlicensed use of medicines). Finally, we will present the results of a few recent drug utilization studies in the paediatric population. It is outside the scope of the chapter to give a complete overview of all available studies, so we have chosen a few large studies to discuss in detail.

Age categories and sample size issues

Sample size is one of the major issues when studying drug use in the paediatric population. In the developed world, the paediatric population is generally small and relatively healthy when compared to, for instance, the over-65s. Children and adolescents account for less than 25% of the population of 0–80 years old only. Thus, the number of paediatric patients in need of treatment is smaller than the adult population.

Each age group has its own characteristics and needs to be studied separately. Therefore, paediatric drug utilization research methods capable of systematically capturing large populations are essential. Rather than conducting many small studies with insufficient power, efforts should be made to organize multinational or multisource database studies that will have the advantage of size and allow for a full evaluation of drug- and dose-specific risks and for comparisons between countries.

Data sources

Depending on the type of research (i.e. descriptive, qualitative or analytical studies), different database parameters are needed. In drug utilization research, a large source population is important to obtaining reliable results. As already described, sample size is one of the major constraints in paediatric medicine research. In this section, we address some of the issues around data sources specific to the paediatric population. A more general discussion of data sources in drug utilization research can be found in Chapter 4.

In 2008, a survey of databases available for paediatric medicine research was conducted among all European databases that were listed on the website of the International Society of Pharmacopidemiology (ISPE) and/or known by an expert group [8]. The survey comprised questions regarding (i) the nature of the database, (ii) the database's size, (iii) demographic, clinical and drug-related data, (iv) cost and (v) accessibility. The assessment comprised 17 databases from 10 different European countries, for a total of at least 9 million children aged 0–18 years. All databases that participated in the survey collect information about prescription drugs and the unit dispensed or prescribed; most also record the dosage regimen, which is particularly important for the paediatric population. Drugs that do not require a prescription (e.g. over-the-counter (OTC) drugs) are recorded in some databases, but only if they have been prescribed by the primary care physician. This is particularly common in the paediatric population, because these drugs are reimbursed by some national health care systems when they are prescribed for children.

Information on drugs that need a prescription but are not reimbursed is usually available in electronic record databases and in some pharmacy-based dispensing databases, but not necessarily in claims-oriented dispensing databases. In many countries, more drugs are reimbursed for use in children than in adults. Consequently, there is the possibility that in claims-oriented databases, more drugs are covered for children; however, the rules vary from country to country, which makes it difficult to compare results from these databases.

Major confounders in pharmacoepidemiological research are indications for prescriptions, severe underlying diseases and contraindications (e.g. allergies etc.). Most of this information is available in the electronic medical record databases. Dispensing databases have the disadvantage that diagnosis and indications are not available. In the survey, 13 out of 17 databases analysed stored patients' diagnoses, and 10 of these were medical record databases. However, only 6 out of the 17 had specific indications for individual drug prescriptions. Table 24.2 presents a summary of the databases

Table 24.2 Databases identified in the survey of Neubert et al. [8] and characteristics of the paediatric populations captured.

Source: Data from[8].

Database name	Country	Starting year	Number of children[a]	Percentage coverage of the paediatric population	Children's person years since the database began
Electronic medical record databases					
The Health Improvement Network (THIN) Data	United Kingdom	1985	501 936	Approx. 4%	5.5 million
General Practice Research Database (GPRD)	United Kingdom	1987	1 146 578	6%	5.1 million
IMS Disease Analyzer UK (IMS-DA UK)	United Kingdom	1991	460 000	5.80%	2.3 million
QRESEARCH	United Kingdom	1988	739 977[b]	8%	8.8 million
Scottish Programme for Improving Clinical Effectiveness in Primary Care (SPICE)	United Kingdom	2000	387356	40%	n.n.
Pedianet	Italy	2000	106 554	n.n.	315 065
Integrated Primary Care Information (IPCI)	The Netherlands	1992	161 108	4%	550 540

Database name	Country	Starting year	Number of children[a]	Percentage coverage of the paediatric population	Children's person years since the database began
IMS Disease Analyzer France (IMS-DA France)	France	1997	190 000	2.90%	1.7 million
IMS Disease Analyzer Austria (IMS-DA Austria)	Austria	1995	30 000	8%	270000
IMS Disease Analyzer (Germany)	Germany	1992	250 000	6%	2.2 million
Claims databases					
PHARMO	The Netherlands	1985	>360 000	14%	2.2 million
InterAction Database (IADB)	The Netherlands	1995	111 960	5%	615 330
The Danish Prescription Database	Denmark	1995	nn	100%	n.n.
Finland Prescription Register	Finland	1994	480 000	100%	NA
Other					
ARNO Observatory	Italy	1987	1 500 000	17%	10 million
Prescription-Event Monitoring (PEM)	United Kingdom	1984	59 490	NA	NA
Swedish Medical Birth Register	Sweden	1973	3 230 794	99% of all births	NA

[a] In 2004. [b] In 2006.

n.n., not named; NA, not applicable.

included in the survey. All databases have previously been used to conduct pharmacoepidemiological research published in scientific papers. Ten of the databases are used in published studies specifically relevant to the paediatric population. Overall, the survey showed that databases are particularly useful for the study of drug utilization because they record either prescriptions or drug dispensing. The results of these utilization studies might be used to generate useful data on age, gender and country patterns of drug use, as well as dosages and durations of use.

Measurement units

Defined daily doses (DDDs) are normally assigned based on use in adults (see Chapter 6). Dose recommendations for use in children vary according to age and body weight, and there is a lot of off-label use (see next section). Thus, the World Health Organization (WHO) International Working Group for Drug Statistics Methodology has concluded that paediatric DDDs are impossible to assign. Prescribed daily dosages and indications in a paediatric population should be used if available and compared with the DDD values. If the paediatric subgroup is difficult to identify, the general DDD should be used as a measuring tool for overall comparisons [9]. Some research groups have proposed defining paediatric DDDs (e.g. [10]). Actual weight or body surface area could be used to calculate the dosages, although in practice such information is often not available/unreliable in databases. The use of treatment period has also been suggested as a measure [11]. In practice, however, not many studies describe volume of consumption. If this is provided, number of prescriptions or number of dispensed drug packages is usually used [12].

Off-label use

Medicines are frequently prescribed to children without being approved for the paediatric population [13,14]. Among medicines that were newly licensed by the European Medicines Agency (EMA) between 1995 and 2005, only one-third were specifically licensed for children [15]. The situation is even worse for the neonatal population [16]. The Paediatric Regulation, which came into force in 2007, requires companies to develop a PIP and grants incentives once a licence for paediatric use has been obtained [6]. In the United States, the passage of the Best Pharmaceuticals for Children Act and the Pediatric Research Equity Act has resulted in improvements, including more than 500 labelling changes [17].

Worldwide, there is no common scientific or regulatory approach to off-label/unlicensed use of medicines and, most importantly, a shared definition is missing

[18,19]. The EU-funded project TEDDY made major efforts to overcome this problem and establish a common definition to be shared among stakeholders in Europe and, ideally, the world, using a two-stage Delphi technique [20]. The project included 34 European experts (scientists, health professionals, pharmaceutical companies and regulatory agencies). Results were shared with the EMA before the final proposal was circulated to participants. Consensus was reached for the majority of questions. The lowest level of consensus was for questions related to alternative formulations and the prescribing of contraindicated drugs. At the final stage, 85% of experts agreed on the proposed definition for 'off-label' and 80% on the definition for 'unlicensed'.

Off-label use was defined as 'all uses of a marketed drug not detailed in the Summary of Product Characteristics (SPC) including therapeutic indication, use in age-subsets, appropriate strength (dosage), pharmaceutical form and route of administration' [20]. 'Paediatric off-label use' specifically includes 'all paediatric uses of a marketed drug not detailed in the SPC', with particular reference to [20]:

- therapeutic indication;
- indication for use in subsets;
- appropriate strength (dosage by age);
- pharmaceutical form;
- route of administration.

Unlicensed use was defined as 'all uses of a drug which has never received a European Marketing Authorisation as medicinal for human use in either adults or children' [20].

A widespread implementation of this definition will facilitate the conduct of studies into unlicensed and off-label drug use, allowing them to provide comparable data. Requisites for such studies are data sources and/or databases that provide indications, dosages and comorbidities which can help identify whether a drug is being used without licence or off-label. It should be emphasised that 'off-label' use of medication as such does not imply an improper, illegal, contraindicated or investigational use. Evidence – not label indication – should be the basis for therapeutic decisions by practitioners [17].

National and international studies report a wide range of prevalence rates of off-label/unlicensed medicine use in children and adolescents. Some of these differences are probably due to differences in definitions [21]. In hospitalized patients, including neonates, the proportion of off-label use varies between 10 and 65% and unlicensed use varies between 3 and 48%. In ambulatory care, the proportions of off-label and unlicensed used vary between 11 and 31% and between 0.3 and 17%, respectively [13]. A recent analysis investigated the impact of the new paediatric regulations on the incidence of unlicensed and off-label use [22,23]. It appears that the situation is on its way to being improved, but there is still a large degree of off-label use in children. There is also some evidence that unlicensed and off-label use is more often related to ADRs than are drugs approved for children [22,24].

Recently, a German study utilized population data from the German Health Interview and Examination Survey for Children and Adolescents (KiGGS) to identify the extent of off-label drug use in children and adolescents [25]. Almost half of the children surveyed had taken medication 7 days prior to the interview, and 30% of all medications were found to be off-label. Most interestingly, underdosing was the most common reason for medicines being considered off-label. This kind of off-label use was more apparent in children with highly educated parents and of upper social class. It is assumed that parents try to minimize the hazard caused by medicines by decreasing the dose; they are not aware that the risk of ADRs remains. In some cases, such as antibiotic use, the development of resistances will be facilitated without the drug even being effective. This study shows that the type of population studied will have a large effect on the degree of off-label use found [25].

Examples of paediatric drug utilization studies

Studies from both primary and secondary care settings indicate that there are significant differences in drug utilization in paediatric populations both across countries and between health care institutions within a single country.

Ambulatory studies

Studies using ambulatory data are currently the most common type of paediatric drug utilization study.

The TEDDY project

Sturkenboom et al. [26] provided probably the most comprehensive overview of primary care prescription patterns in a large multinational European paediatric

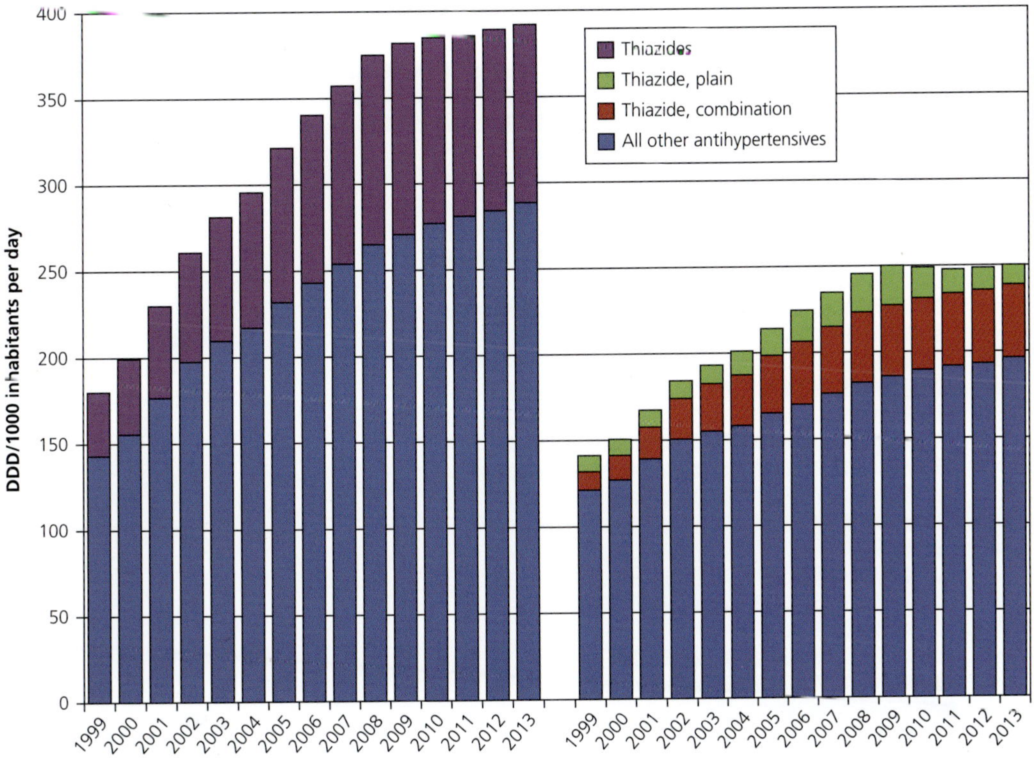

Figure 6.1 Use of antihypertensives. (a) Consumption in a country where only plain products are marketed (if a patient needs two antihypertensives, they must take two products). (b) Consumption in a country where combinations pills (e.g. thiazides combined with other antihypertensives, such as ACEIs or ARBs) are available.

Drug Utilization Research: Methods and Applications, First Edition. Edited by M. Elseviers et al. © 2016 John Wiley & Sons, Ltd.
Published 2016 by John Wiley & Sons, Ltd.

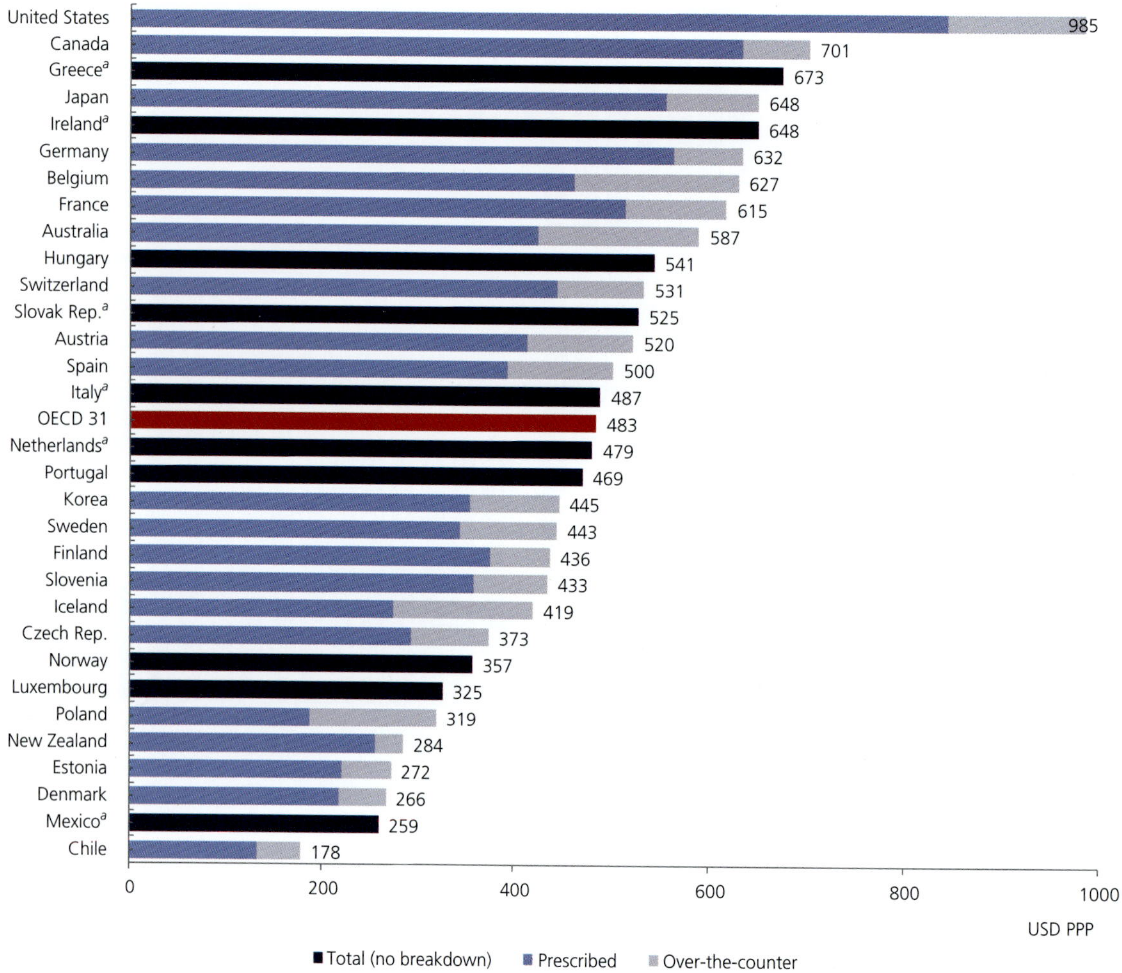

Figure 8.1 Pharmaceutical expenditure per capita, 2011 (latest available year). OECD31: 31 of the 34 OECD countries covered; USD PPP: United States Dollar Purchasing Power Parities.

[a]Includes medical non-durables

Source: Organisation for Economic Co-operation and Development 2013 [6]. Reproduced by permission of OECD Publishing.

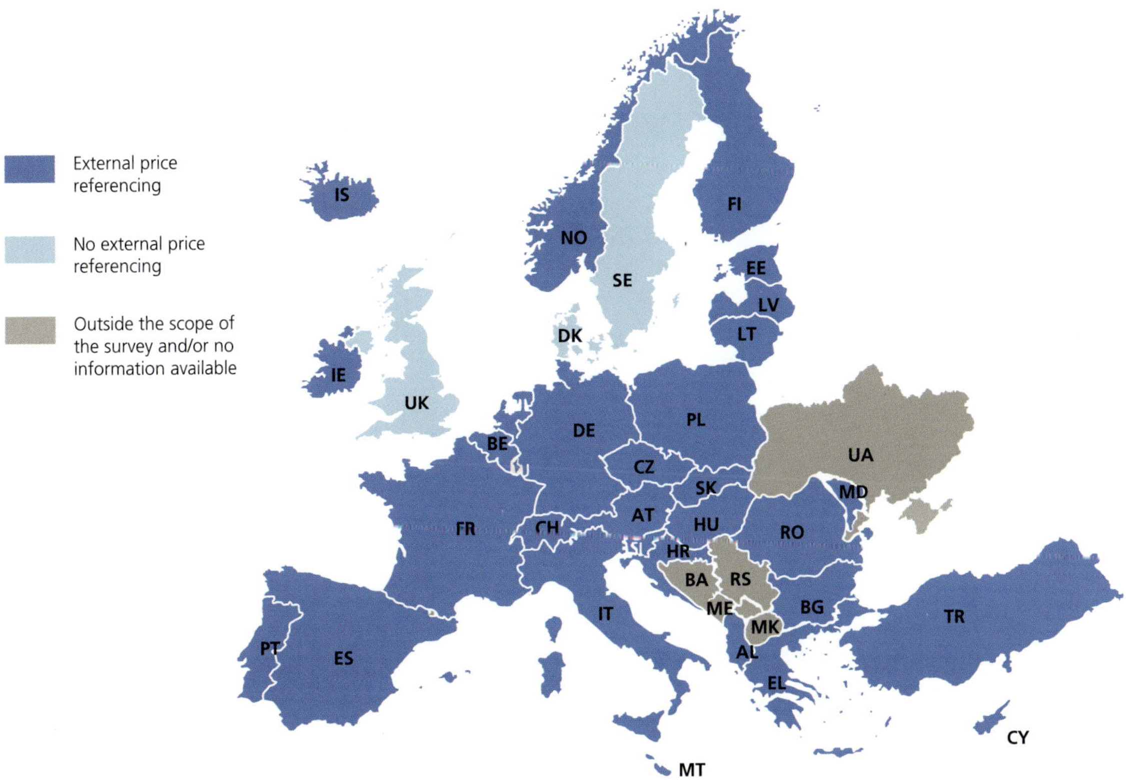

Figure 8.3 External price referencing applied as pricing policy in the 28 EU member states, Albania, Iceland, Moldova, Norway, Switzerland and Turkey.

Source: Data from [15] and [16].

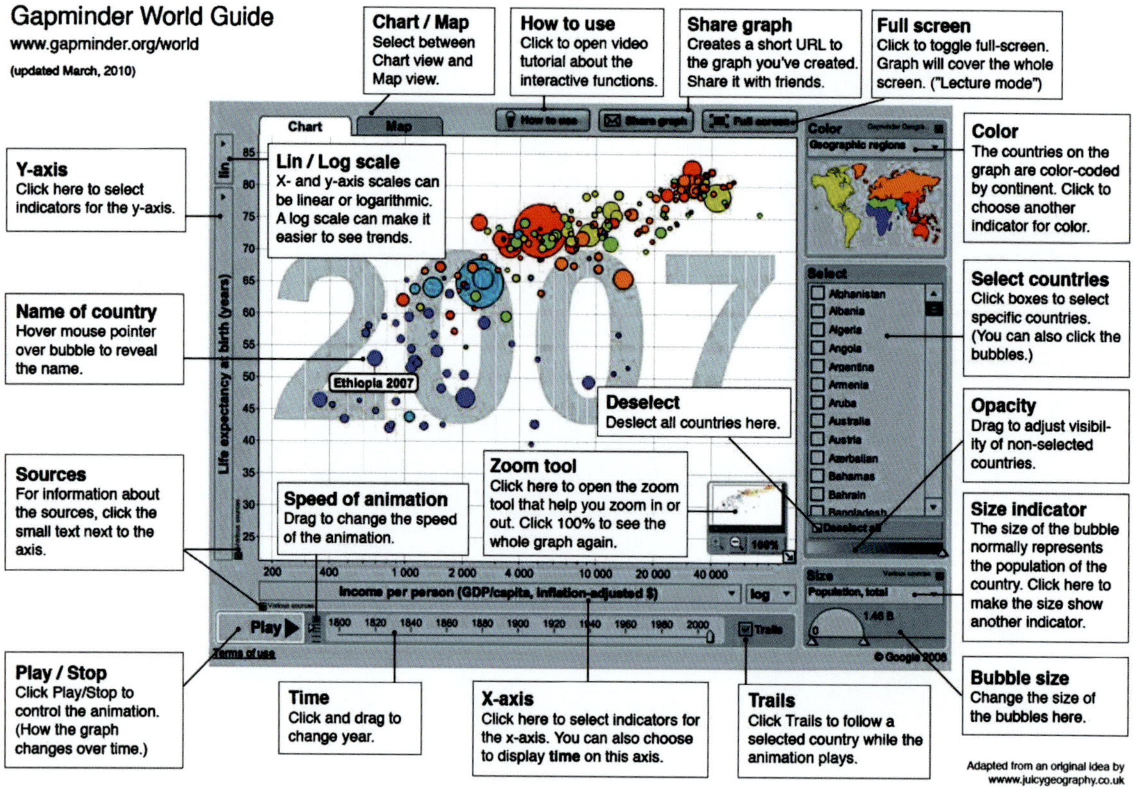

Figure 10.15 Static view of an animated bubble chart. Guide to the Gapminder World – Health and Wealth of Nations. The illustration shows the basic functions of the Motion Chart tool, originally developed by the Gapminder foundation [39,40].

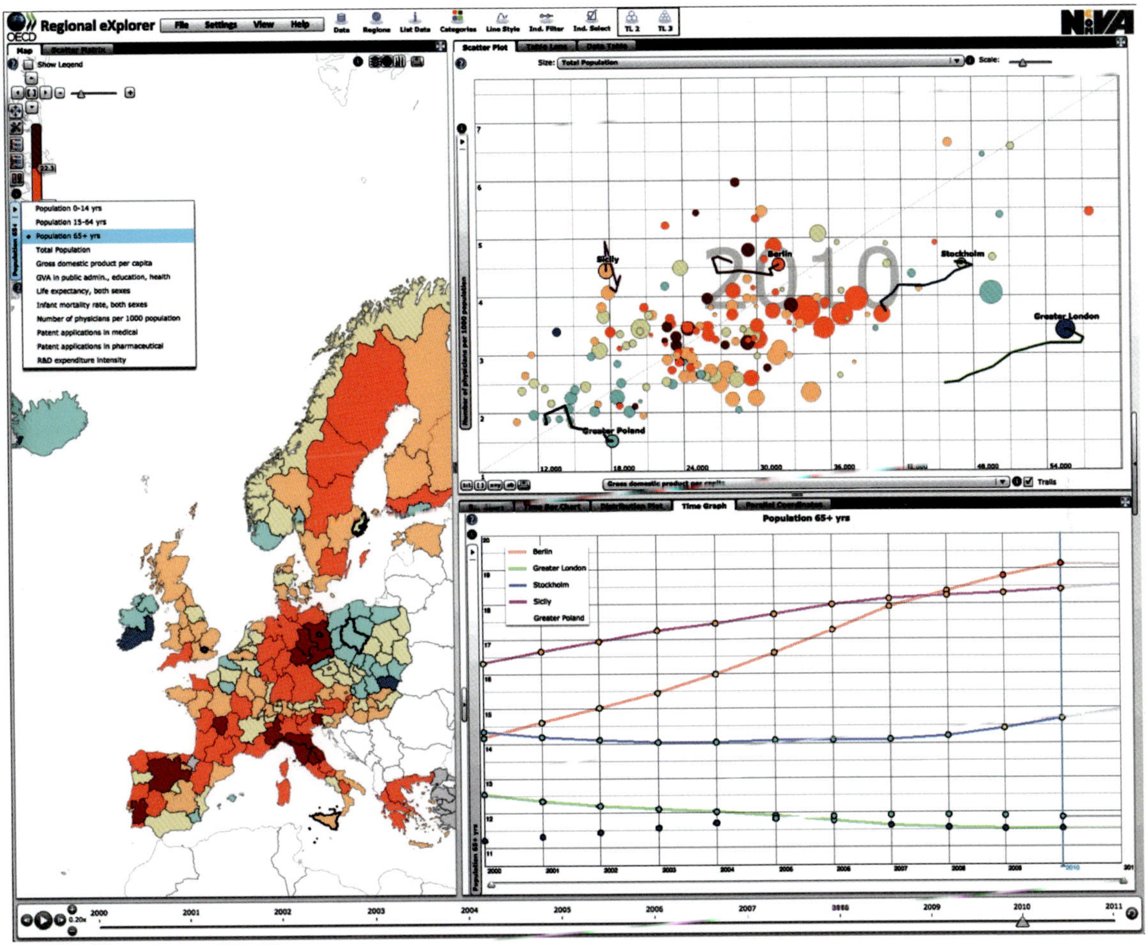

Figure 10.16 Static view from a visualization tool showing data linked between different graphs.

Source: OECD Factbook [41,42].

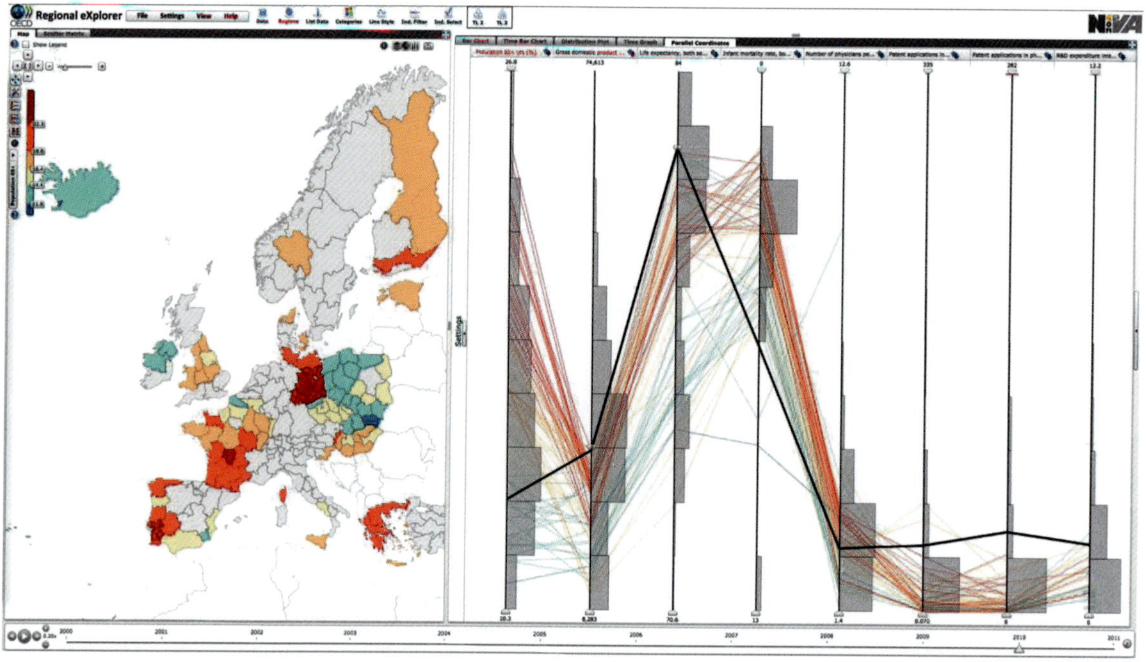

Figure 10.17 Parallel coordinate plot [44] used to filter a multivariate dataset (the same as that in Figure 10.16). By repositioning the sliders on each vertical line, the dataset is successively filtered not only in the parallel coordinate plot, but also in all associated visualizations (in this case, only the map is shown). Each remaining coloured line represents a geographically defined population that fulfils all criteria. Source: OECD Factbook [42].

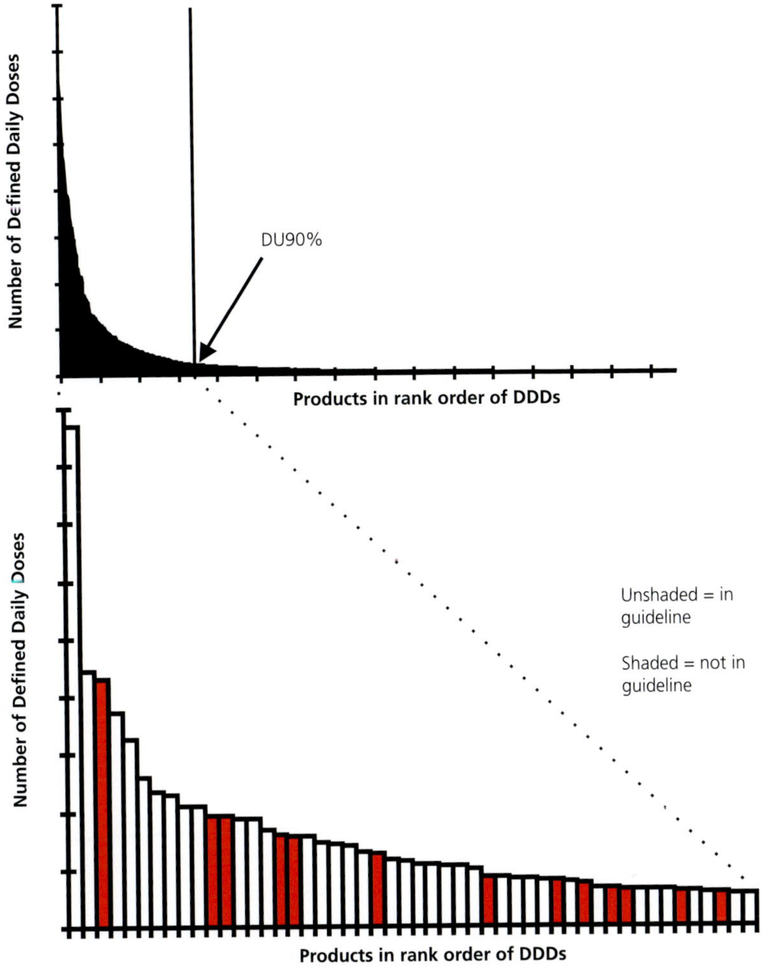

Figure 12.3 Drug utilization 90% (DU90%) method. (a) Number of drugs (products or substances) ranked by volume of DDDs. The arrow indicates the number of drugs accounting for 90% of the DDDs. (b) The DU90% segment enlarged, indicating drugs listed (unshaded) and not listed (shaded) in guidelines.

Source: Bergman et al. 1998 [71]. Reproduced with permission from Springer Science and Business Media.

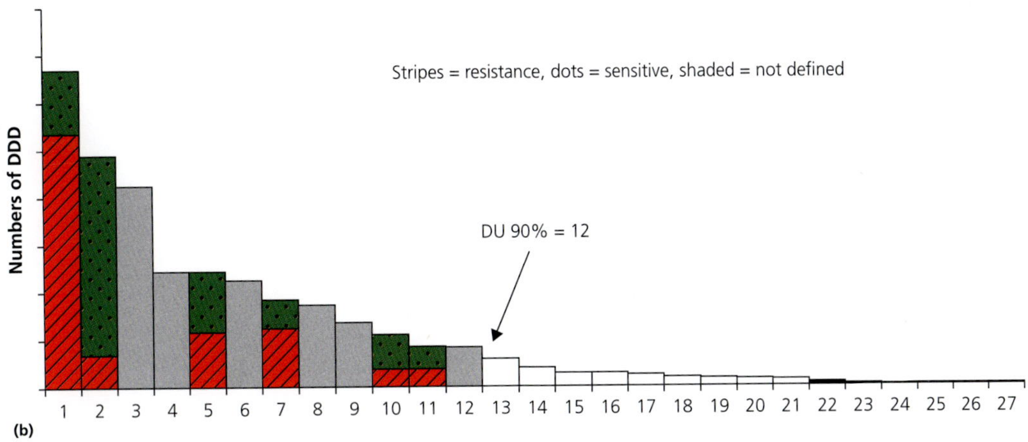

Figure 15.1 (b) DU90% of antibiotics use and cumulative microbial resistance in a Russian hospital: a tool to alert physicians. It is generally agreed that in order to create the DU90% list, cumulative percentage of DDDs must be used, with the last medication in the list being the one that provides attainment of the full coverage of 90% of use, even though the final percentage may become slightly higher.

Sources: Figure 15.1(a) Wettermark et al. 2003 [42]. Reproduced with permission from John Wiley and Sons. Figure 15.1(b) Zagorodnikova K, Goryachkina K. 2013 [62]. Reproduced with permission from Ksenia Zagorodnikova.

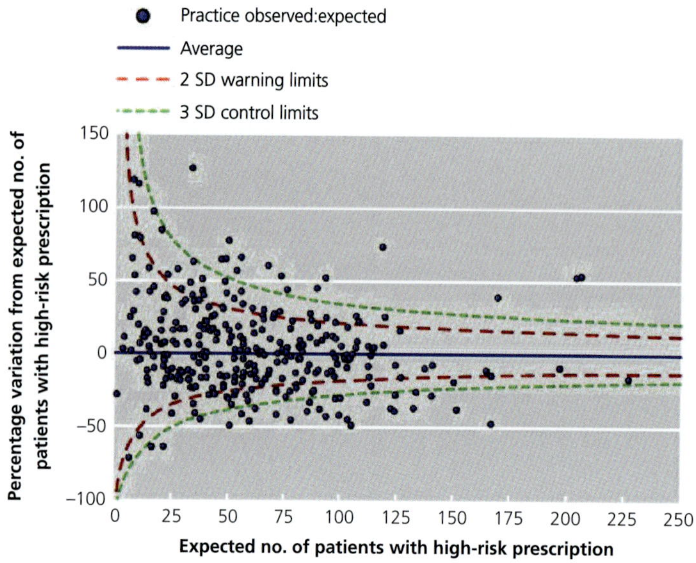

Cross-sectional control chart for observed versus expected number of patients with a high-risk prescription. Practices lying outside 3-SD control limit are statistically significantly different from average

Figure 15.2 Results from a study of 315 general practices in Scotland contributing to the Scottish Programme for Improving Clinical Effectiveness in Primary Care (SPICE-PC). Observed numbers of patients with a high-risk prescription differ from those expected in each practice after adjustment for patient case mix. Variability between practices' prescribing of high-risk medicines is considerable even after prescribing rates are adjusted to account for patient-level variables (age, sex, number of regular drugs). Practices lying outside the three-standard-deviation control limits are statistically different from the average and vary from having half the expected rates of high-risk prescribing to having a 50–125% excess rate.

Source: Guthrie et al. 2011 [45]. Reproduced with permission from BMJ Publishing Group Ltd.

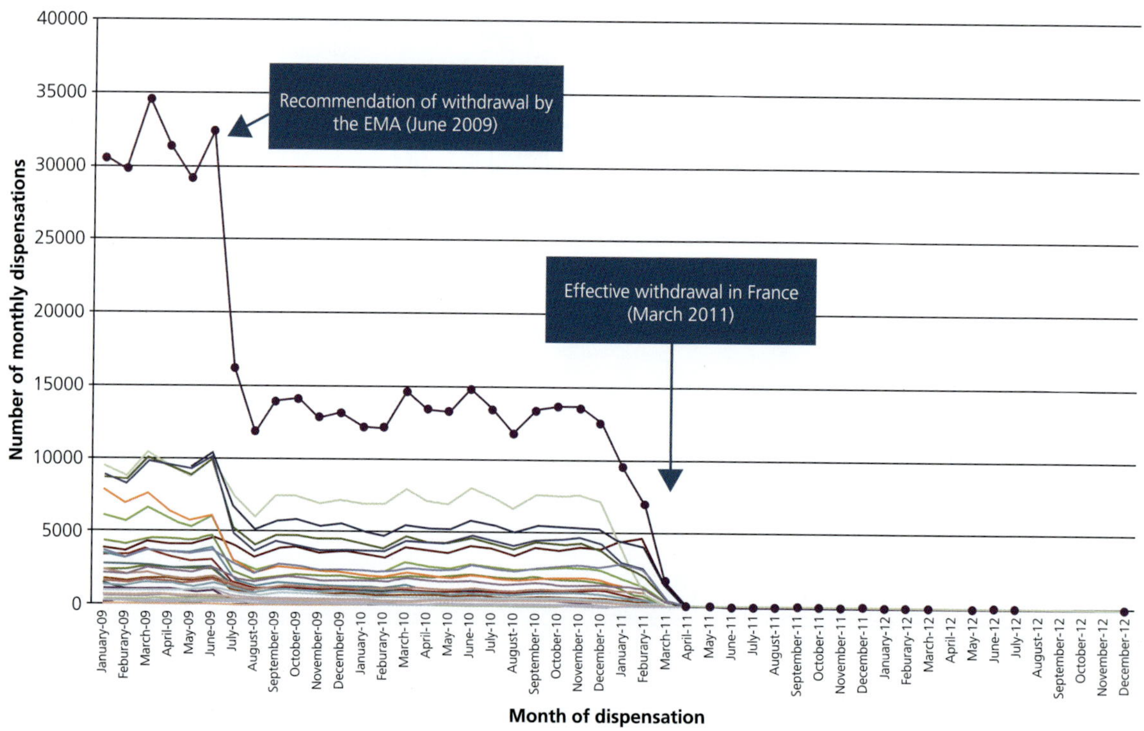

Figure 16.4 Kinetics of DXP withdrawal (dispensations) in French Rhone-Alpes claims data, 2009–2012. Different curves show specific packagings.

Source: Data from Regional claims data (URCAM Rhone-Alpes).

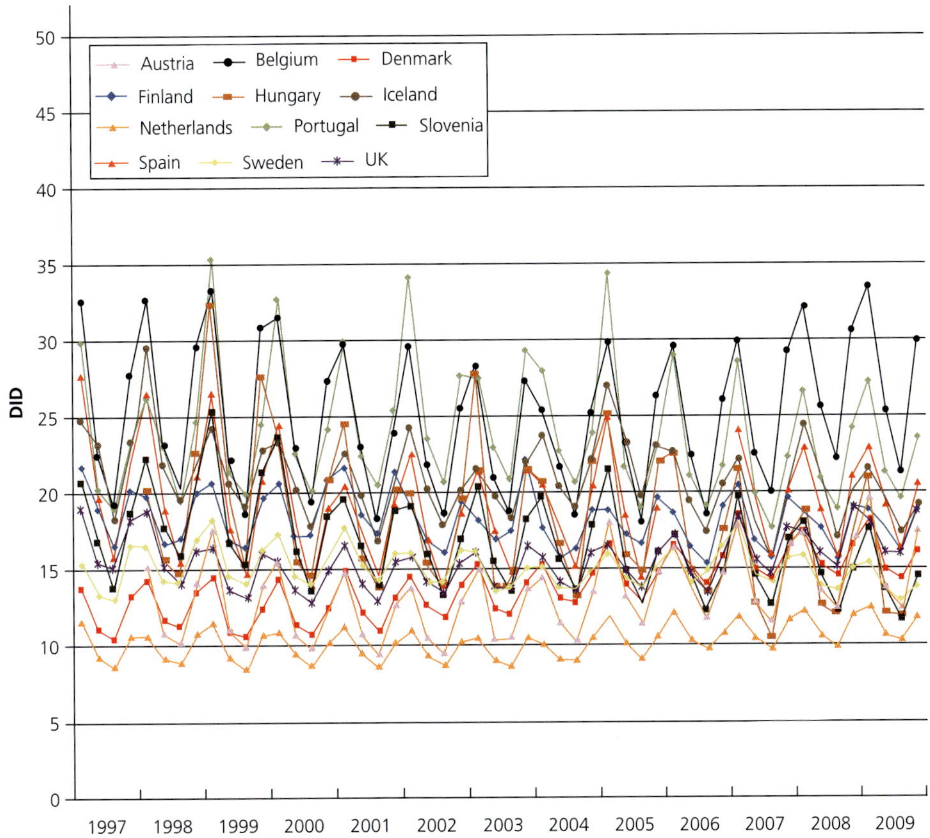

Figure 16.7 Seasonal variation in outpatient antibiotic use in 12 European countries, expressed in DDD/1000 inhabitants/day (DID).

Source: Adriaenssens et al. 2011 [37]. Reproduced by permission of Oxford University Press.

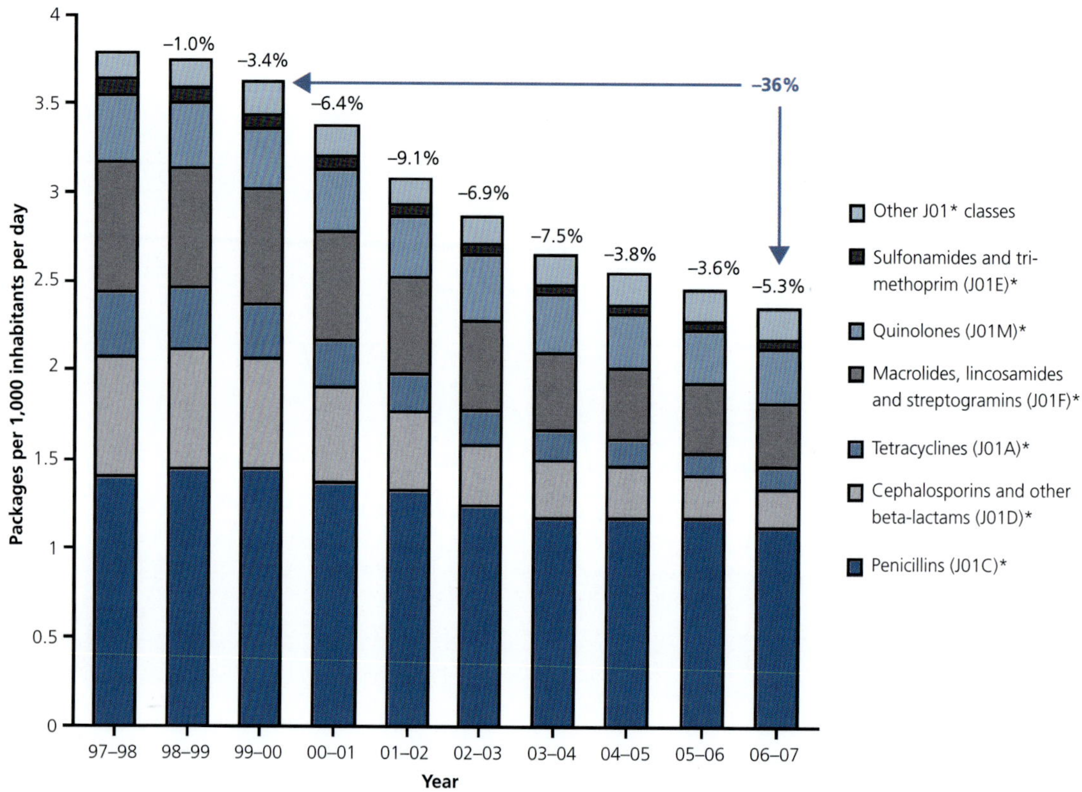

Figure 16.8 Outpatient antibiotic use in Belgium in packages/1000 inhabitants/day, July 1997 to June 2007.

*Anatomical Therapeutic Chemical (ATC) classification code

Source: Goossens et al. 2008 [41]. Reproduced with permission from Eurosurveillance.

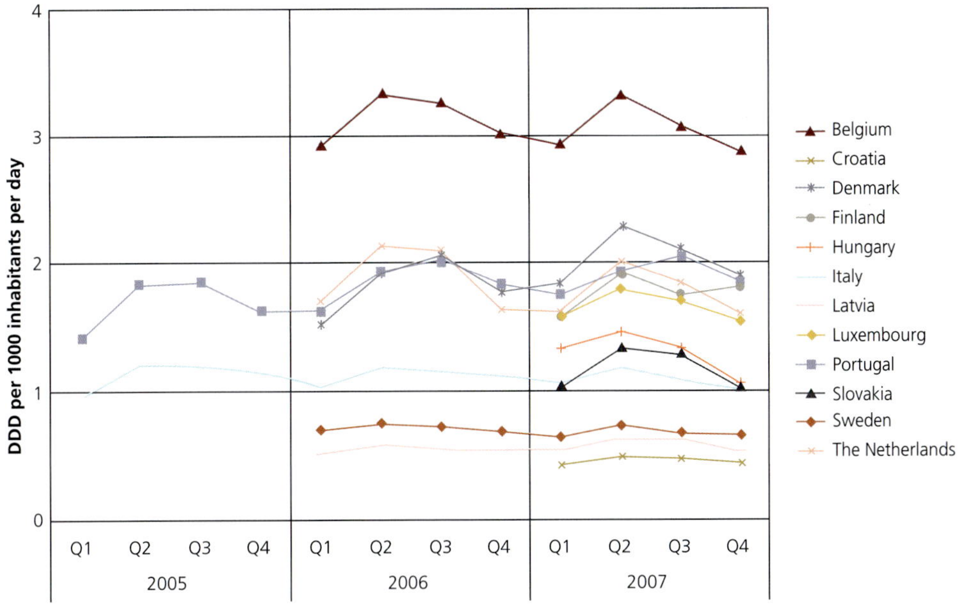

Figure 16.9 Seasonal variation in outpatient systemic antimycotic and antifungal use in 12 European countries. Data by quarter (Q) for 2005, 2006 and 2007.

Source: From Adriaenssens et al. 2010 [42]. Reproduced by permission of Oxford University Press.

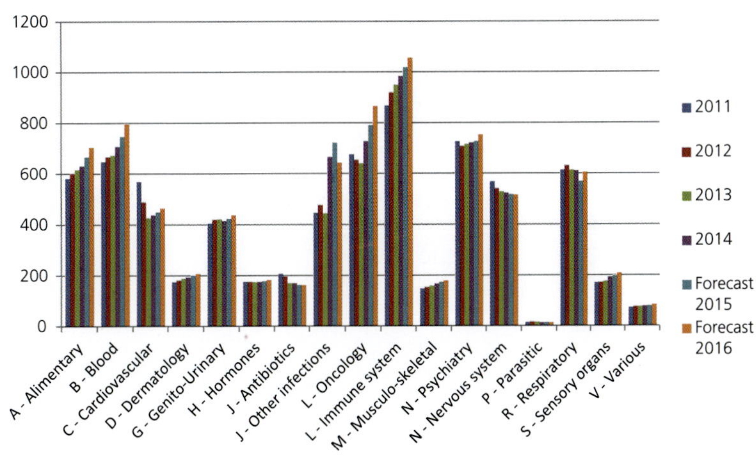

Figure 20.5 Actual and forecasted expenditure on medicines in Stockholm County Council, broken down by ATC class.

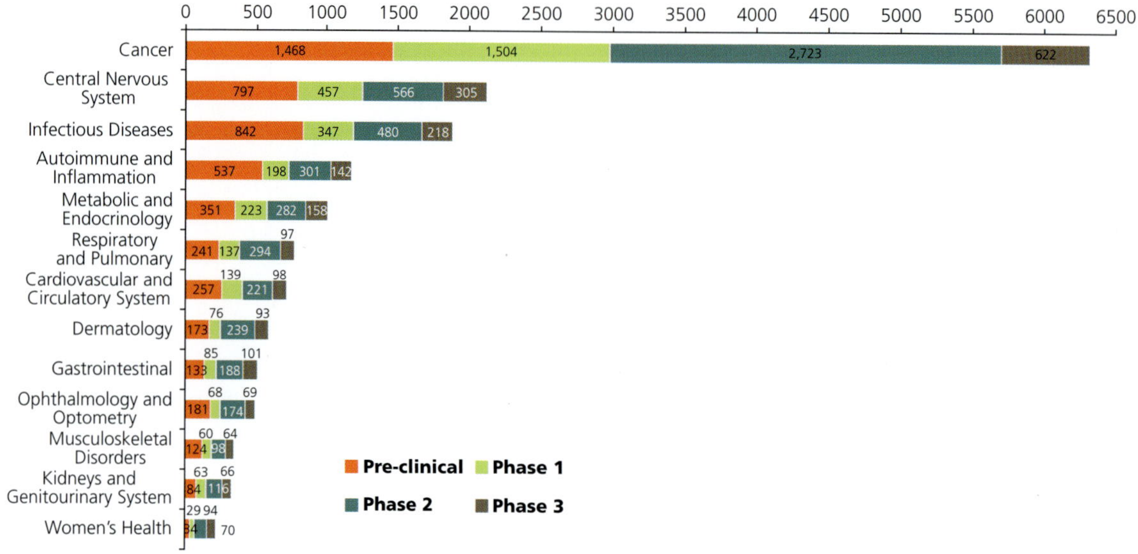

Figure 22.2 Pharmaceutical medicines in development in 2011.

Source: EFPIA. HEALTH & GROWTH – Working together for a healthy Europe. A vision towards a life sciences strategy for Europe [63].

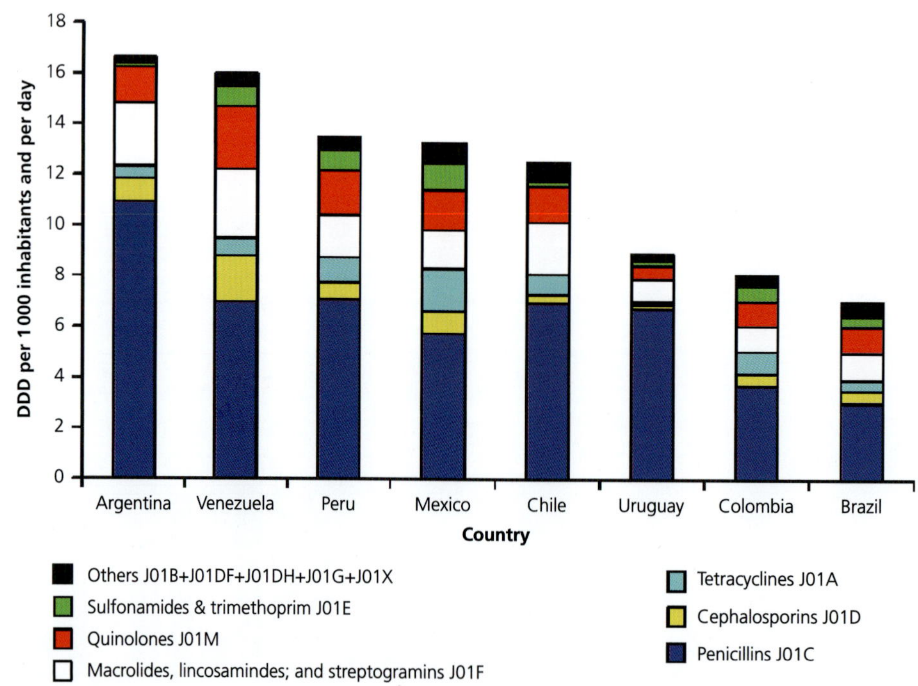

Figure 26.2 Total (ambulatory and hospital care) antibiotic consumption in eight Latin American countries. DDD: Defined daily dose

Source: Wirtz 2010 [42].

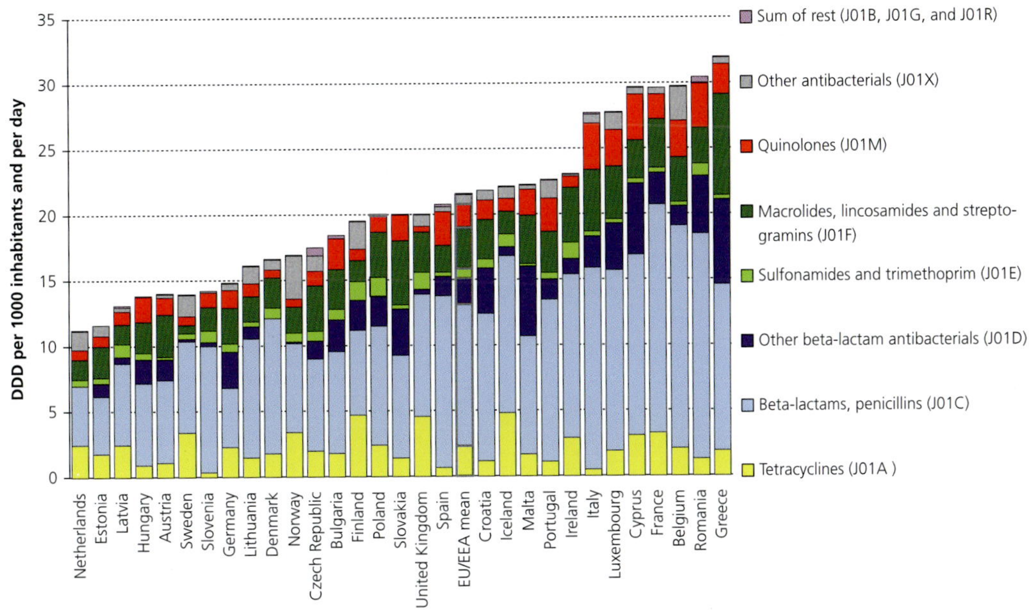

Figure 26.3 Pattern of antibiotic use in ambulatory care in European countries, 2012. Note: data for Cyprus, Iceland and Romania are total care data (i.e. including the hospital sector). Data for Spain are reimbursement data only (i.e. not including consumption without a prescription and other nonreimbursed courses). The EU/EEA mean shows the population-weighted mean. Figure based on national data that were available at the ESAC-Net interactive database in 2015. DDD: Defined daily dose

Source: Courtesy of Maria Matuz.

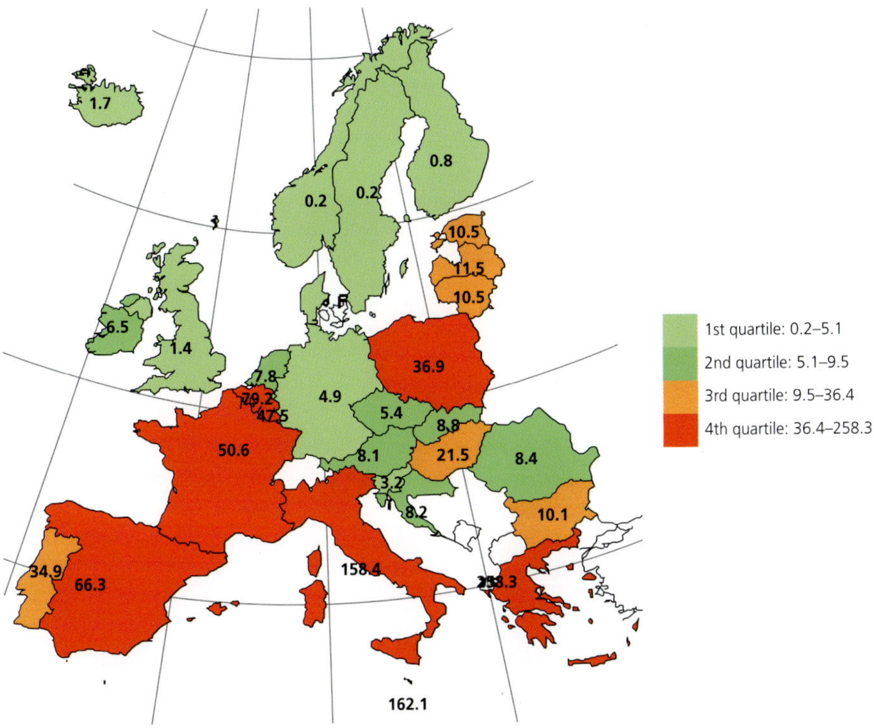

Figure 26.4 Ratio of the consumption of broad- versus narrow-spectrum penicillins, cephalosporins and macrolides in ambulatory care in European countries (B/N ratio), 2012. Broad-spectrum: J01CR, J01DC, J01DD, J01F minus J01FA01. Narrow-spectrum: J01CE, J01DB, J01FA. Figure based on national data that were available at the ESAC-Net interactive database in 2015.

Source: Courtesy of Maria Matuz.

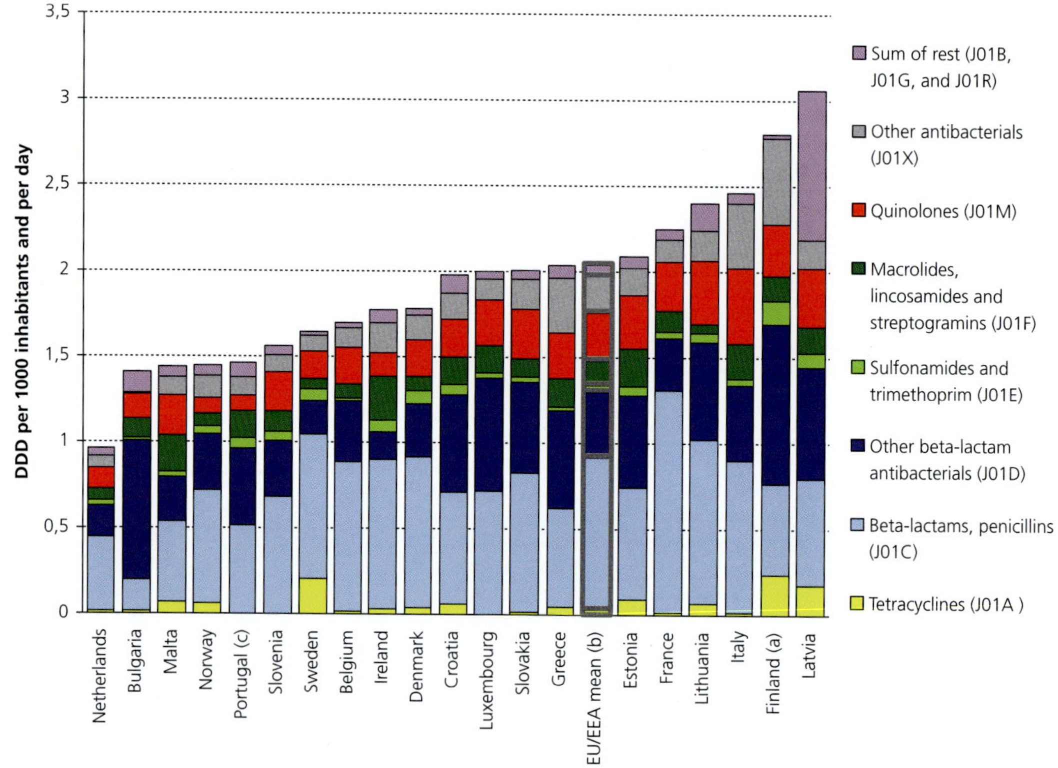

(a) Finland: data include consumption in remote primary healthcare centres and nursing homes

(b) EU/EEA mean refers to the corresponding population-weighted mean consumption based on 20 countries that provided data

(c) Portugal: data correspond to public hospitals only,

Figure 26.6 Pattern of hospital care antibiotic use in European countries, 2012. Data for Finland include consumption in remote primary health care centres and nursing homes. Data for Portugal correspond to public hospitals only. The EU/EEA mean refers to the corresponding population-weighted mean consumption based on 20 countries that provided data. The figure is based on national data that were available at the ESAC-Net Interactive database in 2015.

DDD: Defined daily dose
Courtesy of Maria Matuz

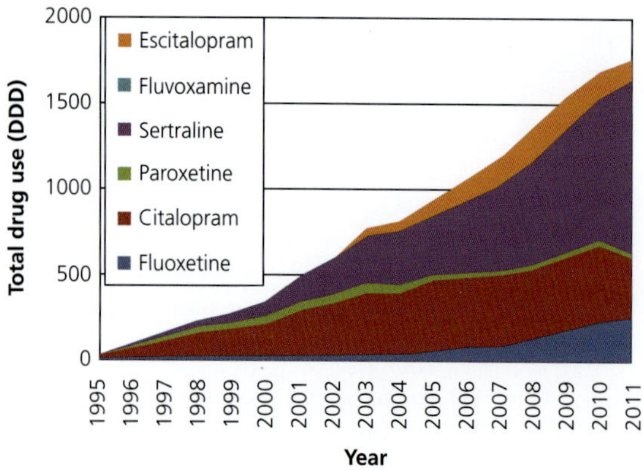

Figure 28.5 Total use of SSRIs, measured in DDDs and specified by drug substance and year, among the total paediatric population (5–18 years) in Denmark in 1995–2011.

Source: Pottegård et al. 2014 [101]. Reproduced with permission from Springer Science and Business Media.

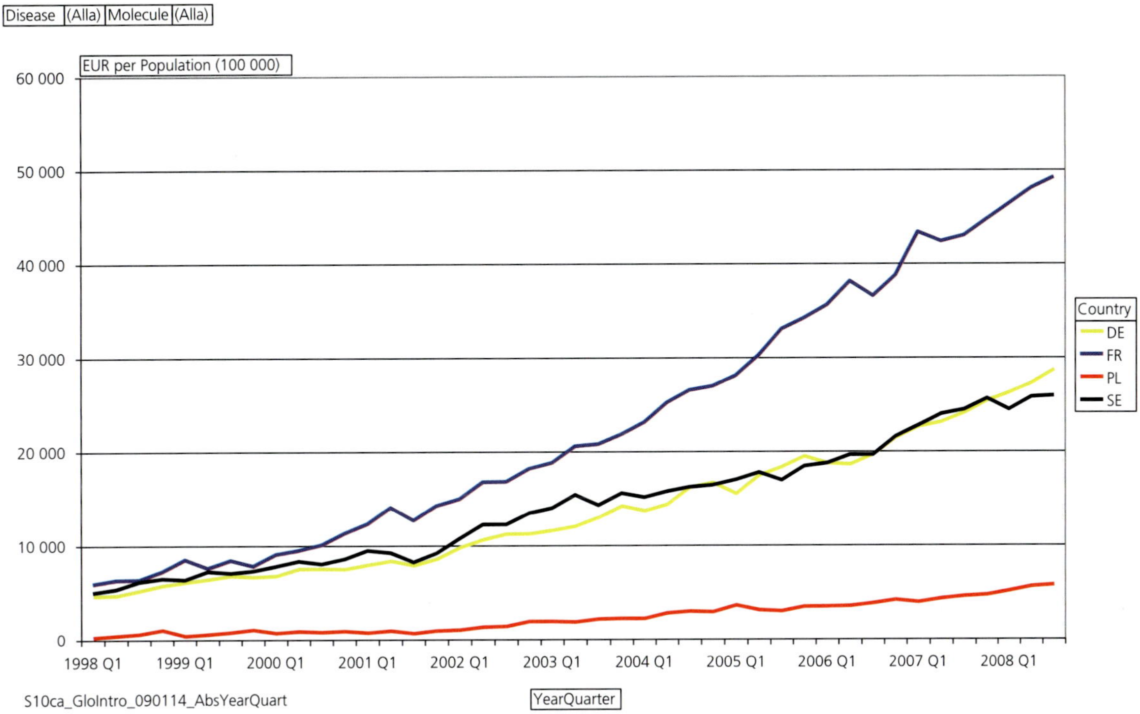

Figure 30.2 Total sales of 24 cancer drugs approved during 1995–2004, expressed in euros per 100 000 inhabitants in Germany (DE), France (FR), Poland (PL) and Sweden (SE).

Source: Data from [65].

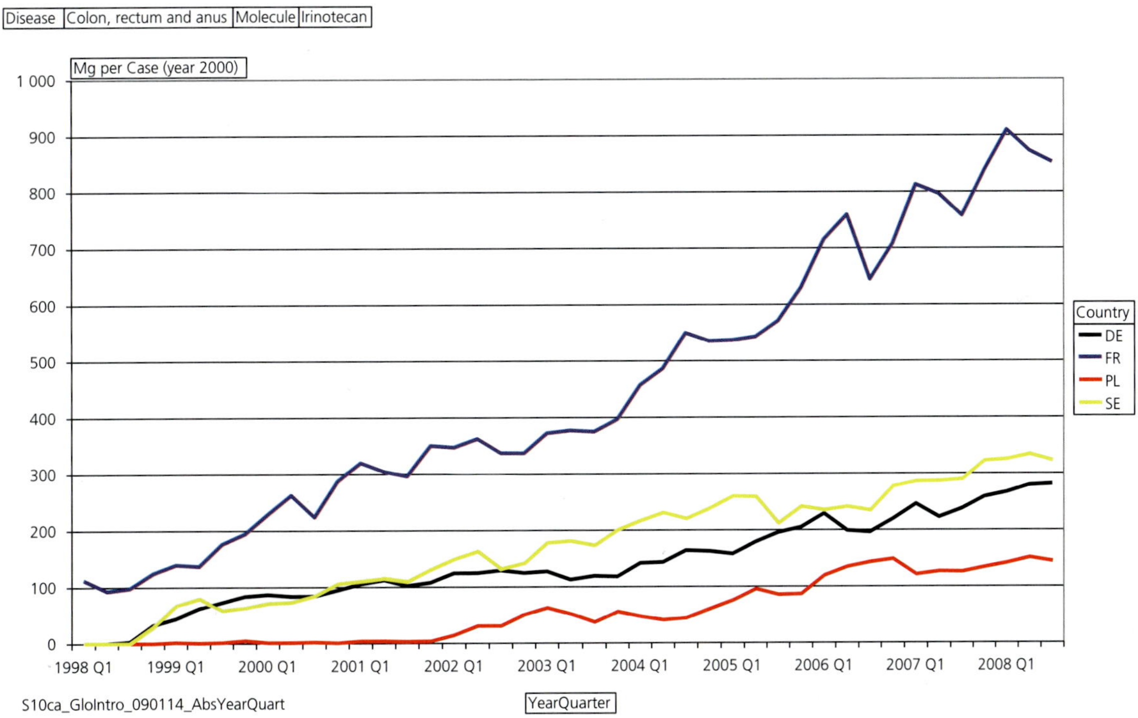

Figure 30.3 Use of irinotecan, expressed in milligrams per mortality case (case = mortality in colorectal cancer in 2000) in Germany (DE), France (FR), Poland (PL) and Sweden (SE).

Source: Data from [65].

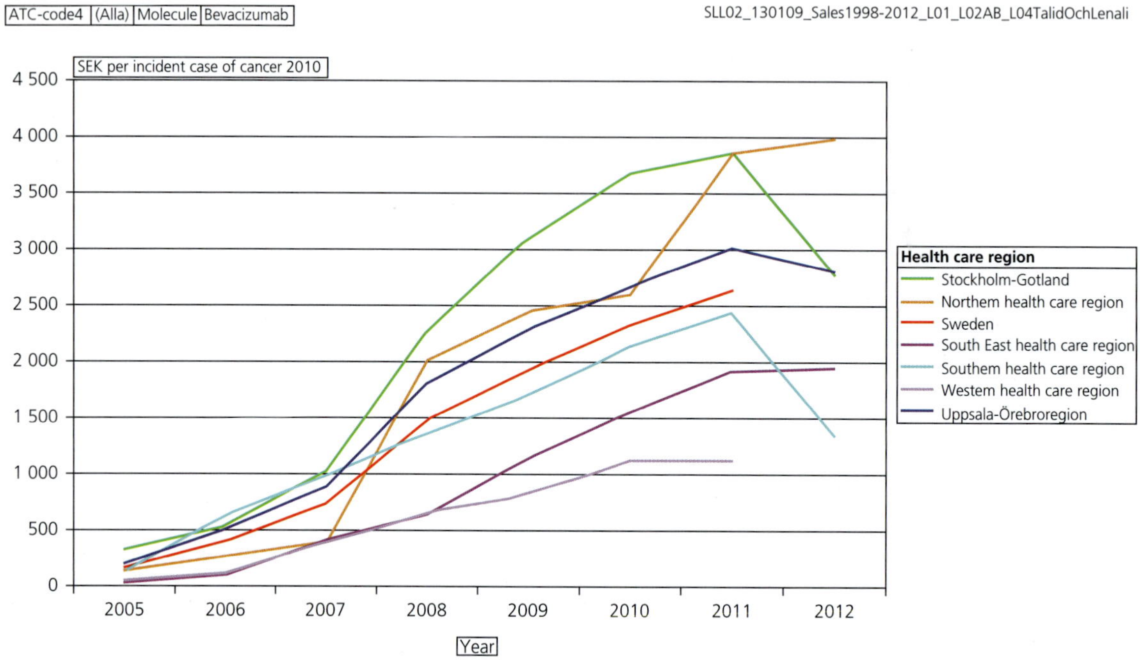

Figure 30.4 Use of bevacizumab, expressed in SEK per incident case (case = incidence in colorectal cancer in 2010) in the six health care regions in Sweden.

Source: Data from [33].

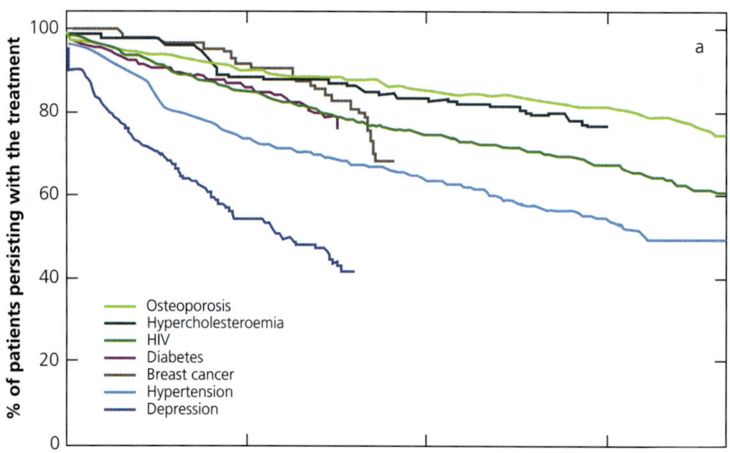

Figure 35.1 Differences in adherence according to different disease conditions, showing noninitiation and short persistence in seven disease conditions based on Kaplan–Meier persistence curves across different therapeutic areas. Note the between-disease differences in the percentage of patients who initiated the prescribed treatment.

Source: Adapted from Blaeschke et al. 2012 [4].

population as part of the TEDDY project (Task-force in Europe for Drug Development for the Young). The same protocol was used to study prescription patterns in three European countries, making use of the Pedianet database (comprising paediatric electronic medical records from 150 paediatricians, gathered since 2000) in Italy, the Integrated Primary Care Information (IPCI) database (comprising adult and paediatric electronic medical records from more than 400 doctors, gathered since 1996) in the Netherlands and the Intercontinental Marketing Services Disease Analyzer (IMS-DA) database (comprising adult and child electronic medical records from 670 doctors) in the United Kingdom. The study population consisted of 675 868 children and 2 334 673 person-years of follow-up. More than 5 million prescriptions were recorded.

Three levels of drug use were distinguished in the study population: high (>10/100 children per year), moderate (1–10/100 children per year) and low (<1/100 children per year) use. For all age categories, antiinfective, dermatological and respiratory drugs were in the high-use group, while cardiovascular and antineoplastic drugs were in the low-use group. Emollients, topical steroids and asthma drugs had the highest prevalence of recurrent use. In the top five highest-prevalence drugs, topical inhaled and systemic steroids, oral contraceptives and topical or systemic antifungal drugs were most commonly used off-label.

Furthermore, this study found that antiinfective and respiratory drugs were the drugs most commonly prescribed to children in the primary care settings in Italy, the Netherlands and the United Kingdom. Although this study found similarities between countries, differences were also observed. In the Netherlands, the prevalence of use of antiinfective drugs was much lower than in the other two countries, but the prevalance of genitourinary drugs such as oral contraceptives was particularly high in adolescent girls. While in Italy respiratory drug use was greater than in the other two countries, the use of drugs for conditions affecting the sensory organs (e.g. levocabastine eye drop) was much lower. In the United Kingdom, the prevalence of drugs used for neurological disorders was much higher than in the other two countries. Table 24.3 shows the 10 most commonly used therapeutic classes in various age categories. A set of studies investigating paediatric drug utilization in different therapeutic areas was generated using the TEDDY data [27–29].

Table 24.3 The 10 most commonly used therapeutic classes in various age categories.

Source: Sturkenboom et al. 2008 [26]. Reproduced with permission from BMJ Publishing Group Ltd.

Therapeutic class (Anatomical Therapeutic Chemical, ATC)	Users/1000 person years
<2 years	
Antibacterials for systemic use (J01)	435
Ophthalmologicals (S01)	175
Corticosteroids, dermatological preparations (D07)	165
Drugs for obstructive airway diseases (R03)	161
Emollients and protectives (D02)	147
Analgesics (N02	134
Nasal preparations (R01)	83
Antidiarrhoeals, intestinal antiinflammatory/antiinfective agents (A07)	67
Stomatological preparations (A01)	59
Corticosteroids for systemic use (H02)	57
2–11 years	
Antibacterials for systemic use (J01)	288
Drugs for obstructive airway diseases (R03)	108
Corticosteroids, dermatological preparations (D07	86
Emollients and protectives (D02)	67
Ophthalmologicals (S01)	64
Analgesics (N02)	63
Other respiratory system products (R07)	63
Nasal preparations (R01)	38
Antibiotics and chemotherapeutics (D06)	37
Antiinflammatory and antirheumatic products (M01)	33
12–18 years	
Antibacterials for systemic use (J01)	194
Sex hormones and modulators of genital system (G03)	82
Drugs for obstructive airway diseases (R03)	71
Other respiratory system products (R07)	67
Corticosteroids, dermatological preparations (D07)	65
Antiinflammatory and antirheumatic products (M01)	57
Nasal preparations (R01)	48
Ophthalmologicals (S01)	47
Anti-acne preparations (D10)	46
Analgesics (N02)	44

NSAIDs and opioids

Prescribing of analgesics and nonsteroidal antiinflammatory drugs (NSAIDs) in paediatric primary care in the United Kingdom, Italy and the Netherlands was assessed by Neubert et al. [27]. Overall, the prescribing prevalence for NSAIDs was lower in the Netherlands than in Italy and the United Kingdom. Ibuprofen by far exceeded the prescribing of any other drug of the anti-inflammatory and antirheumatic (ATC M01A) classes in the United Kingdom (30.6 users/1000 person-years) and Italy (20.8 users/1000 person-years), whereas diclofenac was dominant in the Netherlands (1.7 users/1000 person-years); in Italy, four other products (niflumic acid, morniflumate, ketoprofen and flurbiprofen) were also commonly prescribed, but not to the extent of ibuprofen. Compared with the NSAIDs, the overall prevalence of opioids was very low: codeine and codeine combinations were most commonly prescribed, with only little use seen for other drugs. It appeared that a great variety of different NSAIDs and opioids were prescribed to children in primary care in Europe. This may be attributed to the varying availability of drugs in different countries, but also to differing prescribing attitudes and reimbursement scheme and a lack of data on the effectiveness of individual drugs.

Asthma drugs

Another study investigated paediatric asthma drug use in the United Kingdom, the Netherlands and Italy [28]. The cohort consisted of 671 831 children, of whom 49 442 had been diagnosed with asthma at some point during follow-up. Among all asthma drugs, β2-mimetics and inhaled steroids were the most commonly used, even in children without asthma, but with large variability between countries. β2-mimetics and inhaled steroids had 4.9 and 4.1 users/100 person-years in the Netherlands, 8.7 and 5.3 users/100 person-years in the United Kingdom and 7.2 and 16.2 users/100 person-years in Italy, respectively. Xanthines, anticholinergics, leukotriene receptor antagonists and antiallergics were prescribed in fewer than one child per 100 per year. In patients without asthma, β2-mimetics were used most frequently. Country differences were greatest for steroids (Italy highest) and for β2-mimetics (the United Kingdom highest). Off-label use was low; it was most pronounced for β2-mimetics in children <18 months (Italy) and for combined β2-mimetics + anticholinergics in children <6 years (the Netherlands).

Antiepileptic drugs

A third study investigated antiepileptic drug (AED) prescribing in the same three countries [29]. In 2005, AED prevalence in children (0–11 years) was highest in Italy (3.9 users/1000 person-years), followed by the United Kingdom (3.0 users/1000 person-years) and the Netherlands (2.2 users/1000 person-years). Over the study period (2001–05), prescribing prevalence in 0–11 years old was stable in all three countries. In contrast, a steady rise in AED prevalence was observed in adolescents (12–18 years) in the United Kingdom, but not in the Netherlands. All countries showed a slight increase in prevalence for newer AEDs. Simultaneously, the prevalence of conventional AEDs decreased in the Netherlands and Italy but not in the United Kingdom. In 2005, lamotrigine use was highest in the Netherlands and the United Kingdom, whereas topiramate was favoured in Italy.

Other ambulatory studies

Table 24.4 summarizes a select number of other studies from around the world describing overall prescribing patterns in ambulatory care. Drug utilization of psychotropic medication and systemic antibacterials has been investigated in detail in many studies, a few of which are summarized in the remainder of this section.

Psychotropic medication

The use of psychotropic substances in children has been extensively studied [39,40]. Overall, the use of psychotropic medications in children and adolescents has been increasing over the past 20 years. There is evidence that psychotropic medications are both over- and underprescribed [41]. A range of studies have focused on individual psychotropic substances, including methylphenidate (used to treat attention deficit hyperactive disorder, ADHD) [42,43] and antidepressants [44].

Systemic antibacterials

A review of paediatric drug utilization studies on antibiotics found quantitative and qualitative differences in prescribing between and within countries [45]. The same result was found in a recent study comparing antibiotic usage in different age groups between five European countries [46]. This latter study also showed seasonal peaks during winter months, especially in countries with high utilization. Furthermore, prescription rates were highest among children in the age group

Table 24.4 Overview of studies on drug utilization in paediatrics from around the world.

Reference	Country	Year(s) covered	Setting	Database(s)	Focus	Population characteristics	Top 10 drugs
[30]	United States	2007–10	Ambulatory care	Outpatient prescription fills based on all-payer administrative datasets (commercial insurance and Medicaid)	Variations in prescribing by small geographic area and insurance type	n = 949 827 children	Amoxicillin, methylphenidate, albuterol, azithromycin, amphetamine-dextroamphetamine, fluoride, montelukast, amoxicillin-clavulanate, ethinyl estradiol/norgestimate, clonidine
[31]	United States	2002–10 Results from 2010 are reported here	Ambulatory care	IMS Vector One: National and Total Patient Tracker; two commercial prescription and patient databases, based on dispensing information from outpatient retail pharmacies Data on OTC medication, herbals and supplements are not included	Frequency and pattern of national outpatient drug utilization	n = 263 million prescriptions (total number of children not reported)	Amoxicilline, azithromycin, albuterol, amoxicillin/clavulanate, cefinier, cephalexin, fluticasone, prednisolone sodium phosphate, ibuprofen, montelukast
[32]	Sweden	2007	Ambulatory care	Drug dispensing data from the Swedish Prescribed Drug Register (SPDR): a nationwide study that includes all drug prescriptions to children aged 0–18 years in Sweden	Paediatric drug use, especially off-label prescriptions, in Swedish outpatient care – a nationwide study	n = 2.19 million drug prescriptions for n = 968 465 children	Antiinfectives for systemic use Respiratory system and dermatologicals groups most commonly prescribed No analysis of individual drugs provided
[33]	United States	2006	Inpatients	Link of three administrative databases: Premier Perspective Database; the Pediatric Health Information System data; Kids' Inpatient Database	Multivariable stratified resampling procedure used to generate national-level estimates of drug utilization in paediatric inpatients	n = 530 708 hospitalizations in 52 children's hospitals n = 782 344 hospitalizations in 411 general hospitals	Acetaminophen (paracetamol), lidocaine, ampicillin, morphine, fentanyl, ceftriaxone, ibuprofen, gentamicin, albuterol, potassium chloride
[34]	Sweden	48 hours in May and October 2008	Inpatients	Data on all prescriptions issued in the study period collected by care nurses and physicians using a form 34 paediatric hospitals and paediatric wards in 7 general hospitals	Paediatric drug use, especially off-label prescriptions, at Swedish hospitals – a nationwide study	n = 11 294 prescriptions for n = 2947 children	Paracetamol, carbohydrates, electrolytes, morphine, ibuprofen, furosemide, salbutamol, multivitamins, midazolam, diclofenac

(continued)

Table 24.4 *(continued)*

Reference	Country	Year(s) covered	Setting	Database(s)	Focus	Population characteristics	Top 10 drugs
[35]	Estonia	2008–09	Inpatients	Data collected twice weekly from neonatal intensive care unit records at two hospitals	Drug utilization pattern and off-label use of medicines in Estonian neonatal units	n = 1982 prescriptions for n = 490 neonates	Gentamicin, ampicillin, heparine, simeticone, fentanyl, furosemide, laurylsulphate+sodium, citrate, benzylpenicilline, salbutamol, midazolam (but use varied widely by development stage)
[36]	Brazil	2001	Inpatients	Data collected by interviews and from medical records at one paediatric public hospital	Off-label and unlicensed drug utilization in hospitalized children in Fortaleza, Brazil	n = 1450 prescriptions for n = 272 patients, 56% female Median age was 2 years (range 1 month–14 years)	Metamizole, fenoterol, oxacillin, mebendazole, ceftriaxone, prednisone, benzylpenicillin, furosemide, metronidazole, hydrocortisone
[37]	Mexico	2001–06	Inpatients	Database of dispensing information from the pharmacy department of the National Paediatrics Institute	Frequency of drug consumption and lack of paediatric formulations	n = 7514 dispensed medications (no patient details provided)	Ranitidine, paracetamol, midazolam, dicloxacillin, amoxicillin, furosemide, metamizol, prednisone, phenytoin, phenobarbital
[38]	Nepal	2003–04	Inpatients	Data collected from the medical records of one paediatric ward at a teaching hospital	Prescribing patterns among paediatric inpatients in a teaching hospital in western Nepal	356 children, 36% female, range 0–14 years	Ampicillin, paracetamol, fluid with dextrose, domperidone, ranitidine, cefotaxime, salbutamol, midazolam, cetirizine, gentamicin

≤4 years in all countries, predominantly due to high use of broad-spectrum penicillins. Data suggest that antibiotics are inappropriately used to a large extent, despite a substantial decrease in antibiotic use in children in the last 2 decades (probably caused by campaigns on rational antibiotic use). A recent US-based study found that this trend has now probably levelled, at least in some age groups [47]. In this study, children between 3 months and 3 years were again the highest consumers of antibiotics. Penicillins (including amoxicillin/clavulanate) and azithromycine were the most frequently used antibiotics.

Inpatient studies

In contrast to data from primary care, where the majority of published studies originate, there are limited data relating to paediatric drug use in hospitals, although it appears that there are significant differences in this setting. For example, a survey of the use of ciprofloxacin and fluconazole for sepsis treatment in neonates in 25 European countries found that there was great variability in the use of these two drugs for sepsis within and between the participating countries [14].

In the framework of a large, prospective, multicentre pharmacovigilance study, drug utilization patterns on general paediatric wards in five different countries (the United Kingdom, Germany, Hong Kong, Malaysia and Australia) were analysed [48] using a common protocol and standardized data collection methods and terminologies across study sites. The study population comprised 1278 patients. Data were collected prospectively by local study staff. A total of 5367 prescribed drugs (prescriptions) were recorded in the study cohort. The UK cohort contributed the highest number of prescriptions (38%), followed by Germany (25%), Malaysia (17%), Australia (14%) and Hong Kong (7%)

Four therapeutic drug groups accounted for 56% of all prescriptions; the highest number of prescriptions was for systemic antibacterials (25%), followed by analgesic drugs (17%), drugs for obstructive airway diseases (9%) and antiinflammatory and antirheumatic products (5%). Similar patterns were seen in each country for the systemic antibacterials and analgesics. Drugs for obstructive airway diseases were significantly more common in Malaysia than in the other countries (see Table 24.5 for the top 10 drugs by country).

NSAIDs and analgesics

In the overall cohort, paracetamol was the most frequently prescribed drug (12%), followed by ibuprofen (5%). A similar pattern was seen in each country for paracetamol prescriptions, except in Germany, where ibuprofen was the most frequently used drug. Ibuprofen was the second most frequently prescribed drug in the United Kingdom. Metamizole was only prescribed in Germany, and accounted for 9% of all prescriptions there. Morphine was prescribed in the United Kingdom and Australia only.

Across all countries, 61% of patients received at least one analgesic and 22% received at least one of the antiinflammatory and antirheumatic products. When combining these two groups into analgesics/NSAIDs, exposure rates varied between 84% in the United Kingdom and 35% in Hong Kong. In the overall cohort, there was no significant difference within age groups in the number of patients exposed to this combined group, with similar results in each country.

Drugs for obstructive airway diseases

Across all countries surveyed, 24% of patients received at least one of the drugs for obstructive airway diseases. There was a significant difference in percentage of patients exposed to this therapeutic group between countries, with the highest exposure in Malaysia (34%) and the lowest in Germany (13%). Among drugs for obstructive airway diseases, salbutamol was dominant in all countries. Salbutamol was administered only by inhalation in all countries except the United Kingdom, where it was also given intravenously. Also, in the United Kingdom, ipratropium bromide was almost

Table 24.5 Top 10 drugs (chemical substance) in each country participating in the ADVISE study adopted from [48].

Australia (n = 753)[a]		Germany (n = 1343)[a]		United Kingdom (n = 2010)[a]		Hong Kong (n = 357)[a]		Malaysia (n = 904)[a]		Total (n = 5367)[a]	
Paracetamol	92 (12)	Ibuprofen	120 (9)	Paracetamol	257 (13)	Paracetamol	35 (10)	Paracetamol	156 (17)	Paracetamol	640 (12)
Prednisolone	33 (4)	Metamizole)	115 (9)	Ibuprofen	108 (5)	Salbutamol	17 (5)	Cefuroxime	152 (17)	Ibuprofen	248 (5)
Salbutamol	25 (3)	Paracetamol	100 (8)	Amoxicillin and enzyme inhibitor	78 (4)	Prednisolone	16 (5)	Salbutamol	86 (10)	Salbutamol	226 (4)
Benzylpenicillin	26 (4)	Cefotaxime	54 (4)	Salbutamol	65 (3)	Cefuroxime	13 (4)	Calrithromycin	69 (8)	Cefuroxime	195 (4)
Gentamicin	36 (5)	Prednisolone	48 (4)	Ipratropium bromide	55 (3)	Ampicillin	12 (3)	Prednisolone	47 (5)	Prednisolone	195 (4)
Cefotaxime	21 (3)	Cefotiam	44 (3)	Morphine	53 (3)	Gentamicin	9 (3)	Cefotaxime	45 (5)	Amoxicillin and enzyme inhibitor	145 (3)
Flucloxacillin	21 (3)	Amoxicillin and enzyme inhibitor	34 (3)	Prednisolone	51 (3)	Amoxicillin and enzyme inhibitor	7 (2)	Fluticasone	39 (4)	Cefotaxime	144 (3)
Omeprazole	20 (3)	Salbutamol	33 (3)	Ranitidine	50 (3)	Fomatidine	7 (2)	Benzylpenicillin	38 (4)	Metamizole	115 (2)
Ondansetron	17 (2)	Sodium chloride	27 (2)	Ceftriaxone	49 (2)	Mometasone	7 (2)	Amikacin	27 (3)	Clarithromycin	105 (2)
Ibuprofen	16 (2)	Omeprazole	26 (2)	Sodium chloride	43 (2)	Insulin	7 (2)	Montelukast	24 (3)	Benzylpenicillin	92 (2)

[a]Total number of prescriptions.

Data reported as n (%); percentages are calculated based on number of prescriptions divided by total number of prescriptions.

as frequently prescribed as salbutamol; this was not the case in Germany, Hong Kong or Australia, and in Malaysia it was not prescribed at all. Fluticasone was predominantly prescribed in Malaysia, but it was not prescribed in Germany or Hong Kong.

Systemic antibacterials

Systemic antibacterials accounted for highest number of prescriptions in all countries: at least one antibacterial substance was among the four most frequently prescribed drugs in each case (Table 24.5). Cefuroxime was the second most frequently prescribed drug in Malaysia, after paracetamol. In the United Kingdom, amoxicillin plus enzyme inhibitor was the third most common prescription, after paracetamol and ibuprofen. Overall, 65% of patients received at least one systemic antibacterial; 51% were exposed to one systemic antibacterial, 30% to two different types of antibacterial and 19% to three or more different antibacterials. A similar pattern was observed across the countries, except in Australia, where the highest percentage was patients receiving three or more different antibacterials.

In a large European study of 32 hospitals with 69 paediatric units [49], part of the ESAC project (see also Chapter 26), 32% of hospitalized children (n = 1799; range 17–100%) received one or more antimicrobials (96% were systemtic antibiotics). The majority were administered intravenously and a high proportion of children were given combination therapy, both of which raised concerns about appropriateness of treatment. About 70% of use was therapeutic; the remainder was prophylactic or a combination of therapeutic and prophylactic. Third-generation cephalosporines, aminoglycosides and penicillins with extended spectrum were the most commonly used antibiotic classes in therapeutic indications. Combinations of penicillins and combinations of sulphonamides and trimethoprim were used most commonly for prophylaxis.

A recent worldwide study of 73 hospitals was carried out as part of the European project (www.arepecproject.eu) aiming to standardize the method of surveillance of antimicrobial use in children and neonates. Initial results of this study show a higher prevalence of antibiotic use in non-European versus European countries. Use is consistently lower in neonatal patients versus children. Antibiotic use is highest in haematology/oncology wards and paediatric intensive care units [50].

Conclusion

The majority of paediatric drug utilization studies in ambulatory settings have been conducted using large automatic datasets; international studies allow interesting comparisons of drug utilization patterns between countries and enhance our understanding of paediatric drug use in real life. In contrast, drug utilization studies in secondary care settings have mainly been conducted using intensive data monitoring methods; these studies are very labour-intensive but usually provide rich information on drug utilization. Studies that include a sufficient number of patients remain rare, especially in rare diseases and small patient groups such as neonatal intensive care patients. Greater cooperation among researchers is therefore needed in order to perform larger (international) studies. The results of drug utilization studies in paediatrics should be used to inform outcome research analyses. In particular, efficacy and safety studies are needed around drugs with frequent adverse drug events, off-label use and considerable heterogeneity in use between countries and settings. In planning such studies, drug utilization data could be used to indicate those geographical areas and settings most suitable for effective data collection.

CHAPTER 25

Drug utilization in older people

Katja Taxis[1], David O'Sullivan[2], Shane Cullinan[2] & Stephen Byrne[2]
[1]*University of Groningen, The Netherlands*
[2]*School of Pharmacy, University College Cork, Ireland*

KEY POINTS

- Population ageing is a global phenomenon. Older individuals (above 65 years of age) are the most frequent consumers of medicines among all age groups.
- Polypharmacy is very common in older individuals. Currently, the highest rates are reported from Asian countries.
- Appropriateness of prescribing can be assessed using explicit or implicit criteria, or a mix of both. Beers criteria and STOPP/START criteria are used frequently to assess inappropriate prescribing.
- There is widespread concern about the quality of prescribing in older people.
- Deprescribing is a recently introduced term for 'medication withdrawal', such as withdrawal of preventative medication near the end of life. Studies indicate benefits from this approach, but more research is needed in this area.

Introduction

Population ageing

Population ageing is a global phenomenon. In 1990, older people (≥60 years) constituted 9% of the world's population; in 2013, they made up 12%; and they are estimated to make up 21% by 2050. This growth has been mainly attributed to a decrease in mortality and a decline in fertility levels. It is also forecasted that the proportion of the oldest old (i.e. persons aged ≥80 years) will increase over the next few decades. In general, older women have a higher life expectancy than their male counterparts. In 2013, in the ≥60 years age group, there were 85 men for every 100 women, and in the ≥80 years age group, there were 61 men for every 100 women. In 2013, 40% of older persons globally lived independently (alone/with their spouse), with higher levels of independent living observed in more developed countries. It is forecasted that by 2050, the number of older individuals in developed countries who are no longer capable of living independently (i.e. caring for themselves) will quadruple [1].

Disease burden in older people

The majority of health-related problems and disabilities in older individuals are caused by noncommunicable diseases (NCDs). Globally, in 2008, 85% of people aged ≥60 years died from NCDs, with mortality rates ranging from 92% in the more developed regions to 74% in the less developed ones. For older individuals from high-income countries, the most prevalent diseases are ischaemic heart disease, visual disorders, dementia, cancers and stroke; for older individuals from low- and middle-income countries, they are ischaemic heart disease, stroke, visual impairment and chronic obstructive pulmonary disease (COPD) [2].

Typically, older people suffer from multiple chronic diseases (comorbidity) [3], as well as an array of nonspecific conditions/symptoms that cannot be ascribed to a particular organ or pathology. The latter group of conditions/symptoms is often referred to as 'geriatric syndromes' and is reported to include immobility, instability, incontinence and impaired intellect/memory [4]. An accumulation of impairments in multiple physiologic systems results in frailty, defined as a state of increased vulner-

Drug Utilization Research: Methods and Applications, First Edition. Edited by M. Elseviers et al.
Published 2016 by John Wiley & Sons, Ltd.

ability and reduced ability to recover homeostasis after a stressful event [5]. Age-related physiological changes affect how medicines are handled by the body (i.e. pharmacokinetic parameters change). One of the most important changes is the decrease in renal function, which risks accumulation and toxicity of drugs eliminated by the kidneys. In addition, older people may have altered drug responsiveness (pharmacodynamics); for example, the risk of orthostatic hypotension is greater in older people prescribed vasodilators [6]. Such changes are one reason for the negative risk–benefit ratio of a number of drugs in older people (see later).

Frail older individuals with a high level of physical and functional dependency usually need long-term care, provided either in their homes or in institutional facilities. A large European study of nursing home residents (n = 4156), undertaken by Onder et al. in 2012 [7], found that 68% were cognitively impaired. Urinary incontinence (73.5%), pain (36.0%), depression (32.0%), behavioural symptoms (27.5%), falls (18.6%) and pressure ulcers (10.4%) were also found to be prevalent.

Prescribing patterns in older people

Research on prescribing in older people is a dynamic and rapidly expanding field. A variety of tools and methods have been developed for use in this field, and have been utilized in many studies around the world. Ultimately, this research contributes to the development of strategies for the enhancement of prescribing quality in older people; this is covered in Chapters 45–47. Further information can be found in references [8–11].

Polypharmacy

Drug prescribing is a crucial aspect of the care of older people. Older adults use more medicines than any other age group [12–15]. Moreover, the mean number of medicines used by older adults has increased remarkably in recent decades [16–18]. Prescribing aims to cure and prevent disease, eliminate or reduce symptoms relating to an underlying disease state and improve individuals' functional capacity. Older individuals typically suffer from multiple acute and chronic disease states, which often necessitate the use of multiple concomitant medications (i.e. ***polypharmacy***) [19]. In many cases, polypharmacy is justified as best practice in the management of multiple conditions. It is therefore necessary to distinguish between ***appropriate*** and ***inappropriate or problematic*** polypharmacy [8]. Polypharmacy may also result from a phenomenon known as the ***prescribing cascade***: the prescribing of a medication to treat the symptoms of an adverse effect of another medication, rather than stopping the latter. Examples are the prescription of antihypertensives to treat nonsteroidal anti-inflammatory drug (NSAID)-induced hypertension and the prescription of prochlorperazine to manage drug-induced dizziness [20,21].

Although the term 'polypharmacy' is used often in the literature, it lacks a universally consistent definition. The following have been proposed:

1 The consumption of an arbitrary number of concomitant medications. A variety of different cut-offs have been used, ranging from two to nine concomitant medications. The vast majority of studies report polypharmacy as the use of five or more concomitant medications [8].
2 The unnecessary prescribing of more medications to a patient than is clinically indicated [22,23].

While polypharmacy most commonly refers to prescribed medications, it is important also to consider the number of over-the-counter (OTC) medicines and herbal medicines/supplements used.

The prevalence of polypharmacy varies widely between studies (Table 25.1). Two recent studies from Asia reported the highest prevalence: >80% of older adults using six or more medicines concomitantly [27,28]. Several studies report a steady increase in the prevalence of polypharmacy over recent decades [17,18,24]. Age, comorbidities, hospitalization, gender, socioeconomic position, number of physicians and number of pharmacies have been associated with polypharmacy [8,29]. Although polypharmacy is often justified in the management of multiple conditions, it predisposes older individuals to an increased risk of drug–drug interactions, drug–disease interactions, adverse drug events and potentially inappropriate prescribing (PIP) and has been associated with reduced patient compliance (see later).

Prescribing patterns in community-dwelling older people

Globally, cardiovascular medications, medications for the central nervous system and analgesics are among the most frequently used medicines in older adults (Table 25.1). Among cardiovascular medicines, diuretics and beta-blockers are common, but over time there

Table 25.1 Examples of studies of prescribing patterns in community-dwelling older adults.

Reference	Country, year	Data source	Study design	Number and characteristics of participants	Percentage of patients on polypharmacy	Three most common medications (%)
Jyrkkä et al. [24]	Finland, 1998, 2003	Interviews at home/ outpatient clinic/institution	Longitudinal study of a random sample of community-dwelling and institutionalized ≥75 years (only results from the home-dwelling population in 2003 are given here)	289 Mean age 80, 75% female	67% >5 medicines; 28% ≥10 medicines	86% cardiovascular medication, 70% blood and blood-forming organs, 65% nervous system
Nobili et al. [25]	Italy, 2005	Administrative database of prescriptions covered by the National Health Service, Lombardy region	Cross-sectional study of community-dwelling 65–95-year-olds	1 767 239 Mean age 75, 71% female	81% ≥1 medicine, 46% ≥5 medicines	66% cardiovascular medication, 42% alimentary tract and metabolism agents, 41% antiinfectives for systemic use
Kaufman et al. [12]	United States, 1998–99	Telephone interviews (Slone Survey, data collection till 2007) concerning medicine use, including OTC and herbals, during the preceding week	Random-digit dialling of 2590 community-dwelling persons >18 years old	263 male, 231 female Mean age not reported – all ≥65 years old	Male: 91% ≥1 medicine, 44% ≥5 medicines, 12% ≥10 medicines Female: 94% ≥1 medicine, 57% ≥5 medicines, 12% ≥10 medicines	Men: 39% aspirin, 16% paracetamol, 12% furosemide Women: 27% paracetamol, 23% aspirin, 17% conjugated oestrogens
Quato et al. [26]	United States, 2005–06	In-home interviews of a nationally representative probability sample of the United States	Cross-sectional, 57–85-year-olds	3500	81% ≥1 medication, 29% ≥5 medications	28% aspirin, 16% hydrochlorothiazide, 13% atorvastatin
Kim et al. [27]	Korea, 2010–11	Claims database: Health Insurance Review and Assessment Service – National Patient Sample (HIRA-NPS); gender- and age-stratified random sample of 3% of all Korean patients	Cross-sectional, ≥65-year-olds	319 185 Mean age 74, 60% female	86.4% ≥6 medicines, 44.9% ≥11 medicines, 3.0% ≥21 medicines	Not reported

have been changes in this group, such as an increase in the use of angiotensin-blocking agents [30,31] and a decrease in the use of cardiac glycosides [17]. Hypnotics and sedatives are among the most commonly used psychotropic substances, especially in the very old [32]. In a Finnish study, almost one-third of adults aged ≥75 years were using some anxiolytic or hypnotic and almost one-tenth were using antidepressant or antipsychotic medicines [33]. Paracetamol and NSAIDs are the most commonly used analgesics. One large survey found that paracetamol is used by every third older adult in the United States [18]. Differences among studies for this drug class depend on whether OTC medicines and as-needed (prn) medicines use are included. Over the last few decades, a considerable increase in the use of medicines from the group of blood and blood-forming organs, especially antithrombotic medications (including acetylsalicylic acid: aspirin), has been observed [17]. For example, a Swedish study showed that half of all older adults using five or more medicines used antithrombotics [14].

Pronounced differences in prescribing patterns have been observed for age and gender among old adults. For example, the highest use of central nervous system medicines seems to be among the oldest age groups [32–34]. Women in general use more medicines and receive more cardiovascular medicines and psychotropic medicines than men [17]. A recent study suggests that some of these differences may be explained by gender-related morbidity [35].

Prescribing patterns in hospitalized older people

Hospitalization has been associated with a change in prescribing patterns, although some studies report a substantial increase in the number of drugs used [36,37], while others report a decrease [38]. In an Indian study, antibacterials were the most commonly prescribed medication during hospitalization [39], whereas in a study from Italy, drugs for acid-related disorders and antithrombotic agents were most common [37]. Such differences are probably due to differences in the patient groups studied.

Prescribing patterns in nursing home residents

Admission to a nursing home has been shown to impact on prescribing patterns [40]. Compared to community-dwelling older adults, nursing home patients are considerably older. The average age of nursing home residents in the majority of studies is between 80 and 85 years. Furthermore, approximately 75% of all residents are female. Polypharmacy is reported to be highly prevalent in older nursing home residents, with concomitant use of five to nine drugs being observed in about half of residents and concurrent use of ten or more in about a quarter. Laxatives have been found to be the most frequently used medication, followed by antiulcer drugs, aspirin and other antiplatelet medications. Also, it has been reported that cardiovascular medications are commonly used, with more than a third of residents using diuretics, about a quarter using angiotensin converting enzyme (ACE) inhibitors or beta-blockers and about a fifth using calcium channel blockers and statins. More than a third of residents also use some form of analgesic (paracetamol, NSAIDs or opioids) [7].

Studies consistently report a high use of psychotropic medications in older nursing home residents, with some reporting as much as 75% of all residents using at least one psychotropic medication [41,42]. Between a third and half of all nursing home residents receive a benzodiazepine, antidepressant or an antipsychotic [7,41–44]. Variations in the psychotropic prescribing practices between nursing homes may be a reflection of the underlying 'prescribing culture' [45].

Antibiotics are also reported to be commonly prescribed in older nursing home residents. A cross-sectional study showed that approximately 5% of nursing home residents take at least one antibiotic, with a range of 6–136 defined daily doses (DDDs)/1000 inhabitants across Europe. Penicillin-type antibiotics such as amoxicillin with or without clavulanic acid were among the most frequently prescribed antibiotics in this patient population, while nitrofurantoin and methenamine (in Nordic countries only) were also reported to be commonly used [46].

It is important to note the variation in the terminology used to describe long-term care facilities across the world. For example, facilities providing 24-hour nursing care are described as nursing homes in the United Kingdom, skilled nursing facilities in the United States and aged care facilities providing high-level care in Australia; those providing personal care are described as residential homes in the United Kingdom, assisted-living facilities in the United States and aged care facilities providing low-level care in Australia.

Data sources

A wide range of methods is used to establish drug utilization patterns in older people (Table 25.1), including telephone surveys using random-digit dialling (as in the Slone Survey in the United States) [12], interviews at home and in outpatient clinics [24,26], clinical audits and administrative databases [25,45] and national registers [44,47]. General aspects of validity and reliability around drug utilization data sources are addressed in Chapters 3 and 4. As highlighted in these chapters, analyses based on administrative data cannot establish whether a given medication was actually taken by a patient. This is particularly important in contexts such as analysis of prescribing patterns on the day of death (as carried out by Jansen et al. [48]). Similarly, as has already been highlighted, some analyses are limited by a lack of information on OTC medication, herbal medication or as-required medication. In addition, many studies on drug utilization in older adults are limited by small and selected samples, resulting in a lack of statistical significance and reduced generalizability.

Much recent research has concentrated on the prevalence of inappropriate prescribing (see next section), and there are fewer publications describing overall patterns of use in older adults. In particular, there are only a few recent longitudinal studies. Inconsistencies in definitions (e.g. of 'polypharmacy') and differences among studied populations (e.g. in age categories and other inclusion/exclusion criteria) make it difficult to come to conclusions about the prevalence of drug use in older individuals.

Assessing prescribing quality

Appropriate prescribing is a concept that encompasses a number of different facets of prescribing, including evidence-based prescribing, prescribing that is well tolerated by the majority of patients, prescribing that is cost-effective and prescribing that takes the patient's preferences into account [49]. Prescribing in the older adult population is frequently complicated by factors such as estimated life expectancy, unfavourable risk–benefit ratios and a lack of evidence for the use of a particular medication in this population [50].

Inappropriate prescribing

Inappropriate prescribing is a major area of concern in older individuals. PIP covers a number of different suboptimal prescribing practices:

- **Overprescribing:** The prescribing of medications which, given the patient's clinical status (or life expectancy), are unnecessary or no longer required. Or, the prescribing of medications at doses, frequencies and/or durations greater than required or clinically indicated.
- **Misprescribing:** The prescribing of a medication with a high risk of an adverse event (i.e. where the risk of an adverse event outweighs the potential benefits). It has been shown that certain medications ought to be used with caution in older patients; if safer, equally effective alternatives are available, these ***potentially inappropriate medications*** (PIMs) should be avoided altogether.
- **Underprescribing or prescribing omission(s):** The failure to prescribe a medication which, given the patient's clinical status, is clearly indicated, where there is no reason for it not to be prescribed (i.e. there is no contraindication or caution). These events are commonly referred to as ***potential prescribing omissions*** (PPOs). Examples include not prescribing warfarin for atrial fibrillation, antidepressants for major depression and pain medications and laxatives in the general population.

Appropriateness of prescribing can be evaluated using either explicit or implicit criteria [49]; a number of the PIP screening tools use a combination of both. The aim of a PIP screening tool is to optimize prescribing by assisting the health care professional in identifying PIP instances in the clinical setting, thereby potentially reducing the negative outcomes that may result from PIP [51–53]. This use is different from using PIP tools as prescribing indicators (see Chapters 12 and 43).

Explicit criteria are usually clearly defined statements of potential inappropriateness, often developed from a variety of different sources, including evidence-based guidelines, published reviews, experts' opinions and consensus techniques. Explicit criteria are usually medication- and/or disease-oriented and typically require little to no clinical interpretation or judgement. Therefore, these criteria are quick and easy to deploy and generally exhibit a good level of inter-rater reliability. They usually comprise lists of medications, dosages, drug–drug combinations and drug–disease combinations that should be avoided. However, explicit criteria are usually quite inflexible and generally do not take into consideration all facets of care, patient preference and issues relating to multiple comorbidities [49,51,52,54]. They can nevertheless be useful in international comparisons of prescribing patterns (see e.g. [55]).

Implicit criteria rely on the formulation by health care professionals of clinical judgements relating to the appropriateness or inappropriateness of a specific treatment option based on all of the available clinical evidence. This type of approach is considered more sensitive than the use of explicit criteria, as it is intended to take both the perspective and the preferences of the patient into consideration. However, implicit criteria can often prove quite time-consuming to apply and, as they depend on clinicians' knowledge and attitudes, can be subject to differences of opinion and therefore generally exhibit a poor level of inter-rater reliability. Implicit criteria are also often difficult to apply to administrative databases and national registers [49,51,52,54].

There is no ideal approach to assessing prescribing appropriateness, and both types have advantages and disadvantages which should be taken into consideration when devising or choosing a suitable screening tool. However, due to the time-consuming nature, poor inter-rater reliability and limited application to administrative databases of implicit criteria, the majority of studies that have examined PIP to date have used explicit criteria, even though implicit criteria are considered more sensitive. Much of the assessment of appropriateness of medication use is conducted from a biomedical perspective, and much work has to be done to incorporate the patient's perspective (see Chapter 33).

Table 25.2 presents some criteria for the assessment of prescribing in the older adult population. Two sets have gained international recognition: the Beers criteria and the STOPP/START criteria.

The ***Beers criteria*** were among the first sets of explicit PIP criteria to be developed, first being published in 1991; the most recent revision was issued by the American Geriatrics Society in 2015 [62–65]. The 2015 Beers criteria consist of a list of medications or medication classes that are deemed potentially inappropriate in all older individuals, a list of medications that are considered potentially inappropriate in older individuals who have one of the specified health problems and a list of medications/medication classes that should be used with caution in all older individuals. For each criterion, the quality of the evidence is graded and the clinical significance (severity) is rated. New to the 2015 criteria are a list of drug drug interactions with a high risk of harmful outcome in older people as well as a list of drugs to be avoided/adjusted in individuals with renal impairment. The Beers criteria were based on an extensive literature review, followed by a modified Delphi consensus validation methodology conducted by an expert panel from the United States and Canada. Although the Beers criteria have been very influential and are widely used, they have been criticized for their restricted applicability outside the United States, due to differences in the availability of medication, and lack of criteria assessing underuse of medication [77].

The ***Screening Tool of Older People's Prescriptions (STOPP) criteria*** and the ***Screening Tool to Alert to Right Treatment (START)*** were developed in Ireland in 2008 by Gallagher et al. [71], with an update published in 2014 [72]. The STOPP criteria comprise 80 instances where certain medications or medication classes would be considered potentially inappropriate in older individuals. The START criteria comprise 34 criteria on the issue of underprescribing (i.e. the potential underprescribing of clinically beneficial medications/medication classes that should be prescribed in older individuals with certain underlying medical conditions, unless otherwise contraindicated). Both the STOPP and START criteria are organized according to the physiological system to which each criterion relates (the cardiovascular, respiratory, central nervous, gastrointestinal, musculoskeletal and endocrine systems). Each criterion is accompanied by a brief explanation, outlining why each PIM is considered potentially inappropriate or why a particular condition is underprescribed. When the STOPP and START criteria are used together, they address issues relating to drug–drug interactions, drug–disease interactions, potentially inappropriate duration of treatment, medications which adversely affect older patients at risk of falls, duplicate medications from the same therapeutic class, potentially inappropriate dosages of medications based on recent biochemical data and potential underprescribing of clinically beneficial medications [50,78].

Another approach to the evaluation of medication use in older adults is to determine a patient's anticholinergic load. Medications with anticholinergic properties carry a high potential risk of central and peripheral side effects. Tune et al. [83] developed a method to measure serum anticholinergic activity (SAA), which has been used in some studies (e.g. [84]). Furthermore, a number of different scales/methodologies have been developed

Table 25.2 Summary of potentially inappropriate prescribing (PIP) criteria.

Name and year of publication	Country of origin	Target population	No. of rules/ criteria	Description
North America				
Medication Appropriateness Index (MAI), 1992 [56]	United States	Developed for an older population (≥65 years), but use is not restricted to older people	10	Based on a literature review of studies published between 1982 and 1990
McLeod criteria, 1997 [57]	Canada	Individuals ≥65 years	38	Developed based on (i) a literature review, (ii) the 1991 Beers criteria and (iii) Canada's national drug formularies. The expert panel consisted of 32 members, who used the Delphi consensus methodology
Assessment of Underutilization (AOU) criteria, 1999 [58]	United States	Individuals ≥65 years	26	Based on the clinical experience of the investigators
Improving Prescribing in the Elderly Tool (IPET), 2000 [59]	Canada	Individuals ≥70 years	14	Based on the most common instances of PIP encountered in clinical practice, as identified by McLeod's criteria. Not independently validated
Zhan criteria, 2001 [60]	United States	Individuals living in ambulatory care ≥70 years	33	Developed from the 1997 Beers criteria. A subset of 33 drugs considered potentially inappropriate irrespective of dose, frequency of administration and duration were included in this list. The expert panel consisted of seven members, who used the Delphi consensus methodology
Assessing Care of Vulnerable Elders (ACOVE) criteria, 2001 [61]	United States	Individuals ≥65 years	236 indicators, 68 of which relate to PIP	Derived from a systemic review of the literature, expert opinions and guidance from specialist expert groups
Beers criteria, 2015 [62–65]	United States	Individuals ≥65 years	94	Update of the previously published 1991, 1997, 2003 and 2015 criteria. The expert panel consisted of 13 members, who used the Delphi consensus methodology
Rancourt criteria, 2004 [66]	Canada	Individuals ≥65 years residing in long-term care	111	Developed b an expert panel of four members, who reviewed and amalgamated the Beers criteria (1991, 1997, 2003), the McLeod criteria and the IPET criteria
Healthcare Effectiveness Data and Information Set (HEDIS) criteria, 2006 [67]	United States	Individuals ≥65 years	42	Derived from the experience/opinions of an expert review panel, which reviewed the 2003 Beers criteria independently of a diagnosis list
Europe				
Swedish Prescribing Indicators, 2004 [68]	Sweden	Individuals ≥65 years	33	Based on a review of the 1997 and 2003 Beers criteria
Norwegian General Practice (NORGEP), 2009 [69]	Norway	Individuals ≥70 years in general practice	36	Based on a review of the Swedish and Beers criteria (1991, 1997, 2003), evidence from the literature and the clinical experience of the investigators. An expert panel of 47 expert reviewers agreed these criteria using the Delphi consensus methodology

(continued)

Table 25.2 *(continued)*

Name and year of publication	Country of origin	Target population	No. of rules/ criteria	Description
La Roche French consensus criteria, 2007 [70]	France	Individuals ≥75 years	34	Based on a review of the Beers criteria (1991, 1997, 2003), the McLeod criteria, the 2001 French IM criteria and guidelines developed by the French Medicine Agency. An expert panel of 15 reviewers agreed these criteria using the Delphi consensus methodology
STOPP, 2008 [71], 2014 [72]	Ireland	Individuals ≥65 years	65	Based on clinical experience, the expertise of the investigators and a systematic review of the literature. An expert panel of 18 reviewers agreed these criteria using the Delphi consensus methodology
START, 2008 [71], 2014 [72]	Ireland	Individuals ≥65 years	22	Developed based on clinical experience, the expertise of the investigators and a systematic review of the literature. An expert panel of 18 reviewers agreed these criteria using the Delphi consensus methodology
Priscus List, 2010 [73]	Germany	Individuals ≥65 years	83	Developed by reviewing the Beers criteria (1991, 1997, 2003), the 2007 French criteria, STOPP and the most recent literature. An expert panel of 38 reviewers agreed these criteria using the Delphi consensus methodology
Asia and Australasia				
Phadke's Criteria, 1998 [74]	India	Not restricted to older population	4	Based on the clinical experience of the investigators
Australian National Prescribing Service (NPS) indicators, 2006 [75]	Australia	Not restricted to older population	21	Based on a comprehensive review of the literature and focus group discussions (including general practitioners (GPs), other health care professionals, consumers and policymakers)
Australian Prescribing Indicators, 2008 [76]	Australia	Individuals ≥65 years	48	Based on a review of Australian prescribing practices derived from the Australian Pharmaceutical Benefits Scheme in 2006. These are based on the most common medical conditions presented to consultant medical practitioners

to assist in the calculation of an individual's anticholinergic load. The most important are:

- anticholinergic risk scale (ARS) [85];
- anticholinergic drug scale (ADS) [86];
- anticholinergic cognitive burden (ACB) [87,88].

All of these scales are based on experts' judgements based on in vitro/in vivo and clinical studies from the published literature. There are considerable differences between the different scales regarding the ranking and number of medications included [89]. Recently, a new scale called the drug burden index (DBI) has been developed [90]. The DBI is designed to determine both the anticholinergic and sedative burden of a given individual, taking dose into consideration. Table 25.3 summarizes a number of studies that have found a causal relationship between a high anticholinergic load and several adverse outcomes (cognitive decline, falls and mortality). Note, however, that a number of other studies have failed to show such a relationship. Currently, there is no gold-standard approach to calculating an

Table 25.3 Overview of studies assessing anticholinergic load in older adults.

Reference	Anticholinergic scale used	Country and setting	Study design	Data source	Patient characteristics	Percentage of patients receiving anticholinergics	Associations between higher anticholinergic load and outcomes	Common anticholinergic medications
Kumpula et al. [79]	ARS	Finland, long-term care	Cross-sectional study	Medical records	n = 1004, mean age 81.3 (SD 10.9), 75% female	36% mild anticholinergic load, 19% high anticholinergic load	No association with mortality	Risperidone, mirtazapine, olanzapine, hydroxyzine, haloperidol
Agar et al. [80]	ADS	Australia, palliative care (home and care homes)	Secondary analysis of data from an RCT	Medical records/clinical assessments	n = 461, mean age 71 (SD 12), 50% female	Not reported	Associations with increasing side effects, time to death, decreasing functional status, decreasing quality of life	Oxycodone, morphine, dexamethoase, temazepam, fentanyl, clonazepam
Fox et al. [81]	ACB	United Kingdom, community-dwelling, ≥65 years old	Longitudinal study over 2 years	Patient interview	n = 12 423, mean age 75.2 (SD 6.8), 60% female	48% possible anticholinergics, 4% definite anticholinergics	Association between definite anticholinergics and decline in MMSE; association with greater 2-year mortality	ACB score = 1: furosemide, dextropropoxyphene, atenolol, nifedipine; ACB = 2: carbamazepine; ACB = 3: amitriptyline
Hilmer et al. [82]	DBI	United States, community-dwelling Medicare recipients (70–79 years) (the Health, Aging, and Body Composition (Health ABC) Study cohort)	Retrospective longitudinal study over 6 years	Patient interviews	n = 3075, age 73.6 (SD 2.9), 52% female	25% anticholinergics; 14% sedatives 34% had DBI > 0 at baseline	Association with poorer function, decrease in short physical performance battery, gait speed and grip strength	Not reported

ARS, anticholinergic risk scale; SD, standard deviation; ADS, anticholinergic drug scale; RCT, randomized controlled trial; ACB, anticholinergic cognitive burden; MMSE, mini-mental state examination; DBI, drug burden index.

individual's anticholinergic burden. Different scales give different results, as shown in an Australian study [91]. The differences between the scales may account for some of the mixed results observed in studies examining the causal relations between anticholinergic burden and adverse outcomes [92].

We have seen an evolution of the criteria used to assess appropriateness of prescribing, with new versions taking into account the weaknesses of the older ones [93,94]. Although some studies have been conducted to test the predictive validity of some of these criteria (see e.g. [94,95]), more work is needed in this area.

Prevalence of PIP

Over the last 25 years, a number of studies have reported on PIP and PPO prevalence, determined by a variety of different screening tools across a number of different jurisdictions and health care settings. Prevalence varies widely, from 3 to 96% [94–96]. Throughout the literature, the majority of PIP instances are attributable to a small number of medications/medication classes (i.e. proton pump inhibitors (PPIs), benzodiazepines, neuroleptics, NSAIDs, nonbenzodiazepine hypnotics, calcium channel blockers, antidepressants (TCAs and SSRIs), opioids, anticholinergics (bladder antispasmodics, antihistamines, gastrointestinal antimuscarinics), cardiac glycosides (digoxin), alpha-blockers (doxazosin), muscle relaxants and antiarrhythmics). Underprescribing of beneficial medication is observed for cardiovascular medication (post-myocardial infarction, heart failure, atrial fibrillation), antidepressants and pain treatment, although a limited life expectancy, a negative risk–benefit ratio and a patient's refusal might be reasons not to prescribe a drug [97].

Determinants of PIP and PPO

A number of different factors have been proposed to contribute to PIP and PPO [94–96]:

- age-related changes in pharmacokinetics and pharmacodynamics;
- complex drug regimens;
- increasing number of prescribing physicians;
- increasing desire to be compliant with international disease-specific guidelines;
- presence of multiple comorbidities.

As already stated, a number of papers have reported on the association between polypharmacy and PIP. In a recent Irish study by Gallagher et al. [98], which examined PIP in older hospitalized patients, it was reported that patients receiving more than five medications were three times more likely to receive a PIM than those on five or fewer medications. Similar results have been reported in other studies from across the world [22,66,99]. A number of studies have also reported a negative association between polypharmacy and patient adherence/compliance; poor patient compliance could in turn lead to a reduction in the clinical effectiveness of such medicines (e.g. [100]).

Given the large number of studies that have found an association between polypharmacy and PIP and between polypharmacy and poor compliance, reducing the number of medications a patient takes could lead to an improvement in compliance and a reduction in the prevalence of PIP. This might lower the risk of a patient having an adverse drug reaction (ADR) and thereby reduce drug-related costs [101].

Deprescribing

Deprescribing is a recently introduced term to describe 'cessation of long-term therapy, supervised by a clinician' [102] or, alternatively, 'medication withdrawal in older people' [103]. Reasons for deprescribing include a lack of efficacy, actual or potential ADRs, nonadherence, resolution of the condition, development of a contraindication, introduction of an interacting drug and limited life-expectancy. Presently, only a small number of studies have examined the impact of deprescribing. However, these studies appear to suggest possible benefits and an absence of harm when deprescribing is utilized in older, frailer individuals. Examples of studies where deprescribing has been successfully utilized include one on antipsychotics in older nursing home residents [104] and one on antidepressants in older dementia patients [105]. A systematic review of the withdrawal of antihypertensives in older persons has also been carried out [103]. A number of tools have been proposed to assist in decision-making around deprescribing [106].

To date, there have been few systematic studies investigating the effects of deprescribing in different populations. Shaffer et al. [107] reported an increase in prescribing of medication for symptom relief and a decline in the use of preventive medication (such as statins and osteoporosis medication) with increased probability of death in a large US-based study among community-dwelling older adults. Similar patterns were observed in a population of palliative care patients in Australia [108]. A Norwegian study showed that palliative therapy, including morphine, midazolam, glycopyronium and haloperidol, was prescribed to almost 75% of nursing home residents; about half of those receiving palliative medication also received curative/preventive medicines on the day of death [48].

Conclusion

Of all age groups, older persons are the most frequent consumers of medication. Polypharmacy is common in this group, and a steady increase has been observed over the last few decades. Inappropriate prescribing and poor patient compliance are both a problem in this population. Various measures have been developed to assess inappropriate prescribing, and efforts to optimize prescribing must continue in the future.

CHAPTER 26

Drug utilization research in the area of antibiotics

Ria Benko[1], Marion Bennie[2] & Samuel Coenen[3]

[1]*Department of Clinical Pharmacy, University of Szeged, Hungary*

[2]*Strathclyde Institute of Pharmacy and Biomedical Sciences, University of Strathclyde, Scotland and Information Services, NHS National Services Scotland, Scotland*

[3]*Department of Epidemiology and Social Medicine (ESOC), Department of Primary and Interdisciplinary Care (ELIZA) and Vaccine & Infectious Disease Institute (VAXINFECTIO), University of Antwerp, Belgium*

KEY POINTS

- Antibiotic resistance is a major global risk. Antibiotic use and resistance are causally related and are involved in a vicious cycle, driving the use of more, broader-spectrum, newer and more expensive antibiotics.
- Frequent use, public health consequences and high costs mean that antibacterial consumption has been extensively studied and drives drug utilization research. Meaningful reporting and interpretation of both ambulatory and hospital antibacterial use data requires careful consideration to avoid misleading findings.
- Cross-national comparisons in both ambulatory and hospital settings have demonstrated substantial differences in the level and pattern of antibiotic use. These differences represent a serious quality and health problem, calling for public awareness campaigns and professional interventions.
- As children and the elderly are the most exposed age groups, drug utilization studies and quality improvement programmes should particularly focus on these populations. In the hospital sector, special attention should be paid to high-consumption departments such as the intensive care unit and haemato-oncology.
- Antibiotic use is the result of a complex process influenced by many factors among different stakeholders. Diverse, multifaceted intervention programmes should involve multiple stakeholders in improving antibiotic use.

Introduction

Antibacterial agents (Anatomical Therapeutic Chemical (ATC) group J01) are unique in that their use has consequences for the whole community, through the development of antibiotic resistance. Because of their frequent use, high cost and public health consequences, the consumption of antibacterial agents has been extensively studied. The terms antibacterial/antibiotic and use/consumption are synonyms and used alternately through the chapter.

The 'microbial threat' was first recognized as a widespread problem in the 1990s [1] and is now highlighted as a major global risk by several agencies, including the World Health Organization (WHO) and World Economic Forum (WEF) [2–4]. The WHO has recently produced a global action plan to combat bacterial resistance [5].

Outside the Nordic countries, which have published joint drug statistics since 1979 [6,7], the only international antibacterial surveillance system currently in place is the European Surveillance of Antimicrobial Consumption Network (ESAC-Net; formerly (2001–11) the European Surveillance of Antimicrobial Consumption (ESAC)), run by the European Centre for Disease Prevention and Control (ECDC). Many countries have

Drug Utilization Research: Methods and Applications, First Edition. Edited by M. Elseviers et al.
Published 2016 by John Wiley & Sons, Ltd.

established national surveillance systems, including Denmark, Sweden, Norway, the Netherlands, Canada and Australia [8–13]. The Strategies to Address Antimicrobial Resistance (STAAR) Act was reintroduced in the United States in 2014 with the aim of monitoring antibiotic consumption and resistance data in a similar manner to ESAC-Net [14].

Human, animal and ecosystem health are inextricably linked. The One Health (formerly 'One Medicine') concept is dedicated to improving the lives of humans and animals through the integration of human and veterinary medicine and environmental science [15]. In this chapter, we address antibacterial use in humans; however, when examining the global threat of bacterial resistance, it is important to take all use of antibiotics into account. In addition to human consumption, antibiotics are used extensively in agriculture and in animal husbandry, where they provide disease prevention and growth promotion (note: in some countries, antibiotics are banned as growth promoters). As resistant bacteria can be transmitted from animals to humans, ensuring prudent use of antibacterials in animals is important [8]. The European Surveillance of Veterinary Antimicrobial Consumption (ESVAC) project launched in 2009 to monitor veterinary usage of antibacterials. It published its first report in 2011 [16]. For the first time veterinary and human antibiotic use in Europe have been included in one common report in 2014.

The WHO has proposed criteria to rank antimicrobials according to their relative importance in human medicine, in order to help regulators develop risk management strategies for control of the use of antimicrobials in food-production animals [17]. It has also launched the Advisory Group on Integrated Surveillance of Antimicrobial Resistance (AGISAR) to support these efforts [18].

Antibiotic use in relation to antibiotic resistance

Antibiotic resistance is a major public health problem that is mainly caused by antibiotic consumption. In human care, the highest volume of antibiotics is prescribed and consumed in the ambulatory setting. The causal link between antimicrobial resistance (AMR) and antibiotic prescribing in primary care cannot, however, be derived from (admittedly strong) associations between outpatient antibiotic use and antibiotic resistance data collected at the country level [19–22]. Causality has been shown at the individual patient level in randomized controlled trials (RCTs), [23] including the most convincing RCT to date, which assessed the effect of macrolide use on resistance selection in healthy volunteers [24]. This study also demonstrated resistance selection by macrolides (azithromycin and clarithromycin) that persisted for more than 6 months. Another study (non randomized) suggests shorter (i.e. shorter than 6 month) persistence of resistant bacteria after amoxicillin treatment [25], but these findings require confirmation by an RCT. The exact role of antibiotic consumption in ambulatory care on resistance problems encountered in hospitals is still unclear.

The consequence of antibiotic resistance is the use of more broad-spectrum antibiotics, which creates a vicious cycle that is hard to break. In addition, previous antibiotic use creates expectations in patients that they will be prescribed antibiotics the next time they show similar symptoms [26]. Accumulating literature is providing evidence that vaccination has potential advantages for primary prevention of AMR. However, any strategy that prevents infections has these advantages. Moreover, many vaccines that address bacterial pathogens do not address AMR pathogens. Further concern is that serotype replacement, as observed in pneumococcal strains (increased prevalence of serotypes not included in the vaccine), can undermine long-term vaccine effectiveness [27].

Antibiotic use in ambulatory care

Data reporting for antibiotic use in ambulatory care

Several measures have been proposed for the assessment of outpatient antibiotic use [28] (see Chapter 6). ESAC adopted the most widely recommended: the number of defined daily doses (DDDs). To control for differences or changes in population size between or within countries, utilization data are expressed in DDDs per 1000 inhabitants per day (DID). Recently, in addition to DDDs, other measures have been proposed to measure outpatient antibiotic consumption, including number of packages, number of prescriptions and number of treated individuals [28]. As the number of DDDs per package differs between countries and changes over time, it may be that number of packages is a more appropriate measure than number of DDDs when assessing outpatient antibiotic

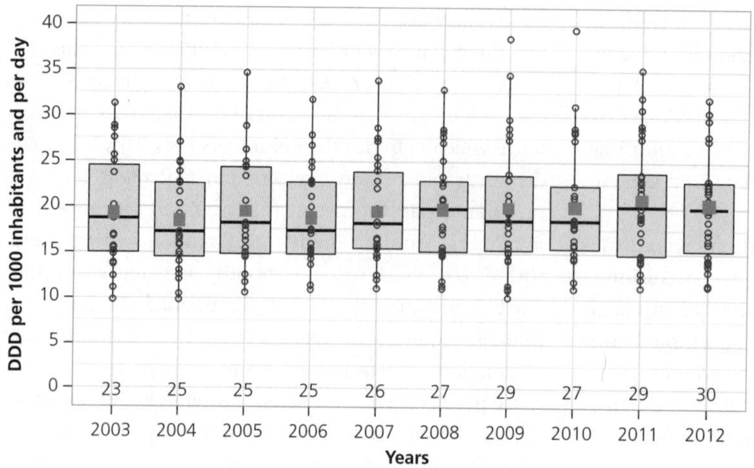

Figure 26.1 Distribution (Tukey-style box and whiskers plot) of ambulatory care antibiotic use in European countries between 2003 and 2012. Note: certain countries reported total care data. Squares: average. Line: median. The numbers over the years show the number of reporting countries in the particular year. The figure is based on national data that was available at the ESAC-Net interactive database in 2015 DDD: Defined daily dose.

Source: Courtesy of Maria Matuz.

use over time, especially in countries dispensing whole packages (in contrast to the few countries dispensing the exact number of tablets from bulk packages). Therefore, caution should be exercised when interpreting trends based only on DDDs [29–31]. For this reason, ESAC began, and ESAC-Net continued, to collect antibiotic use data in packages as well as DDDs. A recent study on global antibiotic use applied the standard unit as an outcome measure. It seems, however, that this measure has similar trends and caveats as DDDs [32].

Since antibiotic use is linked to seasonal influenza epidemics, with peaks early in winter in one year and late in winter in another, one can observe zero, one or two influenza winter peaks in a single calendar year. In order to ensure there is one influenza winter peak per 12-month period, it has been suggested that July-to-June years be used instead of January-to-December years when expressing annual antibiotic use data (in the northern hemisphere). More detailed information on seasonal variation in antibiotic use can be found in Chapter 16.

In addition to the ATC classification, antibacterials can be classified in a number of other ways. The ESAC team has suggested subgrouping for macrolides and quinolones [33,34]. Several methods of distinguishing between narrow- and broad-spectrum antibiotics have been suggested [35,36], but no consensus has yet been established.

Antibiotic exposure in ambulatory care: consumption level, pattern and trends

The average antibiotic consumption in European countries was ~20 DIDs between 2003 and 2012, which equals ~7.3 DDDs per inhabitant per year ((365 × 20)/1000; see also Figure 26.1). Taking 7 days as the average length of antibiotic treatment, this use corresponds to approximately one antibiotic treatment per inhabitant per year.

The use of antibiotics varies threefold between European countries (Figure 26.1), with a general north–south increasing gradient. If the whole European region (42 countries) were included in analyses, difference in total (ambulatory and hospital care) antibiotic consumption would reach fourfold [37,38].

US and Australian outpatient antibiotic use is high compared to that in Europe: in 2004, the United States would place fourth and in 2011, Australia would place third in a ranking of European countries [39–41]. In 2010, Canadian outpatient antibiotic use fell in the middle of the recorded range in Europe [13,41]. Total (ambulatory and hospital care) antibiotic utilization in Latin American countries ranges between 7 and ~16 DIDs (Figure 26.2) [42].

A recent study reported antibiotic use for 71 countries, which means that we still do not have data for the majority of the world's countries [32]. This fact should encourage the setting up of antibiotic use monitoring systems worldwide.

Low antibiotic use may reflect underuse due to limited access to medicines (e.g. in Armenia, Africa, South Asia) [37,38,43].

High antibiotic use can indicate antibiotic overprescription by doctors and/or easy access to antibiotics without prescriptions. Despite the fact that antibiotics are prescription-only medicines almost everywhere in Europe and the United States, self-medication with antibiotics still occurs in these countries (mainly

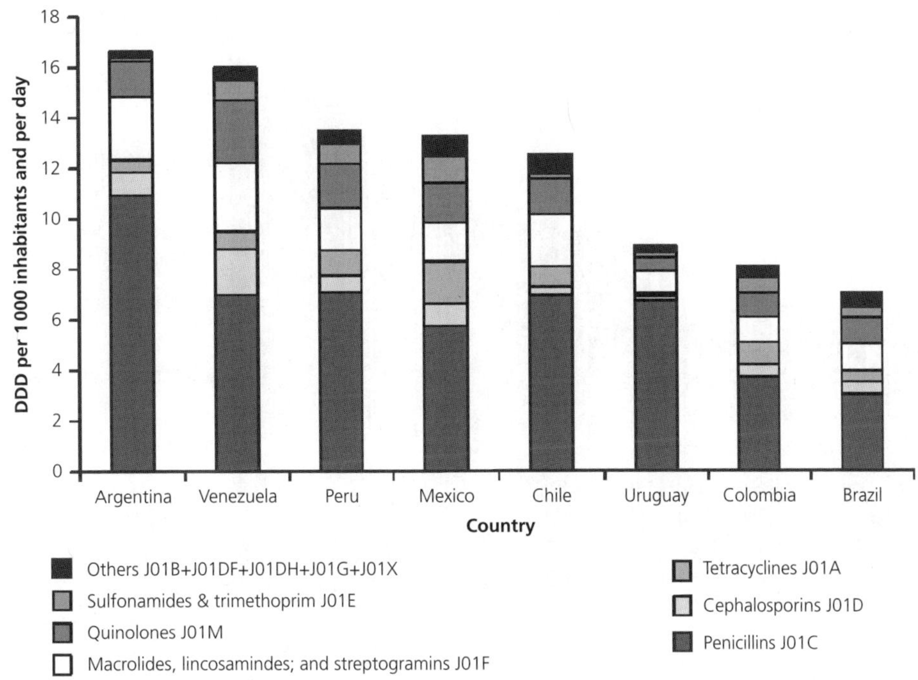

Figure 26.2 Total (ambulatory and hospital care) antibiotic consumption in eight Latin American countries. DDD: Defined daily dose. For colour details, please refer to the colour plates section.

Source: Wirtz 2010 [42].

in Southern or Eastern European countries, due to lack of enforcement of policies) [37,44–47]. Nonprescription antibiotic use outside (Northern) Europe and North America is widespread, accounting for 19–100% of antimicrobial use in different countries [48–50].

The relative use of different antibacterial groups has been shown to vary widely, too [32,51] (see Figure 26.3). Globally, penicillins (J01C), especially those with broad spectrum, are generally the most used antibacterials [32,37,41] – only Scandinavian countries use beta-lactamase-sensitive penicillins (J01CE) in higher proportion [41]. Like the overall use of antibiotics in ambulatory care, the consumption of broad- to narrow-spectrum penicillins, cephalosporins and macrolides (see Figure 26.4) demonstrates a north–south increasing gradient in Europe. Overall, in the last 15 years, there has been a general shift toward newer agents with a broader spectrum of activity (e.g. increased use of fluoroquinolones (J01MA) and of extended-spectrum (J01CA) and combined (J01CR) penicillins [32,41,42,52].

Therapeutic indications for outpatient antibiotic use

Over 90% of antibiotic prescriptions for systemic use are prescribed in primary care [20], with respiratory tract infections (RTIs) and urinary tract infections (UTIs) being the most common indications. The latter has been repeatedly demonstrated in national and international research projects, including the recent European project Appropriateness of Prescribing Antibiotics in Primary Health Care with Respect to Antibiotic Resistance (APRES). Despite the transition from acute to chronic disease management in primary care, RTIs will continue to represent a significant proportion of primary care morbidity and mortality, while ageing of the population will increase antibiotic use for UTIs as well. This can also be concluded from the association between the burden of influenza-like illnesses/flu epidemics, the annual volume of total outpatient antibiotic use (which is inappropriate, because influenza-like illnesses are most often viral and do not benefit from antibiotic treatment) and the continuously increasing use of substances for the treatment and prevention of UTIs [28,53–57,58].

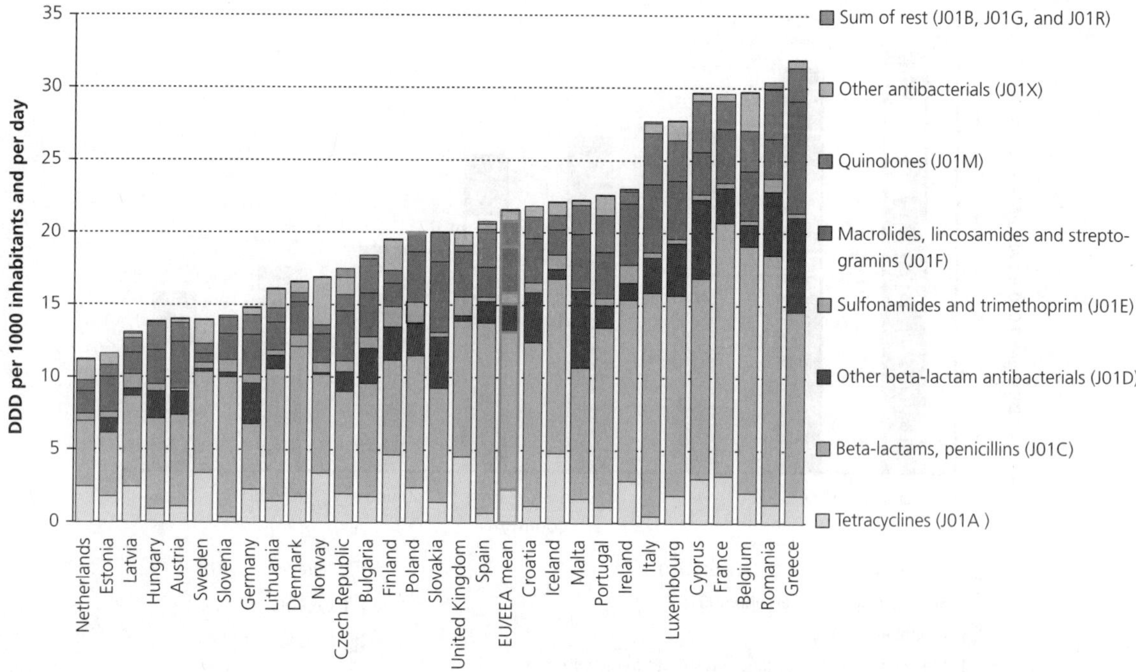

Figure 26.3 Pattern of antibiotic use in ambulatory care in European countries, 2012. Note: data for Cyprus, Iceland and Romania are total care data (i.e. including the hospital sector). Data for Spain are reimbursement data only (i.e. not including consumption without a prescription and other nonreimbursed courses). The EU/EEA mean shows the population-weighted mean. Figure based on national data that were available at the ESAC-Net interactive database in 2015. DDD: Defined daily dose. For colour details, please refer to the colour plates section.

Source: Courtesy of Maria Matuz.

Quality indicators of outpatient antibiotic use

Following quantification of antibiotic use by the ESAC project, validated quality indicators for outpatient antibiotic use in Europe were developed. The so-called drug-specific quality indicators of outpatient antibiotic use were developed first (Table 26.1) [29,36]. These indicators are easily calculable and are available from drug utilization data, so can serve as simple tools for the measurement of the quality of antibiotic use.

ESAC-Net provides up-to-date drug-specific quality indicator values for all EU member states on its website (www.ecdc.europa.eu). The total antibiotic consumption is also included as a quality indicator in the United States by the National Committee for Quality Assurance (NACQ; www.ncqa.org) in the Healthcare Effectiveness Data and Information Set (HEDIS) [59], and the Scottish Government and the Scottish Antimicrobial Prescribing Group (SAPG) have agreed that seasonal variation of quinolone use should be not greater than 5% [60].

However, these quality indicators may not be as relevant for individual prescribers as they are for policymakers. Since clinicians need disease-specific rather than drug-specific indicators, ESAC developed disease-specific quality indicators of outpatient antibiotic prescribing (Table 26.2) [61]. Because most but not all RTIs are self-limiting, the disease-specific indicators are accompanied by a proposed range of acceptable use, based on evidence available in relevant national and European guidelines and agreed upon by topic experts [61]. Although in most European countries antibiotic treatment is recommended for the treatment of UTIs, in the United Kingdom pain relief is recommended in all UTI patients, and it is suggested that antibiotics should not be used in nonpregnant women with mild symptoms of uncomplicated cystitis [61].

For these disease-specific quality indicators, it has been shown that it is feasible to collect data from electronic health records (EHRs) and to calculate their values [62]. Moreover, they have been accepted for

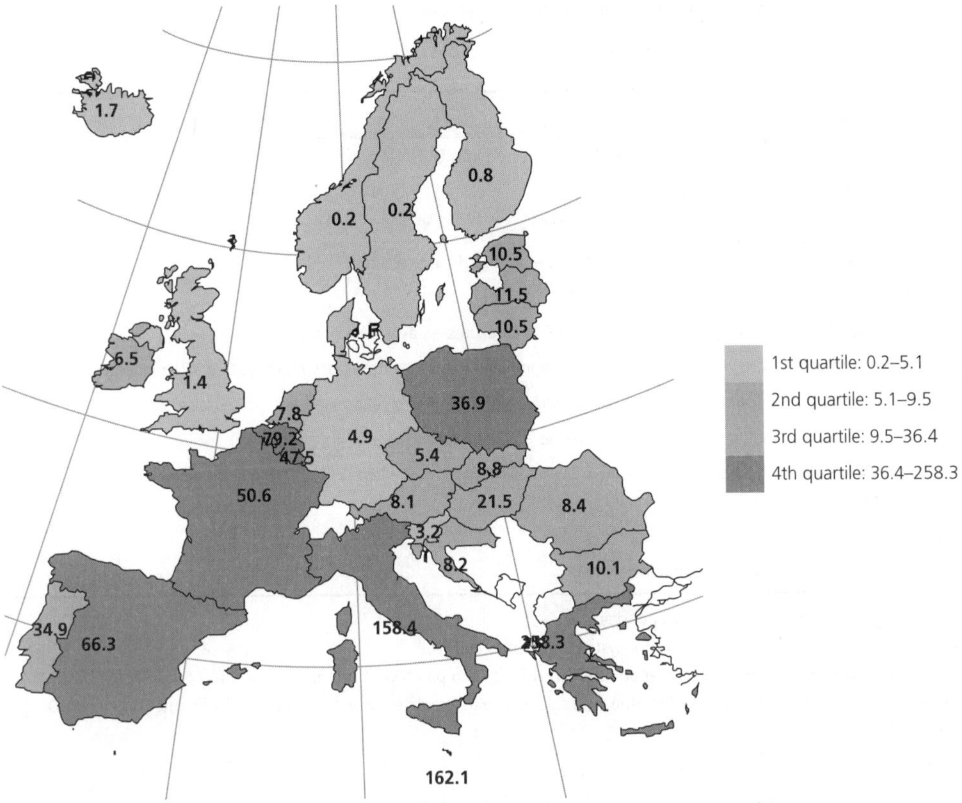

Figure 26.4 Ratio of the consumption of broad- versus narrow-spectrum penicillins, cephalosporins and macrolides in ambulatory care in European countries (B/N ratio), 2012. Broad-spectrum: J01CR, J01DC, J01DD, J01F minus J01FA01. Narrow-spectrum: J01CE, J01DB, J01FA. Figure based on national data that were available at the ESAC-Net interactive database in 2015. For colour details, please refer to the colour plates section.

Source: Courtesy of Maria Matuz.

inclusion as quality indicators by the National Quality Measures Clearinghouse (NQMC; www.qualitymeasures.ahrq.gov) in the United States. These indicators provide a potentially important step in the systematic implementation of standards to further improve the quality of antibiotic use and prescribing.

Ambulatory antibiotic use in special groups: paediatrics and the elderly

Paediatric antibiotic use

Due to their maturing immune system and close proximity to one another (e.g. in daycare centres, classrooms), children are more liable to acquire and transmit infections than are adults [63]. Antibiotics are the most common medicines prescribed to children [63], with those aged under 4 years being the most frequently exposed [64,65] (Figure 26.5).

Despite frequent antibiotic use in children, the primary focus of antibiotic drug utilization research to date has been the adult population [66]. Comprehensive and comparable country-specific paediatric antibiotic use data have only been published for a limited number of countries [64,65,67]. This may partly be due to the lack of a generally accepted method for expressing the volume of antibiotic use in children. To enhance paediatric data reporting, it has been proposed that the proportion of liquid oral drug formulation be analysed as a tool for estimating paediatric antibiotic use [68].

Additionally, a new project (Antibiotic Resistance and Prescribing in European Children, ARPEC) aimed at improving the quality of antibiotic prescribing for children in Europe has recently been conducted [69].

Prevalence rates of ambulatory paediatric antibiotic use in reporting countries range more than fourfold

Table 26.1 ESAC drug-specific quality indicators for outpatient antibiotic use.

Source: Coenen et al. 2007 [36]. Reproduced with permission from BMJ Publishing Group Ltd.

No.	Title
1	Consumption of antibacterials for systemic use (J01), expressed in DID[a]
2	Consumption of penicillins (J01C), expressed in DID[a]
3	Consumption of cephalosporins (J01D), expressed in DID[a]
4	Consumption of macrolides, lincosamides and streptogramins (J01F), expressed in DID[a]
5	Consumption of quinolones (J01M), expressed in DID[a]
6	Consumption of alpha-lactamase-sensitive penicillins (J01CE), expressed as a percentage[b]
7	Consumption of combinations of penicillins, including alpha-lactamase inhibitors (J01CR), expressed as a percentage[b]
8	Consumption of third- and fourth-generation cephalosporins (J01(DD + DE)), expressed as a percentage[b]
9	Consumption of fluoroquinolones (J01MA), expressed as a percentage[b]
10	Ratio of the consumption of broad- (J01(CR + DC + DD + (F-FA01))) to narrow-spectrum (J01(CE + DB + FA01)) penicillins, cephalosporins and macrolides
11	Seasonal variation in total antibiotic consumption (J01)[c]
12	Seasonal variation in quinolone consumption (J01M)[c]

[a] Defined daily doses (DDDs) per 1000 inhabitants per day.

[b] Percentage of total consumption of antibacterials for systemic use (J01), in DID.

[c] Overuse in the winter quarters (October–December and January–March) compared with the summer quarters (July–September and April–June) of a 1-year period starting in July and ending in June the next calendar year, expressed as a percentage: (DDD (winter quarters)/DDD(summer quarters) – 1) × 100.

(percentage of exposed child inhabitants ranges from 14.2% in the United Kingdom (aged ≤16 years) to 63.1% in Ireland (aged ≤15 years)) [64,67]. Similar differences have also been observed in paediatric prescription rates, which peaked in Italy with 1.3 prescription/person/year [67]. The pattern of antibiotic use in children also shows considerable cross-national differences: broader-spectrum agents are prescribed more frequently in countries with higher overall use [67].

The main problem in the paediatric population is the overuse of antibiotics for infections with presumed viral aetiology. Antibiotic prescribing for common cold, acute purulent rhinitis, otitis and other RTIs remains high worldwide [70–76] despite limited or no evidence of benefit [77]. Because of these problems, the European Antibiotic Awareness Day (EAAD; see later) gives especial prominence to paediatric antibiotic use.

Elderly/nursing home antibiotic use

Older people have an increased susceptibility to infection due to their increasing prevalence of chronic diseases and declining immunological response, bad nutritional status and physical immobility [78,79]. The result is increasing use of antimicrobials with age, peaking in the frail elderly (Figure 26.5), leading to an increased risk of AMR and other adverse effects [78,79]. As people live longer, they become frailer, and consequently with the rising elderly population, the demand for supported care in nursing homes is increasing [80]. Such environments further magnify the potential risk of infection acquisition and AMR development [81]. (Note: Some may debate the affiliation of nursing homes, as they can belong to either ambulatory or hospital care. Because in most European countries nursing homes belong to ambulatory care and general practitioners (primary care physicians) are the main prescribers of drugs, we have chosen to discuss antibiotic use in nursing homes in this section.)

Some pioneering studies have assessed antimicrobial use in nursing homes at the country level and found substantial differences between settings [82] and individual patients [83]. In 2011, the ESAC group published the first pan-European point-prevalence study (PPS) on antibiotic use in nursing homes [84], showing a greater than 10-fold difference in antibiotic prescribing (from

Table 26.2 ESAC disease-specific quality indicators for outpatient antibiotic use.

Source: Adriaenssens et al. 2012 [61]. Reproduced with permission from BMJ Publishing Group Ltd.

No.	Title	Range of acceptable use
1a	The percentage of patients ***aged between 18 and 75 years with acute bronchitis/bronchiolitis (ICPC-2-R: R78)*** prescribed antibacterials for systemic use (ATC: J01)	0–30%
1b	= 1a receiving the recommended antibacterials (ATC: J01CA or J01AA)	80–100%
1c	= 1a receiving quinolones (ATC: J01M)	0–5%
2a	The percentage of patients ***older than 1 year with acute upper respiratory infection (ICPC-2-R: R74)*** prescribed antibacterials for systemic use (ATC: J01)	0–20%
2b	= 2a receiving the recommended antibacterials (ATC: J01CE)	80–100%
2c	= 2a receiving quinolones (ATC: J01M)	0–5%
3a	The percentage of ***female*** patients ***older than 18 years with cystitis/other urinary infection (ICPC-2-R: U71)*** prescribed antibacterials for systemic use (ATC: J01)	80–100%
3b	= 3a receiving the recommended antibacterials (ATC: J01XE or J01EA or J01XX)	80–100%
3c	= 3a receiving quinolones (ATC: J01M)	0–5%
4a	The percentage of patients ***older than 1 year with acute tonsillitis (ICPC-2-R: R76)*** prescribed antibacterials for systemic use (ATC: J01)	0–20%
4b	= 4a receiving the recommended antibacterials (ATC: J01CE)	80–100%
4c	= 4a receiving quinolones (ATC: J01M)	0–5%
5a	The percentage of patients ***older than 18 years with acute/chronic sinusitis (ICPC-2-R: R75)*** prescribed antibacterials for systemic use (ATC: J01)	0–20%
5b	= 5a receiving the recommended antibacterials (ATC: J01CA or J01CE)	80–100%
5c	= 5a receiving quinolones (ATC: J01M)	0–5%
6a	The percentage of patients ***older than 2 years with acute otitis media/myringitis (ICPC-2-R: H71)*** prescribed antibacterials for systemic use (ATC: J01)	0–20%
6b	= 6a receiving the recommended antibacterials (ATC: J01CA or J01CE)	80–100%
6c	= 6a receiving quinolones (ATC: J01M)	0–5%
7a	The percentage of patients ***aged between 18 and 65 years with pneumonia (ICPC-2-R: R81)*** prescribed antibacterials for systemic use (ATC: J01)	90–100%
7b	= 7a receiving the recommended antibacterials (ATC: J01CA or J01AA)	80–100%
7c	= 7a receiving quinolones (ATC: J01M)	0–5%

ICPC-2-R: revised second edition of the International Classification of Primary Care [154].

ATC, Anatomical Therapeutic Chemical classification; J01, antibacterials for systemic use; J01AA, tetracyclines; J01CA, penicillins with extended spectrum; J01CE, beta-lactamase sensitive penicillins; J01EA, trimethoprim and derivatives; J01M, quinolone antibacterials; J01XE, nitrofuran derivatives; J01XX, other antibacterials.

~1.4 to 19.4%) and usage (from ~16 to 120 DIDs) across 301 nursing homes in 17 countries. The reasons for between- and within-country differences are currently unknown and need further research [84].

The most common infections observed in the elderly, irrespective of health care setting, are UTIs, RTIs, skin and soft tissue infections and gastrointestinal infections [79]. Two key areas of inappropriate use in the elderly are the prescribing of antibiotics with Gram-negative and anaerobe spectra, which affect the gastrointestinal flora (e.g. fluoroquinolones, clindamycin and penicillin combinations), increasing the risk of *Clostridium difficile* infection, and the repeated use of antibacterials for medical prophylaxis, most commonly in UTIs [85,86]. The United Kingdom has a prominent national programme focused on reduction of broad-spectrum antimicrobials in a drive to reduce *Clostridium difficile* infection, which has achieved significant reductions [87].

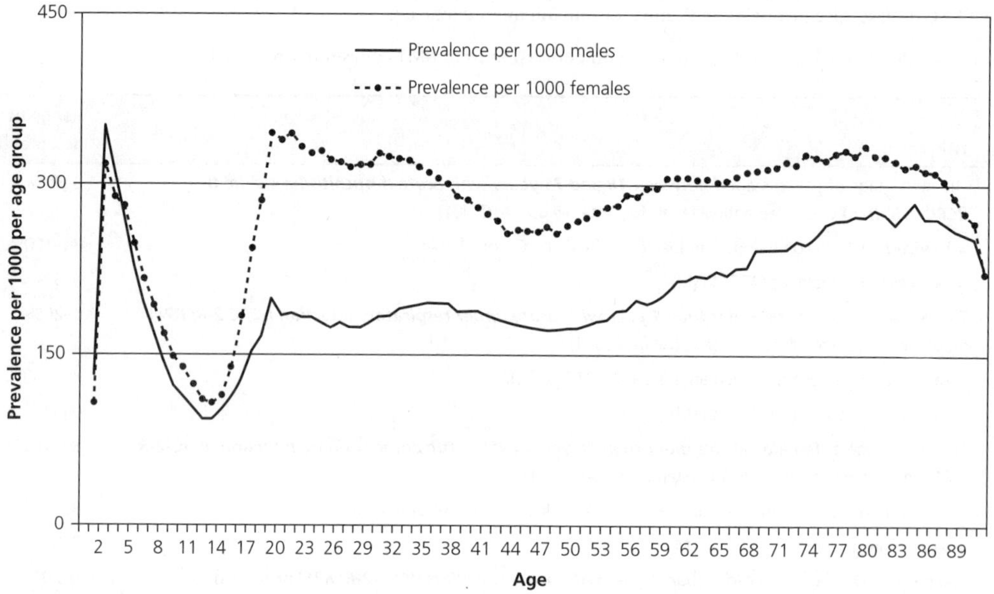

Figure 26.5 Age- and gender-specific population prevalence of patients using antibacterials in the Norwegian population in the period 1 July 2005–31 June 2006 [54]. Note: antibacterials for systemic use include ATC group J01, vancomycin (A07AA09) and metronidazole (P01AB01). Methenamine (J01XX05) is excluded.

Source: Blix HS et al [65]. Reproduced with permission from Oxford University Press.

Determinants of antibiotic use in ambulatory care

In order to enhance the prudent use of antibiotics, the determinants of use should be identified [88]. In most countries, antibiotics are available on prescription only, highlighting the crucial role and responsibility of prescribers (mainly physicians). A recent systematic review of qualitative studies on antibiotic prescribing differentiated between intrinsic and extrinsic factors that influence antibiotic prescribing and proposed a theoretical framework to describe the interconnection between them [89].

Among the intrinsic factors, physicians' attitudes, such as complacency (mainly linked to patients' expectations of or demand for antibiotics) and fear of complications, were identified as major influences on antibiotic prescribing [89]. Patient-related factors (e.g. signs, symptoms and expectations), health care-system related factors (e.g. time pressure) and cost savings (to the patient or health care system) were the most common extrinsic factors cited [89].

Many modifiable factors (e.g. smoking, high body mass index (BMI), alcohol abuse), but also chronic diseases (e.g. chronic obstructive pulmonary disease, COPD), have been shown to be risk factors for acquiring infections (e.g. pneumonia) [90–97]. A high prevalence of these states/conditions in the population might result in higher antibiotic use.

False patient (or parent) expectations or demand for antibiotics – a factor associated with inappropriate antibiotic use – can also derive from a lack of patient knowledge [98]. Results of a special Eurobarometer survey in 2013, which assessed knowledge about antibiotics among European citizens, found that the general public still has misconceptions: every second European believes that antibiotics kill viruses and thinks they are effective against colds and flu. These results are consistent with a previous survey from 2009 [99]. However, it has been reported that doctors frequently overestimate parent expectations, leading to a specific diagnosis being made secondary to the decision to prescribe antibiotics for their child [100].

Further factors, such as active marketing by the pharmaceutical industry and cultural factors (how people label illnesses and their coping strategies), have also been identified as influencing antibiotic use [98,101]. In view of the wide range of influencing factors, intervention programmes to improve antibiotic use should be equally diverse and should involve multiple stakeholders [98,102].

Interventions to improve antibiotic use in ambulatory care: antimicrobial stewardship

The European Antibiotic Awareness Day (EAAD) (18 November; http://ecdc.europa.eu/en/eaad) is a European public health initiative being led by the ECDC [103]. Since 2008, the EAAD has been used as a platform to raise awareness about the threat to public health posed by antibiotic resistance and to communicate the importance of prudent use of antibiotics. The EAAD builds on successful awareness campaigns promoting appropriate antibiotic use run at a national level by various EU member states, including France [104] and Belgium, where the One Health approach has been adopted, targeting outpatient, hospital and veterinary antibiotic use [105,106]. An extensive overview of the characteristics and outcomes of public campaigns aimed at improving the use of antibiotics in outpatients in high-income countries, both at the national and regional levels, and both in and outside Europe, was recently published [107]. In addition to targets and the One Health approach, it is recommended that social marketing activities be applied when developing public campaigns [108]. Given that respiratory infections are the main indications linked to outpatient antibiotic use, most public campaigns explicitly focus on reducing inappropriate antibiotic use for these conditions.

Whereas public campaigns affect consulting behaviour and reduce antibiotic prescribing, professional campaigns may also focus on the choice of prescribed antibiotic [109]. One of the more elegant professional interventions, focusing on inappropriate antibiotic use for respiratory infections, includes the use of point-of-care tests to deal with primary care prescribers' diagnostic uncertainty and the training of primary care prescribers' communication skills (supported by an interactive patient information leaflet) to deal with patient expectations [110–112]. When considering any evaluation of professional intervention, it is important to recognize that this will involve longitudinal data analysis and modelling of data from patients clustered by prescribers, requiring careful consideration of clustering in the design and analysis plan [113].

The first antibiotic stewardship programme (ASP) in Europe was the Swedish Strategic Programme for the Rational Use of Antimicrobial Agents and Surveillance of Resistance (STRAMA) [114,115]. This multidisciplinary and multisectorial programme started in 1994 and contributed to a sustained reduction of antibiotic use without measurable negative consequences [114,115].

Besides public and professional interventions, multifaceted interventions, including various regulatory measures [116], improved regulation of nonprescription antibiotic use [117] and pure reimbursement restrictions (restricted benefit, prior authorization of prescribing; see details in [118]), have proved to be effective in reducing/rationalizing antibiotic use. In a Korean study, regulatory intervention to prohibit antibiotic dispensing by physicians resulted in a dramatic reduction of inappropriate antibiotic use [119]. Such interventions may work in other Asian countries where physicians not only prescribe but also dispense medicines.

Antibiotic use in hospital care

Although antibacterial use in hospitals accounts for only 5–15% of total use, it remains a key driver for AMR, especially in those groups of antibiotics generally reserved for severe infections, such as carbapenems [120,121].

Data reporting for antibiotic use in hospital care

Different aggregate measures can be used to describe hospital medicine use generally (see Chapter 6), and these are applicable for antibacterial use. In the absence of better metrics – at the international level – DID is used to quantify antibacterial consumption [51,122]. However, the DID metric cannot be used to quantify antibiotic use at the hospital level. Many studies have been published on individual hospital consumption data, but, with variable definitions of metrics, it is difficult to compare results [123]. Consequently, in 2008, a standard for reporting hospital antibiotic use data was proposed, advising the parallel use of DDDs per 100 bed days and DDDs per 100 admissions and suggesting a precise definition of denominator calculations [123]. (Note: In the United States, days of therapy (DOT) per 1000 patient days is the recommended metric for measuring antibacterial use in hospitals; this requires patient-level data [124].) The ESAC confirmed the need for denominator calculations in both bed days and admissions to reflect variations in hospital clinical activity [125]. Moreover, the lack of an international standardized hospital categorization system is a major obstacle to the benchmarking of antibiotic use in different hospitals, especially across different countries [126]. Selection of an appropriate comparator is crucial, and consequently the specifics of each individual hospital (e.g. level of care, types of unit) and the patient case mix should be revealed [127–130].

In general, DDDs for antibacterials are based on their use in moderately severe infections in adults [122]. However, in the hospital setting, severe infections are also treated, resulting in the DDD being potentially lower than the actual prescribed dose (PDD) in many cases (most significantly for penicillins). Consequently, consumption data are higher when expressed in DDDs per 100 bed days compared to PDDs per 100 bed days. As access to PDD data is often limited, use of a hospital-adjusted defined daily dose (haDDD; based on recommended doses in guidelines) [129] or of a PDD proxy (averaging the prescribed doses found in PPSs) is recommended in addition to DDDs per 100 bed days in national and local studies [131].

Globally, there is limited information on antibiotic use in hospitalized children [132]. In order to improve the accuracy of reporting and facilitae an international comparison of neonatal and paediatric antibiotic prescribing in hospitals, a new algorithm has been proposed; this is currently awaiting validation [133]. Development of a simplified version of the adult DDD is warranted [132].

To support the description of antibiotic utilization patterns in hospitals – beyond the ATC classification and subgrouping of macrolides and quinolones (see earlier) – the term 'hospital-specific antibiotics' was introduced [120]. The use of these agents (third- and fourth-generation cephalosporins, carbapenems, monobactams, aminoglycosides and glycopeptides) can be used as a quality indicator of hospital antibiotic prescribing (see later).

Antibiotic exposure in hospital care: level, trends and patterns

The first retrospective cross-national study of hospital antibiotic use, encompassing 15 European countries in 2002, identified a roughly threefold variation in systemic use, ranging from 1.3 DIDs in Sweden and Norway to 3.9 in Finland and France [120]. In 2012, continued variation in use was reported across Europe, without clear geographical gradient [51] (Figure 26.6).

Interpretation of such data needs careful consideration, as variation may be in part attributable to differences in health care structures (e.g. inclusion of antibiotic use in nursing homes into reported hospital utilization data, as in Finland; variation in number of hospital bed days) and data sources (these can vary from wholesaler data to sample hospital data extrapolated for national use). Individual reports from different countries/continents show substantial regional and between-hospital differences in antibiotic use [134–139]. For example, in public hospitals in France, the total antibiotic use ranges between 19.6 and 73.7 DDDs per 100 patient days (median 39.5) and between 180 and 792 DDDs per 100 admissions (median 34.1) [137].

A snapshot of European data in 2012 identified penicillins (J01C), other beta lactams (J01D) and quinolones (J01M) as the most frequently used antibacterials (Figure 26.6). As important as the most frequently used antimicrobials (i.e. cephalosporins and penicillins) are 'hospital-specific' antibiotics. Interestingly, no change over time in total consumption of antimicrobials across 15 countries was reported, but on closer examination an increase in use of carbapenems, glycopepetides and third/fourth-generation cephalosporin was detected – these are important signals in understanding changing AMR internationally [120]. Currently, the use of carbapenems and glycopeptides is significantly increased in many European countries [51].

Antibiotic exposure in hospital care: indication and quality problems

The limited availability of electronic prescribing and staff resources in hospitals often prohibits continuous surveillance of antibacterial use. Consequently, the use of PPSs as practical surveillance tools has been widely adopted [140]. PPSs have been used for over 20 years to add information on indication and dose to routine consumption data [141], but studies are inconsistent in many aspects [142]. The ESAC sought to standardize PPS methodology in order to support cross-national comparisons and quality improvement initiatives. The first ESAC PPS, in 2006, covered 20 hospitals, while a Web-based PPS (WebPPS) in 2009 captured data on 25 countries (mainly in Europe), incorporating 172 hospitals. In the 2009 survey, 29% of patients were prescribed antibacterials, most receiving monotherapy. Antibacterials were most commonly prescribed for RTIs (27.2%), followed by skin, soft-tissue, bone and joint infections (19.0%), gastrointestinal infections (17.2%) and UTIs (12.9%) [127,140].

The key value of a PPS is that it can identify targets for quality improvement [140]. Several 'general' quality

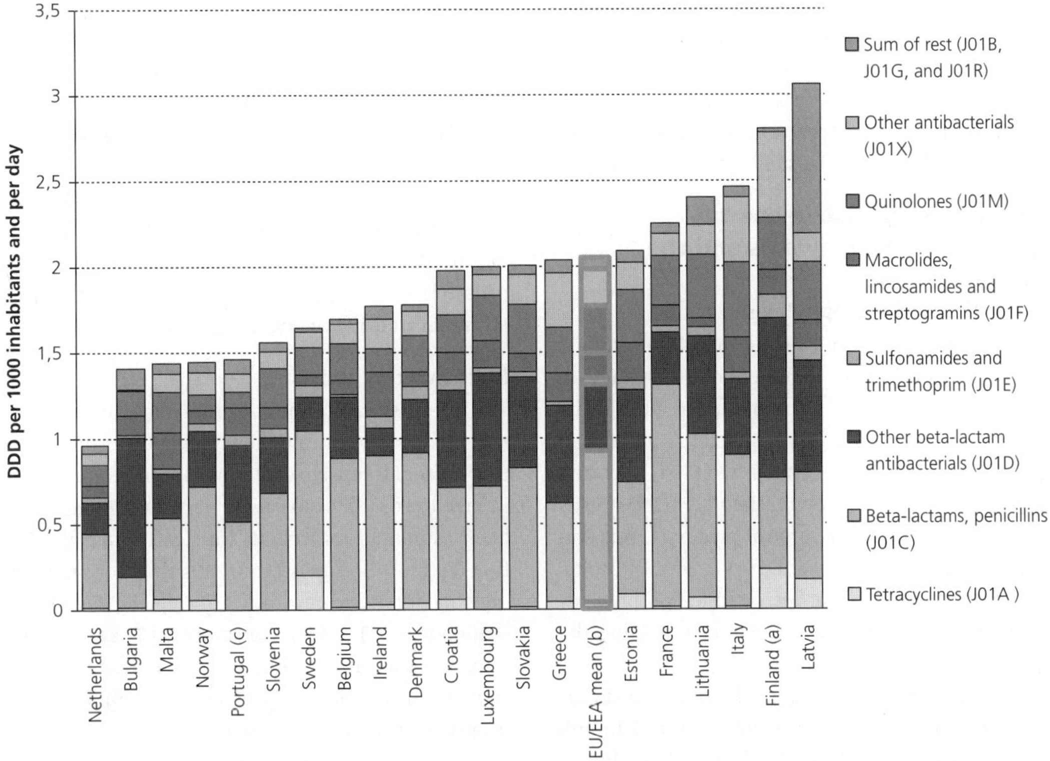

(a) Finland: data include consumption in remote primary healthcare centres and nursing homes
(b) EU/EEA mean refers to the corresponding population-weighted mean consumption based on 20 countries that provided data
(c) Portugal: data correspond to public hospitals only,

Figure 26.6 Pattern of hospital care antibiotic use in European countries, 2012. Data for Finland include consumption in remote primary health care centres and nursing homes. Data for Portugal correspond to public hospitals only. The EU/EEA mean refers to the corresponding population-weighted mean consumption based on 20 countries that provided data. Figure based on national data that were available at the ESAC-Net interactive database in 2015. For colour details, please refer to the colour plates section.

DDD: Defined daily dose
Courtesy of Maria Matuz

indicators for monitoring of antibiotic prescribing have been proposed: (i) proportional use of parenteral therapy, (ii) extent of combination therapy, (iii) proportion of narrow spectrum agents, (iv) proportion of hospital-specific antibiotics, (v) number of drugs accounting for 75% of drug use (DU75%), (vi) number of drugs accounting for 90% of drug use (DU90%), (vii) adherence to local guidelines, (viii) documentation of the reason for starting antibacterial treatment in case notes and (ix) duration of surgical prophylaxis (see later) [127,143,144].

As an example of quality issues, the ESAC 2009 PPS found suboptimal guideline adherence (mean 62%) and a suboptimal documentation rate (mean 75.7%) [127]. A recent US study revealed even more startling results: two-thirds of patients started on empirical antibiotics did not have clinical signs of infection, most regimens were unchanged by the fifth day of therapy and culture and imaging were often not obtained [145].

For many of the indicators mentioned in this section, optimal range depends on hospital/unit type and patient case mix; others can be used universally (e.g. rate of documentation). The SAPG adapted two of these indicators to drive improvements, aiming to achieve a documentation rate over 95% and guideline-compliant antibiotic use over 95% [146]. Quality indicators have also been developed and assessed for specific diagnoses, such as community-acquired pneumonia [147] and, recently, sepsis [148]. Further structural and care-quality indicators (including many diagnosis-specific indicators) require piloting and feasibility studies [149].

Hospital antibiotic use in special groups: surgical prophylaxis and the intensive care unit

Surgical antibacterial prophylaxis

Antibiotic prophylaxis is the use of antibiotics before, during or after a diagnostic, therapeutic or surgical procedure to prevent infectious complications [150]. The efficacy of antibiotic prophylaxis in reducing surgical-site infection has been clearly established [151,152], and several guidelines have been published [151,153,154].

The use of antibiotics for surgical prophylaxis is significant; a recent report showed 16.3% of all hospital antibiotic prescriptions in Europe were for prophylaxis [155]. Drug utilization studies aimed at describing the appropriateness of surgical antibiotic prophylaxis are usually conducted by measuring adherence to different guideline criteria. In studies conducted to date, full adherence ranges from 4.5 to 84.9% [156–160], but as the definition of full adherence differs between them (adherence to two, three, four, five or six criteria), meaningful comparison of results is limited.

When evaluating different elements of the guideline recommendations, the appropriateness of timing usually performs best, while duration of therapy performs worst (Table 26.3).

The 2011–12 ECDC surveillance report found that surgical prophylaxis was prolonged for more than 1 day in 59.2% of cases [155], despite the evidence that prophylaxis beyond 24 hours offers no additional benefit and can drive the development of AMR [161,162].

Intensive care units

The intensive care unit is a designated ward of a hospital that deals with critically ill patients. One study reported that 51% of intensive care unit patients were considered infected [163], and intensive care unit infections have been estimated to account for nearly half of all infections in most hospitals [164]. It is therefore not surprising that intensive care units are epicentres of hospital antibiotic use. The high consumption of antibacterials in intensive care units, while to some extent unavoidable, remains an important focus area for minimizing inappropriate antibiotic use [165].

In a European study, antibiotic consumption in intensive care units varied 14-fold, with a median of 125.4

Table 26.3 Recent studies of adherence to surgical antimicrobial prophylaxis guidelines.

				Adherence to various elements of appropriate antibacterial use in surgical antimicrobial prophylaxis					
Reference	Country	Year	Number of enrolled patients/ procedures	Antibiotic choice (%)	Timing (%)	Dose (%)	Duration (%)	Indication (%)	Full adherence (%)
[156]	Germany	2008–09	5064	NR	NR	NR	29.9	NR	4.5–84.9
[184]	Japan	2004, 2005	2373	53–84	NR	NR	38–68	NR	NR
[185]	Greece	2000	898	70	100	NR	36.3	81	36.3
[186]	Brazil	2009–10	748	80.9	62.5	97.6	4.8	60.5	4.8
[187]	Singapore	2008	216	64	83	100	44	NR	NR
[158]	Italy	2009–12	382	25.5	53.4	NR	NR	NR	18.1
[159]	France	2001–07	8029	83.3	76.6	NR	35	NR	NR
[188]	Iran	2010	365	25.4	61.1		29.4	35.4	10.13
[189]	United States	2009	143	97	73	77	NR	99	48
[190]	The Netherlands	2000–01	1763	92	50	89	82		28

NR, not recorded.

DDDs per 100 patient days [166]. This usage rate is two times higher than the reported median of 49.6 DDDs per 100 patient days found in a pan-European study of hospital antibacterial use [167] and means that, theoretically, every patient receives a minimum of 1 DDD of antibiotic per day during their entire intensive care unit stay.

Mathematical models and clinical findings have shown that heterogeneous antibiotic use (balanced use of all of the different antimicrobials available) is desirable in reducing the selection pressure in antibacterial resistance [168–170]. Two common parameters – the DU90% [144] and the number of agents used – show considerable differences across both adult [171] and neonatal intensive care units [172], which may reflect too-monotonous antibiotic prescribing in some settings. Other quality issues, such as suboptimal dosage regimens, incorrect empiric treatment, failure to de-escalate therapy and a lack of clear documentation concerning indication, are reported to be common problems in intensive care units [173,174].

Determinants of hospital antibacterial use

The determinants of hospital antibiotic use are not well understood. The number of antibiotics used [167] and the level of care have been shown to correlate with total hospital antibiotic use [175] or patterns of use [136]. A number of cultural, contextual (lack of diagnostic resources, lack of time, patient characteristics) and behavioural factors can be possible determinants of hospital antibiotic use [176]. Uncertainty avoidance – a sociocultural factor – has been found to be an important driver for prolonged surgical antibacterial prophylaxis [177]. A recent qualitative study found that doctors' antibiotic prescribing behaviour was governed by a set of unwritten but widely accepted cultural rules ('prescribing etiquette'), with professional hierarchy (a decisive role for seniors/leaders) and autonomous decision-making (accepted nonadherence to policy and noninterference with the prescribing decisions of colleagues) playing an important role in shaping antibiotic use [178].

Interventions to improve antibiotic use in hospital care: antimicrobial stewardship

Antimicrobial stewardship programmes (ASPs) are multifaceted, interdisciplinary approaches to the use of antimicrobial agents employed in order to achieve optimal outcomes [179–181]. The role of ASPs is to strike a balance between the potent ability of antibiotics to help individual patients and their potentially hazardous effects. Guidelines for stewardship identify several potential strategies. The scientific literature is overloaded with reports of hospital care interventions around antibiotic use, but the vast majority have flawed methodology and so do not provide interpretable data [181]. A recent Cochrane Review of interventions to improve antibacterial prescribing in hospital care reviewed 89 studies from 19 countries over 5 continents and found restrictive interventions (restriction of the freedom of prescribers to select some antibiotics) to be more successful in the short term, but restrictive and persuasive interventions (dissemination of educational resources, reminders, audit and feedback) to be equally effective after 6 months [181]. This review found few studies comparing different types of interventions, however, and most provided minimal insight into the sustainability and unintended consequences of the interventions described [182]. Moreover, the effectiveness of interventions may be suboptimal, as all ASPs to date have failed to consider contextual, cultural and behavioural determinants despite evidence from qualitative research [182,183]. Participatory action research (PAR) – a new collaborative process intended to bring about change in social situations – is a promising solution [183] that may address all relevant determinants.

Conclusion

Growing concern over antibiotic resistance and the downward trend in the development of new antibacterials necessitate the judicious use of antibiotics, in order to maintain their effectiveness. The scale and diversity of the issues discussed in this chapter should promote research into antibiotic use aimed at identifying areas of improvement and evaluating the effectiveness of interventions.

CHAPTER 27

Drug utilization research in the area of cardiovascular medicines

Elisabetta Poluzzi[1] & Maarit Jaana Korhonen[2]

[1]*Pharmacology Unit, Department of Medical and Surgical Sciences, University of Bologna, Italy*

[2]*Department of Pharmacology, Drug Development and Therapeutics, University of Turku, Finland*

KEY POINTS

- The use of cardiovascular drugs has been on the increase in recent decades, due to improvements in diagnostic and therapeutic procedures, an ageing population and the emergence of innovative new drugs. This has a positive impact on population health but also causes health care expenditures to rise.
- Despite consolidated strong evidence and widespread international guidelines, drug utilization studies show a wide variation in drug choices between countries, even on the same continent. Lack of adherence to chronic treatments represents an additional clinical concern, since it is estimated that half of patients are nonadherent to these therapies.
- There are a number of specific challenges in using drug utilization methodology to measure antihypertensive use. Additional indications for many agents and dosages (e.g. heart failure, angina, arrhythmia), frequent use of polytherapy (either as fixed or extemporaneous combinations) and ambiguous use of Anatomical Therapeutic Chemical (ATC) codes all make it difficult to evaluate population exposure, assess adherence and compare usage between countries and regions.
- Drug utilization studies indicate that both lipid-lowering drugs and acetylsalicylic acid (ASA) are underused among secondary prevention patients and overused in primary prevention populations and elderly patients. This overuse represents a health care concern.
- Drug utilization studies on oral anticoagulants are important, both due to increasing demand for these drugs as a result of an increasing prevalence of atrial fibrillation and due to the rapid adoption of novel oral anticoagulants (NOACs) into clinical practice.

Introduction

Cardiovascular disease (CVD) is the leading cause of death and disability worldwide [1], representing a major burden to societies and populations. Leading risk factors for the burden of disease in Europe are lifestyle-related; they include high blood pressure, obesity and high blood cholesterol [2]. Evidence from randomized controlled trials (RCTs) supports the routine use of several classes of cardiovascular drugs for both primary and secondary prevention of CVD (reviewed in [3]). Practice guidelines emphasize the use of cardiovascular medications in secondary prevention patients, such as patients with coronary heart disease (CHD), cerebrovascular disease or peripheral arterial disease (PAD). Gradually, they have broadened their recommendations to primary prevention as well [3]. However, the use of lipid-lowering drugs and acetylsalicylic acid (ASA) in the primary prevention setting has long been debated, and recommendations for their use vary across guidelines [4,5]. In light of the high number of drug classes and the multiplicity of indications of use for many cardiovascular drugs, drug utilization studies represent an important basis for verifying whether a population is taking advantage of medicines in cardiovascular disorders. Most drug utilization studies on cardiovascular therapies focus on

Drug Utilization Research: Methods and Applications, First Edition. Edited by M. Elseviers et al. © 2016 John Wiley & Sons, Ltd.
Published 2016 by John Wiley & Sons, Ltd.

(i) trends in the prevalence of use and cross-country comparisons, (ii) adherence to recommendations, both in terms of drug choice and in terms of continuity of use, and (iii) assessment of possible inequities in drug treatment access (by age, gender, social status, etc.).

This chapter starts with an overview of trends in the utilization of cardiovascular drugs and of the main scopes of drug utilization studies in the field of cardiovascular drugs. It then looks at the utilization of antihypertensive, lipid-lowering, and antithrombotic drug therapy, with examples from different countries and settings. For each drug class, the main methodological strategies and challenges for drug utilization studies are also discussed. Finally, the important topic of cardiovascular polypharmacy is touched upon.

Trends in utilization of cardiovascular drugs

Use of cardiovascular drugs has seen a steady increase over the last few decades. The largest increase in utilization has been documented for HMG-CoA reductase inhibitors (better known as statins) and agents acting on the renin–angiotensin system, as shown by surveys on trends in cardiovascular drug use performed in European countries [6–10], North America [11] and Australia [12]. Rather than population ageing, increases in treatment intensity and prevalence seem to have driven the observed trend, especially an increasing tendency to cardiovascular polytherapy and declining discontinuation [10]. Changes in the prescribing and purchasing of cardiovascular drugs reflect uptake of clinical guidelines [6] and changes in reimbursement policies [13].

Antihypertensive drugs

Among drugs used for the treatment and prevention of CVDs, antihypertensives are the most prevalent, reflecting the high number of therapeutic classes and drugs for this indication and the frequent use of antihypertensive polypharmacy. These characteristics highlight the importance of drug utilization analyses in supporting health authorities in planning health expenditure and clinicians in improving the appropriateness of prescription. Prescription of antihypertensives mainly occurs in ambulatory care; hospital use represents a low fraction of the overall antihypertensive utilization and concerns only acute therapies. The prevalence of antihypertensive use varies widely among countries, averaging 16% in the adult population; data collected in 2003–09 show a range from 5.6% in Bangladesh to 32% in Brazil and Poland [14]. In 2003 the use of antihypertensives ranged from 150 to 250 defined daily doses (DDDs) per 1000 inhabitants per day (DID) in Central and Northern European countries [15].

When individual demographic characteristics were analysed, the mean age of patients starting therapy was about 60, and women were more frequently treated than men (F/M = 1.4/1) [16]. Age-specific analyses reported that more than 50% of the population over 60 received antihypertensives [17,18]. Antihypertensive utilization in children and adolescents is increasingly seen, however, due to the growing prevalence of childhood obesity and the increased cardiovascular risk factors in this population. A study by Liberman et al. [19] found an increasing awareness of the need to treat cardiovascular risk factors in obese youths; 1.5 per 1000 6–18-year-olds in the United States received antihypertensives, particularly diuretics and beta-blockers.

Population coverage and agreement with recommendations

Current areas of interest in drug utilization analyses of antihypertensives are (i) population coverage (discrepancies between undiagnosed, diagnosed, treated and controlled hypertension), (ii) agreement with recommendations (especially in terms of first choice in the naïve patient) and (iii) adherence to treatment. These areas all fall under the heading of evaluation of appropriateness, and a single drug utilization study will usually deal with more than one of them.

Two main aspects should be considered in assessing the appropriateness of cardiovascular drug use: reliable identification of eligible patients for treatment (i.e. quantification of over- and undertreatment) and choice of drug class. Regarding the first aspect, in a recent survey covering several countries, Chow et al. [14] showed that overall at least one-third of severe hypertensive subjects do not receive pharmacological treatment and about one-third of treated patients have well-controlled hypertension. This kind of study requires diagnostic information on treated and nontreated patients and appropriate prescribing quality indicators (PQIs; see Chapter 43) [20]. To date, electronic health records (EHRs) provide the most suitable source of data, but claims databases (containing information on diagnoses) are sometimes also used. A main issue in defining eligible patients for antihypertensive treatment is to identify when the patient becomes sick. Even more importantly, trends in blood pressure values and other cardiovascular risk factors should be considered in the assessment of antihypertensive appropriateness. A lack of clinical data for untreated hypertensive patients hinders the complete identification of undertreated patients.

As regards the choice of drug class, evaluation of the appropriateness of the prescribed treatment upon initial diagnosis can be carried out by comparing patient-level prescription data (if available) with relevant practice guidelines. When diuretics were the standard first choice of therapy for the initial treatment of uncomplicated hypertensive patients [21], drug utilization studies to assess drug appropriateness was quite easy to perform. Indeed, findings from many European countries are available: in Bosnia, Italy and Norway, descriptions of the antihypertensives used in the population and relevant agreement with guidelines were provided by analysing sales data, prescription data from claims databases and clinical records, respectively [22–24]. In the United Kingdom, Sofat et al. [25] showed important changes in the number of antihypertensive prescriptions made following a revision of British guidelines in 2006 to recommend angiotensin-converting enzyme (ACE) inhibitors or calcium channel blockers as the first-choice treatment. Recent guideline recommendations have been expanded to include several classes of antihypertensive drugs as first-line therapy, making it difficult to identify a suitable reference [15,26], although negative indicators remain applicable. For instance, angiotensin II receptor blockers (ARBs) as a first choice represent a negative indicator in some countries [27]. In fact, patients with comorbidities and with a long history of treatment account for the majority of antihypertensive users, which makes the assessment of appropriateness even more difficult. As a general rule, when planning cross-country studies on the appropriateness of antihypertensives, comparisons among populations with similar epidemiological features (prevalence of hypertension and of associated additional cardiovascular risk factors) are warranted. Where high-quality electronic clinical records are available, additional diagnostic or other clinical information can help in applying validated PQIs.

Adherence to antihypertensives is still a challenge in the rational use of health resources. See later in this chapter and Section F.

Challenges in researching the use of antihypertensive drugs

There are two important considerations in the analysis and interpretation of published data on antihypertensive use. The first is to define which ATC codes should be used in data collection and how to group them to distinguish antihypertensives by class. Many antihypertensive classes are currently available on the market, with a wide spectrum of indication of use. Overall, the following second levels contain all antihypertensives: C02, agents acting on alpha-adrenergic receptors; C03, diuretics; C07, beta-blockers; C08, calcium channel blockers; and C09, agents acting on the renin–angiotensin system (including ACE inhibitors and ARBs). However, each of these can be further classified into levels III or IV to distinguish drugs mainly used for hypertension from those with other principal indications. For example, C03 (diuretics) contains C03A and C03B (low-ceiling diuretics), used mainly for hypertension, and C03C (high-ceiling diuretics), used mainly for heart failure. As examples of the two approaches, three different sudies [22,23,28] used level II classification, whereas Selmer [24] used level III and excluded some classes due to their frequent use in other indications (e.g. high-ceiling diuretics and nondihydropyridine calcium channel blockers). Both methods are acceptable (the former is easier to apply and the second is more accurate), but the lack of a single accepted approach represents an obstacle to comparison of results across different countries and periods. Selmer [24] also collected information on diagnosis, showing that only 30% of subjects starting a beta-blocker had hypertension as the indication for use; conversely, thiazides and ARBs were used for this indication in at least 90% of cases. Table 27.1 lists the main additional indications of various antihypertensive agents. An important case is represented by group C02 (alpha-blockers), which is in fact primarily used for prostate disorders; cotreatment of this group with other antihypertensive drugs can represent an indicator of inappropriateness, because of the risk of hypotensive episodes (see later, in the section on polypharmacy).

The second important consideration concerns the use of the DDD methodology to study utilization of antihypertensives. The range of recommended doses for

Table 27.1 Additional indications of antihypertensive drugs.

ATC level II	ATC level III (most used groups)	Main clinically recognized indications for chronic use
C02: agents acting on alpha-adrenergic receptors	C02A: antiadrenergic agents, centrally acting (e.g. methyldopa)	
	C02C: antiadrenergic agents, peripherally acting (including C02CA: alpha-adrenoreceptor antagonists (prazosine, doxazosine))	Prostate disorders
C03: diuretics	C03A/C03B: low-ceiling diuretics	Heart failure, hypercalciuria
	C03C: high-ceiling diuretics	Heart failure (especially in acute conditions)
	C03D: potassium-sparing agents	Aldosteronism, cirrhosis
C07: beta-blockers	C07AA: beta-blocking agents, nonselective	Post-AMI, essential tremor, migraine (prophylaxis), cardiac dysrhythmia
	C07AB: Beta-blocking agents, selective	Heart failure, post-AMI, angina, migraine (prophylaxis)
C08: calcium channel blockers	C08C: selective calcium channel blockers with mainly vascular effects (including C08CA: dihydropyridine derivatives)	Angina
	C08D: selective calcium channel blockers with direct cardiac effects	Angina, cardiac dysrhythmia
C09: agents acting on the renin–angiotensin system	C09A/C09B: ACE inhibitors	Heart failure, post-AMI, diabetic nephropathy
	C09C/C09D: angiotensin II antagonists	Heart failure, post-AMI, diabetic nephropathy

Note: not all active substances included in the single class have all additional indications listed in the last column.

Post-AMI, post-acute myocardial infarction.

antihypertensive agents according to different guidelines and drug monographs is wide, and so are the actual prescribed daily doses (PDDs). The highly variable dosing for antihypertensive agents results in considerable discrepancies between DDDs and PDDs. For instance, beta-blockers generally have high DDDs compared to PDDs, while the ACE inhibitors tend to have low DDDs compared to PDDs. The need for individual dose titration throughout the course of treatment represents an additional obstacle. The use and interpretation of DIDs requires caution, therefore: DDD values should be used as measurement units when only aggregated data are available [15]. Prevalence, persistence and intensity of use should be calculated when more specific data are available (e.g. doses and durations of use actually prescribed by physicians – a sort of PDD) [16,29]. Alternatively, when only administrative data are obtainable, more conservative approaches – rather than those based on DDDs – can be considered. For instance, Poluzzi et al. [23,30] defined minimal daily doses for the treatment of hypertension for each drug and used them as measurement unit to evaluate patient adherence: the percentage of patients under the threshold represent the lowest estimation of nonadherence in the population, since many prevalent patients receive higher doses than the minimum.

Lipid-lowering therapy

The use of lipid-lowering drugs has increased tremendously since the introduction of statins in the late 1980s and the publication of landmark statin trials in the 1990s, and it continues to rise today. Recommendations and indications for lipid-lowering therapy have broadened from the prevention of recurrent events after myocardial infarction to primary prevention of CVD events in those with risk factors [3,13]. Different guidelines recommend different thresholds of estimated cardiovascular risk for the initiation of lipid-lowering medication. During the past 2 decades, guidelines have also shifted towards setting lower low-density lipoprotein (LDL) cholesterol targets based on individual cardiovascular risk [5]. In this section, trends, patterns and targeting of lipid-lowering medication according to cardiovascular risk are presented based on studies employing various drug utilization research designs.

Drug utilization studies using the ATC/DDD methodology have demonstrated considerable increase and variation in lipid-lowering drug utilization across European countries, Australia and Canada. An early international comparison based mostly on sales data covering the years 1990–94 documented a steady increase in lipid-lowering drug utilization in four European countries and Australia, although differences in the level of utilization remained large, with Australia ranking the highest [31]. Conversely, a study using pharmacy claims data on predominantly older populations from Queensland, Australia and Nova Scotia, Canada reported comparable levels of and similar fourfold increases in statin use (in DID) in both countries during 1997–2001 [32]. Data from administrative and commercial databases (e.g. IMS Health [33]) showed that, in Europe, the prevalence of statin use increased at a median rate of ~35% per year during 1997–2003. This rate varied considerably across the 13 countries included, as did the prevalence of use of statins and other lipid-lowering medications. In most European countries, lipid-lowering drugs other than statins (mostly fibrates) made up less than 10% of total DID in 2003, the maximum proportion being 25%. A review of more recent studies in Europe suggests that the cross-country variation in statin use persisted and the increase continued during 2001–07, although at a slower rate on average [34]. However, these variations in the level or trend of statin utilization appear to have no relation to those in CHD mortality, a proxy for population coronary risk [35].

Data from the largest public drug benefit programme in Canada indicate a large (greater than sevenfold) increase in statin utilization measured in DID during the 10-year period 1997–2007; however, the increase roughly halved when utilization was calculated as days of treatment or as tablets dispensed per population [37]. As in other countries [32,33], average PDDs for most statins increased over time. Thus, variation in PDDs partly explains the growth – as well as cross-country and within-country variations – in statin utilization [38].

Jackevicius et al. [11] provided further evidence for a steep increase in statin use in Canada, expressed as number of dispensed prescriptions per 100 000 population. Similar aggregate-level data (IMS Health) show comparable levels of overall lipid-lowering medication utilization in the United States during the first decade of the 2000s; however, within the lipid-lowering drug class, utilization patterns diverged between these two countries, with different clinical guidelines, pharmaceutical marketing strategies and drug policies [39,40]. Specifically, the number of statin prescriptions per population increased at a slower rate in the United States than in Canada [40], while use of fibrates increased in the United States but remained stable in Canada [39]. Use of ezetimibe-containing products increased faster in the United States than in Canada until 2008, when the negative surrogate outcomes evidence from the ENHANCE trial was published [40]. Unexpectedly, ezetimibe use continued to increase in Canada but decreased rapidly in the United States. Future drug utilization research will show whether the 2014 conference presentation of the IMPROVE-IT trial results (on the beneficial effects for clinical end points of adding ezetimibe to statin therapy following acute coronary syndrome (ACS)) [41] and the subsequent publication of the full trial report affect utilization patterns of lipid-lowering medications.

More accurate information concerning lipid-lowering medication use in the population has been obtained from studies based on individual-level data drawn from nationwide drug dispensation databases and representative surveys allowing for calculation of rates per age and gender. In the whole Danish population aged ≥40, the annual prevalence (proportion with at least one statin dispensation during the observation year) increased from 0.7 to 18.7% between 1996 and 2009 [13]. Similarly, the cross-sectional National Health and Nutrition Examination Survey (NHANES) in the United States showed a steady increase in the age-adjusted point prevalence of lipid-lowering medication use from 5 to 23% in the noninstitutionalized population aged 40–74 between surveys in 1988/94 and 2007/10 [42]. The increase was greatest among older people. Dispensation data from Denmark and Finland show that about one in four statin users was aged ≥75 by the end of the first decade of the 2000s [13,43].

In Denmark, a constant increase in the incidence of statin use across age and indication groups was seen until 2008, but a very different picture emerged in Israel during the years 2000–10 [13,44]: the incidence of statin use peaked at 4% in 2005 and started to decline thereafter. Differences in the definition of an incident user are a likely explanation for this discrepancy: the Israeli study considered only incident users with no previous statin dispensations, while the Danish study defined incident users as individuals without statin dispensations within 365 days prior to each observation year. The Israeli study points to a diminishing pool of individuals who have never used statins: less than 10% of the population with CHD and ~20% of that with diabetes were statin-naïve in 2010.

Agreement with recommendations

Various drug utilization studies have demonstrated an association between implementation of clinical guidelines and increasing statin utilization [13,45,46]. Changes in statin choices and in the characteristics of incident users in response to changes in reimbursement rules and other official or unofficial recommendations have also been shown [13,44,47]. Typically, however, studies on the appropriateness of drug utilization require individual-level prescription or dispensation data with linkage to the reasons for the prescription. Statins in high-cardiovascular risk patients represent one of the most widely assessed (disease-oriented) PQIs, with good clinimetric results in terms of face/content validity, reliability and feasibility reported across settings [48].

Along with the expansion of statin utilization, underuse of lipid-lowering medication among patients with established CVD has declined over time, but studies suggest continued suboptimal prescribing of lipid-lowering medications in cardiovascular populations. The EUROASPIRE I, II and III surveys collected cross-sectional data on the use of cardioprotective medication from patients with coronary revascularization or acute myocardial infarction/ischaemia in the same selected geographical regions and hospitals across eight European countries at four time points [6]. The prevalence of lipid-lowering medication 6 months after hospital discharge increased on average from 32 to 89% between 1995/6 and 2006/7; however, there was considerable variation in lipid-lowering medication use across countries, and almost half of patients studied did not meet the lipid targets recommended by the Joint European Societies' guidelines. Another study, based on data from a computerized primary care database in the United Kingdom, documented a similar increase in the proportion of patients prescribed statins within 6 months after their first myocardial infarction, from 37 to 92%, between 1997 and 2006 [49]. Younger age, affluence, revascularization after myocardial infarction, presence of hypertension or diabetes and absence of congestive heart failure predicted initiation of statin therapy. A US study based on data from nationally representative samples of patient visits to physicians' offices and hospital outpatient departments in the years 1998/99 and 2008/09 reported a more modest increase in statin use: from 27 to 59% among patients with CHD and from 12 to 36% among patients with diabetes [50].

An important topic for drug utilization studies dealing with underuse of lipid-lowering medication, especially in secondary prevention of CVD, is the intensity of therapy. An analysis of >65 000 hospitalizations for ACS in 344 hospitals participating in the Get With the Guidelines (GWTG-CAD) initiative in the United States provides an example [51]. This study included admissions with an ACS diagnosis in 2005–09 and collected data from hospital records on patient demographics, medical history, in-hospital treatment and procedures, discharge treatment and lipid levels at admission. At hospital discharge, <40% of the patients were treated with the guideline recommended high-intensity lipid-lowering therapy, defined as therapy likely to achieve a >50% reduction in LDL cholesterol. The likelihood of receiving high-intensity lipid-lowering therapy actually decreased towards the end of the observation period, as prescribing of ezetimibe declined rapidly after the publication of the ENHANCE trial results [40].

Statin use has expanded to the primary prevention setting for patients without existing CVD. According to the Danish study linking data from nationwide drug dispensation and hospitalization registers [13], less than one-third of prevalent statin users had myocardial infarction or CHD, while another third were free of myocardial infarction/CHD but had other risk factors for CVD (i.e. history of stroke, PAD, other potential atherosclerotic CVD or diabetes). About one-third of users did not have any register markers for CVD, and received statins for questionable indications. Overall, this shift in statin use towards asymptomatic and older populations has raised concerns about overtreatment of people who are unlikely to benefit from lipid-lowering therapy. In

2007, UK clinical guidelines recommended that statins should be part of the primary prevention management strategy for patients at high risk of developing CVD (10-year risk ≥20%). A study covering the years 1993–2011 and based on the primary care records of almost 4 million general population patients and ~300 000 statin initiators aged 35–74 without pre-existing CVD or diabetes reported that the proportion of high-risk patients receiving statins increased after 2007 (from 7 to 30%); however, there was a mismatch in targeting of statin therapy, as only ~50% of statin initiators were at high risk [52]. Another UK study, which included patients with diabetes, reported that in total 14% of patients free of CVD initiated statins over a 2-year follow-up in 2008–10 [53]. The proportion was 26% among patients eligible for treatment according to UK guidelines, and 10% among those deemed ineligible; that is, less than half of the initiators were eligible. Predictors of statin initiation in this primary prevention population included older age, male gender, presence of diabetes, use of antihypertensive drugs, frequent blood pressure measurements, high total and low high-density lipoprotein (HDL) cholesterol levels, family history of CHD and smoking, reflecting guideline recommendations.

Challenges in researching the use of lipid-lowering therapy

In addition to variation in PDDs, differences between databases (administrative versus commercial) and changes in prescribing and reimbursement rules (if not the main focus of the study) may hamper international comparisons and trend analyses of lipid-lowering medication utilization based on aggregate data. A dosage assumption of one tablet per day may be preferable to DDD in individual-level studies where no information is available on dosage instructions or number of days of supply, as validation studies have shown that for >95% of statin prescriptions, the instruction is one tablet daily [36,37].

Results concerning the appropriateness of prescribing of lipid-lowering medication obtained from ad hoc studies and registries of hospitalized patients, such as EUROASPIRE and GWTG-CAD [6,51], may not be generalizable to those secondary prevention patients treated in nonparticipating hospitals even in the same country, because the participation of hospitals, physicians and patients is voluntary. Specifically, such non-population-based studies may tend to provide an overestimation of drug use. On the other hand, studies relying on more representative administrative data often lack information (e.g. laboratory data) essential to classifying patients' cardiovascular risk for all [13] or a substantial proportion of the population [52].

Antithrombotic drug therapy: oral anticoagulants

Anticoagulation therapy is used to prevent thromboembolic events in people with a range of different conditions. Vitamin K antagonists (VKAs), especially warfarin, have been the mainstay of oral anticoagulant therapy since the 1950s. Atrial fibrillation is by far the most common indication for VKAs (e.g. ~40–60% of warfarin users), followed by venous thrombosis, pulmonary embolism and mechanical prosthetic valve replacement [54,55]. In patients with atrial fibrillation, the guidelines recommend that the choice between a VKA and ASA be made based on their baseline stroke risk, as calculated by $CHADS_2$ or CHA_2DS_2VASc scoring systems; moderate- to high-risk patients are recommended to receive oral anticoagulants [56,57]. As a recent drug utilization study in Denmark reported, VKA therapy may often be initiated in hospital, but maintenance therapy is almost completely handled by primary care physicians [58].

Despite its effectiveness, VKA treatment is challenged by the risk of bleeding, potential food and drug–drug interactions and routine monitoring requirements. In fact, warfarin has been implicated as the most common cause of emergency hospitalizations for adverse drug reactions (ADRs) in older people [59]. The challenges related to the use of VKAs have motivated the development of novel (non-VKA) oral anticoagulants (NOACs). Dabigatran and rivaroxaban entered the market at the end of the first decade of the 2000s, originally for use in patients undergoing orthopaedic surgery [60]. In the early 2010s, they were approved for use in atrial fibrillation. Currently, dabigatran, rivaroxaban and abixaban are recommended as an alternative or first-line therapy for stroke prophylaxis in atrial fibrillation in many countries [61]. Accordingly, drug utilization studies have documented rapid increases in the utilization of NOACs [62]. For example, a nationally representative audit of office-based providers in the United States showed that prescribing of oral anticoagulants shifted from warfarin to dabigatran during 2010–11 [54]. In the last quarter of 2011, dabigatran visits made up almost 20% of all visits in which oral anticoagulants were prescribed, and direct expenditures (as the retail value of dispensed medications) on dabigatran exceeded those of warfarin. Another drug utilization study based on dispensation records in Ontario, Canada found that the number of prescriptions for NOACs, including dabigatran and rivaroxaban, increased over 20-fold in the 2 years following dabigatran's market approval [60]. In Denmark, rapid uptake of dabigatran was documented using national registers. Within the first 4 months after its market entry, 40% of all patients with atrial fibrillation who initiated oral anticoagulation therapy received dabigatran [63].

Agreement with recommendations

Several qualitative drug utilization studies in a number of different countries, subpopulations and settings and using different quality indicators have demonstrated the inappropriateness of warfarin use in atrial fibrillation patients. According to a systematic review, less than 60% of atrial fibrillation patients with high risk of stroke are on oral anticoagulants [64]. A US study based on two nationally representative surveys of visits to ambulatory care practices suggested an improvement in the use of anticoagulation therapy between 1999 and 2009: the number of visits in which patients were prescribed anticoagulants (numerator) as a proportion of all visits by patients with atrial fibrillation but without contraindications (denominator) increased from 46 to 72% [50].

Prior to the era of NOACs, a UK study of atrial fibrillation patients at 400 general practices, which employed the $CHADS_2$ and CHA_2DS_2VASc scoring systems, reported both under- and overuse of warfarin [65]: 55% of high-risk patients and 37% of low-risk patients were on warfarin. A recent Swedish study of atrial fibrillation patients in the Stockholm region, comprehensively identified through inpatient, specialist ambulatory and primary care records, supported the view that there is considerable under- and overuse of warfarin [66]. However, while this study reported common use of ASA (instead of warfarin) in high-risk atrial fibrillation patients, a further investigation suggested that 50% of those patients had either relative or absolute contraindications to oral anticoagulant therapy, such as dementia, alcohol abuse, renal disease, anaemia, earlier severe bleeding or frequent falls [67]. This example highlights the care needed when assessing the appropriateness of drug utilization using databases that do not include information on relevant patient characteristics and comorbidities. Accordingly, a meta-analysis of 28 observational US studies conducted in inpatient and outpatient settings in 1989–2007 suggests that the decision to prescribe warfarin in atrial fibrillation is affected by multiple patient characteristics [68]: in addition to absolute contraindications, alcohol/drug abuse, perceived barriers to adherence, dementia, history of falls, gastrointestinal or intracranial haemorrhages, hepatic or renal impairments, race (African American) and advanced age predicted decreased use of warfarin. The characteristics predicting increased use of warfarin versus non-use included history of stroke, congestive heart failure and male gender.

Recently, several studies using patient registries and active monitoring in different countries have documented discrepancies between clinical trial populations and real-world patients receiving NOACs (reviewed in [62]), which may bring into question the applicability of trial results to clinical practice. A nationwide register-based study including all atrial fibrillation patients who initiated oral anticoagulant use in Denmark during 2011–13 showed that initiators of rivaroxaban and apixaban had a higher predicted risk of stroke and bleeding than initiators of warfarin and dabigatran [63]. In contrast, a US study of atrial fibrillation patients from one commercial health plan demonstrated preferential prescribing of NOACs to healthier patients in 2010–13: higher predicted stroke and bleeding risks, as well as female sex and lower income, were associated with lower likelihood of receiving a NOAC compared to warfarin [69]. Importantly, NOACs accounted for ~60% of new prescriptions but 98% of anticoagulation-related drug costs in 2013.

The preceding findings call for qualitative drug utilization studies of NOACs, studies on the comparative safety, effectiveness and cost implications of NOACs versus VKAs and evaluations of policy models governing the entry of new drugs into the market [62]. Early comparative safety and effectiveness studies are likely to be confounded by differences in baseline stroke and bleeding risks between patients initiating or switching to various NOACs and patients receiving VKAs [69,70].

Antithrombotic drug therapy: acetylsalicylic acid

Aspirin is one of the most widely used drugs worldwide. Low-dose ASA (B01AC06) is used for the prevention and treatment of CVD [4]. A recent register-based study covering the whole population of Denmark indicated a steady increase in the 1-year prevalence of low-dose ASA use (from 4 to 7% between 1999 and 2012), with 40% of those aged 80 and over being exposed in 2012 [71]. Comparing sales statistics and dispensation data, the study demonstrated a considerable increase in the proportion of low-dose ASA use that is prescribed and thus detectable through dispensation records (from 62 to 92%); therefore, the increase in ASA use is partly apparent.

Agreement with recommendations

Along with agents acting on the renin–angiotensin system, beta-blockers, other antihypertensive drugs and statins, antiplatelet agents are widely recommended for secondary prevention of CVD. ASA and antiplatelet medication in high-cardiovascular risk patients belong to the most widely assessed PQIs, with good clinimetric properties shown in different settings [20].

According to the Prospective Urban Rural Epidemiology (PURE) study, on average, every third patient aged 35–70 years with prevalent CHD and almost every second patient with history of stroke is not on antiplatelet therapy in high-income countries, including Sweden, Canada and the United Arab Emirates; however, underuse of even low-cost ASA is several times more common in low-income countries, such as Zimbabwe and Pakistan [72]. A country's economic status was found to explain two-thirds of the variation in drug use. The PURE project collected data on community-living people in different countries and obtained data on indications (CVD) and drug use from self-reports; therefore, quality of data may vary across communities.

In contrast, in low-risk populations, there is evidence of overuse of ASA from both Europe and North America, although recommendations vary across different guidelines [4]. A recent cross-sectional analysis of the EHRs of >16 000 American adults with no clinical indication for ASA showed that 19% were regular ASA users [73]. Overuse was more common among older people and males. A specific challenge in studying overuse of ASA is its wide over-the-counter (OTC) use, which leads to underestimation of the population exposure.

Patient adherence to cardiovascular drugs

Among cardiovascular drugs, the lowest adherence is found for statins, followed by antihypertensives. Adherence to other classes, such as ASA and antidiabetics, appears to be better, without major differences among them [74]. Chowdhury et al. [75] estimated that 9% of all CVD events can be attributed to nonadherence to cardiovascular medication. A definition of adherence indicators is provided in Section F. Of the large number of patient-related variables studied, fewer comorbidities (primary prevention, not having hypertension), new use, fewer lipid tests, greater out-of-pocket costs and lower income have been most consistently identified as predictors of statin nonadherence [76]. A meta-analysis of 53 mostly register-based studies confirmed that women and non-white individuals have an increased risk of nonadherence [77]. In addition to sociodemographic characteristics associated with low adherence (e.g. low income and low education), polypharmacy is an obstacle to the correct use of chronic cardiovascular medications (see next section).

Adherence to VKA therapy seems suboptimal, with low adherence associated with lower proportions of time spent at the therapeutic interval and worse morbidity and mortality [78]. Specifically, ~20–40% of patients with atrial fibrillation discontinue warfarin therapy within the first year of treatment [78,79]. Early studies have reported lower or equal rates of anticoagulation therapy discontinuation among patients initiating with NOACs versus VKAs [79]; however, in a Danish study, 51% of new NOAC users were found to have switched to VKAs within 6 months after initiation [58]. These observations further highlight the need for drug utilization studies to identify potential problems in the use of NOACs and to promote optimal use of oral anticoagulants.

The predictive power of models based on administrative data in explaining adherence seems poor [80,81]. Better identification of barriers to adherence and effective interventions remain important topics for drug utilization studies. Accordingly, in register-based studies assessing the association between adherence and health outcomes, a bias known as the 'healthy user' or 'healthy adherer' effect is a challenge. This bias may account for a considerable (but unknown) proportion of the beneficial health effects attributed to preventative cardiovascular medication in observational studies [82].

Cardiovascular polypharmacy

CVDs resulted in the greatest increase in the average number of medications both in primary care and among in-hospital patients [83–85]. Treating hypertension *per se* can require more than one medication: 4 years after the start of treatment, more than one-quarter of Norwegian patients were treated with three or more drug combinations [24]; while in Portugal, where diuretics represent the most common antihypertensive drug class, only 37% of patients on treatment reached target blood pressure values and more than 30% took at least four drugs [86]. Heart failure and post-acute myocardial infarction (post-AMI) represent a typical scenario requiring cardiovascular polypharmacy (ACE inhibitors and beta-blockers for heart failure; ACE inhibitors, beta-blockers, antiplatelets and statins for post-AMI). As a consequence, the use of at least five cardiovascular drugs is not rare. The appropriateness of cardiovascular polypharmacy is difficult to evaluate, since many patients require multiple cardiovascular drugs depending on existing diseases and risk factors. In fact, most medications should be chronically used and, for each therapy, only adherent patients can obtain expected benefits.

The influence of cardiovascular polypharmacy on adherence to individual therapies is not easy to interpret. On the one hand, patients who have more than one risk factor for cardiovascular events (i.e. patients who receive the relevant therapy) show higher adherence to medications [30], probably because of their awareness of disease. On the other, it is difficult for a patient with increasing numbers of medications to be adherent to all of them. Among older adults with CVD, the high prevalence of polypharmacy, coupled with age-associated physiological changes and comorbidities, is a major challenge to adherence, predisposing this population to adverse events [87].

In the early 2000s, the idea of improving adherence by administering a multiple cardiovascular drug therapy in a single tablet was advocated: the so-called 'polypill'. So far, evidence on the overall risk–benefit profile of the polypill is still uncertain: it shows high adherence and efficacy in reducing blood pressure and cholesterol levels, but also high risk of an adverse event, due to the difficulty of changing the dose of a single agent throughout chronic treatments [88–91]. Drug utilization studies will be very useful in defining the specific populations that should be treated with polypills.

More recently, in order to optimize risk–benefit and cost-effectiveness profiles, the strategy of deprescribing has been proposed [92] (see Chapter 25). As for cardiovascular medications, findings from observational studies can be very useful in identifying drugs that, in the light of low adherence in clinical practice, do not provide their expected benefit. Such is the case, for example, with beta-blockers in post-AMI therapy [93] and with antihypertensives in older patients [94]. Less useful drugs should probably be withdrawn in order to improve adherence to others and to reduce the risk of drug–drug interactions and side effects.

From a methodological point of view, drug utilization studies in patients receiving chronic polypharmacy require additional efforts, especially to distinguish co-medications from switching between therapies. Appropriate windows of observation are needed for this purpose.

Conclusion

Drug utilization research in the field of cardiovascular classes represents a rich topic that continuously provides new challenges. Apart from their crucial role in clinical practice (preventing CVD in the population), these drugs also provide a useful reference when planning pharmacoeconomic and outcome research studies (see Chapters 41 and 42). The most common aim of drug utilization research on cardiovascular drugs is to compare amount of use, adherence to therapy and the impact of generics on prescription habits among countries and regions. Methodological approaches should take into account the peculiarities of each drug class, especially concerning measurement units (DDDs versus tablets), multiple indications (e.g. beta-blockers, diuretics, ACE inhibitors) and switching between analogues.

Evidence is appearing at a consistently higher rate for the effects of drugs on CVD as compared to other clinical areas. This translates to faster and more frequent guideline changes, and shows the importance of drug utilization studies in this area: both those applying already developed methodologies and those finding ways of improving the quality of data sources and harmonizing the use of cutting-edge approaches in as many countries as possible.

CHAPTER 28

Drug utilization research in the area of analgesics and psychotropics

Helga Zoëga[1], Alesha Smith[2] & Nadia Barozzi[3]

[1]*Centre of Public Health Sciences, Faculty of Medicine, University of Iceland, Iceland*

[2]*School of Pharmacy, University of Otago, New Zealand*

[3]*Healthy4Life, Basel, Switzerland*

KEY POINTS

- The use of pain medications and psychotropic drugs, including antipsychotics, hypnotics, sedatives, antidepressants and psychostimulants, is increasing worldwide, although many people with mental health conditions and pain continue to be undertreated.
- It is estimated that over 50% of patients are nonadherent to prescribed treatment with psychotropic drugs.
- Off-label use of antipsychotics and antidepressants is increasing in both adults and children worldwide.
- Abuse of opioids, benzodiazepines and psychostimulants is a pronounced and growing problem in many countries.

Introduction

Psychotropic drugs, used in the treatment of mental health conditions and pain, are among the most commonly used drug classes worldwide. In this chapter, we describe the main analgesic and psychotropic drug groups, their most common indications and the characteristics of patients treated. We also describe clinical and therapeutic problems and concerns regarding the quality of use of these drugs and provide examples of relevant drug utilization studies.

The chapter is divided into sections on ***pain medications***, ***psycholeptics*** and ***psychoanaleptics***. Pain medications include paracetamol (acetaminophen), nonsteroidal antiinflammatory drugs (NSAIDs) and centrally acting agents such as narcotic analgesics (opioids), antidepressants and anticonvulsants. In the Anatomical Therapeutic Chemical (ATC) drug classification system, psycholeptics (ATC group N05) include antipsychotics, anxiolytics and hypnotics/sedatives and are broadly defined by the calming effect they provide. Psychoanaleptics (ATC group N06) include antidepressants and psychostimulants and are defined by a stimulating effect exerted on brain activity.

Pain medications

Pain is a common symptom. It can range from minor acute episodes to more severe chronic aches, and it is a frequent reason for someone's seeking medical assistance. Chronic pain is often defined as any pain lasting more than 12 weeks. The prevalence of chronic pain ranges from approximately 19 to 34%, depending on the characteristics of the population studied and on the how pain has been defined or assessed [1,2]. Medications indicated for the treatment of pain are among the most commonly used drug classes [3]. A number of pharmacologic treatments are available for the treatment of acute and chronic cancer-related and nonmalignant pain. Pharmacologic treatments typically include peripherally acting agents such as paracetamol

Drug Utilization Research: Methods and Applications, First Edition. Edited by M. Elseviers et al.
Published 2016 by John Wiley & Sons, Ltd.

and NSAIDs and centrally acting agents such as opioids, antidepressants and anticonvulsants. NSAIDs (e.g. ibuprofen, diclofenac, naproxen) and paracetamol are normally administered orally and are mainly used for short-term acute pain. Other, more effective NSAIDs (e.g. diclofenac, indomethacin, naproxen and tolfenamic acid) may also be prescribed by physicians for more severe conditions, such as rheumatoid arthritis and osteoarthritis [4]. Drugs acting at opioid receptors (e.g. codeine, morphine, oxycodone, hydromorphone, fentanyl and methadone) are used to treat both cancer-related and nonmalignant acute or chronic pain. Tricyclic antidepressants (TCAs) exhibit synergic analgesic efficacy in a number of chronic pain conditions (e.g. diabetic neuropathy, tension headache, migraine, atypical facial pain, fibromyalgia and low back pain) [5]. Certain anticonvulsants (e.g. carmazepine, gabapentin, oxacarbazepine) also exhibit analgesic action in neuropathic pain by reducing neuronal excitability [5].

Pain treatment can be initiated in both primary and secondary care settings. Physicians in primary care commonly prescribe analgesics, including opioids, after an injury or trauma and for low back pain, diabetic neuropathy, degenerative joint disorders and headache [7]. Self-medication with over-the-counter (OTC) medications such as NSAIDs and paracetamol, without prior medical consultation, is also common [6]. In addition, analgesics represent one of the most frequently administered drugs in hospitals; it has been estimated that between 40 and 80% of inpatients experience intermittent pain during their hospital stay [8]. Inpatients may obtain opioids around the time of an operation or during invasive diagnostic procedures.

Characteristics of patients using pain medication

Chronic pain is heterogeneously distributed within the population, although higher occurrence is observed in particularly vulnerable subpopulations [9]. There is generally a higher prevalence of chronic pain in older people, due to the greater frequency of other medical conditions in this age group (e.g. musculoskeletal disorders, cancer) [10]. Pain also appears to be more recurrent in women, as the modulation of pain seems to be related to oestrogen levels [11,12]. Patients suffering from psychological conditions seem to be more at risk of experiencing pain [13]. Anxiety and depression have been associated with higher occurrence of chronic pain [7,14]. This may suggest that depression and anxiety augment pain perception. An additional factor characterizing pain patients is their individual genetic profile [15]. Chronic pain occurrence has been also correlated to socioeconomic status, being higher in people from lower socioeconomic classes [9].

Drug utilization of pain medication

Medication nonadherence is a frequent problem in chronic conditions, and both under- and overuse of medications have been reported [16]. It has been estimated that up to approximately 50% of patients with pain are nonadherent to their therapies; of these, approximately two-thirds underuse and one-third overuse the prescribed medications [16]. Both over- and underuse of pain medications can lead to significant health consequences. Overuse of NSAIDs, especially those available over the counter, is a well recognized problem internationally [6]. The ease of accessibility increases the risk of NSAID users experiencing adverse events [17]. It has been calculated that in the U.S. for each dollar spent on NSAIDs, approximately the same sum is needed to manage their side effects [18]. Paracetamol is considered much safer and equally effective for a number of indications that are more often treated with NSAIDs, but patients perceive it as less effective and it is often underutilized [19].

Under- and overuse of narcotic analgesics is also a reason for concern. Consensus exists that prescribing opioids for chronic pain caused by cancer is appropriate. Much more controversial is their use for other types of chronic condition, such as back pain, migraine and musculoskeletal disorders. Opioids put patients at risk of dependence and drug abuse. Consequently, narcotic analgesics have often been stigmatized for their potential to lead to addictive behaviour and their use may be feared by many patients [20]. Additionally, strict regulations, penalties following inappropriate opioid prescribing and fear of causing harm put medical professionals under pressure when initiating pain therapies, and many would refrain from prescribing opioids [21]. Patients with mental disabilities such as dementia and patients who are unable to communicate appropriately with caregivers are also at risk of undertreatment of pain [22]. Potential underutilization of pain medication has also been reported in women [11]: the higher pain sensitivity of women is frequently underestimated, and dosages are often not adjusted accordingly [11].

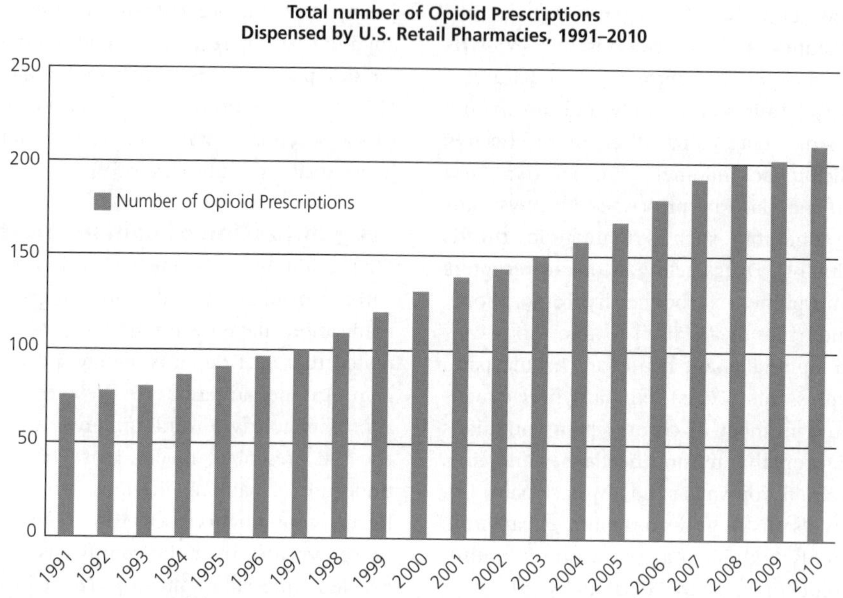

Figure 28.1 Total number of opioid prescriptions dispensed by U.S. retail pharmacies, 1991–2010.

Source: Data from National Institutes of Health, Prescription Drug Abuse. https://d14rmgtrwzf5a.cloudfront.net/sites/default/files/prescriptiondrugrrs_11_14.pdf. Last accessed 18 November 2015.

A global rising health care problem is the nonmedical use of centrally acting drugs such as opioids, benzodiazepines and prescription stimulants [23]. In 2008, the Drug Abuse Warning Network (DAWN) estimated that approximately 1 million visits to emergency departments were due to prescription or OTC drugs used nonmedically (e.g. too high or too frequent dosages, intentional use to become euphoric, coadministration with alcohol or illicit drugs). The most common drug categories involved were opioid and psychotropic drugs, mainly sedatives and antidepressants. The populations that are particularly vulnerable to drug abuse and nonmedical use of medications are older adults, women and adolescents [23]. Older people tend to use several medications and may be experiencing declining cognition; they are therefore more susceptible to accidental misuse or abuse [24]. Women have a higher risk than men of experiencing depression, anxiety or physical or emotional abuse [25]. Adolescents are vulnerable to negative peer influence and substance abuse initiation [26]. A high prevalence of prescription drug abuse may also result from high availability. The number of prescriptions for some of these medications has increased dramatically since the early 1990s [27]. In fact, the number of opioid prescriptions dispensed by U.S. retail pharmacies increased from 76 to 210 million in the period 1991–2010 (Figure 28.1).

The health consequences of prescription drug abuse are a problem that deserves attention. There is a need to improve the balance between analgesia and adverse effects. Enhancement in opioid prescribing could be achieved through research and educational interventions targeting physician and appropriate patient subpopulations. Identification of risk factors and optimization of guidelines to achieve satisfactory outcomes and reduce the risks associated with abuse and addiction are also essential steps.

Psycholeptics: antipsychotics, anxiolytics and hypnotics/sedatives

The psycholeptics include three subgroups within the ATC drug classification system: antipsychotics, hypnotics/sedatives and anxiolytics.

Antipsychotic drugs are used to provide relief from symptoms such as hallucinations, delusions and abnormal behaviour/thought, and for their sedative and tranquillizing effects in very disturbed or aggressive patients [28]. Although they are indicated in acute and chronic psychoses (e.g. schizophrenia) and bipolar disorder, they are often used in low doses as hypnotics and for behavioural disturbances in dementia patients. Antipsychotics are increasingly being prescribed off-label for a variety of disorders (e.g. autism in some countries) [28,29]. Antipsychotics are classified as first-generation (typical; e.g. chlorpromazine, haloperidol) or second-generation (atypical; e.g. olanzapine, clozapine, risperidone, quetiapine). However, such classifications are not clinically helpful or accurate, as these are a heterogeneous group of drugs with different mechanisms of action, properties and adverse effect profiles.

The initiation and monitoring of antipsychotic drugs is usually the prerogative of specialists in hospital settings, but an increasing trend has been demonstrated for these medicines to be initiated and managed by family physicians and/or mental health teams within the community [30].

While there is no first-line antipsychotic drug which is suitable for all patients [31], second-generation antipsychotics are now usually prescribed as first-line therapy and have generally replaced the use of first-generation antipsychotics, as shown in Figure 28.2 [32,33].

The adverse effects caused by antipsychotics are common, may be irreversible and require continuous monitoring. These include cardiovascular effects, sexual dysfunction, hyperglycaemia, hypotension and neuroleptic malignant syndrome, and they contribute significantly to nonadherence. Extrapyramidal symptoms occur most frequently with first-generation antipsychotics, which has partly driven the shift towards the use of the atypical antipsychotics, although these are associated with higher risk of metabolic effects [34].

Continuous antipsychotic therapy is recommended to limit disease severity in those with schizophrenia. However, nonadherence with oral antipsychotic medication is high (estimated in the range of 50–75% [35]). Partial compliance (taking some but not all medication as prescribed) is even more prevalent, occurring in approximately 90% of patients [36].

Long-acting injectable antipsychotics (depots) are used for maintenance therapy, especially when adherence to oral treatment is unreliable. They are administered at intervals of 1–4 weeks. A study including over 3500 patients with schizophrenia in the U.S. found that approximately 15% of patients on long-term antipsychotic therapy used depots [37]. Debate exists as to whether depots are associated with improvements in disease severity and functioning and with decreased psychiatric hospitalizations compared to oral dosing [38,39]. Anxiolytics are used to control symptoms and improve social functioning as second line to, or in combination with, psychological therapy for short-term relief of severe anxiety, panic disorders, social phobia and obsessive compulsive disorder (OCD) [28]. Benzodiazepines, both long-acting (e.g. diazepam) and short-acting (e.g. temazepam), are the most commonly prescribed anxiolytics. Buspirone (a partial agonist of serotonin receptors), beta-blockers (e.g. propranolol), some antidepressants (e.g. fluoxetine) and short-term use of some second-generation antipsychotics (e.g. quetiapine) are also indicated for anxiety and related

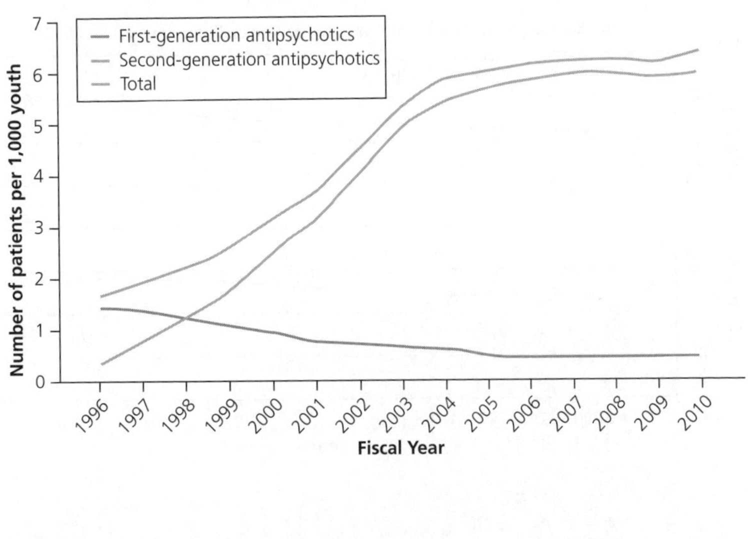

Figure 28.2 Trends in antipsychotic prescription by type for patients aged 18 or younger in British Columbia from 1996 to 2010.

disorders, although they are rarely used [40]. Antihistamines are often prescribed for anxiety, but this is usually not indicated or appropriate [41]. Indications vary among countries.

Hypnotics are primarily prescribed for insomnia and before dental and surgical procedures. Hypnotics include benzodiazepines, nonbenzodiazepines (Z-drugs, e.g. zopiclone) and antihistamines.

Prescribing of benzodiazepines/Z-drugs is widespread in all health care settings, but the largest use occurs in primary practice [42]. Although these drugs are fast-acting and well tolerated, they do have a concerning adverse effect profile, which includes sleepwalking and related behaviour, such as sleep-eating and sleep-driving (Z-drugs only), drowsiness, confusion, impaired judgment and memory, increased reaction time, ataxia, dependence and tolerance. Rapid withdrawal may produce convulsions, delirium or psychosis [31].

Characteristics of patients using psycholeptics

A systematic review of the incidence of schizophrenia across 33 countries between 1965 and 2001 calculated a median value of 15.2 per 100 000 persons, generally occurring at a higher rate in men than in women [43]. The use of antipsychotics is higher in younger individuals (20–55-year-olds have the highest prevalence for both schizophrenia and bipolar disorder) and in patients over 65 years old with dementia (typically, older women) [44,45]. It has also been reported that those affected by chronic medical conditions are more likely than others to receive psycholeptic medications [46].

Recently, the use of antipsychotics has increased in populations such as children and adolescents [32], pregnant women [47] and hospitalized patients [44], but it seems it has decreased in Dutch cancer patients [48].

Hypnotics and anxiolytics are used by a large percentage of all populations [33,49–51]. In France, for example, 15–20% of the population uses them, making then the most commonly used drugs in that country [50]. Figure 28.3 demonstrates high use in two further jurisdictions. The use of benzodiazepines is associated with older (>65 years) females with poor health status, despite lower rates of anxiety in the elderly and very old [51,52]. Data from some geographical areas show that utilization of benzodiazepines in older adults may in fact be decreasing, however [53].

Drug utilization of psycholeptics

There has been a significant increase in psychotropic polypharmacy over the last decade, particularly in older adults, which is concerning because of the adverse drug reactions (ADRs) that can occur with multiple drug use [54]. Concomitant antipsychotics (except in periods of 'crossover' from one drug to another) and the use antipsychotics for nonpsychotic illnesses (e.g. in anxiety or for sedation) should be avoided [41].

There has been a marked increase in the use of antipsychotics in a number of countries over the last 10 years [40,55], which does not reflect the relatively stable schizophrenia prevalence [56], suggesting considerable off-label use. In a U.S. study, 29% of nursing home residents received an antipsychotic, of which 32% had no identified clinical indication [57]. Many older patients

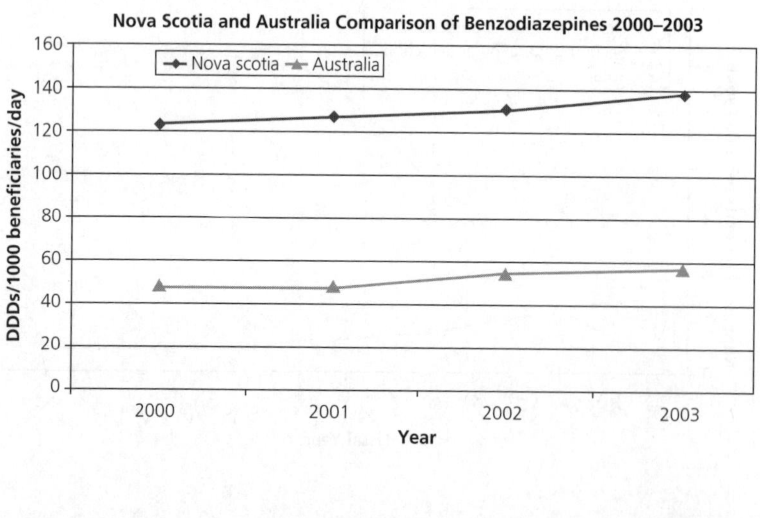

Figure 28.3 Overall use of benzodiazepines among Pharmacare beneficiaries in Nova Scotia and Australia, 2000–03. DDD; defined daily dose.

also receive long-term antipsychotic regimens that do not follow current recommendations regarding dosage or medication choice for behavioural and psychological symptoms of dementia [58]. The increasing use of antipsychotics in the paediatric population is somewhat controversial because of a lack of high-quality data on long-term outcomes to inform evidence-based clinical practice recommendations [59].

The adverse effect profile of benzodiazepines suggests that these drugs should be reserved for short courses of no longer than 4 weeks to alleviate acute conditions [28]. There has been a focus on reducing benzodiazepine use over the past 25 years, and while interventions have had some success [60], the inappropriate use continues to rise in many jurisdictions, especially in long-term use, with one study finding 50% of new prescriptions were for 4 weeks or longer [42,61]. This is particularly concerning in older individuals, who are more vulnerable to the neurological adverse effects and in whom use is associated with least a 50% increase in the risk of a hip fracture. Older adults should rarely be prescribed benzodiazepines/Z-drugs [62], but prescribing in this age group is still prevalent, especially in those who are residents of long-term care facilities [52,63].

The use of Z-drugs, which were originally marketed as a safer alternative to benzodiazepines, has also increased substantially since their introduction in the late 1980s. One example of this is demonstrated by the use in the United Kingdom, where zopiclone is now the most commonly prescribed hypnotic [53,63,64].

Psychoanaleptics: antidepressants and psychostimulants

Antidepressants were introduced in the late 1950s. Their use was relatively limited, in part due to the poor side-effect profiles of older agents (e.g. amitriptyline and imipramine), until the 1980s, when selective serotonin reuptake inhibitors (SSRIs) were introduced. Antidepressants are now used in the treatment of an increasingly wide array of medical syndromes, including depression, anxiety disorders, nocturnal enuresis, chronic pain, eating disorders and Tourette's syndrome. SSRIs (e.g. citalopram, sertraline, escitalopram, fluoxetine and paroxetine) are the most commonly prescribed class of antidepressants. They are used as a first-line treatment for depression, over the older classes (i.e. TCAs and monoamine oxidase inhibitors (MAOIs)), as they have less extensive adverse effects and are less likely to be harmful if taken in an overdose [65,66]. The efficacy of SSRIs in treating depression is not necessarily greater than that of the older antidepressants, however, and their onset of action is similar [66]. The initiation and monitoring of antidepressant treatment occurs in both primary and specialty care. Treatment duration depends upon the indication. Gradual discontinuation of antidepressant treatment is recommended, especially when patients have been treated long-term, to avoid withdrawal symptoms.

Psychostimulants are among the oldest, most researched and most widely used drugs in psychiatry. They were first used in clinical practice for behavioural disorders in children in 1937 and became the mainstay of treatment for those conditions in the 1960s. Randomized clinical trials have consistently shown positive effects for psychostimulants, such as amphetamines and methylphenidate, as well as the nonstimulant atomoxetine, in reducing the core symptoms of attention deficit hyperactive disorder (ADHD) in children [67] and young to middle-aged adults [68]. Data on drug efficacy in older patients and on long-term outcomes of drug treatment are, however, lacking [69,70]. Other indications for psychostimulants include narcolepsia (modafinil) and, in some instances, depression and fatigue. Short-acting psychostimulant formulations (e.g. Ritalin, Equasym XL and Amfetamin) have a duration of action of up to a few hours and require multiple daily doses. More recently, long-acting or extended-release formulations (e.g. Concerta, Ritalin LA and Adderall XR) have been marketed. Issues of adherence and abuse seem to be less frequent with these products [71]. Atomoxetine, while classified as a psychostimulant, is in fact a specific noradrenergic reuptake inhibitor. It is indicated for individuals who do not tolerate or do not respond well to stimulants and for those with comorbidities, including substance abuse [71,72].

The initiation of psychostimulant treatment is usually the prerogative of specialists in outpatient settings (e.g. child and adolescent or general psychiatrists and paediatricians), but follow-up treatment may be monitored by family physicians or general practitioners. Combined treatment of psychostimulants with other psychotropic drugs, such as antidepressants and antipsychotics, is relatively common in individuals with ADHD [73], especially those dealing with comorbidities.

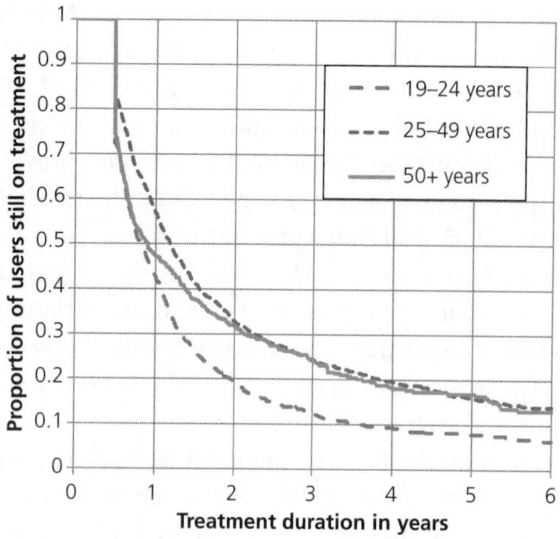

Figure 28.4 Duration of ADHD drug treatment among the total adult population of Iceland (2003–12) according to age at time of treatment start. Treatment was considered terminated when 180 days had passed without an ADHD drug prescription fill.

Source: Data from the Nationwide Medicines Registry in Iceland.

Early discontinuation and/or nonadherence to psychostimulant treatment is relatively common and may be related to factors such as adverse effects, lack of treatment response, societal stigma associated with the use of stimulants and the patient's underlying ADHD or psychiatric comorbidities [74–76]. Figure 28.4 shows that only about half of all new adult psychostimulant users in Iceland were still receiving treatment 1 year after prescription; after 5 years, only 8–17%, depending on age group, were still on treatment [77].

Psychotimulants are generally well tolerated, but common adverse effects include decreased appetite, insomnia, headache and stomach ache [67]. Approximately 20–30% of patients with ADHD experience adverse drug effects or a lack of treatment response [68,78]. Unresolved safety issues such as cardiovascular risk and sudden death [79,80] have kindled controversy over their use. More recent evidence, however, indicates that current use of psychostimulants is not associated with an increased risk of serious cardiovascular events [81].

Characteristics of patients using psychoanaleptics

Depression and anxiety disorders are the primary indications for antidepressants. Depression is a broad and heterogeneous condition, characterized by depressed mood and/or loss of pleasure in most activities, resulting in impairment in multiple areas of functioning. It affects individuals of all ages, ethnicities and socioeconomic circumstances and is a leading cause of medical disability [82]. The natural history of depressive disorders can be remitting–relapsing, with episodes lasting anywhere from months to years. The lifetime risk for major depressive disorder ranges from 5 to 12% for men and from 10 to 25% for women, with an estimated 1-month point prevalence of 2–3% for men and 5–9% for women, occurring at higher rates during and after pregnancy [83,84]. In older adulthood, depressive and anxiety disorders commonly co-occur with neurological disorders, such as dementia and Parkinson's disease, as well as with other chronic illnesses [85,86]. Only a few antidepressants (e.g. sertraline, fluoxetine and fluvoxamine) are currently labelled for use in children; these are indicated to treat major depressive disorder, OCD and enuresis. A number of antidepressants are prescribed off-label to both adults and children, however.

Psychostimulants have mainly been used to treat symptoms of ADHD. ADHD is a neurodevelopmental disorder, characterized by behavioural symptoms of inattention, hyperactivity and impulsivity. The prevalence of the disorder is estimated to be 5–10% among school-aged children, boys being about three to four times more likely than girls to be diagnosed [87]. In recent years, adults have increasingly been diagnosed with ADHD, with an estimated prevalence of 2–4%, and with a smaller gender difference than is found among children [69,88]. In general, the use of psychostimulants reflects the underlying epidemiology of ADHD, although use has been shown to vary considerably between countries and geographic areas, as well as with socioeconomic status, ethnicity and children's relative age in class [87,89–92]. Unlike most other psychotropic drugs, psychostimulants have mainly been used in the treatment of children, with prescribing to adults mostly off-label. However, atomoxetine recently became the first classified psychostimulant to be approved for the treatment of ADHD in adults, and since then a few other psychostimulants have followed.

Drug utilization of psychoanaleptics

The use of antidepressants is widespread. An increased awareness of the nature of depression and the development and marketing of new drugs (e.g. SSRIs in the

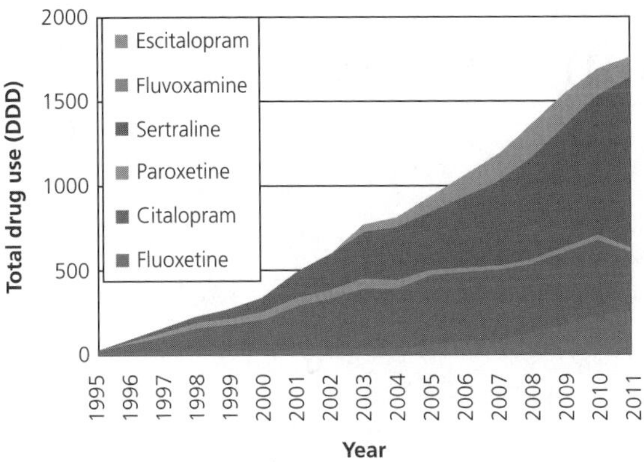

Figure 28.5 Total use of SSRIs, measured in DDDs and specified by drug substance and year, among the total paediatric population (5–18 years) in Denmark in 1995–2011. For colour details, please refer to the colour plates section.

Source: Pottegård et al. 2014 [101]. Reproduced with permission from Springer Science and Business Media.

1980s) have contributed to an enormous growth in their prevalence worldwide [65]. It is debatable whether this development has succeeded in reducing the overall burden of depressive disorders [93]. In 2011, antidepressants were the most commonly prescribed drugs in the U.S. followed by lipid regulators [94]. Data suggest the overuse of antidepressants, but underuse has also been demonstrated. In fact, while the proportion of antidepressants prescribed without a psychiatric diagnosis seems to be growing [95], only about half of patients with major depressive disorder receive medical care [96].

The prescribing of SSRIs in children became the subject of controversy with the publication of several studies in 2003–04 that linked the use of SSRIs to suicidal thoughts and behaviour in youth [97]. Warnings and new guidelines were issued by several regulatory authorities (e.g. in the U.S. and Europe). The association between suicide and antidepressants is complex, however, and to date, data are not conclusive [98,99]. Figure 28.5 shows the growing use of SSRIs, measured as number of dispensed defined daily doses (DDDs), among the Danish paediatric population [100].

In parallel with the increasing prevalence of ADHD diagnosis in both children and adults, the use of psychostimulants has grown notably over the past 2 decades [101–103]. Nevertheless, not all individuals diagnosed with ADHD receive or benefit from psychostimulant treatment. National survey data from the U.S. indicate that, in 2007–11, two-thirds of children with ADHD were being treated for ADHD [89]. Concerns about the growing use of psychostimulants, in relation to overuse, abuse and uncertain long-term outcomes, are widespread. Recent evidence indicates that psychostimulant treatment may provide a protective effect against development of substance abuse [104]. In addition, it seems to lower the risk of criminality [105] and accidents [106] among individuals with ADHD. On the other hand, misuse and abuse of psychostimulants is a pronounced and growing problem in many communities, especially among students and young adults, who use them to enhance academic performance or for recreation purposes [107]. Thus, clinicians need to remain highly alert to the potential problem of misuse and diversion when prescribing psychostimulants.

Conclusion

Psychotropic drugs constitute one of many therapeutic options to be considered in the treatment of mental health conditions and pain. Considerable and growing proportions of individuals worldwide are currently using these drugs, with many studies reporting overuse, inappropriate use and misuse. Differences in the utilization of this heterogeneous group of drugs are not surprising, as wide variations exist between health care systems around the world, particularly when focusing on mental health [108].

Given the serious burden of pain and mental health conditions on those affected, their families and society, the promotion of optimal treatment and rational use of psychotropic drugs is of major public health importance. Drug utilization studies serve as important tools in describing patterns of psychotropic drug use across population demographic and health conditions, geographical areas and calendar time, and may, as such, enhance health policies, leading to increased overall treatment success.

CHAPTER 29

Drug utilization research in the area of biologicals

Carlo Piccinni[1], Luigi Naldi[2] & Martin Neovius[3]

[1]*Pharmacology Unit, Department of Medical and Surgical Sciences, University of Bologna, Italy*

[2]*Unità Complessa di Dermatologia, Azienda Ospedaliera Papa Giovanni XXIII and Centro Studi GISED (Italian Group for Epidemiologic Research in Dermatology), Italy*

[3]*Clinical Epidemiology Unit, Department of Medicine, Karolinska Institutet, Sweden*

KEY POINTS

- Biologicals are a heterogeneous group of drugs, including antibodies and fusion proteins, that specifically target immunological pathways relevant to the pathogenesis of immune-related diseases.
- Patient registries are systematic collections of information on (all) cases of a particular disease or other health-relevant conditions. Data obtained from registries may be useful in understanding drug use in clinical practice.
- Experience of using registry data for drug utilization analyses is still limited. Registries may represent an important tool in promoting the appropriateness of biological use and in obtaining additional information on the risk–benefit profile of biologicals.
- Future harmonization of study procedures and standardization of registry data will allow data pooling and combined analyses.

Introduction

The term 'biologicals' refers to a heterogeneous group of antibodies and fusion proteins that directly target specific steps in the purported immunologic process. Unlike traditional small molecules, which can penetrate the cell membrane and have a broad spectrum of activities, biologicals remain outside the cell and modulate specific functions of the immune system. Therefore, these drugs are used in various disorders involving the immune system, such as autoimmune diseases and cancers (see Chapter 30). Given the specific features of these agents and their high costs (biosimilars now have been introduced in many countries but their 'reduced' price is still expensive), drug utilization research could provide important information concerning the characteristics of subjects receiving biologicals and the impact of these products on health system resources.

The Agency for Healthcare Research and Quality (AHRQ) defines a patient registry as 'an organized system that uses [an] observational study method to collect uniform data (clinical and other) to evaluate specific outcomes for a population defined by a particular disease, condition, or exposure, and that serves one or more predetermined scientific, clinical, or policy purpose[s]' [1]. If the inclusion of patients into a registry is based on diagnosis, we call it a disease registry; if it is based on exposure to a certain drug/product, we call it a drug (or product) registry (see Chapter 4). Register(s) and registry(ies) are synonym terms and are used alternately through the chapter.

Patient registries can be used for various purposes: to observe natural disease history, to understand variations in treatment and outcomes, to monitor long-term safety and harm, to describe the care patterns (including appropriateness of care) and to examine factors that influence prognosis and quality of life [2]. Therefore, a registry can be useful as a bridge to the efficacy–effectiveness gap resulting from randomized controlled trials (RCTs), as argued by Eichler et al. [3]. Generally, disease

Drug Utilization Research: Methods and Applications, First Edition. Edited by M. Elseviers et al.
Published 2016 by John Wiley & Sons, Ltd.

Box 29.1 Registries as a source of observational data. Usage of different stakeholders.

- Professional organizations can use registries to assess adherence to evidence-based treatment guidelines and approved indications or to compare clinicians' prescribing patterns.
- Policy makers/payers (i.e. health insurers) can establish reimbursement policies by using registry information on how procedures, devices or pharmaceuticals are actually used and on their effectiveness in different populations. Drug approval bodies (e.g. the European Medicines Agency (EMA) or the US Food and Drug Administration (FDA)) can use data on the long-term safety and effectiveness of drugs to make decisions.
- Drug or device manufacturers can promote registry-based studies to demonstrate product performance in clinical practice or to identify patient populations that will be useful for product development, clinical trial design and patient recruitment.
- Physicians can incorporate safety data derived from registries into electronic health records (EHRs) in order to flag patients at risk of adverse effects, supporting their decision-making process.

and related outcomes are collected rapidly for a large number of patients, thereby producing a real-life picture of the natural history of a disease, of current treatment practices and of outcomes. Some uses of registry data for different stakeholders are given in Box 29.1.

In summary, the potential of registries is very high, and in the future these tools will probably enable us to overcome the limitations of RCTs, as suggested by some authors [4] after the publication of results deriving from the first registry randomized clinical trial (RRCT), conducted in Sweden in 2013 [5]. In this scenario, patient registries – in addition to representing an important tool in promoting the appropriateness of drug use – will allow additional information to be acquired on the risk–benefit profile of a given drug. In fact, theoretically, a registry should function as a support system to increase the number of patients who benefit from a given therapy and, concurrently, to reduce the population experiencing unfavourable effects or missing benefits (Figure 29.1).

In order to underline the importance of these tools and their differences from electronic health records (EHRs), this chapter is divided into four parts: the first three describe the impact of registries in different diseases, while the last concerns the potential uses and pitfalls of registries in drug utilization research. As registries are created primarily to monitor the use, safety and effectiveness of biologicals, we focus on this drug class and related drug utilization data. The diseases we discuss are multiple sclerosis (MS), rheumatoid arthritis (RA) and psoriasis, as the advent of biologicals has radically changed the treatment strategies in these diseases and a large proportion of patients have been started on biologicals.

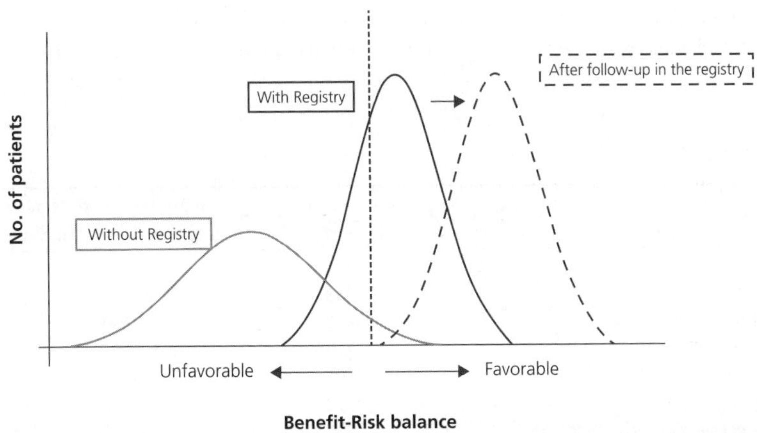

Figure 29.1 Theoretical influence of registries in promoting the appropriateness of drug use. The presence of a registry should enable the population with the best risk–benefit balance (black line) to be selected, rather than a population with a poor one (grey line). On follow-up (dashed line), subjects reporting a more favourable benefit-risk profile should be identified.

Source: Courtesy of Dr Nello Martini, Research & Development Director of the National Academy of Medicine (Accedemia Nazionale di Medica), Italy.

Multiple sclerosis

MS is an autoimmune disease of the central nervous system. In 2013, approximately 2.3 million people were affected by MS around the world, and it is the most common cause of neurological disability in young adults (30–40 years old), especially women (2 : 1 ratio of women to men). Reported incidence and prevalence vary considerably across regions and populations and over time [6]. Two distinct disease-modifying drug (DMD) groups are used in the treatment of MS: biologicals (beta-interferons, glatimarer acetate, natalizumab, ocrelizumab, ofatumumab, alemtuzimab and daclizumab) and small molecules (fingolimod, liquinimod, teriflunomide and dimethyl fumarate). A number of new drugs have recently been approved or are about to be launched [7]. On the one hand, this increases therapeutic options, but on the other, it poses new challenges for the continuous/long-term and safe use of these drugs. The majority of this new therapeutic arsenal consists of biologicals: the first line of treatment consists in beta-interferons and glatiramer acetate, while natalizumab is among the second-line agents.

Patient registries and related drug utilization research

A number of national databases have been developed to improve our knowledge of MS, such as the Danish MS Registry, the Swedish MS Registry and the Italian MS Database [8,9]. International databases also exist, such as the European Database for MS (EDMUS) [10] and the MSBase Registry [11]. An overview of some of the available databases and their characteristics is presented in Table 29.1. All are disease registries, and all collect data on the clinical course and therapeutic history of patients with MS.

The literature contains several examples of drug utilization studies performed using MS registries (see examples in Table 29.2). These provide a detailed pattern of DMD use, with information on (i) initiation of therapy, (ii) switching among different drugs, (iii) adherence/persistence of therapy (see Section F) and (iv) discontinuation of therapy. Moreover, correlating the sociodemographic and clinical characteristics of patients entered into a registry with information on their treatment history allows possible predictors of treatment choice and modification of therapy to be identified.

A number of drug registries have also been developed recently, mainly for natalizumab, which requires strict monitoring due to safety concerns and its high cost. The history of natalizumab (see Box 29.2) demonstrates the usefulness of registries in investigating and improving drug use in MS. In 2006, natalizumab was approved by the European Medicines Agency (EMA) as monotherapy in highly active relapsing–remitting MS for (i) patients with high disease activity despite treatment with beta-interferon and (ii) patients with rapidly evolving severe relapsing–remitting MS. Subsequently, the Italian Medicine Agency (AIFA) founded the Italian neurological expert panel, which established more restrictive criteria for dispensing and reimbursing natalizumab and developed a national Web-based registry for monitoring its use

Table 29.1 Multiple sclerosis (MS) registries.

Registry	Start	Number of patients at latest available update	Reference
National EU registries			
Danish MS Registry	1948	>20 000	[12]
Norwegian National MS Registry	1998	>3000	[13]
Swedish National MS Registry	1997	>12 000	[14]
Italian MS Database Network (MSDN)	2001	>5000	[15]
German MS Registry	2002	>10 000	[8,16]
NARCOMS (North American Research Committee MS)	1996	>36 000	[17]
MS Ontario (Canada) database	1972	>1000	[18]
British Columbia (Canada) MS Database	1980	>6000	[19]
International registries			
EDMUS (European Database for MS)	1990	>30 000	[20]
MSBase Registry	2004	>29 000	[21]

Table 29.2 Drug utilization studies of biologicals and other disease-modifying drugs (DMDs) in MS.

Reference	Focus	Design
Jokubaitis 2013 [22]	Treatment persistence and predictors of treatment discontinuation and switching	Longitudinal observational study using the MSBase Registry
Fox 2013 [17]	Patient-reported reasons for discontinuation of injectable disease-modifying therapy	Cross-sectional study using the NARCOMS database
Wong 2011 [23]	Adherence to various disease-modifying therapies	Historic cohort study using the MS Ontario database
Sorensen 2006 [24]	Use of immune-modulatory therapies in Denmark	Longitudinal observational study using the Danish MS Registry
Trojano 2009 [25]	The optimal time at which to initiate interferon (early versus delayed)	Prospective observational study using the Italian MS Database Network
Lebrun 2008 [26]	Different effects of disease-modifying therapies in patients according to their ethnic origins	Descriptive population-based study using EDMUS

and safety. This registry contains the following electronic forms: centre registration, patient registration, treatment eligibility, follow-up during therapy, drug withdrawal, adverse drug reaction (ADR) report and follow-up after drug withdrawal. In these forms, a number of sociodemographic, clinical and therapeutic characteristics can be collected (e.g. previous drugs, disability expressed as Expanded Disability Status Scale (EDSS) values, number of relapses, lesions on magnetic resonance imaging (MRI); see Table 29.3 for a complete list).

Box 29.2 The history of natalizumab.

> Natalizumab (Tysabri Biogen Idec) is a humanized antibody that blocks the transmigration of leukocytes form blood to the central nervous system [27]. In November 2004, the drug was approved [28–30] by the US Food and Drug Administration (FDA) for the treatment of relapsing–remitting MS on the basis of two phase III clinical trials (the AFFIRM trial [28] and the SENTINEL trial [31]). In February 2005, only 4 months after approval, natalizumab was withdrawn from the US market due to three reports of progressive multifocal leucoencephalopathy (PML) in patients receiving natalizumab in addition to other immunomodulatory/immunosuppressive drugs. In June 2006, natalizumab was resumed in the United States as monotherapy under a specific monitoring programme called TOUCH [32], in which patients treated with natalizumab are monthly evaluated for symptoms consistent with PML. In the same year, the European Medicines Agency (EMA) approved natalizumab on the basis of a post hoc subgroup analysis of the AFFIRM trial and established restrictive measures for risk minimization [33]. Based on a review of safety and efficacy data, natalizumab was approved in Europe as monotherapy in highly active relapsing–remitting MS for (i) patients with high disease activity despite treatment with beta-interferon and (ii) patients with rapidly evolving severe relapsing–remitting MS.

Analyses of the collected information are useful for various objectives. First, these data allow monitoring of adherence to specific criteria established by regulators. For example, natalizumab can be prescribed with reimbursement only in patients with relapsing–remitting MS, with restrictions in terms of EDSS values and number of MRI lesions, and with an adequate washout period after discontinuation of previous treatment. The latter is important in ensuring the safe use of the drug, as during RCTs, three patients receiving immunomodulatory/immunosuppressive treatments in addition to natalizumab were affected by progressive multifocal leucoencephalopathy (PML), a rare and a potentially fatal viral disease. Therefore, it is crucial to verify that subjects have discontinued previous treatment for a sufficient time before they start natalizumab treatment. Regarding safety, the registry allows the recording of data on adverse events and early identification of subjects with clinical parameters predictive of serious adverse events, such as PML and other undetected safety issues. In addition, since the PML risk increases with the number of infusions, particularly after 2 years of treatment [34], it is important to investigate the duration of therapy and any cause of discontinuation by analysing the patient's prescription history. For example, upon analysing data on 198 patients from the Emilia Romagna region entered in the Italian Registry from January 2007 to June 2010, it emerged that the frequency of interruption was low in the first 2 years of therapy, but that in the third year the rate of treatment discontinuation statistically increased [35] (Figure 29.2).

Table 29.3 Forms and required items of the Italian Natalizumab Registry.

Form	Items
Centre registration	Location, centre name, head physician, medical staff
Patient registration	Name and surname, gender, birth date and place
Treatment eligibility	MS onset date, MS diagnosis date, 12-month previous treatments, MS course, number of relapses in previous 12 months, relapses with clinical consequences, EDSS score (recorded at three points: start of therapy, before last relapse and 12 months before treatment start), number of MRI lesions (T_1 gadolinium enhanced and T_2), presence of infections, immunosuppression and immunodeficiency, white blood cell count, pregnancy, use of contraceptive methods, previous disease-modifying treatment (start and end date), other treatments
Drug (natalizumab) request	Request date, number of previous administrations, number of vials, date of first administration
Follow-up during therapy (filled in quarterly)	Follow-up date, patient status (alive, dead, lost to follow-up), change of MS course, number of relapses, relapse therapy, EDSS score, MRI lesions, natalizumab therapy (withdrawn or continuous), cause of death, date of death, ADRs
Drug withdrawal	Date of withdrawal, reason for withdrawal, number of administrations, switch to different DMT, death, cause of death
ADR report	Date of onset of ADR, clinical description, degree of severity, reaction outcome, clinical management, rechallenge, dechallenge, concomitant drugs, reporter information
Follow-up after drug withdrawal (filled in 6-monthly)	Date of withdrawal, reason for withdrawal, number of administrations, death, cause of death, date of death

MS, multiple sclerosis; EDSS, expanded disability status scale; MRI, magnetic resonance imaging; ADR, adverse drug reaction.

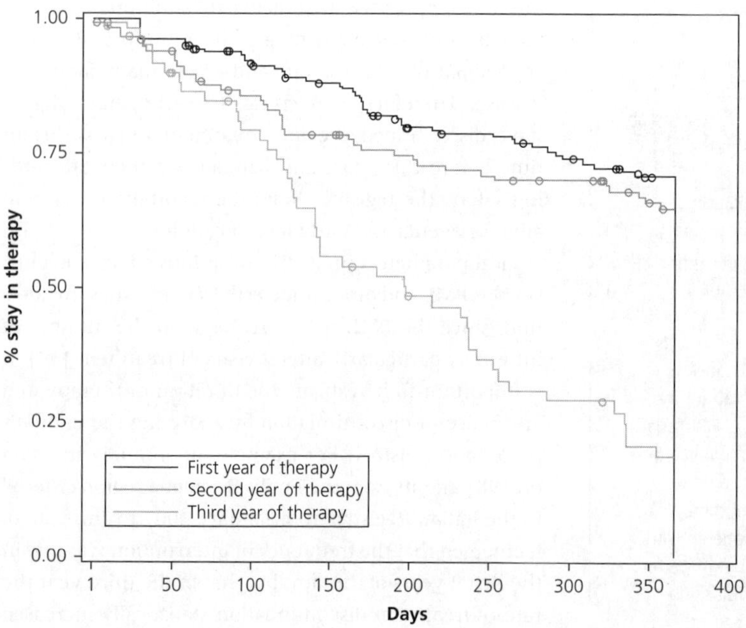

Figure 29.2 Duration of natalizumab treatment in a cohort of Italian patients in the Emilia Romagna region from January 2007 to June 2010. The three Kaplan–Meier curves refer to the entire cohort of patients observed in the three different years of therapy. The individual curves represent the duration of therapy during the first year (black), second year (dark grey) and third year (light grey).

Source: Data presented during the ISPE/EuroDURG meeting on Better Public Health through Pharmacoepidemiology and Quality Use of Medicine, 30 November—3 December 2011, Antwerp, Belgium [35].

Table 29.4 Comparison of patient characteristics between the Italian Natalizumab Registry (data extracted from Mancardi et al. 2011 [38]) and subjects assigned to treatment group in the AFFIRM trial [28].

	Italian Natalizumab Registry (n = 2554)		AFFIRM trial
Characteristics	**Group A (n = 2230)**	**Group B (n = 324)**	**Natalizumab group (n = 627)**
Age – years			
Mean	36.2	33.0	35.6
Gender – number of patients (%)			
Male	691 (31)	107 (33)	178 (28)
Female	1539 (69)	217 (67)	449 (72)
Disease duration – years (a = mean, b = median)			
	10[a]	5.3[a]	5.0[b]
Number of relapses in previous year – Number of patients (%)			
0	5 (<1)	0 (<1)	6 (<1)
1	301 (24)	2 (<1)	368 (59)
2	599 (47)	77 (52)	197 (32)
>=3	366 (29)	68 (46)	56 (9)
Missing data	6 (<1)	1 (<1)	
Mean	2.2	2.9	1.5
EDSS score			
Mean	3.5	3.5	2.3

Group A: patients not responding to beta interferons or glatiramer acetate.
Group B: patients with a rapidly evolving severe MS not treated previously with immunomodulating drugs.
EDSS, Expanded Disability Status Scale.

Second, the sociodemographic and clinical characteristics (duration of disease, baseline EDSS, number of relapses) of patients treated in clinical practice can be compared with those enrolled in RCTs [36–38] (Table 29.4).

Other registries established to collect information on MS patients treated with natalizumab include the Tysabri Observational Program [39], the Swedish Tysabri Registry (IMSE) [40] and the French Tysabri Registry (TYSEDMUS) [41]. Clinical data collected in these databases have been presented to the EMA in order to support the extension of indication for natalizumab [42] and to discuss the risk of PML (and other opportunistic infections) related to natalizumab [43], and probably to all monoclonal antibodies [44].

Rheumatoid arthritis

RA is a chronic inflammatory disease with an estimated worldwide prevalence of 0.1–1.0% [45]. The prevalence increases with age, and is two to four times higher in women than men, depending on age group [46].

Currently, there is no cure for RA, and until the 1990s treatment was focused on pain relief with antiinflammatory drugs. In the 1990s, synthetic disease-modifying antirheumatic drugs (DMARDs) were introduced, and towards the end of the 1990s biological DMARDs were introduced. These drugs have revolutionized treatment and changed the treatment goals from pain relief to inducing remission.

In RCTs, biological drugs have been shown to be more efficacious than monotherapy with methotrexate, a nonbiological DMARD that was previously the standard first-line treatment [47]. However, safety concerns still exist due to the immunomodulatory action of biologicals, with serious infections and certain malignancies at the top of the list [48]. Also, their cost is very high: approximately €10 000–15 000 per patient per year [49–51]. When introduced in the late 1990s, the use of biologicals was generally restricted to those patients with the most severe disease. Over time, however, they have been initiated in patients with less severe disease and earlier in the disease course [51] (Figure 29.3).

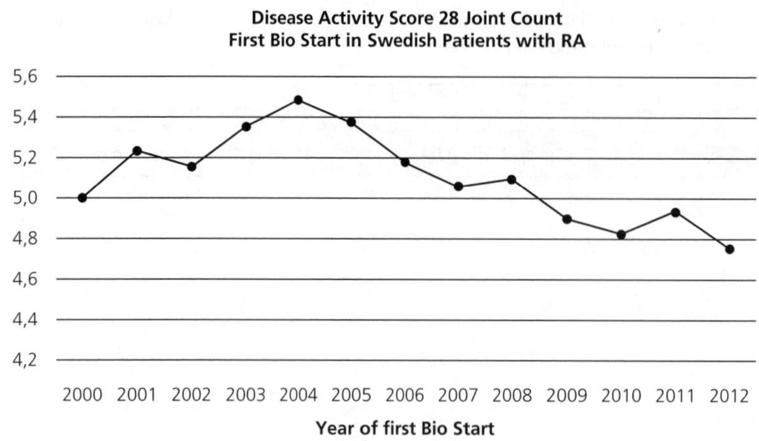

Figure 29.3 Age-standardized disease activity score 28 joint (DAS28) count at first biological start in Swedish patients with rheumatoid arthritis (RA).

Patient registries and related drug utilization research

Given the superior efficacy but uncertain long-term safety profile of biologicals compared to methotrexate monotherapy, several countries have started national or regional registries to monitor patients with RA treated with biologicals, including the United Kingdom, Germany, Spain, Switzerland and Denmark [52] (Table 29.5). These national registries share many similarities, but also tend to have some distinct features. All were started mainly for the purpose of monitoring safety, but several are now being used for effectiveness and health economic analyses.

Table 29.5 European rheumatology biological registries.

Country	Name	Type	Comparator
United Kingdom	BSRBR	Cohort study	DMARD cohort
Germany	RABBIT	Cohort study	DMARD cohort
Sweden	ARTIS	Routine registration	RA and admin registers
Spain	BIOBADASER	Cohort study	Historical RA cohort
Denmark	DANBIO	Routine registration	RA and admin registers
Norway	NOR-DMARD	Cohort study	DMARD starts
The Netherlands	DREAM	Cohort study	–
Switzerland	SCQM	Routine registration	DMARD patients
Czech Republic	ATTRA	Routine registration	DMARD patients

DMARD, disease-modifying antirheumatic drug; RA, rheumatoid arthritis.

From 1999, and before their market approval in 2000, tumour necrosis factor (TNF; formerly TNF-α) inhibitors could be prescribed in Sweden, but on license prescription [53]. This meant that doctors needed specific approval from the Medical Products Agency to prescribe them with reimbursement (only for named patients). Mainly due to safety concerns regarding serious infections and malignancies, prescribing doctors were obliged to enter all patients initiating treatment into the Anti-Rheumatic Treatment in Sweden (ARTIS) register, allowing patient characteristics, treatment, adverse events and clinical effectiveness to be followed. This was accomplished partly through information entered into the register by physicians, nurses and patients and partly through nationwide register linkage to other health registers kept by the Swedish National Board of Health and Welfare and other agencies (Figure 29.4). The ARTIS register has since been used extensively both for academic research and for regulatory follow-up. Even though it is no longer mandatory to enter data into the register, approximately 90% of all patients with RA on biologicals in Sweden are entered and monitored for effectiveness, safety and cost [54,55].

In addition to the ARTIS register, which was started and is still run by the profession (i.e. the Swedish Rheumatology Association), all prescription drugs dispensed in ambulatory care in Sweden can be tracked on a patient level in the nationwide Prescribed Drug Register, kept by the National Board of Health and Welfare [56] (Figure 29.4). Each dispensing can be tracked via

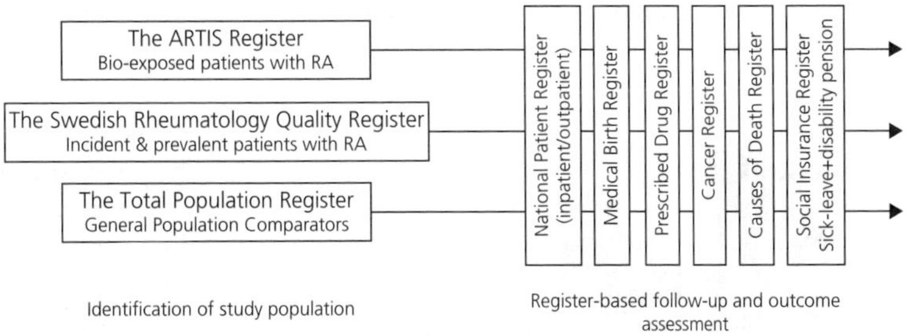

Figure 29.4 Nationwide health registry infrastructure for registry-based identification of patients and outcome assessment in patients with rheumatoid arthritis (RA).

this register, including date of prescription and dispensing, Anatomical Therapeutic Chemical (ATC) code, drug name and cost (total, out-of-pocket and reimbursed). However, a limitation of this registry from the perspective of biologicals is that infliximab and other infusion biologicals are mainly used as in-hospital drugs. This means that they are generally not dispensed from pharmacies directly to patients, but ordered at the department or clinic level and administered in inpatient care, and therefore not traceable via the Prescribed Drug Register [56]. This makes for a complementary interplay between the ARTIS registry and the Prescribed Drug Register: ARTIS contains a large number of patients treated with infusion biologicals that it is not possible to capture via the Prescribed Drug Register, while the Prescribed Drug Register adds some patients on non-infusion biologicals not covered by ARTIS. A third source of data on drug use is EHRs, which have been used in a pilot study in Stockholm county [57].

Through linkage of ARTIS data to, for example, the Swedish Cancer Register, the National Patient Register and the Causes of Death Register, adverse events such as malignancies, severe infections and deaths can be followed at low cost with virtually complete follow-up of all patients ever registered until death (or emigration; see Figure 29.4) [58–61]. Also, drug utilization and economic analyses can be performed using the same registry data infrastructure (Table 29.6).

In 2000, total TNF inhibitor sales in Sweden constituted 0.8% of prescription drug sales (including all indications, not just RA). This had increased to 5.0% by 2009 [62]. Determinants of use included sex, age and county of residence. In the prevalent RA patient population, women tended to be prescribed biologicals to a greater degree than men, although age was a much stronger determinant, with a fairly stable drug penetration in patients of working age but much lower use in the elderly (Figure 29.5). This may partly be explained by there

Table 29.6 Examples of drug utilization, safety and economic studies of biologicals in rheumatoid arthritis (RA) using the Swedish ARTIS registry.

Reference	Focus	Design
Eriksson et al. 2015 [63]	Costs of drugs, health care and work loss in prevalent and incident patients with RA	Cross-sectional and longitudinal observational study
Neovius et al. 2011 [46]	Penetration of biological and nonbiological DMARDs	Cross-sectional study
Neovius et al. 2015 [29]	Head-to-head comparison of drug survival on different biological drugs	Longitudinal observational study
Eriksson et al. 2013 [66]	Effect on work loss of biological versus non-biological therapy in early RA	Register-enriched RCT
Eriksson et al. 2015 [67]	Cost-effectiveness analysis of biological versus non-biological therapy in early RA	Register-enriched RCT
Askling et al. 2009 [30]	Lymphoma risk in patients with RA treated with biologicals	Longitudinal observational study
Neovius et al. 2011 [62]	Small-area variation in use of biologicals	Cross-sectional study

RCT, randomized controlled trial.

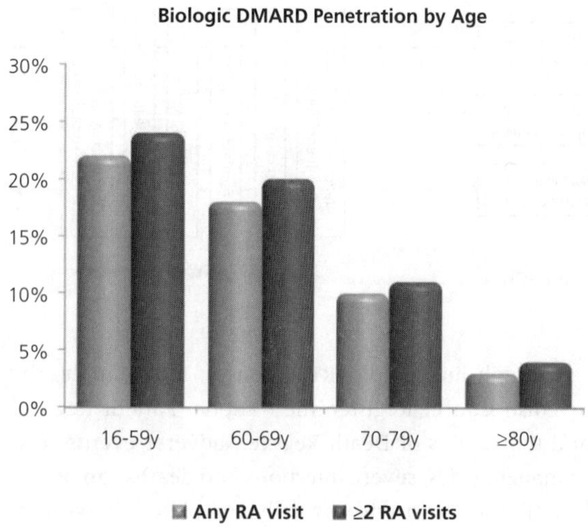

Figure 29.5 Biological disease-modifying antirheumatoid drug (DMARD) penetration by age in Swedish prevalent patients in 2008 with rheumatoid arthritis (RA), based on two register-based definitions (any visit listing an RA diagnosis versus at least two visits listing an RA diagnosis)[46].

being more contraindications for the use of biologicals (e.g. malignancies, severe infections) in elderly patients. It may, however, also reflect health economic considerations, as the productivity gains in working-age patients are likely greater. Furthermore, younger patients usually have shorter disease durations and therefore potentially less permanent joint damage, which means that disease remission is a realistic treatment target.

In terms of variations by county of residence, a twofold difference in biological drug penetration in the RA population has been described in Sweden [62]. This small-area variation remains when restricting the analysis to the three largest counties, where small numbers and chance have less impact on biological drug penetration estimates. These variations are likely to be largely explained by different policies (through different interpretation of national treatment guidelines) for biological drug use in the respective counties.

Although the ARTIS register and similar biological drug registries in other countries have mainly been used for follow-up of adverse events, the nationwide registries available in Sweden also provide opportunities to monitor economic consequences [63,64,67] (Table 29.6). For example, costs of inpatient and non-primary outpatient care can be followed via the National Patient Register, which includes visit and discharge dates, main and contributory diagnoses and surgical procedures. Drug costs, for both antirheumatic drugs and all other prescription drugs, can be followed via linkage to the Prescribed Drug Register, while data on sick leave and disability pensions can be collected from the Social Insurance Agency [63] (Figure 29.4).

Specific interest has been given to productivity losses in RA in relation to the high cost of TNF inhibitor treatment and the fact that work loss constitutes the greatest cost in patients with RA [63]. The high treatment cost is sometimes justified by the positive effect on work loss and reductions in health care and other drug use. Long-term observational and randomized data on the consequences of TNF inhibitor treatment for work loss and health care costs are scarce.

At present, there is a growing interest in the comparison of TNF inhibitor treatment with synthetic DMARD combination treatment, both for efficacy and for economic outcomes [65, 68–70]. Most trials have compared TNF inhibitors with methotrexate monotherapy and not combination DMARD therapy, which has been shown to result in better efficacy and work loss outcomes than mono-DMARD therapy [71,72]. Combining the strengths of RCTs, patient registries and nationwide registries, a recent randomized trial was conducted using The Swedish Rheumatology Quality Register as a platform and building upon it with economic outcome data on drug and health care use, as well as work loss, collected from nationwide registries [66–68]. The registry-enriched randomized SWEFOT trial showed similar work loss and quality of life outcomes over 2 years, but markedly higher drug costs in the TNF inhibitor treatment arm compared to the combination DMARD arm.

Psoriasis

Psoriasis is a chronic inflammatory skin condition with an immune-related pathogenesis and a genetic background that may be triggered by several environmental factors, such as smoking. Psoriasis affects about 2–3% of the general population, with about 15–20% of patients suffering from moderate to severe psoriasis needing systemic therapy or phototherapy. Treatment options are traditionally classified into topicals, ultraviolet light-based (or phototherapy) and systemic agents, the latter including conventional and so-called 'targeted' therapies, which are mainly represented by biologicals [73]. The biologicals currently used to treat psoriasis belong to three major groups: antagonists of TNF and antagonists of the p40 subunit of interleukins (ILs) 12 and 23 and antagonists of IL-17.

Inhibition of TNF can be achieved using a monoclonal antibody such as infliximab or adalimumab or with a circulating receptor fusion protein such as etanercept. The only antagonist of the p40 subunit of ILs-12 and -23 currently available is the antibody ustekinumab and secukinumab is the first antagonist of IL17 to enter the market. Although the introduction of biologicals was a significant advance in the management of psoriasis, their place in the hierarchy of systemic therapies is not exactly defined, partly because they are expensive: depending on the drug and the dose, they can cost from $10 000 to $30 000 a year. In Europe, most of the biologicals are approved for the treatment of patients with moderate to severe chronic plaque psoriasis for whom phototherapy or conventional systemic treatments have been inadequate or inappropriate. Only secukinumab has been approved as a "first line" therapy. In the United States, the indications include, broadly, patients with moderate to severe plaque psoriasis who are candidates for systemic therapy or phototherapy.

Patient registries and related drug utilization research

Registries of psoriasis patients treated systemically are active at local, regional, national and international levels. A collaboration among some of these registries is ongoing, in the so-called 'Psonet collaboration' (Table 29.7).

An example of a national disease registry is the Italian Psocare registry, promoted by the AIFA and managed in collaboration with the main Italian dermatological societies and patient associations [75]. The innovative aspects of this project are its promotion directly by a governmental body (i.e. AIFA), its restriction of the prescribing of biological drugs to a predefined network of psoriasis reference centres (i.e. the Psocare centres) and its registration of all patients receiving a first-ever prescription of a new systemic agent, including conventional and biological drugs. The objectives in setting up this registry were: (i) to assess patterns of drug use in clinical practice; (ii) to evaluate and compare the long-term outcomes of different systemic treatments, with particular interest in patients not eligible for enrolment in RCTs (e.g. patients with comorbidities, children, pregnant women) and to identify groups at high risk for adverse events; and (iii) to assess the application of clinical guidelines in practice and to identify areas of uncertainty as a starting point for future research. Unfortunately, after 2010, the Psocare project was temporarily suspended, with the AIFA expressing a desire to change it from a disease registry to a series of individual drug registries [76].

In addition to academic registries, company-driven registries also exist. One example is the Psolar registry, which focuses on the safety of infliximab and ustekinumab compared with other biologicals and with conventional treatment for psoriasis. The Psolar registry is expected to enrol and follow up a total of 12 000 patients [77].

At this stage, only limited data are being published by psoriasis registries, since data collection and follow-up are still limited (see Table 29.8). Analyses of the Spanish BIOBADA-

Table 29.7 Registries participating in the Psonet collaboration.
Source: Data from Ormerod et al. [74].

Country	Registry	Year started	Number of patients on biological (as of January 2010)
Australia	Australian Psoriasis Registry	2008	130
Denmark	DermBio	2007	1200
France	PSOBIOTEQ	2012	Not available
Germany	PsoBest	2008	540
Israel	Clalit Health Service registry	2007	≈500
Italy	Psocare	2005	≈8300
Spain	BIOBADADERM	2008	510
Sweden	PsoReg	2007	≈580
Switzerland	SDNTT	2011	Not available
The Netherlands	PRESTON	2005	140

Table 29.8 Examples of registry-based and other types of drug utilization study in psoriasis.

Reference	Focus	Design
Carretero et al. 2015 [79]	Comparison of the safety of biologicals with that of classic systemic treatment	Prospective observational cohort study (Spanish BIOBADADERM registry)
Svedbom et al. 2015 [80]	Estimation of drug persistence, switching and augmentation and of insufficient treatment result in psoriasis patients	Observational longitudinal cohort study (Swedish administrative registers)
Ahlehoff et al. 2014 [81]	Examination of the rate of cardiovascular events in patients with severe psoriasis treated with systemic antiinflammatory drugs	Observational longitudinal cohort study (Danish administrative registries)
Gisondi et al. 2014 [82]	Estimation of the nationwide prevalence of latent tuberculosis infection in psoriatic patients candidate to a systemic treatment	Observational longitudinal cohort study (Italian Psocare registry)
Papp et al. 2015 [83]	Evaluation of the incidence of various adverse events of interest in psoriasis treatment	Observational longitudinal cohort study (PSOLAR multicentral registry)
Augustin et al. 2012 [84]	Profiling of treatment received by 34 728 insured patients diagnosed with psoriasis in Germany, plus cost assessment	Cross-sectional analysis of prescription data
Lebwohl et al. 2014 [85]	Comparison of treatment received by a random sample of 3426 people with a confirmed diagnosis of psoriasis in North America and Europe	Telephone survey of treatment received
Armstrong et al. 2013 [86]	Analysis of trends in prescriptions of systemic therapies for psoriasis in 5604 patients with psoriasis or psoriatic arthritis, surveyed by the National Psoriasis Foundation USA	Analysis of data from a series of cross-sectional studies conducted from 2003 to 2011
Ragnarson Tennvall et al. 2013 [87]	Comparison of prescriptions of systemic therapies for psoriasis in 404 patients attending dermatological services in Scandinavian countries	Cross-sectional analysis of prescription data

DERM registry have shown that patients ineligible for RCTs make up an important proportion (30%) of those receiving systemic therapy for psoriasis. These patients have a higher risk of severe adverse events. Moreover, the risk–benefit ratio in ineligible patients receiving biologicals may be different from that in eligible patients [78].

Interestingly, a pooled analysis of data from registries participating in the Psonet collaboration (n = 20 232 patients) showed large between-country heterogeneity in the clinical profiles of treated patients and in access to treatment [88]. Percentages of patients with moderate to severe psoriasis at the beginning of therapy ranged from 10.0% in Australia to 40.7% in Spain for conventional systemic drug therapy and from 0.5% in Australia to 31.8% in Germany for biologicals. The percentage of patients with arthritis in the registry ranged from 13% in Spain to 39% in Australia. Data on previous therapy before starting the drug prescribed at entry, reflecting cumulative therapy at a given time point in the disease course, also showed large differences, with the percentage of patients who received biologicals as a first-line systemic therapy ranging from 0% in the Netherlands to 35.5% in Italy. Variability in the history of previous therapy was much larger than variability in the characteristics of patients likely to influence the selection of therapy.

Besides being useful in analysing heterogeneity in prescription patterns, registries can help identify non-responders and possible determinants of poor response to treatment. Data from the Psocare registry in Italy show that being overweight or obese affects early clinical response to systemic treatment, irrespective of the systemic treatment being administered, suggesting the importance of adopting a more holistic approach to the management of psoriasis [89]. Analyses of data from the Psocare registry also indicate that clinical response in patients who switch from one anti-TNF agent to another is significantly reduced when the switching is due to a primary inefficacy of the first anti-TNF [90].

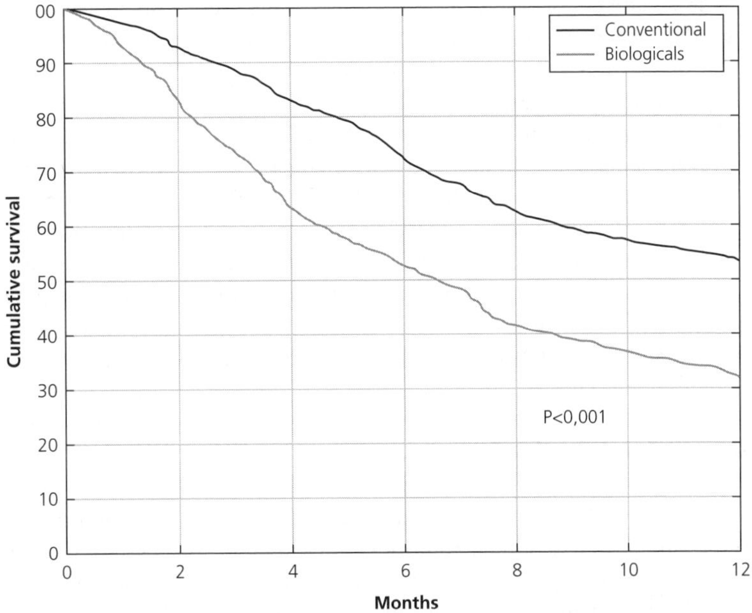

Figure 29.6 Kaplan–Meier curves of patients starting a conventional (n = 13 017) versus a biological (n = 7034) drug for psoriasis. Patients were followed up for the first 12 months after starting treatment and were removed from the study upon shift to another drug or drug withdrawal.

Drug 'survival' (i.e. persistence of drug use) can also be assessed using registries. In the Psocare registry, follow-up data up to week 52 after entry show that drug persistence is better for biologicals than for conventional treatment (see Figure 29.6).

Registries enable outcomes to be tracked and compared across different treatment groups. For example, a comparison by Fonia et al. [91] showed hospitalization rates per year were reduced in patients receiving biologicals (0.1%) as compared conventional treatment (0.5%).

Safety concerns can influence prescription of biologicals, particularly as they relate to infection defence mechanisms and cancer immune surveillance. Safety data are derived from a variety of sources, including systematic reviews of RCTs [92] and registry data [74].

Registry data do not necessarily have to cover large populations. If clinical information is combined with carefully obtained biological data, such as serological markers or human leukocyte antigen (HLA) phenotyping, based on a specific, clearly defined hypothesis, then even a small sample size will be informative. A good example of such an approach is the documentation of the prognostic value of antibodies against adalimumab in patients treated with this drug. In a study involving 80 patients, the presence of such antibodies strongly correlated with adalimumab blood concentration and greatly influenced clinical response [93].

Potentials and pitfalls of using registries in drug utilization research

The strengths and weaknesses of biologicals registries vary both by country and by registry design. Countries differ in their health data infrastructure, possibilities for linkage between different registries and the design and content of national clinical registries. This section highlights some important aspects of registry coverage, duration of follow-up, scope of data collection and possibilities for registry linkage.

Registry coverage

The patient population coverage of a registry (i.e. how complete is the registration of patients by clinicians) is important whether it is used as a data source in its own right or to enrich other data sources. Patient population coverage refers both to the actual pool of patients with a certain disease/treatment captured in the registry [54,55] and to the degree of long-term follow-up (if the registry is focused on a chronic disease, which biologicals registries tend to be). Coverage analyses should be performed routinely and regularly, although this is difficult in many countries due to a lack of nationwide registries (prescriptions, health care contacts, residency/death) that can be used to benchmark patients in the patient registry versus the real number of treated patients.

It is of interest to record drug coverage in disease registries, as different biologicals can be captured in different databases, which may be used to complement one another (see the section on RA for an example, as well as the linkage section later in the chapter).

For chronic diseases, the duration of follow-up should be lifelong and should include not only data on the specific disease and disease activity, but also data on comorbid conditions and events which may be related to the disease or its treatment. Linkage to data on work loss and other social outcomes may be of interest to both patients and other stakeholders, such as pricing and reimbursement agencies.

Scope of data collection

Most data are entered into a registry by physicians, but some can be collected by patient questionnaires. Due to the administrative burden and risk of questionnaire fatigue, most registries limit the volume and detail of data collected at the clinical encounter. Additionally, questionnaire data can be problematic, as patients may not know or remember their exact diagnoses in other health care contacts, or which specific drugs (and doses) they use. Such data may be better collected via nationwide registries of health care contacts and prescription drugs. Missing data is another common obstacle associated with questionnaires: a problem that may be circumvented by linkage to nationwide registries. Incomplete coverage over time is yet another problem that can make questionnaire-based data suboptimal for research use. Some data must be collected from the patient, however: patient-reported outcomes, such as health-related quality of life, can usually not be found in any national register. Health-related quality of life is not only important in its own right, but can also be used in economic evaluations for pricing and reimbursement agencies.

Registry linkage possibilities

Countries with well developed health data infrastructure, such as Denmark, Finland and Sweden, have several major advantages over those that lack such infrastructure on a nationwide scale. Advantages pertain to both research questions and data quality assessments, as well as to analyses of registry coverage.

Using registry linkage, researchers can enrich their own patient registry (which ideally will contain highly granular clinical data) with nationwide and virtually complete data on dispensed prescription drugs, in- and outpatient health services, cancer and mortality [53].

Linkage allows both cross-sectional and longitudinal analyses to be performed (e.g. on drug utilization, costs, off-label use and adverse events). Such analyses can be carried out both forward in time to assess the course of treatment and backward to investigate changes/patterns of drug or health care use before diagnosis or treatment intensification. The follow-up is also lifelong, or until a patient emigrates (which can be ascertained via national registers in some countries).

Registry linkage is not confined to observational research designs, but can be used for outcome assessment in randomized trials [4,5,66, 67].

The validity of data collected from nationwide registries may need to be confirmed through random selection of a number of medical records or, when analysing rare outcomes, deliberate extraction of all medical records for patients with the specific outcome [94].

Conclusion

Biological drugs represent medicines available for the care of several diseases, which often lacked effective therapeutic strategies in the past (e.g. as discussed in the chapter, MS, RA and psoriasis). These drugs are prescribed by different specialists and, often, dispensed in hospital settings.

In order to monitor patient response, in terms of both benefits and side effects, it is necessary to collect laboratory and clinical information. The classical drug utilization studies were performed mainly using prescription databases, which are often limited to outpatient prescriptions and do not collect clinical information. Therefore, as shown by the examples in this chapter, registries have greatly improved our knowledge of the prescription of biological drugs in specific settings and have demonstrated that patients treated with these therapies often differ from those enrolled in clinical trials. These findings are useful in generating evidence of the effectiveness and safety of biological drugs and thus in guiding regulatory decisions on their appropriate prescription. Registries should be considered an important tool by drug utilization researchers and their involvement in drug utilization studies should be encouraged, especially given the massive market entry of new biologicals and biosimilar drugs.

CHAPTER 30

Drug utilization research in the area of cancer drugs

Nils Wilking[1], Thomas Hofmarcher[2], Ulla Wilking[3] & Bengt Jönsson[4]

[1]Department of Oncology, Skåne University Hospital Lund/Malmö, Sweden

[2]Department of Economics, Lund University, Sweden

[3]Department of Oncology-Pathology, Karolinska Institutet, Sweden

[4]Stockholm School of Economics, Sweden

KEY POINTS

- Increased biological understanding of cancer diseases has resulted in a paradigm shift in the medical treatment of cancer. Despite encouraging advances, most cancer types are still incurable and cancer is the second most common cause of death in developed countries.
- The high price of cancer drugs is a major challenge to equal access and puts heavy strains on public health care payers. After sharp increases in the 2000s, total expenditures on cancer drugs have levelled off due to patent expiration of many expensive and widely used drugs.
- Cancer drug utilization studies cover a great variety of topics. Four main research areas are patient adherence, physician adherence to guidelines, effectiveness and safety (outcomes research) and access (market uptake).
- Most cancer drugs are classified under Anatomical Therapeutic Chemical (ATC) group L. The use of defined daily dose (DDD) as a measurement unit is feasible for oral cancer drugs. As most cancer drugs are administered as infusions or injections at hospitals, usage is commonly measured in milligrams.
- Drug utilization research in the area of cancer is faced with a lack of data. Comparisons are challenging, as prices and population bases vary across regions. The linkage of registries and health care databases that include cancer drug usage will create improved opportunities in the future.

Background

Cancer epidemiology and development of cancer drug usage

An estimated 14 million new cancer cases and 8.2 million cancer deaths occurred worldwide in 2012, with 57% of new cases and 64% of deaths occurring in the less developed regions. The most commonly diagnosed cancers worldwide are lung (1.8 million, 16.7% of total), breast (1.67 million, 11.9%) and colorectal (1.36 million, 9.7%) cancer. The most common causes of cancer death are lung (1.82 million, 22%), stomach (723 000, 8.8%) and liver (746 000, 9%) cancer [1].

In Europe, cancers of the female breast (464 000 cases), colorectal system (447 000), prostate (417 000) and lung (410 000) represented half of the overall cancer incidence in 2012. The most common causes of death were cancers of the lung (353 000 deaths), colorectal system (215 000), breast (131 000) and stomach (107 000) [2,3]. This makes cancer the second most common cause of death after cardiovascular diseases (CVDs) [2,3].

Cancer therapies have been developed for more than 100 years, from the use of oophorectomy for hormone deprivation in breast cancer to the first chemotherapy – similar to mustard gas – in the mid-20th century (cyclophosphamide, still in use). The increased use of antitumour

Drug Utilization Research: Methods and Applications, First Edition. Edited by M. Elseviers et al.
Published 2016 by John Wiley & Sons, Ltd.

agents seen over the last few decades was a paradigm shift, as many cancers became treatable and even curable. Today, the use of cancer drugs has become the standard therapy in most cancers, both as adjuvant treatment with curative intent and as a palliative approach in metastatic disease.

Chemotherapy was long the standard treatment, alongside surgery and radiation therapy. Chemotherapeutic agents aim at inhibiting the ability of rapidly dividing cancer cells to replicate their DNA. However, some normal cells also divide rapidly (e.g. in the digestive tract and bone marrow), so chemotherapies often have severe side effects, which can prevent administration of the optimal doses.

Noncytotoxic agents have been developed since the 1980s, including targeted drugs that block cancers by interfering with specific molecules involved in cell proliferation mechanisms (Table 30.1). Targeted cancer therapies include tamoxifen (targeting hormone

Table 30.1 Targeted drugs approved for use in oncology.

Source: Data from [7–9].

Trade name	INN	Year of first EMA approval	Year of first FDA approval	Therapeutic indication(s)
Rituxan, MabThera	Rituximab	1998	1997	Non-Hodgkin's lymphoma, CLL, RA
Herceptin	Trastuzumab	2000	1998	Breast cancer, metastatic gastric or gastroesophageal junction adenocarcinoma
Mylotarg	Gemtuzumabozogamicin	NA	2000	AML
Campath	Alemtuzumab	2001	2001	B-cell chronic lymphocytic leukaemia
Zevalin	Ibritumomabtiuxetan	2004	2002	Non-Hodgkin's lymphoma
Bexxar	Tositumomab and iodine 131 tositumomab	NA	2003	Non-Hodgkin's lymphoma
Avastin	Bevacizumab	2005	2004	Metastatic colorectal cancer, NSCLC, metastatic breast cancer, glioblastoma multiforme, metastatic renal cell carcinoma
Erbitux	Cetuximab	2004	2004	Head and neck cancer, colorectal cancer
Proximium	Catumaxomab	2005	2005	Head and neck cancer
Vectibix	Panitumumab	2007	2006	Metastatic colorectal carcinoma
Removab	Catumaxomab	2009	NA	Malignant ascites in patients with EpCAM-positive carcinomas
Arzerra	Ofatumumab	2010	2009	CLL
Blincyto	Blinatumomab	2009	2014	ALL
Arzerra	Ofatumumab	2009	2014	CLL
Adcetris	Brentuximab	2012	2011	Hodgkin's lymphoma, systemic ALCL
Xgeva	Denosumab	2011	2011	Prevention of skeletal-related events in patients with bone metastases from solid tumours
Vervoy	Ipilimumab	2011	2011	Melanoma
Perjeta	Pertuzumab	2013	2012	Breast cancer
Gazyva	Obinutuzumab	NA	2013	CLL
Kadcyla	Trastuzumabemtansine	2013	2013	Breast cancer
Beleodaq	Belinostat	2013	2014	Lymphoma
Imbruvica	Ibrutinib	2014	2014	Mantle cell lymphoma, CLL
Zydelig	Idelalisib	2014	2014	CLL
Vargatef	Nintedanib	2014	2014	NSCLC
Gazyvaro	Obinutuzumab	2014	2013	CLL
Lynparza	Olaparib	2014	2014	Ovariancancer
Cyramza	Ramucirumab	2014	2014	Gastric cancer
Mekinist	Trametinib	2014	2014	Melanoma
Opdivo	Nivolumab	2015	2014	Melanoma
Keytruda	Pembrolizumab	2015	2014	Melanoma
Zykadia	Ceritinib	2015	2014	NSCLC

INN, international nonproprietary name; EMA, European Medicines Agency; FDA, US Food and Drug Administration; NA, not approved; CLL, chronic lymphocytic leukaemia; RA, rheumatoid arthritis; AML, acute myeloid leukaemia; NSCLC, non-small-cell lung cancer; ALL, acute lymphocytic leukaemia; ALCL, anaplastic large-cell lymphoma.

receptors in breast cancer) and monoclonal antibodies such as trastuzumab (targeting the HER2 receptor in breast and stomach cancer), as well as immunotherapy, such as ipilimumab (targeting the CTLA-4 receptor in malignant melanomas) [4–6].

Targeted therapies have been shown to have different – and often minor – side effects compared to chemotherapeutic agents. The combined use of targeted therapy and chemotherapy provides minor negative synergistic effects and thus results in better treatment effects (optimized dosing) and improved quality of life [10,11].

In this chapter, we discuss the availability of new cancer drugs and briefly describe the overall cost of cancer care. We review both country-specific and international studies covering four main areas in cancer drug utilization research, which serve as examples in the discussion of methodological aspects of drug utilization research in cancer.

Availability of new cancer drugs

Just like other drugs, cancer drugs have to be tested in clinical studies before they can receive marketing authorization. A certain number of cancer drugs are subject to early regulatory approval based on limited clinical data and not on randomized controlled trials (RCTs). The reason behind this is that cancer drugs may provide effects in small cancer populations, and therefore obtain the designation 'orphan drugs' [12,13]. An important aspect of cancer drug evaluations in the pivotal clinical studies is the use of surrogate end points such as progression-free survival (PFS). There are ongoing discussions in relation to the use of surrogate end points. Data show also that there is often poor correlation between PFS and overall survival, especially in long-term survivors [14,15].

Historically, safety was the central aspect in the process of drug approval and marketing authorization. From the early 1970s, demonstration of efficacy was included in the criteria. Later, the quality of life aspect was added. In the European Union and the United States, these three aspects are centrally assessed by the European Medicines Agency (EMA) and the Food and Drug Administration (FDA), respectively. As health budgets have become tighter, the cost aspect was added. Evaluation of value for money (cost-effectiveness) is usually carried out by national or regional reimbursement health technology assessment (HTA) agencies, although not all countries have formalized HTA processes to guide decisions about funding and use (e.g. the United States does not).

Figure 30.1 shows the number of cancer drugs launched within 3-year periods from 1990 to 2013. In recent years, the introduction of new cancer drugs has increased rapidly. Around 40% of drugs in development are intended for use in cancer, which is by far the largest development area [16].

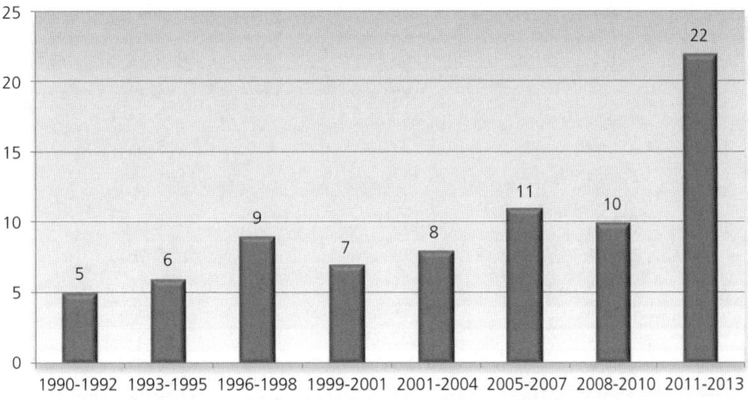

Figure 30.1 Number of cancer drugs (ATC code L01, L02A and L02B) launched between 1 January 1990 and 31 December 2013. Launch between 1990 and 2005 is defined as the date on which a product or pack is first made available for general release by the manufacturer worldwide [17]. For drugs launched between 2006 and 2013, the European Medicines Agency (EMA) authorization date was used.

Source: Data from [18].

Cost of cancer

European countries spend different proportions of their health care budgets on cancer care. A recent study showed that Denmark spends the lowest proportion in the European Union, with 2%, and that Estonia, Poland and Romania spend the highest proportion, with 6% [19] (see Table 30.2). Another study showed that Germany and Sweden spend the highest proportion (both 7.2%) and Eastern European countries the lowest (3–5%) [17]. For the whole European Union, estimates range from 4.0 to 6.3%. In the United States, cancer costs account for about 5% of health care spending [20]. Purchasing power-adjusted per capita spending on cancer differs even more between countries, and is more than five times greater in most Western European countries than in the Baltic states as well as Bulgaria and Romania. EU average amounts are €102–148 per capita.

Costs of cancer drugs

There have been enormous increases in expenditures on cancer drugs in recent years, but they still account for less than 1% of health care expenditure worldwide, and about 20–30% of total health expendi-

Table 30.2 Estimated health care cost of cancer in the European Union.

	2009 [19]		2007 [17]	
Country	Cancer-related share of total health care expenditure	Health care cost of cancer per capita (PPP adjusted) (€)	Cancer-related share of total health care expenditure	Health care cost of cancer per capita (PPP adjusted) (€)
Austria	4%	119	6.4%	207
Belgium	3%	71	6.4%	181
Bulgaria	5%	54	4%	29
Cyprus	4%	47	–	–
Czech Republic	5%	104	5.0%	72
Denmark	2%	69	6.4%	185
Estonia	6%	82	3–5%	36
Finland	5%	127	4.4%	95
France	3%	97	6.6%	205
Germany	5%	171	7.2%	216
Greece	5%	128	6.4%	158
Hungary	5%	80	5.0%	61
Ireland	4%	88	6.4%	193
Italy	5%	96	6.4%	144
Latvia	5%	53	3–5%	37
Lithuania	3%	33	3–5%	35
Luxembourg	3%	141	6.4%	342
Malta	4%	59	–	–
The Netherlands	3%	123	5.6%	170
Poland	6%	78	5.0%	41
Portugal	3%	61	6.4%	122
Romania	6%	52	3–5%	22
Slovakia	5%	103	3–5%	48
Slovenia	4%	90	3–5%	75
Spain	4%	96	6.4%	141
Sweden	3%	92	7.2%	207
United Kingdom	3%	92	5.6%	132
Total European Union[a]	4%	102	6.3%	148

PPP, purchasing power parity.

[a]Wilking et al. [17] include Iceland, Norway and Switzerland in this estimate.

tures on cancer [17,21]. The cost of cancer drugs is driven by increases in price per treatment over time and by longer treatment periods. In the United States, for instance, 12 of the 13 new cancer drugs approved by the FDA in 2012 were priced above USD100 000 per year. Private health insurance helps patients to pay for the medical expenses, but copayments of up to 20% are not unusual, which makes many drugs unaffordable even for well-insured patients [22,23]. The high price of cancer drugs is a major challenge to equal access. It goes without saying that the effect of high drug prices on access becomes particularly pronounced in countries with lower incomes and lower health care spending.

The high cost of new cancer drugs is attributed to numerous factors:

- The conduct of clinical studies to gain regulatory approval is resource-intensive [24]. Other reasons include the high failure rate in drug development and small indications (few patients). The average cost of getting a cancer drug to the market (including the cost of failures) has been estimated at USD1.3 billion, although this has been criticized as largely overestimated [22].
- The patent right granted to a new cancer drug creates a monopoly, which gives the pharmaceutical company significant market power and – at least in theory – allows for high prices. An analysis of cancer drugs approved by the FDA between 2000 and 2010 indicates that the market prices of new drugs are not related to their clinical benefit [25]. Moreover, the recent increased mergers and acquisitions activity in the pharmaceutical sector strengthens oligopolistic market structures and augments the risk of companies forming cartels.
- The very nature of cancer (seriousness) makes patients and/or health authorities willing to pay the high drug price even for marginal improvements in outcome [24].
- In clinical practice, treatments are often given across years (adjuvant), and during the palliative phase of the cancer disease, many patients receive different anticancer treatments over several years. Most cancer patients are treated with combinations or sequences of drugs. Previously used drugs may also be used again at a later date.

In the European Union, the share of cancer drug expenditure among total health care expenditures on cancer care was estimated at 27% in 2009, but this varied considerably between countries [19]. For France, it has been estimated that the cost of new cancer drugs increased from €335 million in 2003 to €714 million in 2006; that is, it more than doubled in 4 years [26]. Similarly in Sweden, the cost of cancer drugs increased from SEK640 million to SEK2450 million between 2000 and 2007, corresponding to an average annual growth rate of 21% [27]. This increase was not solely attributable to the use of newly introduced and more expensive drugs, as a concurrent increase in the number of cancer patients receiving drug treatment was observed. Based on the expenditures in 2007, drug costs in Sweden were projected to grow by an average annual rate of 5% to SEK4.8 billion in 2022 [27], due to patent expiration on many expensive and widely used cancer drugs during the 2010s, providing significant savings [26,28].

Savings when a patent expires can be very significant. After docetaxel and paclitaxel came off patent, price decreases of 76–87% were seen in Australia [29]. In Sweden, several of the drugs used in breast cancer that have gone off patent (including docetaxel, paclitaxel and the aromatase inhibitors) are now available at 3–10% of prime prices (Nils Wilking, pers. comm.). Some small molecules, such as imatinib, are going off patent in the near future. In this case, generic drugs will probably be introduced at price levels in line with those of other nonbiological drugs.

Biosimilars (also known as follow-on biologicals) to targeted therapies also present opportunities for savings [28]. Over the next 5–6 years, several biological drugs (rituximab, trastuzumab, cetuximab, etc.) will go off patent. It is difficult to predict what the effects on pricing will be, but only modest reductions are expected [30]. This is partly linked to the difficulties in manufacturing biosimilars, which involves very complex and expensive processes. Similar problems were predicted in relation to the patent expiration of small biological molecules (e.g. granulocyte-colony stimulating factor, G-CSF), but in reality price levels came down significantly [31]. Biosimilars (e.g. trastuzumab) have already been introduced to the Indian market, but this has led to legal actions from the producers of the original drugs [32].

Recent reports have confirmed the anticipated end to the ever-rising expenditures on cancer drugs. In Sweden, total sales have been stable at around

SEK2.8 billion between 2008 and 2011 [33]. In Switzerland, per patient expenditures on cancer drugs decreased between 2007 and 2012, although overall spending on cancer drugs increased due to an increase of prevalent cases in this period [34].

Several factors have to be considered in the discussion of future cancer drug expenditures, aside from an expected increase due to population ageing:

• The introduction of new and potentially more effective drugs does not necessarily increase total cancer-related health care costs. More effective drugs may lead to a decrease in relapses, improve patients' health-related quality of life and lower the demand for other medical services, such as inpatient care [35]. Cancer-related indirect costs (i.e. productivity loss due to mortality, sick leave and early retirement) may decrease due to increased survival, which relieves public budgets outside of the health care sector [26]. However, it is worth noting that many new cancer drugs only provide small and uncertain benefits over currently used drugs [36].

• A new drug's incremental cost-effectiveness plays a critical role in the decision by the health authorities on whether to grant reimbursement for it. Analysis of the incremental cost-effectiveness entails a comparison between the new drug and a comparator, usually the current standard treatment. If the comparator drug has come off patent, the new drug is compared with generic drug price levels. This makes it harder to prove a superior cost-effectiveness, and reimbursement may be denied or heavily restricted. This is particularly true if the new drug provides no or only marginal added value compared to the existing treatment(s). Different conclusions may be drawn by different authorities from the same data [37]. Furthermore, the price of a follow-up targeted drug may be lower than that of the first drug in its class (e.g. vemurafib and dabrafenib in malignant melanoma).

• Approval trends and characteristics provide valuable information for drug developers and regulators that ultimately impacts on clinicians and patients. The approval process has become more challenging over time, although evidence from the United States indicates that this is not true everywhere [15], suggesting gaps between practice and development in potentially suboptimal indications. Molecular specifications promise to enhance development, but widespread use in label indications has not yet been achieved [23].

• Given the high prices of new cancer drugs, payment mechanisms, called patient access schemes (PASs) (also known as risk-sharing schemes/agreements or managed-entry agreements (MEAs)), have been developed to allow for (restricted) market access. These aim to reduce uncertainty about the value of a new drug and to allow it to be used within finite health care budgets [38,39]. Within the European Union, country experiences with PASs are mixed and adequate evaluations are scarce [40]. In the United Kingdom, for instance, several schemes are used for cancer drugs (e.g. bortezomib, sunitinib, erlotinib), which have increased the administrative burden and led to discontent among health care staff [41].

Drug utilization studies in oncology

Drug utilization studies enable/contribute to the assessment of:

1 patient adherence with treatment;
2 physician adherence to guidelines;
3 effectiveness and safety (outcomes research);
4 access (market uptake).

Table 30.3 provides five selected examples of country-specific drug utilization studies from these areas and details their outcome measures. Table 30.4 provides an overview of three selected international studies.

Patient adherence with treatment

Nonadherence with treatment restrains efforts to improve health outcomes. It is therefore important to evaluate dosing and patient adherence.

The majority of cancer drugs are hospital drugs, administered as infusions or injections. This means that there is no issue with adherence. Any nonadherence is usually related to side effects/toxicity of treatment. Dosing of drugs is also linked to toxicity, and dosing is adjusted related to the level of toxicity (dose reduction).

In oral cancer therapy, patient adherence can be problematic, as patients can take this at home instead of under the surveillance of hospital staff. Studies have shown that adherence may vary between 16 and 100% [48]. We illustrate this using two examples: oral hormonal adjuvant treatment of breast cancer and oral treatment of chronic myeloid leukaemia (CML). These

Table 30.3 Overview of national studies on cancer drug utilization.

Country/Reference	Outcome measures
Australia [42]	Changes between 1996 and 2008 in patients with breast cancer: • Usage of endocrine therapies measured as DDD/1000 incidence cases/day (incidence of breast cancer in 2005) • Usage by endocrine therapy group (aromatase inhibitors vs tamoxifen) • Total expenditure (in AUD) for endocrine therapies
Sweden [33]	Changes (mostly) between 1998 and 2012 in: • Sales (in SEK) of cancer drugs per 100 000 inhabitants • Sales of cancer drugs (mature drugs (i.e. launched before 1998) vs new drugs (i.e. launched after 2002)) per 100 000 inhabitants • Sales of cancer drugs per incident case (incidence of specific cancer type in 2010) • 20 highest-selling cancer drugs • Usage of selected drugs measured as sales in milligrams per case of cancer mortality (mortality of specific cancer types in 2000) • Usage of selected drugs measured as sales in SEK per incident case (incidence of specific cancer types in 2010) • Usage of new cancer drugs for specific cancer types measured as sales in SEK per mortality case (mortality of specific cancer types in 2010)
Switzerland [34]	Changes between 2007 and 2012 in: • Share of sales of cancer drugs among total drug sales • 10 highest-selling cancer drugs • Share of targeted cancer drugs vs chemotherapy drugs • Average cancer drug expenditures per prevalent case, age group and sex • Share of cancer drugs used in ambulatory care in different regions
Taiwan [43]	Changes between 1998 and 2007 in patients with CML: • Share of (newly diagnosed) patients being treated with any kind of guideline-recommended therapy • Proportion of patients treated with imatinib, conventional therapies (i.e. busulfan, hydroxyurea, IFNα and Ara-C, alone or in combination) and hematopoietic stem cell transplantation • Persistence of therapy with imatinib (i.e. share of patients taking imatinib for ≥18 months without interruption)
United States [44]	Characteristics of patients with NSCLC receiving either adjuvant therapy for stage I–IIIa disease or first-line therapy for stage IIIb–IV disease between July 2009 and June 2010: • Rates of guideline adherence by physicians (use of recommended vs nonrecommended regimens) • Impact of guideline adherence on length of follow-up • Share of patients treated with regimens with median treatment costs equal to or lower than those of the top 11 regimens used • Share of patients receiving a two-drug regimen • Share of patients treated with cisplatin-containing vs carboplatin-containing regimens • Share of patients treated with the top five drug combinations

DDD, defined daily dose; CML, chronic myeloid leukaemia; NSCLC, non-small-cell lung cancer.

have been selected because they are both long-term treatments. In one study, by the end of the first year of adjuvant hormonal treatment for breast cancer, a majority of patients (~80%) was adherent (see Section F). The adherence was much lower (<30%) at the end of the normally recommended 5-year adjuvant treatment period. Nonadherence was more often seen in elderly women [49]. In another study, 50% of patients stopped before the recommended 5-year adjuvant treatment period [50]. A CML study from Taiwan reported that around 40% of patients were compliant with imatinib therapy after 18 months of treatment, but less than 8% were compliant after 5 years of treatment [43].

Table 30.4 Overview of international studies on cancer drug utilization.

Number of countries/Reference	Outcome measures
28 countries [45]	Share of sales of new cancer drugs (i.e. launched between 1999 and 2007) among total cancer drug sales in euros per 100 000 inhabitants between 1998 and 2007
	Speed of usage of selected drugs from 1998 (or start of launch) until 2007, measured as sales in milligrams per 100 000 inhabitants
	Level of usage of selected drugs in 2007, measured as sales in milligrams per mortality case (mortality of specific cancer type in 2000)
14 countries [46]	Drug volume sold (in milligrams) per capita between April 2008 and March 2009, compared separately for three groups of cancer drugs (i.e. drugs launched within the last 5 years, 6–10 years, 10+ years) and a fourth group of hormonal drugs
27 countries [47]	Share of sales of innovative cancer drugs (i.e. launched between 2001 and 2012) among total cancer drugs sales in euros in the fourth quarter of 2012 (note: only a selection of drugs launched between 2001 and 2012 was considered 'innovative')

A major contributing factor to low adherence with oral therapy recommendations is patient copayment, in countries where this is required (e.g. the United States) [51]. The term 'financial toxicity' has recently been applied to the situation arising from the copayment of cancer treatment in the US health care system [52,53]. We know from recent studies that cancer patients in the United States are more likely to have financial problems and to file for bankruptcy than are non-cancer patients [54]. Much of the problem is linked to the cost of treatment, and especially the cost of cancer drugs. Low income, and the consequently lower ability to pay for health care, is a major component of the unequal access to cancer drugs in many other health care systems [21].

Physician adherence to guidelines

Given the importance of cancer to health care systems, treatment guidelines for different cancer types are commonly drawn up by health care authorities and organizations of medical professionals. Ideally, clinical guidelines are based on solid evidence on the effectiveness of different drugs or drug combinations to ensure maximum health benefit for patients. Physician adherence to guideline-recommended therapy has been the subject of numerous studies. In the previously mentioned CML study in Taiwan, the share of newly diagnosed patients being treated with guideline-recommended imatinib increased from 12% in 2002 to 36% in 2007, whereas the share of patients receiving conventional CML therapies decreased from 41 to 25% during this period [43]. In the United States, a study reviewed adherence to national evidence-based guidelines in patients with NSCLC who started adjuvant therapy for early-stage disease or first-line therapy for advanced and metastatic disease between 2009 and 2010. Rates of guideline adherence were 75.0 and 61.3% for the first-line and the adjuvant treatment groups, respectively [44]. In breast cancer therapy with trastuzumab, clinical guidelines recommend pretreatment cardiac function assessment and 3-monthly reassessment during therapy to examine cardiotoxicity. In Australia, 37.7% of patients were assessed pretreatment, 50.4% during therapy and 26.4% both before and during therapy between 2001 and 2010 [55].

Effectiveness and safety (outcomes research)

Real-life utilization of and adherence to cancer drugs can be analysed through the use of prescription registries (see Chapter 4). Such registries have been in place in the Nordic countries for several years: Denmark first set one up in 1990, followed by Finland (2003), Norway (2004) and Sweden (2005) [56]. The Nordic registries contain unique personal identifiers for each individual, making linkage between them possible. Similar registries in the Netherlands have been utilized by a number of studies [57], and there are several registries in the Asia-Pacific region that combine drug utilization and cancer registry data [58]. The development of data registries in which drug usage is linked to expanded cancer registry data, including data on the efficacy and toxicity of a given treatment, will be a future cornerstone in evaluating effectiveness and safety in real clinical practice. This research area is termed 'outcomes research' [59].

A current example of an outcomes research study from the Netherlands illustrates how difficult it can be to assess (incremental) effectiveness or cost-effectiveness in everyday practice versus clinical trials, due to the smaller patient numbers, greater patient heterogeneity, missing data, extensive treatment variation and other such issues [60]. Efforts are currently under way to set up comprehensive registries that can capture the complete chain of care. Examples are an initiative by the American Society of Cancer (ASCO) [61] and a UK initiative with the National Cancer Intelligence Network (NCIN) [62].

Access (market uptake)

Studies on access to cancer drugs analyse usage (also called market uptake) in a particular geographical area during a specific period of time. Figures 30.2 and 30.3 show examples of how access to cancer drugs varies across countries. Figure 30.4 illustrates that even within a single country, big regional discrepancies can exist. The different amounts of resources devoted to cancer drugs is only one explaining factor for theses variations [21,63,64]. Other factors include payment mechanisms, reimbursement systems and prescribing incentives, access to cancer specialists, the capacity within a health care system for diagnosis and treatment, national disease priorities, specific policies and guidelines, results from clinical trials, attention from key opinion leaders, pharmaceutical marketing, physician adherence to guidelines and patient adherence with treatment [46].

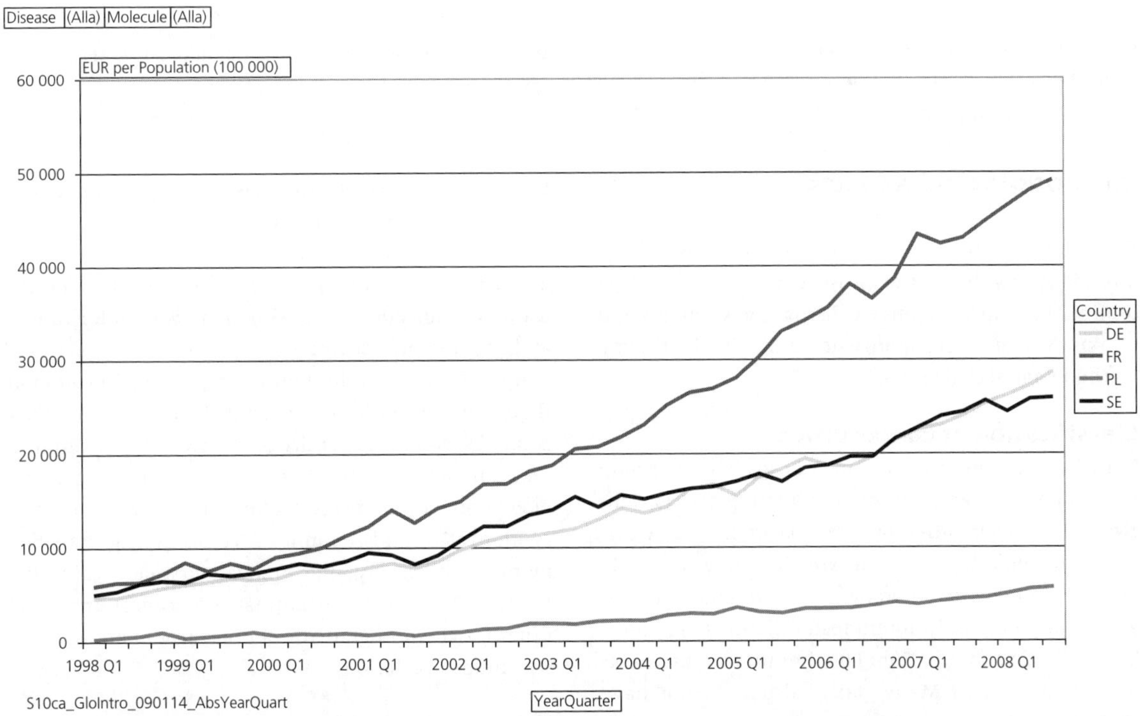

Figure 30.2 Total sales of 24 cancer drugs approved during 1995–2004, expressed in euros per 100 000 inhabitants in Germany (DE), France (FR), Poland (PL) and Sweden (SE). For colour details, please refer to the colour plates section.

Source: Data from [65].

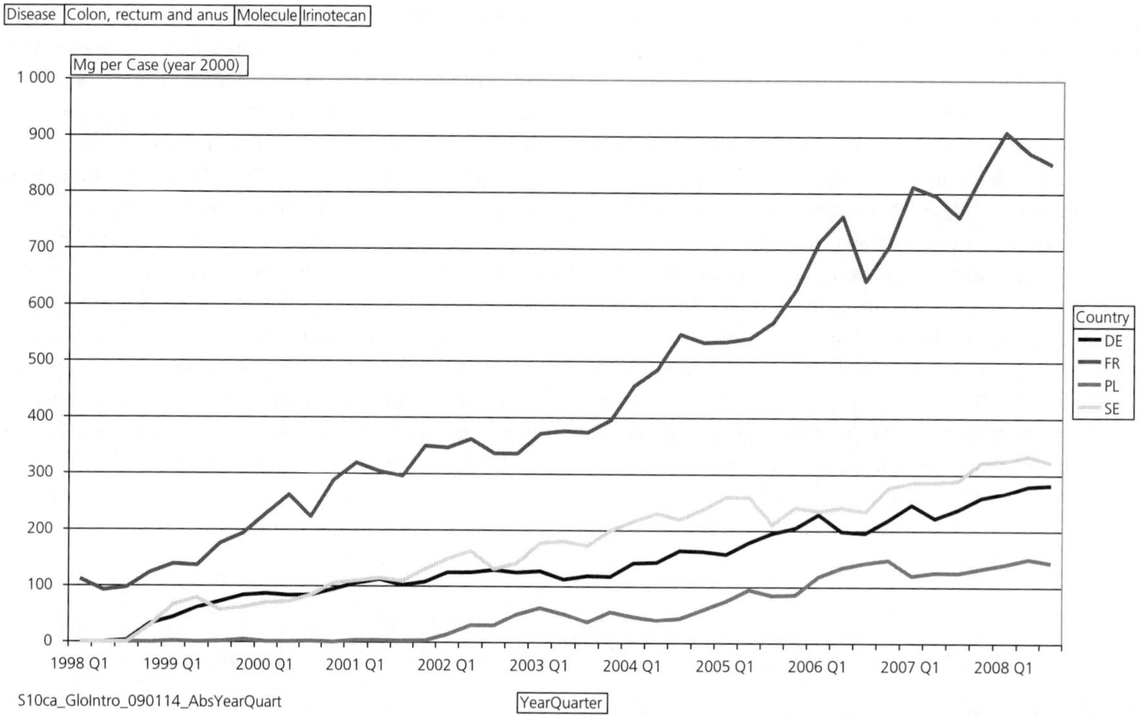

Figure 30.3 Use of irinotecan, expressed in milligrams per mortality case (case = mortality in colorectal cancer in 2000) in Germany (DE), France (FR), Poland (PL) and Sweden (SE). For colour details, please refer to the colour plates section.

Source: Data from [65].

Methodological aspects

The examples provided in Tables 30.3 and 30.4 detail possible approaches to the measurement of cancer drug utilization. In this section, we discuss the strengths and weaknesses of these approaches and highlight some methodological challenges.

Classification of cancer drugs

In the ATC coding system, cancer drugs fall into group L: antineoplastic and immunomodulating agents; subgroup L01, chemotherapy (e.g. paclitaxel) and targeted cancer drugs (e.g. rituximab); subgroup L02, drugs for endocrine therapy (e.g. aromatase inhibitors); subgroup L03, immunostimulants (e.g. interferon alpha); and subgroup L04, immunosuppressants (e.g. thalidomide). Many cancer drugs do not have exclusive indication for the treatment of cancer. For instance, in Switzerland, an estimated 75% of sold units of rituximab, and only 20% of interferon alpha, are used for cancer treatment; the remainder is used for the treatment of other diseases [34]. This needs to be taken into account in order to provide a correct analysis of cancer drug sales. In some countries, such as Australia, the coding system allows for the identification of indications (e.g. rituximab is used for cancer and rheumatoid arthritis).

Apart from the utilization of single drugs, a common theme in the studies reviewed in Tables 30.3 and 30.4 is the division of cancer drugs into two or more groups. This can take the form of a comparison of mature/older and newer drugs (defined by year of launch), of innovative and noninnovative drugs (e.g. classified by means of the five-tier innovation scale used by the French HTA agency [66]), of targeted cancer drugs and drugs for chemotherapy or of drugs from different ATC subgroups [34,46,47].

Value versus volume

The usage of cancer drugs can be measured in value terms (e.g. in euros) or in volume terms (often in milligrams, sometimes in DDDs) (see Chapters 6 and 8).

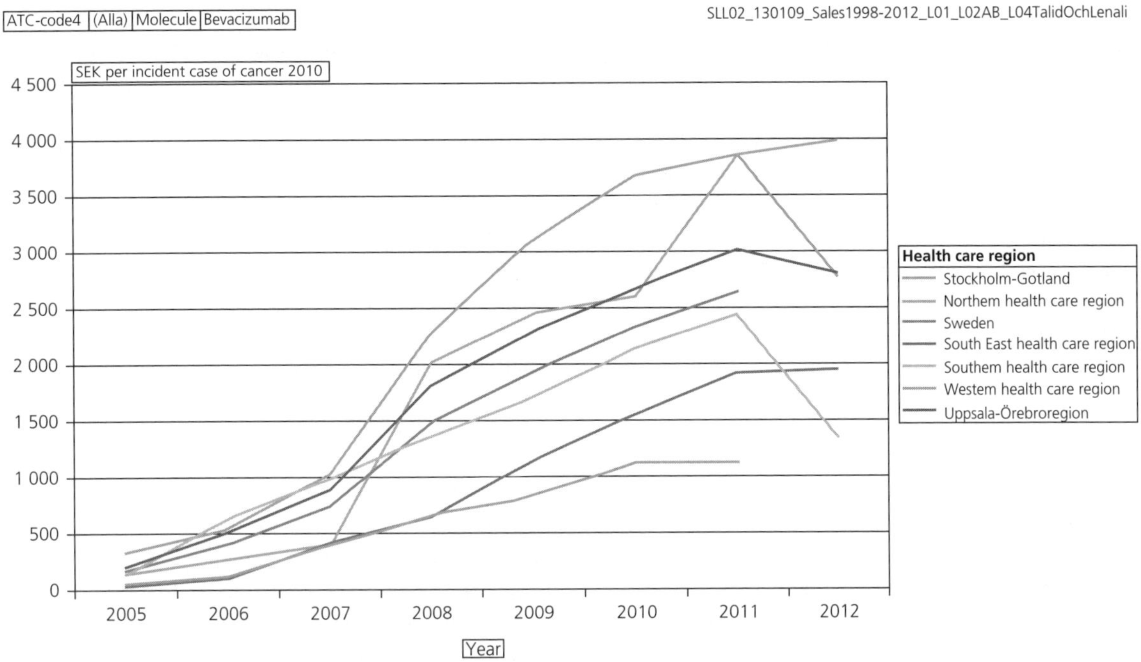

Figure 30.4 Use of bevacizumab, expressed in SEK per incident case (case = incidence in colorectal cancer in 2010) in the six health care regions in Sweden. For colour details, please refer to the colour plates section.

Source: Data from [33].

Using value as the measure of usage will allow for aggregation into total spending for all cancer drugs or drugs used for a specific indication (see Figure 30.2). It also allows for comparisons of spending on cancer drugs in relation to other resources used for cancer care. But this advantage comes with some shortcomings. Using value terms is problematic in international comparisons, due to the need for a common currency basis and fluctuations in exchange rates. Even in countries with a common currency (e.g. the euro area), the prices of a single drug can differ, and a higher usage in a particular country might simply reflect higher drug prices, rather than higher usage in volume terms. This point is equally valid for country-specific studies, if reimbursement prices are determined at a regional and not a national level (e.g. in Sweden). Since most cancer drugs are hospital drugs, their true price may be unknown due to confidential rebates, and patient access schemes can further complicate the determination of the true price. Caution is also required when older and newer cancer drugs are compared, as older drugs (e.g. paclitaxel) that are off patent are sold at much lower prices, making their share of total drug sales small even if their share in volume terms is considerable. One way of dealing with this in studies that measure usage in value terms is to display the number of patients treated with each drug [34,67].

Drug usage is preferentially measured in volume terms in international comparisons, so as to eliminate price effects (see Figure 30.3). This means that each drug must be compared separately. The use of DDDs, which are the gold standard for drug usage, is only possible with oral cancer drugs [42]. Since most cancer drugs are administered as infusions or injections, usage is often measured on a weight basis, in milligrams. However, the use of milligrams comes with at least two drawbacks. First, differences in dosage might explain some of the cross-national variations in usage, as country-specific treatment guidelines for the same drug can differ. Second, it gives equal weighting to large- and small-volume cancer drugs [46]. Further, the volume size(s) of vials of a single drug can differ between countries. Large-volume vials may not be used completely, as drug doses are administered according to the body surface area or weight of the patient, leading to waste of expensive drugs. For instance, in Australia, an estimated 24% of trastuzumab dispensed between 2001 and 2005 was discarded. The use of an additional vial size would have reduced the waste to 6% [68].

Since each of the two methods – value and volume – cancels out some of the other's disadvantages and each method yields informative results, a comprehensive analysis should apply a pragmatic approach and use both [33]. Independent of the method chosen, it is not advisable to display the results of an international comparison solely in the form of country rankings, as this leaves out important information on the extent of differences between countries [46].

Choice of standardization unit

One important puzzle piece in preparing a sound comparison of usage data is the question of the most appropriate unit of standardization. The two options are general population size and epidemiologic cancer data (prevalence, incidence or mortality cases).

Standardization by population size takes the form either of currency per 100 000 inhabitants or of milligrams per 100 000 inhabitants (see Figure 30.2). However, this kind of standardization ignores the epidemiologic profiles of different countries. Countries with older populations typically have a higher number of cancer cases. Given equal drug usage per cancer case, the country with the higher number of cases will appear to have a higher drug usage per 100 000 inhabitants.

When adjusting for variations in the incidence of cancer, the number of current cancer patients (i.e. prevalent cases) can be used for standardization [34]. However, this kind of measurement has its shortcomings, countries in which more cases are diagnosed, due to high screening intensity, tend to have a higher number of less malignant cases in need of little or no drug treatment, so the use of drugs per cancer case differs and countries with a high number of prevalent and non-treatment-intensive cases will appear to have lower levels of drug usage. If specific cancer drugs are compared, it is advisable to standardize by the prevalence of the cancer type to mitigate against this effect. The same arguments hold if incident cases are used for standardization rather than prevalent cases (see Figure 30.4) [33].

Another approach that has been used is to standardize usage by the number of cancer mortality cases [17]. This approach has several downsides. Survival rates – and hence also mortality rates – of specific cancer types (e.g. prostate cancer) differ greatly between countries. In countries with high survival rates (and few mortality cases), a presumably high number of cancer drugs (which may be one reason for high survival rates) will be related to a small number of mortality cases, yielding high rates of usage. By contrast, in countries with low survival rates (and many mortality cases), a presumably small number of cancer drugs will be related to a high number of mortality cases, yielding low rates of usage. Hence, this approach potentially overestimates differences between well- and poor-performing countries. Another point advocating against the use of mortality cases is that while not every mortality case will have been treated with drugs, every prevalent (and every incident) case has the potential to be treated.

If epidemiologic data are used for standardization, they should ideally correspond to the year of usage [34]. If instead usage data covering several years are standardized by, for example, incident cases in a certain reference year, year-to-year changes in usage may only reflect changes in incident cases, rather than changes in usage. In times of increasing cancer incidence, the use of incident cases of a single reference year will bias usage rates downwards/upwards in all years before/after the reference year (see Figure 30.4, where data from 2006 to 2012 are standardized by the number of incident cases in 2010). The magnitude of the bias will differ between countries if their respective increase in cancer incidence differs.

Other issues in international comparisons

If specific drugs are compared between countries (see Chapter 23), variations in usage might be explained by different approved indications. For instance, sunitinib was initially approved by the EMA for use in two indications (gastrointestinal stromal tumour and metastatic renal cell carcinoma) in July 2006 and received a third indication (pancreatic neuroendocrine tumours) in October 2010. Not all European countries reimbursed sunitinib for all indications, and the time between EMA approval and first drug sales differed across countries [65].

Different time points of market introduction of a drug should be taken into account in international comparisons. This means that usage should preferably not be compared on the basis of sales in a certain month or quarter, but instead according to the time passed since the drug was introduced in each respective country [21]. However, if the discrepancy between the dates of market authorization is small and/or if sales are measured in per-year terms, this issue is of less importance. This is also the case for more mature drugs, such as irinotecan: the influence of the date of introduction was tiny in 2008, as the drug had been used for more than 10 years in all countries (see Figure 30.3).

Conclusion

Despite encouraging advances, most cancers are still incurable and – in developed countries – are the second most common cause of death after CVDs. Furthermore, the absolute number of cancer patients will continue to increase in the foreseeable future, mainly due to population ageing. The high prevalence of cancer results in high health care expenditures, and cancer drugs represent a considerable share of total cancer-related medical costs. Many countries experienced sharp increases in total expenditures on cancer drugs during the 2000s. This effect seems to have levelled off, at least in some countries, in the early 2010s, mostly as a result of patent expiration of many expensive and widely used drugs.

In the cancer area, drug utilization research is confronted with an insufficient availability of data, such as usage of drugs administered at hospitals. The incomplete registration of the burden of disease (e.g. prevalence, survival) and the very poor registration of individual patient data (e.g. side effects) make research challenging. Today, we have little knowledge of the outcome of cancer drug usage in clinical practice (both concerning effectiveness and cost-effectiveness). In order to be able to support the evidence from clinical trials, the utilization of cancer drugs should be followed in terms of outcome and of value to patients and to society. The use of population-based cancer registries linked to drug dispensing databases will enhance the possibilities for future outcomes research in the cancer area.

CHAPTER 31
Health system perspectives

Paul Spivey[1] & Brian Godman[2,3]
[1]Independent international pharmacy consultant
[2]Division of Clinical Pharmacology, Karolinska Institutet, Karolinska University Hospital Huddinge, Sweden
[3]Strathclyde Institute of Pharmacy and Biomedical Sciences, Strathclyde University, Glasgow, Scotland

KEY POINTS

- The prescribing and utilization of medicines are determined by a complex range of interrelated factors, including health financing (incorporating out-of-pocket expenditure), available human resources, health information, service delivery and marketing authorization.
- Medicines are typically made available through a combination of public and private supply routes and subject to regulations regarding their quality, sale and supply.
- There are a variety of methods and systems for financing health services, including compulsory taxation, health insurance and private/out-of-pocket financing. Out-of-pocket expenditure on health care can be considerable in low- and middle-income countries.
- Essential medicine lists improve affordability and outcomes. Guidelines are being developed by medical speciality societies and professional associations to improve patient care.

Introduction

The use of medicines is determined by a complex range of interrelated factors, from the way in which the individual end user (patient) regards their medicines, through differences in the practices of prescribers/suppliers and local, regional and national health systems/policies to international influences (Figure 31.1). This section describes the key influences, starting with health systems/policies. Subsequent chapters in this section cover influences on prescribers and patients.

It is recognized that there are 'complex relationships between medicines and health financing, human resources, health information and service delivery' [1]. This chapter considers these 'macro' influences, particularly at the national level, where government policies and systems determine which products are registered, how they are made accessible to users, who may prescribe them and how they will be paid for.

Access to medicines

Although there are many factors which influence the choice and prescription of medicines in the process of finalizing treatment and care regimens, ultimately in order for them to be used, the 'users' must have access to prescribed or recommended medicines. 'Access to medicines' has become a common and popular concept in the area of pharmaceutical policies, health systems and pharmaceutical markets, used to describe the availability and affordability of medicines, particularly from the perspective of the end user (patient/medicine purchaser).

Drug Utilization Research: Methods and Applications, First Edition. Edited by M. Elseviers et al.
Published 2016 by John Wiley & Sons, Ltd.

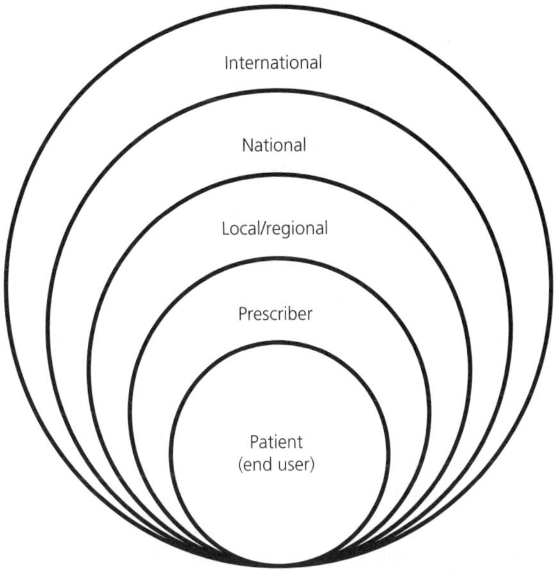

Figure 31.1 Levels of influence on patient use of medicines.

Universal access to affordable essential medicines is an international goal and an objective of national health systems and policies [2]. The selection of 'essential medicines' reflects the national and local context, based on the World Health Organization (WHO) concept that the range of medicines required to meet the health needs of the majority of the population can be identified on the basis of epidemiological data and evidence about the safety, efficacy and cost-effectiveness of treatments.

Access – whether a medicine can be obtained by an individual end user – is influenced by general availability in the country and locality, affordability from the perspective of the country and the individual and acceptability to both the prescriber/supplier and the end user. There have been a number of models that have analysed, described and illustrated the elements and determinants of access to medicines, as well as the barriers to achieving access to medicines [1,3,4].

Medicines in most countries are made available to patients through a combination of both public and private supply routes. These supply routes are normally subject to legislation at the national level, which regulates the range and quality of medicinal products permitted in the market through registration and licensing procedures, and to regulations that govern the prescribing, sale and supply of medicines. In low-income countries, the implementation of regulations is often inadequate, and as a result a large range of products can be purchased over the counter in both legitimate (e.g. pharmacies, licensed drug sellers) and illegitimate (e.g. market stalls) outlets. In addition, there is the problem of counterfeit and substandard products, estimated by the WHO to make up 25% of all products in less developed countries in 2007, but with considerable variation between countries [5]. Illicit supply and counterfeit or substandard products can result in serious adverse events, reduced treatment efficacy and drug resistance. Supply of medicines through unlicensed or untrained providers results in poor professional practice, further affecting the safe, rational and correct use of medicines.

Availability in public-sector health systems is further influenced by the existence and level of implementation of policies (including financial) and systems which control and manage the procurement and supply of medicines. In the private sector, availability is influenced by market forces and user (including prescriber) preferences and demand.

Affordability is influenced in the public sector by health care financing policies and in the private sector by the prevailing market forces, both nationally and internationally. International influences range from the influences of the pharmaceutical industry to the policies and practices of donor organizations for lower- and middle-income countries. In addition, affordability is a factor of the economic circumstances of the individual customer, particularly when purchasing from the private sector, either by choice or by default as a result of public sector system supply failure.

Finance and affordability

The financial factor affects the use of medicines in all countries, regardless of their economic status. If medicines are not affordable, either through the health system or by the end user, then their use will be limited.

The budget allocation spent by any individual government on medicines is an important factor influencing availability. Health systems in all countries have had to face the reality that without some method of managing budgets for new and existing medicines, it will be impossible to meet the increasing cost of health technologies and the rising demand for health care. This situation will only escalate in view of the appreciable number of new drugs in development, including new biological drugs [6–8], irrespective of whether health care systems are funded directly by taxation or through compulsory health insurance. Examples of policies relating to new and existing medicines are given in Section B.

The situation is even more challenging in countries where pharmaceutical expenditure already accounts for a high proportion of total health care expenditure. This is the case in low-income countries, where medicine costs can be up to 66% of total health care costs [9,10], and in transitional countries, where they can be up to 30% [10]. By comparison, the average proportion of medicines expenditure (prescribed and over-the-counter (OTC)) in Organisation for Economic Co-operation and Development (OECD) countries is 17% [11], with some, such as the United Kingdom, spending considerably less (11% in the United Kingdom). Despite the high proportion of health expenditure on medicines, up to 90% of the population in low-income and transitional countries purchases medicines using its own resources (out-of-pocket payments), making medicines typically the largest family expenditure item after food [9].

Health financing and health insurance schemes

There are a variety of methods and systems for financing health services. The most common ones are government general revenues, social insurance financing, private insurance financing and out-of-pocket payments.

Since medicines and other health technologies can be easily costed and charged, they are a tangible and an easy item to use to raise revenue in order to recover some of the costs of health care provision. This is true whether the health care provision is public or private. If the sale of medicines contributes to institutional or private income, it can provide a perverse incentive to overprescribe, resulting in unnecessarily high or skewed utilization patterns [12].

Where health financing uses government-generated revenues, there is usually some element of control that will influence or restrict the use of medicines. In high-income countries, the influence may be minimal, or at least evidence-based. In low-income countries, the influence or restriction is more often unintentional, resulting in limited financing and supply failure; the use of medicines may then be dependent on the ability of patients/users to purchase them from the private sector. Where responsibility for the health budget is decentralized, local decisions may influence the availability and provision of some medicines.

Social insurance financing may also influence the use of medicines by restricting provision under the insurance scheme to a selected list of medicines and requiring copayments for medicines from insured persons, again introducing the influence of affordability. For example, there is significant variation in access to both biologic and synthetic disease-modifying antirheumatic drugs across European countries in terms of the contribution required from the patient, which ranges from zero to full cost [13].

Private insurance financing is probably the least likely method to influence the prescription and consumption of medicines, and consequently is likely to be the most expensive in terms of premiums.

Out-of-pocket payments, as already noted, may not influence the choice and prescription of medicines but may well influence adherence to professional advice on the basis of affordability. As with any out-of-pocket payment for medicines, there is a well-documented risk of partial provision and incomplete consumption of prescribed courses of treatment, resulting in reduced efficacy and, in the case of antimicrobials, proliferation of resistant organisms and public health risks [14].

Health policies affecting affordability

Health policies have been developed to improve affordability from a national perspective, which include providing lists of essential medicines, encouraging the use of generic products and restricting the availability of single-sourced (patented) medicines (especially as some European and other countries no longer fund new premium-priced drugs) [6,7].

Developing lists of essential medicines that can treat the majority of illnesses seen in ambulatory care is the core element of the 'essential drugs concept', which was endorsed by World Health Assembly in 1975 as a recommended approach by which low-income countries could focus available resources on those medicines which would meet the health needs of the majority of the population. The first WHO Model List of Essential Drugs in 1977 identified 208 individual medicines which could provide safe, effective treatment for the majority of communicable and noncommunicable diseases in these countries [10]. It was principally intended for primary health care situations, both to ensure that scarce resources were focused on cost-effective medicines of relevance to the majority of the population and to stop secondary and tertiary institutions from using up medicine budgets on sophisticated and expensive medicines for the minority.

The essential drugs concept has also been used in high-income countries. Restricting prescribing choices enhances physicians' familiarity with the medicines they prescribe, improving cost-effectiveness and reducing potential adverse drug reactions and drug–drug interactions [15]. This was the philosophy behind the development of restricted formularies, initially for hospital prescribers and later for both primary and secondary care, pioneered in Scotland [16,17]. Similar initiatives are developing elsewhere, such as the 'Wise List' in the Stockholm Metropolitan Healthcare Region [15]. High adherence rates with these initiatives are enhanced by the involvement of prescribers in the selection process (contributing to trust in the guidance) and regular communication, including feedback [15,18].

Encouraging generic prescribing and purchasing is an alternative and additional policy promoted to maximize scarce resources, since generic products are normally appreciably cheaper than innovator products [19–21] (see Section B). This policy can be effective and safe where generic products are well regulated and carefully procured, but has risks where procurement of generics is not quality-assured and price is the main driver [21]. Initial policies on generics were not welcomed by the pharmaceutical industry. A court case brought in South Africa in relation to antiretrovirals and patents was particularly significant. The outcome in favour of the South African government contributed to the pharmaceutical industry reconsidering its response to, and involvement in, the provision of affordable medicines for major public health problems. Moreover, there has been a tendency towards mixed pharmaceutical companies in recent years, through mergers and acquisitions [21]: many companies now have both originator and generic divisions, so that their revenues do not fall after patent expiry. For instance, Novartis has its own generic division with Sandoz, while Daiichi Sankyo bought Ranbaxy Laboratories [21].

Health authorities have taken steps to address provider and patient concerns over the use of generics, including providing education on quality control, and have done all they can to benefit from the increasing availability of low-cost generics, such as incentivizing pharmacists to substitute generics for originators [19,20].

Subsequent to the essential medicines concept, the WHO encouraged the development of hospital and national drug and therapeutic committees (DTCs) and published guidelines for their development and function (see Box 31.1) [22]. Such committees not only influence the use of drugs but frequently also have responsibility for monitoring drug use in relation to their recommendations. Guidelines are normally focused on individual diseases/conditions; for example, the WHO issues model guidelines for the treatment of acquired immunodeficiency syndrome (AIDS), tuberculosis and malaria (among others), and many countries have adapted these for their own use. In England, the National Institute for Health and Care Excellence (NICE) encourages auditing against national guidelines and provides criteria for this purpose, thereby facilitating drug utilization research.

Health systems that encourage the use of locally 'approved' treatments on an evidentiary basis will also, by definition, affect the use of medicines in their institutional or geographical area of influence. However, where budgets are devolved to regions, neighbouring health authorities may reach different conclusions and approve different treatments. In the United Kingdom, this has led to development by the media of the term 'postcode prescribing'. In response, initiatives around the managed entry of new drugs have been introduced to reduce regional variations [23]. One such initiative is the technology appraisal process used by NICE, which uses evidence on efficacy and cost-effectiveness to provide recommendations on whether to prescribe individual products, which must be adopted by all local health organizations, with all NICE-approved drugs included

Box 31.1 Ideal attributes of drug and therapeutic committees (DTCs).

- Multidisciplinary in nature.
- Contain members from both primary and secondary care.
- Include patient/public input.
- Make evidence-based decisions, with full declarations of interest from members.
- Provide a limited role for 'key opinion leaders'.
- Apply decisions/recommendations equally in primary and secondary care, with no 'carte blanche' for specialists. However, some medicines may be limited to use on specialist advice (or even require a specialist prescription).
- Publish minutes on the website of a pertinent health organization.

in any local formularies. This is in contrast to clinical guidelines, which are recommendations for good practice. All such initiatives inevitably have an influence on prescribing patterns. However, differences in drug utilization still persist [24]. For more on good prescribing practice, see Section B.

Where health care is provided through the private sector, either alongside government provision or alone, cost of treatment may be less visible to health policy-makers as a factor that influences the prescribing and use of medicines. However, the costs of medicines in this situation are still a major factor in actual use.

Supply and availability

Availability of medicines is a significant issue in low- and middle-income countries, particularly in rural areas. Obviously, if a product is not available, it cannot be used. There are many reasons why health supply systems fail to provide medicines or limit availability.

One reason is a lack of adequate finance in national health budgets. In-low income countries, the government budget allocation for medicines may be as little as USD5 per capita per annum, compared to USD1000 in high-income countries [25]. The variation in the proportion of government health expenditure allocated to medicines is a reflection of the sizes of overall health budgets.

Another reason is the mechanism for supply. As already mentioned, across the world, a variety of systems affect the distribution and supply of medicines to public sector health institutions, which have been shaped by historical, economic and political forces. At one extreme is total state responsibility for medicine supply and at the other is absolute dependency on the private sector. State responsibility for health care and medicine supply continued to be a feature of most socialist political systems in Europe until the end of the 20th century, but changes in politics and economies have resulted in the dismantling of most state supply systems, with a sudden expansion of, and reliance on, the private sector.

In low-income countries, the private sector medicine supply is normally concentrated in major urban centres, where pharmacies can be viable businesses. Hence, there can be differences in drug utilization between urban and rural localities. In such circumstances, the government must be seen to take responsibility for the equitable provision of accessible health care. As a result, many low-income and transitional countries continue to employ a policy of government responsibility for medicine supply for the public sector, although the coverage is frequently poor due to inadequate budgeting, procurement and supply systems. Most available medicines are distributed or sold against prescriptions from busy hospital outpatient clinics, with some available through community health clinics. Where supplies are limited, the balance of medicines must be purchased by the patient from the private sector (whether a pharmacy or another provider), and it is in such cases that the resulting burden of medicines expenditure falls primarily on the individual, as out-of-pocket expenditure [9].

Middle- and high-income countries increasingly favour using the private sector to supply medicines to public health institutions, either using centrally negotiated price contracts (e.g. South Africa, the United Kingdom) or by reimbursing costs to patients from the government health budget (e.g. UK primary health care prescriptions via contracted community pharmacies). Elsewhere, the private sector is contracted directly for the supply of medicines in both the public and private health sectors, often through health insurance schemes (e.g. France, Switzerland, the United States).

Health policies affecting availability

Policies of relevance here relate to the governance of suppliers through the registration of individuals qualified to supply medicines and of the premises from which they do so, which are usually monitored through inspection. In many low-income countries, rural and primary care services may not require – or be able to attract – medical doctors and professional pharmacies may not be viable. In theory, this limits the range of medicines available for use. Alternative sources in such situations are licensed medicine sellers and licensed drug stores. These suppliers may have no or minimal medical or pharmaceutical training, yet can make available a surprisingly wide range of medicines.

In addition to restrictions on prescribing, many countries categorize medicines into different groups for supply or prescribing purposes, resulting in variations in accessibility. International and national legislation normally covers the medicines most likely to be misused, such as opioids and other psychoactive medicines, but may also restrict supply to the order of a qualified and registered prescriber: 'prescription-only' medicines. In countries with strict regulation of medicine prescribers and suppliers, access to commonly prescribed or essential medicines is often improved by the deregulation of products from prescription-only to 'pharmacy-only' status, thus providing some level of restriction, usually for safety purposes, but widening access through private supply. Such changes in regulation can result in significant changes in drug utilization. For example, the availability of 10 mg simvastatin for purchase through pharmacies in the United Kingdom corresponded with a decrease in prescribed simvastatin of both 10 mg and 20 mg doses [26].

In countries with a strong economy, the private market can make licensed medicinal products available within a short time and with guaranteed quality, whether it is supplied to the end user directly or through a public or private institution. However, in low-income countries, the government health system is often inadequately funded and the infrastructure of medicines supply (usually a government system) is, as a consequence, not able to ensure consistent availability of medicines, even basic and essential ones. Health systems which cannot make medicines consistently available inevitably restrict prescribing and the consumption of medicines, which is not in the best interest of any stakeholder group.

The expansion of the Internet as a source of health information and medicines supply is convenient for the consumer but brings with it many risks. A WHO evaluation revealed that 'countries vary substantially in their regulations on the sale and promotion of medicines via the Internet' [27]. The existence of counterfeit and substandard products is widespread in some countries, and 'blind' purchasing via the Internet by uninformed individuals provides an increased opportunity for the inappropriate use of medicines and for manipulation and extortion by criminal elements. The WHO and regulatory authority websites in the United Kingdom and United States all warn of the dangers. An online presence is an increasingly important factor in the ability of pharmaceutical companies to raise public awareness of available products, especially in countries where direct-to-consumer advertising (DTCA) is not permitted. In one study, all 10 companies examined had Facebook pages, Twitter/Friendster feeds, sponsored blogs and really simple syndication (RSS) feeds, and most had dedicated YouTube channels and mobile applications. They also had dedicated websites, dedicated Facebook pages, health communications-related Twitter and Friendster feeds and DTC advertisements on YouTube for individual drugs [28]. Such promotion is widely regarded as leading to inappropriate medication use, overutilization and increased spending on expensive branded drugs, with potential to endanger public health due to promotion of potentially dangerous products.

Policies about the advertising of medicines and the level of control over advertising also influence medicines use. In most high-income countries, it is illegal to advertise medicines available only on prescription, but in some there is no restriction on advertising, resulting in patient pressure on prescribers to prescribe medicines on demand (see Chapter 32). In a private sector environment, prescribers can cave into such demands, often leading to irrational use (see Chapter 33).

Policies on regulation

In addition to the integrity of the supply system and the competencies of the prescriber/supplier, the availability of medicines is dependent on their authorization for supply and use within a country and its market. Most countries now have some system for the registration and regulation of medicines, by which marketing authorizations are issued and medicinal products are made available.

Whether a product is legally allowed to be distributed in a particular country or region is determined by its safety, quality and efficacy. It is the responsibility of the national regulatory authority to determine this, and such an authority may, on the basis of its own assessment of the evidence, decline to licence a product for use even though it is licensed in other countries.

Post-authorization pharmacovigilance systems, found in most countries, can result in the withdrawal of products if there are concerns over their safety in routine clinical practice. For example, 19 medicines were withdrawn from the European market between 2002 and 2011, with case reports cited in 95% of cases (18/19) [29]. Cardiovascular complications were the most common reason given (9/19), followed by hepatic disorders (4/19) [29]. Examples include valdecoxib in 2005, due to cardiovascular and cutaneous disorders; rimonabant in 2008, due to psychiatric disorders; and sibutramine and rosiglitazone in 2010, both due to cardiovascular disorders [29]. Rofecoxib was withdrawn in 2004 following evidence of increased cardiovascular events [30]; it was found to be one of the most selective COX-II inhibitors, producing minimal COX-I activity [31], which reduced the cardioprotective effect of COX-I inhibition. This effect is similar to that of low-dose aspirin [32]. A reduction in the risk of thrombotic cardiovascular events was found in patients treated with naproxen compared to rofecoxib [33,34]. The VIGOR study [34] led to a caution being placed on the rofecoxib product label in May 2002 [35], while the APPROVe study [32] led to its withdrawal [29,30]. There are ongoing debates about whether withdrawal might have been avoided if there had been fewer marketing activities, including considerable DTCA in the United States, promoting the safety of the COX-II inhibitors [36].

Policies for health worker regulation in high-income countries often require registration with a professional/accreditation body, which ensures adequate knowledge about medicines. The competency of health staff to safely prescribe and handle or administer treatment determines whether and how a product is used. Policies frequently also cover the registration of individuals permitted to prescribe medicines, which is a further factor affecting availability. A medical doctor and a health assistant or nurse prescriber have different training and different competencies and are therefore permitted to prescribe different medicines. In most high-income countries, strict regulations cover prescribing and supply, with the result that typically only a limited number of medicines are available for purchase through a wide range of outlets. In recent years, high-income countries have begun to train prescribers from different professions (e.g. pharmacy and nursing) in order to facilitate use of medicines and treatment of particular health issues (e.g. childbirth, chronic health problems, pain control). This enhances access to medicines and treatment. Where laws affecting the supply of medicines are strictly observed and training is provided, the use of medicines is theoretically enhanced by expanding prescribing responsibility to other professionals working within agreed limits according to their competencies (see Chapter 32).

International influences

While WHO policy has had a major impact on the availability of essential medicines, both international guidance and donor practices influence the care and treatment of global public health problems (e.g. human immunodeficiency virus (HIV)/AIDS, tuberculosis, malaria, maternal and child health). Consequently, they also influence the use of medicines in these areas [37].

The emergence of some health issues as being of concern to international public health has resulted in the large-scale gathering of evidence. This has led to the publication of international guidelines and protocols for treatment. There are a number of different motives for producing these guidelines, which are designed for use in all countries, regardless of economic status. One is to avoid the development of resistance and tolerance to particular medicines (e.g. antimalarials, tuberculostatics). Another is to share best practice and avoid misuse and waste.

International policies and guidelines can and should influence use of medicines in treatment. However, where a switch to follow international recommendations occurs in many countries concurrently, it can result in unanticipated demand on raw materials and shortages of finished products (e.g. antimalarials and antiretrovirals) [38].

Many guidelines developed in one country (e.g. by medical specialty societies and professional associations) are often recognized by others. However, when a country adopts guidelines developed somewhere else, it may pay inadequate attention to the other country's development processes. One recent study has shown that panel members producing guidelines sponsored by nongovernment sources in the United States and Canada were significantly more likely to have conflicts of interest (e.g. industry sponsorship) compared with those working on government-sponsored guidelines [39]. The US Institute of Medicine has recommended that guideline panels should be as conflict-free as possible, to ensure the credibility and evidence-based nature of the clinical practice guidelines produced. There is international agreement on how guidelines should be developed (the AGREE criteria) [40].

There are also other ways in which the pharmaceutical industry can influence medicine use and government policy, both locally and internationally. The most obvious is industry lobbying. Many countries wish to support local manufacturing, but this can create conflict between availability of medicine and maximization of profits. International pharmaceutical companies tend to concentrate on product development that will maximize profits, and may neglect research into diseases with low return on investment [41]. Industry pricing policies play a major part in product availability. Premium prices are commanded for novel products, which can lead companies to stop producing older medicines (see Chapter 24). In addition to DTCA, pharmaceutical companies may engage in 'disease-mongering': medicalizing conditions in order to increase 'awareness' and sales [42–45]. There are also concerns that pharmaceutical companies have corrupted the practice of medicine and medical knowledge through their influence over what drugs are developed, how they are tested and how they are marketed [44].

Conclusion

The evidence-based, safe and cost-effective use of medicines is an objective of most health systems and health policies. To achieve this goal, medical products and technologies which meet the required quality specifications must be accessible to both prescribers and end users. Efficient and appropriate health systems and health financing should be geared towards ensuring the continuous and convenient availability of affordable medicines and treatment. Only then can trained health care professionals fulfil their intended potential and the population receive the treatment it needs.

CHAPTER 32

Prescriber perspectives

Colin Bradley[1], Kathleen Holloway[2] & Janet Krska[3]

[1]*University College Cork, Ireland*

[2]*World Health Organization Regional Office for South-East Asia*

[3]*Medway School of Pharmacy, Universities of Greenwich and Kent, United Kingdom*

KEY POINTS

- Prescribers are central to determining the usage patterns of medicines and are influenced by a wide variety of factors. Prescribers include a range of health professionals. Drug utilization research studies frequently focus on influencing medicines use through changing prescribing practice.
- Education is a key factor influencing prescribers, and much medical education encourages rational prescribing through restricted core drug lists. Evidence-based medicine is an important influence in many countries and is heavily promoted to prescribers through guidelines and formularies.
- Prescribing processes in many high-income countries have become computerized. This brings with it the potential for improvements in prescribing quality and reductions in medication errors, although this potential has not been widely realized.
- Key influences on prescribers are patients, peers, the pharmaceutical industry and third-party payers.
- In many low-income countries, systems designed to promote good-quality prescribing are not well developed, and the pattern of factors that influence prescribing differs between high- and low-income countries.

Introduction

While medicines are ultimately consumed (or not) by patients, key decisions relating to their use are often made by others – specifically, health care professionals with prescribing privileges. Thus, the attitudes of prescribers are quite central to the utilization of most medicines. If prescribers are enthusiastic about medicines, more are likely to be consumed; if they are circumspect about the benefits, fewer are likely to be consumed. Where prescribers sit on this spectrum will depend on such factors as their education and training, their understanding of patients' health problems, their cumulative experiences and issues such as prescribing incentives.

Prescribers' attitudes are also influenced by their peers and mentors, and either directly or indirectly by the marketing endeavours of the pharmaceutical industry. In the health care systems of most high- and some middle-income countries, medicines are paid for in whole or in part by third parties, including the state and health care insurers. These third-party payers have an interest in how the medicines they pay for are used, so they will usually seek to influence prescriber behaviour. This can be achieved by setting policy, through the remuneration system or by prescriber education. In 2007, Canadian researchers proposed a long list of factors that might influence prescribers (Figure 32.1) [1], based largely on the work of Denig et al. [2], Haaijer-Ruskamp & Hemminki [3] and Wirtz et al. [4]. It is clear from Figure 32.1 that prescribers are also influenced by patients, on whom there are a wide range of influences in turn (see Chapter 33).

For most people in high- and upper middle-income countries, access to prescribers also facilitates access to medicines. Thus, the number of prescribers, their locations and their accessibility will also influence

Drug Utilization Research: Methods and Applications, First Edition. Edited by M. Elseviers et al.
Published 2016 by John Wiley & Sons, Ltd.

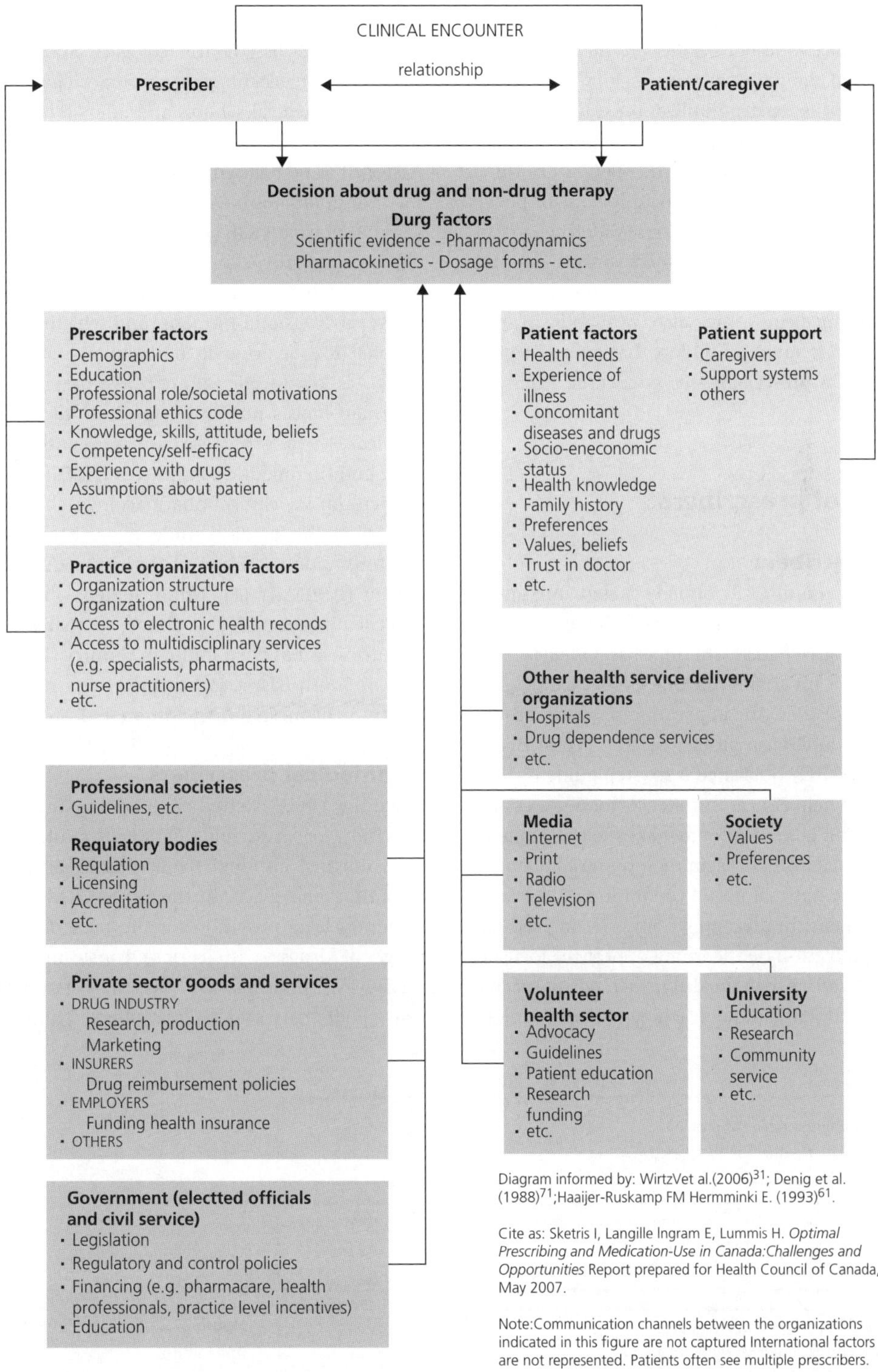

Figure 32.1 Influences on prescribers in their encounters with patients.

Source: Sketris et al. 2007 [1]. Reproduced with permission of Health Council of Canada.

overall medicines consumption. Prescribers and their prescribing choices and behaviours are therefore major determinants of the patterns of medicines use and are an important focus for drug utilization studies. In low-income countries, the regulatory and policy frameworks within which health systems operate are much weaker and medicines are often paid for out of pocket by patients in the private sector. These differing circumstances change the degree to which various determinants of the patterns of medicines use operate.

Of course, medicines are also available to purchase from a wide range of outlets that do not require access through a prescriber; this is covered briefly in Chapter 33.

Education of prescribers

Medical prescribers

Education and training, as already stated, are major influences on prescribing practices. Although there is no universally agreed curriculum for basic medical education, curricula invariably include pharmacology followed by therapeutics (the application of pharmacological knowledge to clinical problems). The World Health Organization (WHO) published a six-step guide in 1994 [5], designed to help educators to teach good prescribing (Figure 32.2).This guide sought to make medical students aware of potential influences on their prescribing and to help them make optimal use of the information available to them, to ensure their prescribing was appropriate and used a problem-based learning approach, focusing on the patient, rather than the drug. Such an approach is widely used in undergraduate teaching of pharmacology and therapeutics, basing these subjects around clinical cases. The British Pharmacological Society (BPS) has reviewed the teaching of pharmacology and prescribing in UK medical schools and offers a core curriculum for safe and effective prescribing [6]. This curriculum is designed to be focused on outcomes, ensuring that new medical graduates have core competencies which allow them to prescribe safely and effectively.

Internationally, clinical pharmacology – the scientific discipline that involves all aspects of the relationship between drugs and humans, and which focuses on the rational use of drugs in both individuals and populations – is key to safe and effective prescribing. Clinical pharmacologists not only contribute to undergraduate medical teaching but are also frequently members of drug and therapeutic committees (DTCs). A model core curriculum for clinical pharmacology, therapeutics and prescribing for medical students has been published by the International Union of Basic and Clinical Pharmacology (IUPHAR) [7]. Unfortunately, the discipline of clinical pharmacology is absent in many low-income countries, as has been found in country situational analyses in South East Asia [8] (http://www.searo.who.int/entity/medicines/country_situational_analysis/en/).

Nonmedical prescribers

Since the 1960s, some health care systems have made provision for 'prescribing' by health professionals other than doctors, although what this involves has varied over time and place. In the United Kingdom, there is currently legal provision for the prescribing of a wide range of drugs (with certain constraints) by nurses, midwives, pharmacists, optometrists, physiotherapists, podiatrists and radiographers. The education of

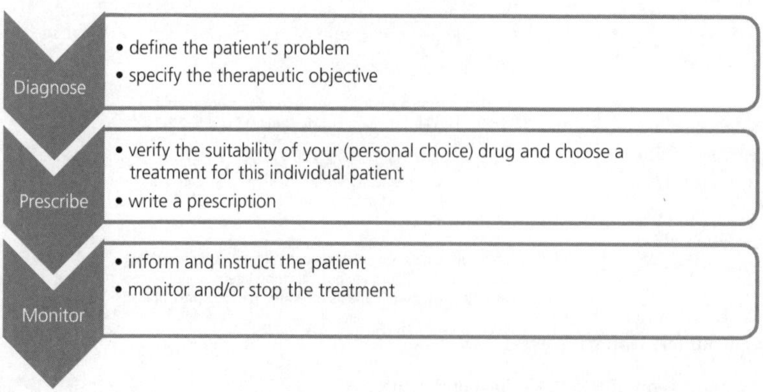

Figure 32.2 Processes involved in good prescribing.

Source: Adapted from De Vries et al. 1995 [5]. Reproduced with permission from World Health Organization.

nonmedical prescribers has been developed in parallel with the extension of prescribing rights to these professionals. Although initially developed for nurse prescribers, the training curriculum now follows a broadly similar pattern for all relevant health professionals. It includes a university-based component and a period of practice-based learning under the supervision of a clinical mentor relevant to the trainee prescriber's scope of practice [9]. Thus, nonmedical prescribers acquire both the necessary knowledge of disease diagnosis and management (including the safe and effective use of medicines) and prescribing skills. The latter include:

- conducting consultations;
- selecting appropriate medicines;
- writing prescription forms;
- monitoring the safety and efficacy of prescribed medicines.

A growing number of other countries have introduced some form of nurse prescribing, including Australia, Canada, Ireland, New Zealand, Sweden, the United States, the Netherlands and Spain, although this varies from independent prescribing to prescribing within strict conditions under the supervision of physicians [10]. A significant part of the rationale behind extending prescribing rights to other health professionals is the need to increase patient access to medicines, particularly in remote and rural areas and areas with shortages of medical staff. While most studies exploring the impact of nonmedical prescribing are from the United Kingdom, some demonstrating potential benefits have come from low- and middle-income countries, including Botswana and Zimbabwe [11–13]. All show that nonmedical prescribing is widely accepted and viewed positively by patients and professionals.

Making prescribing decisions

Early studies of decision-making suggested that when a doctor makes a diagnosis, they immediately think of a number of pharmacotherapeutic possibilities (termed the 'evoked set'), which can range from 1.7 to 5 different options [14]. A model of therapeutic reasoning was proposed in 2009 by Bissesseur et al. [15], based on existing literature covering clinical reasoning. These authors suggested that a 'therapy script' appears in the doctor's brain once a diagnosis is determined, based on existing associations developed through prior experience. Choice of therapy is then based on simultaneous use of both nonanalytical (including pattern recognition, evoked sets) and analytical (such as evidence-based medicine) reasoning processes.

However, in making prescribing decisions, medical practitioners are influenced by a range of other factors, including their view of what the patient wants and what might be in the patient's best interest, their view of what their peers might regard as appropriate prescribing and many other emotional, psychological and social factors [16]. Overall attitude to medicines plays an important role. Many doctors are 'therapeutic enthusiasts', an attitude which may be absorbed during training through observation of clinician teachers prescribing to their patients: the 'hidden curriculum' [17]. Importantly, financial incentives play a key role in prescribing decisions for many prescribers, particularly where they are also the provider of medicines and generate income from this provision, as is the case in many countries.

Evidence-based medicine

In many countries, both students and practitioners are taught and encouraged to use treatments that are evidence-based and to avoid those of no proven effectiveness (but see Chapter 31). However, applying evidence-based medicine requires an interpretation of evidence, rather than its unthinking application in situations where it does not necessarily apply. This is an increasingly important issue, particularly in preventive medicine. Thus, for example, evidence suggests statins reduce the risks from cardiovascular disease (CVD). Does this mean they should be prescribed to large tranches of the population? The most recent guidance from the National Institute for Health and Care Excellence (NICE) in England recommends that statins be given to people with an estimated 10% or greater risk of CVD [18]. There are currently approximately 7 million people in the UK taking statins, at an estimated annual cost of £285 million. This guidance, if followed, could reduce CVD deaths, but it would also dramatically increase both the number of people taking statins and the associated costs.

The proponents of evidence-based medicine highlight the fact that evidence should be critically appraised and that in deciding on whether or not a treatment is merited, consideration should be given to both numbers needed to treat (NNT) and numbers needed to harm (NNH). Moreover, even in 1996, the potential for clinical practice to become 'tyrannized' by evidence was recognized, since even the best evidence may not be applicable to individual patients [19]. However, the application of these concepts to prescribing decisions is not always apparent, and medicines are sometimes prescribed for much wider groups of the population than the evidence supports. Furthermore, making comparisons between different treatments regarding what is a sufficiently low NNT or high NNT requires clinical judgment.

Evidence does, of course, contribute extensively to local formulary development (see Chapter 31 and Section B), as well as to national guidelines. Doctors are encouraged to contribute to formulary development and to develop and use their own personal formularies in everyday practice. IUPHAR encourages medical schools to identify a core list of drugs (as appropriate for local circumstances) they will teach students about (e.g. mechanism of action, indications, route(s) of administration, important contraindications and adverse effects) [7]. Such a core list could be viewed as a student formulary, which might encourage continued rational prescribing after qualification. Pharmacy schools often adopt a similar approach to learning. The WHO Guide to Good Prescribing also advocated this approach, teaching medical students to develop a set of first-choice drugs (their P(ersonal) drugs) as standard treatment for common disorders, while following existing national and international treatment guidelines and formularies [5]. General practitioners have described using a personal 'head-held' drug formulary in deciding whether and what to prescribe, which is often established during their medical training, but is subsequently shaped by colleagues, patients, policy and personal experiences [20].

Prescribing processes

The conventional model of the prescribing process envisages a doctor reaching a diagnosis on the basis of a history provided by the patient and the results of the doctor's examination and/or investigation, and, on the basis of this diagnosis, selecting and prescribing a medicine or medicines. However, this model is about the assessment and treatment of a newly presented problem; both medicines to control long-term or chronic illnesses and preventive medicines to control risk factors for diseases (especially CVD) result in patients using long-term medicines that require only ongoing monitoring. Partly because of new drug developments and the increasing evidence base for their use, there are more medicines available to treat a wider range of patient conditions than ever before. In addition, the population is increasingly ageing, leading to greater comorbidity, which is increasing polypharmacy (with all its consequences) and patient demand. All these factors contribute to the need to make prescribing processes easier.

Computerized prescribing (computerized provider order entry) systems

In a number of countries, prescribers in both primary and secondary care settings use computerized methods to generate drug prescriptions. Most of these systems offer predefined options for the selection of formulations, quantities and doses, once the initial drug choice has been made. Many systems also incorporate alerts or prompts highlighting potential drug–drug interactions, drug–disease interactions and overdoses, which can either require action or simply provide information [21]. These systems help to reduce errors and certainly reduce problems with illegibility of prescriptions [22]. However, there is recent evidence that despite the universal use of electronic prescribing systems in general practices in England, there is still a high proportion of errors, which may reduce the effectiveness of drug use [23].

Some electronic systems include clinical decision-support features and local formularies, both of which should in theory help to improve clinical decision-making and result in potentially more evidence-based or guideline-adherent prescribing decisions, as well as reduce prescribing errors. A recent systematic review of electronic health interventions that included these systems concluded, however, that there was weak evidence for behaviour change, which did not always translate into improved care [24]. One potential cause is overreliance on decision support or overestimation of its functionality, resulting in decreased practitioner performance [23].

Repeat prescribing systems

In some countries, such as the United Kingdom, Norway and the Netherlands, individuals register with a single primary care physician, who acts as gatekeeper for most of their health needs. To support the continuing provision of long-term medicines that don't require a face-to-face consultation, indirect prescribing processes or 'repeat prescribing systems' have been developed. These indirect prescriptions make up an increasingly high proportion of medicines use in primary care [25]. In England, recent work shows that the proportion of medicines prescribed as repeat items has remained unchanged over the last 2 decades, at around 77%, but the number of repeat prescription items issued per patient per year has doubled from 5.8 to 13.3 [26], while the mean number of acute prescription items is 3.8 per patient per year.

Access to repeat supplies of long-term medicines is important, given the increase in noncommunicable diseases worldwide. Systems that can facilitate this while providing a degree of monitoring are therefore essential. Repeat prescribing systems reduce doctor workload and increase patient convenience, but they may not always provide sufficient control to ensure that every repeat prescription is appropriate, effective, well tolerated and optimally used by the patient [27]. Effective medicines management requires the deployment of a safe and effective repeat prescribing system – one which facilitates access to necessary medicines but does not allow them to be too readily available without assessment or review.

One widely used mechanism introduced in recent years to increase convenience for prescribers, pharmacists and patients, while minimizing errors, is direct electronic transfer of prescriptions from the prescriber to the pharmacy. There is some evidence for improved organizational efficiency and more accurate communication resulting from such systems, but less evidence for improvements in patient-level outcomes, including medication errors [24]. Obviously, the systems for prescribing and dispensing vary substantially between countries, and the existence and extent of both repeat prescribing and repeat dispensing will also vary. For example, in remote areas of South Africa there are nurse-run clinics that provide repeat supplies of medicines, taking recourse to medical review only when required [28].

Review of prescriptions

Drug utilization review as it was originally developed (see Chapter 1) is an important mechanism which enables patterns of poor prescribing to be highlighted. Drug utilization research studies are still widely used for this purpose in North America, together with intervention studies aimed at improving prescribing. Elsewhere, clinical audit serves the same purpose. However, good prescribing practice requires that all prescriptions be reviewed, particularly for long-term medicines, and that patients be involved in the review process. Inadequate or infrequent reviews of repeat or regular prescriptions can result in drug-related problems and drug wastage, which are simply reflected as increased use in drug utilization studies.

Medication reviews conducted by pharmacists (or a multidisciplinary team including a pharmacist and a physician) have been shown to reduce drug-related problems (see Chapter 45), but prescribers should also conduct regular reviews themselves. Pharmacists can assess the continued need for/use of medicines during the dispensing process [25]. However, some pharmacies operate collection and delivery services for repeat prescribed medicines, aimed at reducing patient inconvenience, which can mean there is no pharmacist–patient contact. This can contribute to drug-related problems and medicine waste.

Influences on prescribers

As shown in Figure 32.1, a variety of nonmedical pressures and influences can affect doctors' prescribing decisions. Age, gender, urban versus rural location of the practice, experiences at medical school and specialty versus generalist care can all play a role [1]. Studies note that doctors are subject to pressure from patients to issue prescriptions when they might otherwise not, and that they often feel uncomfortable when they do so [29]. Workload and time pressures contribute to the speed with which prescribing decisions are made and may result in less than rational prescribing. There can also be pressures – real or perceived – from a range of sources to avoid prescribing where it is not strictly necessary (e.g. through campaigns to reduce antimicrobial prescribing) [30]. Pharmaceutical manufacturers devote considerable resources to persuading doctors to prescribe their products, while third-party payers have a vested interest in minimizing the costs of health care, and so have developed various policies and mechanisms to discourage excessive or unnecessarily costly prescribing (see also Chapter 31). The potential to profit personally from prescribing in general, prescribing particular medicines or prescribing certain quantities of medicines must not be ignored.

Patients

Patients frequently have views on whether they want a prescription, and sometimes they have a view on what medicine(s) they would or would not like to be prescribed [29] (see Chapter 33). Patient preferences for using medicines, the extent to which they are willing or able to express these preferences and the means by which they communicate them all vary. Some patients are inherently averse to medicines in general [31], but some may expect a prescription when they see a doctor and may feel disappointed or dissatisfied if one is not given. That said, many patients place a higher priority on other outcomes, such as receipt of advice and information, while doctors may over-anticipate patients' desire for a medicine and prescribe when no such desire exists [32]. This has been found in both high- (England) and low-income (Indonesia) countries [32,33].

Several initiatives aimed at increasing patient involvement in decision-making during the doctor–patient consultation have been developed, and much research and debate have been devoted to the topic [34]. A recent systematic review suggests that a variety of interventions aimed at both patients and doctors serves to enhance the patient experience and patient knowledge, but there is little evidence that these lead to improvement in service use or health outcomes [35].

Workload

Some studies, particularly in the area of antibiotic prescribing (which may account for up to 25% of general practitioner (GP) consultations), suggest the time available for a consultation and the doctor's desire for a quick fix may influence prescribing, such that busier doctors prescribe for a higher proportion of patients attending [36]. A lack of willingness to explain prescribing decisions to patients may also result from time constraints, and this can result in inappropriate antimicrobial prescribing [37].

Peers

There is little doubt that doctors influence one another's prescribing. Indeed, peer pressure, through provision of feedback on prescribing patterns and comparison with a 'norm' or 'ideal', is a widely used means of encouraging changes in physician prescribing habits.

Hospital doctors influence primary care prescribing both through initiation of medicines in hospitals and outpatient clinics and, more generally, through their involvement in GP education at all levels [38]. The views of specialists on the use of medicines within their speciality, understandably, carry considerable weight with nonspecialist colleagues. Even among specialists, some are perceived to have more influence than others over their colleagues – including fellow specialists – and these are identified as 'key opinion leaders'. The views of opinion leaders are often canvassed for the support of rational prescribing [39]. Research-active doctors and opinion leaders may also exert influence on prescribing through their own publications and by participation in local guideline development through DTCs (see Chapter 31).

Within primary care, doctors also influence one another's prescribing when they share care of individual patients and observe the outcomes of medicines initiated by colleagues. It has been shown, for instance, that the greater the number of doctors in a practice, the larger the variety of drugs prescribed [40]. Additionally, observation of changes upon initiation of medicines in secondary care can lead primary care physicians to initiate new drugs themselves.

Pharmaceutical manufacturers

Prescribing behaviour is obviously a major concern to the pharmaceutical industry, whose profits are critically dependent on the prescribing of their products. It is little wonder, therefore, that the industry applies considerable resources to trying to influence prescribers, through a multitude of means (Figure 32.3). It uses all the standard marketing means at its disposal, including straightforward advertising, detailing (face-to-face promotional activities), product placement, providing 'free' samples and entertaining potential customers. The industry is also deeply involved in the funding of prescriber education and medicines research. This involvement may include influencing the content of educational materials and research. Academic institutes and their general research programmes are often funded by the industry (see also Chapter 22).

In 2012, the pharmaceutical industry spent more than $27 billion on drug promotion in the United States, of which more than $24 billion was spent on marketing to physicians [41].

Most studies of prescriber exposure to information provided directly by pharmaceutical companies have found it is associated with higher prescribing frequency, higher costs or lower prescribing quality, although some

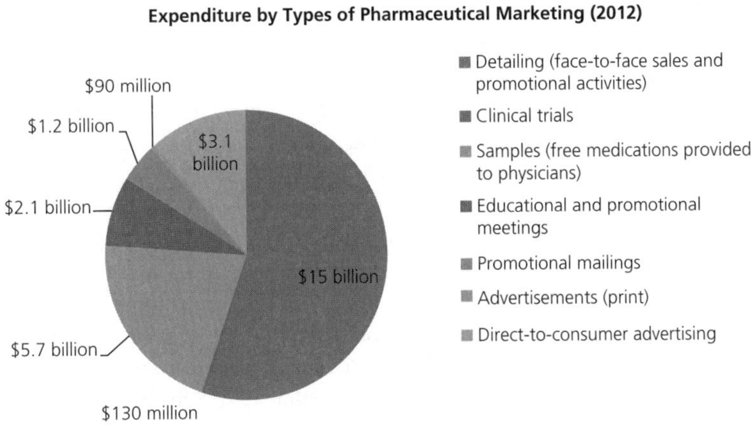

Figure 32.3 Expenditure on promotional activities by type of pharmaceutical market.

Source: Cegedim Strategic Data 2013.

have found no associations [42]. It is for this reason that DTCs recommend prescribers avoid exposure to information from pharmaceutical companies. However, while this is clearly feasible for those with good access to independent information, in many countries the industry is still the most frequent or even the only source of information about medicines. Indeed, in some low-income countries, there may be as many as one representative for every five doctors [43].

Because medicines are regarded as a particular type of commodity, requiring tight regulation of supply, there have long been concerns about industry marketing practices. The WHO introduced Ethical and Scientific Criteria for Pharmaceutical Advertising in 1988, setting out criteria for the detail that should be provided in any advertising material. In a recent study in India, none of the drug promotional literature reviewed fulfilled all the WHO criteria, with most lacking information on indications, correct dosage regimens, dose adjustments in special situations, adverse drug reactions, drug interactions, precautions or overdosage. In addition, false claims were given in 86% of the literature reviewed [44]. Different countries place different restrictions and codes on the marketing of medicines, although the legislative force and, no doubt, adherence to these codes also vary from jurisdiction to jurisdiction.

In an attempt to reeducate prescribers about the potential benefits of collaborating with the pharmaceutical industry, a document was developed by a mix of organizations within the United Kingdom offering guidance to prescribers working with the industry [45]. However, influential others were against close working [46], based on the extensive evidence already cited that pharmaceutical company marketing strategies impact on the quality and volume of prescribing [42]. Overall, the various interventions shown to be effective in controlling or countering the influences of promotion are: government regulation, training of students (both before and after graduation), media exposure of abusive promotion and free and abundant provision of reliable, noncommercial therapeutic information to professionals and the public [47]. Health Action International (HAI) has recently published a guide on teaching students in schools of both medicine and pharmacy to recognize and respond to pharmaceutical promotion at an early stage in their careers [47].

Payers

Three types of payer predominate: the state (which incurs the costs of medicines to some extent in virtually all systems), health care insurers and patients (or their families). While all have a vested interest in ensuring value for money, the first two are generally in a much stronger position to influence prescribers. They use a variety of mechanisms to try and reduce the costs of medicines – or the proportion of the costs of medicines that they incur. At the state level, they may engage directly with manufacturers and wholesalers to negotiate more favourable or reduced costs through 'risk-sharing' schemes [48].

Other mechanisms involve influencing prescribers by either mandatory or persuasive means (see Chapter 31 and Section B); for example, by restricting what may be prescribed, or, more commonly, which medicines will be reimbursed. Alternatively, payers may set a reference price above which they will not reimburse or stipulate that only cheaper forms of medicines (typically, generic medicines or biosimilars) will be reimbursed. They may also restrict the quantities that can be prescribed.

As already indicated, payers may also seek to influence prescribers by providing feedback on their prescribing, often using medical or pharmaceutical advisors to supplement the feedback with academic detailing, whereby the advisor engages prescribers in discussions about their prescribing data, which may be supplemented by incentive schemes (see Section B). Payers may also invest more generally in ensuring prescribers have guidance on cost-effective prescribing by funding the production and supply of independent medicines information and therapeutic guidance.

Third-party payers also seek to reduce prescribing expenditure in high-income countries, by shifting the cost on to other payers – particularly patients – through copayments. The perceived benefit is that copayment elicits the patient's interest in the cost and cost-effectiveness of their medicines and reduces waste. However, copayment may reduce consumption of essential medicines or of medicines whose benefits are remote (in time), and thus the costs of other forms of care or future costs may be increased (beyond any savings made on the medicines). There is also the potentially negative effect of patient demand for nonessential medicines or unnecessarily expensive medicines leading to increased drug costs.

An example of a copayment scheme is the Pharmaceutical Benefits Scheme in Australia, which provides subsidized prescription drugs to the population with the aim of ensuring access to affordable essential medicines [49]. Since patients receive these drugs at reduced cost, this scheme influences both prescribers and patients with regard to what drugs are prescribed. In addition, Australia has an extensive national Medicine Policy [50], a major objective of which is quality use of medicines. The Australian National Prescribing Service [51] was set up in order to achieve quality use of medicines and runs programmes promoting the rational use of medicines, targeting both prescribers and consumers. In Europe, in recognition of the multiple factors influencing the use of medicines, multifaceted campaigns have been run in many countries, targeting both prescribers and consumers to improve the use of antibiotics [30,52].

Organization of health care

The extent to which prescribers can profit personally or pass on profits to their patients or their organization is a factor that can influence both the quantity and the quality of prescribing. Most Organisation for Economic Co-operation and Development (OECD) countries ban physician dispensing, but the United States, the United Kingdom, Japan, the Netherlands and parts of Switzerland allow medical doctors to dispense drugs. If physicians are allowed to sell drugs to patients, they may prescribe more drugs or (if the drug pricing system allows it) select more expensive prescriptions in order to generate additional income [53]. Some work suggests that antibiotic prescribing is reduced when physicians do not dispense and that physician dispensers select more branded products, leading to increased overall drug expenditure [54].

A wide variety of governmental strategies aimed at incentivizing good prescribing or reducing overall drug costs through incentive schemes have been developed. Direct schemes can be either positive (e.g. bonuses for meeting an objective or payments for preferred prescribing) or negative (e.g. withholding money or imposing fines for not meeting stated objectives). Indirect mechanisms allow involvement in decision-making; these have the capacity to either generate 'savings' or reduce costs. The trend in England is towards prescribers having greater involvement in designing the delivery of health services, including prescribing policy and practice.

Additional issues in low-income countries

Many of the influences described in this chapter exist in both high- and low-income countries, but their strength can vary between settings due to very different health systems and different levels of infrastructure. In addition, many countries lack policies aimed at promoting rational use of medicines (Figures 32.4 and 32.5), and this policy gap is greater in low-income countries, where implementation of existing policies is also weak [55,56].

In low-income countries with weak regulatory and policy frameworks, while qualified prescribers play a major role in determining patterns of medicine use, other factors are also very influential [57,58]. First, prescribing may be carried out by informal and unqualified prescribers and drug sellers. Such 'prescribers' often lack

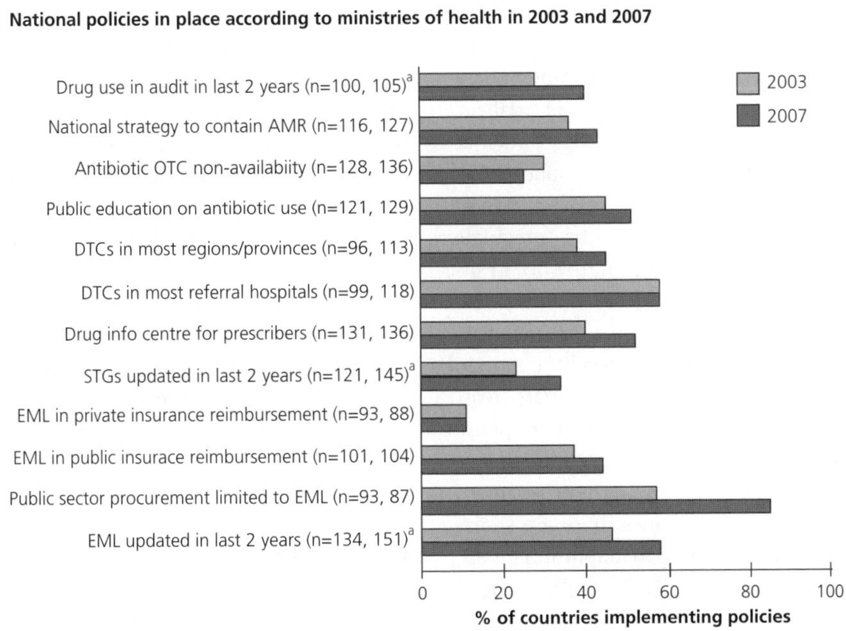

Figure 32.4 National policies in place in 2003 and 2007, according to various ministries of health. AMR, antimicrobial resistance; DTC, drug and therapeutic committee; EML, essential medicines list; OTC, over-the-counter; STG, standard treatment guidelines.

Source: Holloway and van Dijk 2011 [59]. Reproduced with permission from World Health Organization.

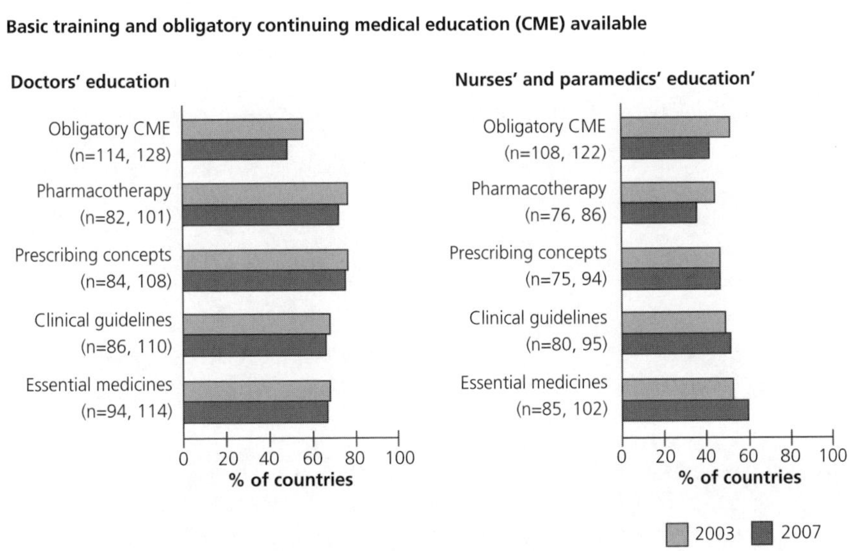

Figure 32.5 Availability of basic training and obligatory continuing medical education (CME).

Source: Holloway and van Dijk 2011 [59]. Reproduced with permission from World Health Organization.

knowledge and are heavily influenced not only by the prescribing practices of qualified or more senior doctors in nearby clinics and hospitals but also by patient demand and profit motivation. Second, prescribers' access to and use of independent information, such as clinical guidelines or drug bulletins, is often suboptimal. Pharmaceutical promotion may be unethical, and most regulatory authorities are unable to monitor or regulate such activities [56]. Third, prescribers often work in situations of inadequate infrastructure. For example, some prescribers must see more than 100 patients per day, with only 1 minute per consultation – too little time to make an adequate diagnosis and give appropriate treatment. Dispensers are sometimes constrained to dispense medicines in a matter of seconds – too little time to give patients proper instruction [58]. Often, there are insufficient diagnostic facilities. Sometimes there are shortages of essential medicines, leading to inappropriate use of other, nonessential medicines [59]. Fourth, in countries where patients must pay for their medicines, many poor patients have to go without, and thus affordability and availability are the major determinants of use (see Chapter 31). Prescribers and patients are heavily influenced by their own views on the need for medicines within the specific social context. For example, in a study in Nepal – where many patients have to travel, often by foot, for some hours to reach health facilities – both prescribers and patients concurred that patients only came to health care facilities when they had at least three problems, because they expected each would require at least one medicine; patients preferred to pay a flat rate for a prescription, regardless of the number of medicines it contained, even though such a system would be more expensive if only one or two medicines were needed [60]. Finally, poor regulation can lead to an excessive number of products being on the market, poor post-marketing surveillance, the selling of prescription-only medicines over the counter and unethical drug promotion – all of which can influence how medicines are used [61,62].

Conclusion

The influences on prescribers are many and varied, and are closely interlinked with both health systems/policies and patients. Attempts to influence prescribers have also been many and varied, and, as the prescriber is a key decision-maker affecting drug use patterns, such attempts will no doubt continue in the future.

CHAPTER 33

Patient perspectives

Janine Traulsen[1], Nicky Britten[2] & Janet Krska[3]
[1] Section for Social and Clinical Pharmacy, Department of Pharmacy, University of Copenhagen, Denmark
[2] University of Exeter Medical School, United Kingdom
[3] Medway School of Pharmacy, Universities of Greenwich and Kent, United Kingdom

KEY POINTS

- Patients view medicines and their risks and benefits differently from health professionals, which influences the way they use them and their attitudes towards them.
- Self-medication is the most common form of medicine use worldwide. It is mostly used for self-limiting conditions in high-income countries, but it can also be used for chronic conditions in many countries.
- Information provision is key to enabling decision-making, but information about the risks and benefits of medicines is generally not well conveyed by health professionals, and patients frequently seek information from a wide range of sources. A patient's understanding of information about medicines is influenced by their health literacy.
- Perceptions about generic medicines or formulations influence medicines use, as do cultural and religious beliefs.
- Researching the patient perspective is important to drug utilization research, and usually requires qualitative techniques.

Introduction

While in theory drug utilization research seeks to quantify, understand and evaluate the processes of prescribing, dispensing and consuming medicines, rather than focus on end-user or patient perspectives and experiences, much research has focused on the provision and regulation of medicines and on efforts to improve the quality of prescribing [1]. In this chapter, we argue for the importance of understanding and researching the patient perspective as an essential component of successful intervention studies and rational drug use. The patient or end user is the key determinant of use in most situations, affecting both whether a medicine is used at all and whether it is used appropriately.

Previous chapters have discussed determinants of drug utilization from both health system and prescriber perspectives. However, both are influenced by the perspectives of the end user, and they in turn are influenced by health systems and prescribers. In this chapter, we will attempt to answer the following questions: Why is the patient perspective important? What are the relevant issues? What do people do with their medicines? What is the 'patient rationale'? Why is researching the patient perspective necessary for drug utilization research? We hope that by reading this chapter, the reader will gain an insight into and appreciation of how individuals experience and interpret their medicine treatment and how patients' perspectives affect utilization.

Importance of the patient perspective

There is a huge gap between how health systems and health professionals interpret and understand rational use of medicines and how patients (or the public) perceive it. It is essential for both policymakers and health professionals to recognize and accept that no policy or intervention involving treatments, care and services

Drug Utilization Research: Methods and Applications, First Edition. Edited by M. Elseviers et al.
Published 2016 by John Wiley & Sons, Ltd.

will be successful unless the patient perspective is recognized, acknowledged, respected and understood – even when so-called 'scientific rationality' appears absent.

The two basic things that drug utilization research researchers need to understand regarding patient perspectives on medicines are:

1 That medicines are perceived differently by lay people than by experts – this includes patients' definitions of 'medicine', their knowledge and understanding about medicines and their perceptions of medicine risks and benefits. This differing perception leads to differences in what is seen as rational and appropriate use.
2 That medicine is not on most people's 'wish list'. In fact, for the majority of the population, a medicine is a product they do not want, and often people will go to extremes in order to delay and/or avoid using medicines. Despite this, most people value the fact that there are medicines available, and a minority of people with life-threatening diseases will actively lobby for access to the latest drugs.

Patient perceptions of medicines

It is important that health professionals and researchers be aware of the variety of definitions and interpretations of the terms 'drugs' and 'medicines' that exist among lay people [2]. Misunderstandings as to what is and is not a medicine are common. Patients' definitions often contrast with 'official' definitions (i.e. those found in pharmacopeia, drug information handbooks, guidelines and legislation). For health professionals, understanding the patient perspective requires not only awareness of this difference [2], but also the knowledge that the prevalence and use of complementary/alternative medicines is increasing [3]; this can present problems when asking patients about their medicine use – important information when planning therapy – as they may not report such treatments, or medicines bought over the counter (OTC). Moreover, in many countries, traditional medicines are of greater significance than allopathic products. In general, medical pluralism – the coexistence of different systems of traditional and Western medicine – is a common phenomenon [4].

Risk perception is inevitably a key determining factor in whether or not a product is used, but perceptions of the risks associated with prescribed medicines, OTC products and alternative treatments vary greatly between lay persons and experts. Sociological and cultural theories of risk have provided insights into these different perceptions and into differences between these two groups [5]. Much research indicates that the public perceives allopathic medicines as 'unnatural' and as having the potential to cause adverse effects but sees products manufactured from plants and other natural products as being without risk [6]. Such differences are found not only for existing drugs but also for newly developed ones. One study exploring lay perspectives on future drugs showed a high level of scepticism and a low level of risk acceptance [7].

From a cultural perspective, anthropologists researching risk point out that definitions of risks must be seen in the context of people acting within social groups, where 'social principles' determine which 'real dangers' are selected for attention. Within these social groups, we find certain risks are downplayed and others are emphasised. This is a means of managing the unknown, and at the same time of maintaining and controlling the group. It is the group that is concerned with how to manage and how to negotiate risk in a society [8]. This approach can help explain differences in approaches to policy decisions between countries and other geographic areas.

In making decisions about whether or not to use medicines, patients must balance their perceptions of the risk against their perceptions of the potential benefits, as well as against the risks associated with illness. A wide variety of factors then come into play, but it is important for health professionals to recognize that these are patient perceptions, and that they may differ from their own. A study using the Health Beliefs Model (HBM) showed that doctors frequently erroneously consider patients' beliefs to be aligned with their own [9]. Ideally, professionals should help patients make assessments of potential benefits and harms in a process of shared decision-making. Dowell et al. [10] have set out several models of shared decision-making in their work on patient-centred prescribing. In a systematic review of 115 studies, Chewning et al. [11] found that in nearly two-thirds the majority of patients preferred sharing decisions with physicians to delegating decision-making to the physician. However, it must be recognized that some patients – particularly older people – do not believe they should question doctors or other health professionals [12].

Patient perceptions of the appropriateness or rationality of medicines may also differ from those of health professionals. Methods for assessing the appropriateness of medicines are almost entirely derived from the biomedical perspective (see Chapters 25 and 32), which may not align with that of patients [7,13,14]. Some authors have proposed definitions of good prescribing that take patients' perspectives into account [15,16], but a recent key report aimed at identifying steps in reducing inappropriate polypharmacy (an increasingly global issue of concern) made little mention of the patient perspective [18].

Patient attitudes towards medicine use

If given the choice, most patients would prefer not to take medicine. This is especially true of chronically ill patients: many describe medicines and the daily regime of medicine-taking as a 'necessary evil' [14,19]. Patients display coexisting accounts of positive and negative attitudes and experiences with medicine use [20]. Studies reveal the complexity of being at once grateful that a medicine provides relief of symptoms (and in many cases extends life), anxious about adverse effects and sceptical about the total net benefit [14,21,22]. People may also fear dependency and addiction [23]. All of these factors contribute to decisions about medicine use.

Key issues in medicine use

Self-medication

Self-medication, defined as the selection and use of medicines by individuals to treat self-recognized or self-diagnosed conditions or symptoms, is the most common form of medicine use worldwide [24]. The extent to which individuals are able to self-medicate is dependent on the regulation of medicines availability where they live (see Chapter 31). In high-income countries, self-medication is usually restricted to treatment of self-limiting conditions, but it is still widespread. For example, a community-based survey in the United Kingdom found that 42.7% of people with a range of long-term health problems, such as back pain and menstrual problems, had used OTC medications in the preceding 6 months [25]. Use of the Internet as a source of medicine supply has resulted in increased medicine use and has enabled individuals to circumvent regulations [26]. For example, people can buy pharmaceuticals (or what are sold as pharmaceuticals) that are restricted or illegal in their own country without a prescription or the authority of a pharmacist.

In other parts of the world, people may be largely self-sufficient in terms of health care until they suffer a major crisis [4]. In many countries, purchase of medicines without a prescription from pharmacies, street markets and other outlets is the main method of supply. Issues of affordability then come into play, along with provision of information and advice on product selection.

Decisions regarding treatment and self-care include choosing to use OTC treatments, seeking complementary and alternative therapies, self-adjusting prescribed therapies and engaging in self-diagnosis. Self-medication results in increased access to medicines, with attendant management of medical conditions, but also allows individuals to play an active role in their own health care. In theory, it can lead to more effective use of doctors' and pharmacists' skills and to reduced government expenditure on medicines. However, self-medication is not without risk, including incorrect self-diagnosis, incorrect choice or use of product, adverse reactions and interactions, use of medicines against recommendations [27], delay in seeking medical advice and masking of underlying serious conditions [28].

Self-diagnosis is itself not without problems. Especially where there is direct-to-consumer advertising (DTCA), it can lead to physicians being pressured by patients to prescribe medicines. In situations where a desired medicine is not available without a prescription, the patient may seek a medicine for off-label use. A recent example is students' use of attention deficit hyperactive disorder (ADHD) medicine to enhance study time [29].

Generics

As described in Chapters 21 and 31, there are many initiatives in many countries designed to increase the use of generic medicines. However, in spite of the general acceptance of generic products as clinically bioequivalent to the branded versions by health professionals and health organizations, these products often differ in their excipients, resulting in variations in efficacy and adverse effects and in their physical characteristics (e.g. size, shape and colour). Although it may be considered irrational by health professionals, these differences have been shown to affect patients' understanding and acceptance. A recent study concluded that some patients who receive generic medicines that vary in colour are over 50% more likely to stop taking them, increasing the odds of nonpersistence and leading to potentially important and adverse clinical effects [30].

Patients' confidence in and knowledge of generic medicines in general have increased over recent years in high-income countries, due to widespread educational initiatives and improved communication by health professionals [31]. In low- and middle-income countries, however, views are often more negative, with generics being seen as inferior and less acceptable [32]. A recent literature review concluded that although generic substitution is well accepted by the majority of patients, approximately one-third report negative experiences, which can end in poor adherence and medication errors [33]. In addition to policies advocating generic substitution, there are increasing numbers of programmes being developed in many high-income countries aimed at therapeutic substitution through switching policies. Very little work has explored patient perceptions of such policies or practices [34], but the general view is that no harm arises from switching drugs, such as statins. There may be some recognition that it can be inconvenient for patients and that switching can conflict with patient choice. One study illustrated the genuine negative experiences of patients on the receiving end of such switches: 54% did not understand the reason for the switch despite being sent an information sheet with a letter, 18% experienced an increase in adverse effects and 10% claimed they never received any information, only learning of the change to their medicine when filling their prescription [35].

Cultural influences

In addition to generic formulations, a range of other factors (which health professionals may dismiss as irrational) influence which medicines are seen as acceptable in particular countries and cultures. In developing countries, although the biggest problem is access to health care and medicines, cultural factors also play an important role in medicine use.

The form in which a medicine is administered (injection, tablet or liquid) and its colour can both affect acceptability and thus adherence to prescribed therapy [36]. For example, large stocks of ferrous sulphate went unused in Zambia in the late 1980s, reportedly due to the sugar-coated tablets being coloured black (a 'bad' colour); red-coloured tablets would have been perfectly acceptable, haematinics being the same colour as blood (Spivey, pers. comm.).

This 'cultural reinterpretation' of medicines is described by Van der Geest et al. [37]. The increasingly multicultural nature of societies globally suggests that it is not just a factor in low-income or traditional societies.

Beliefs about the superiority of injections over oral medicines are a major influence on drug use in some countries, resulting in the proportion of injectables prescribed becoming a key indicator for rational use (see International Network for the Rational Use of Drugs (INRUD) indicators in Chapter 1).

Research also shows that religion affects personal beliefs and choices, often playing a defining role in drug use. Religious beliefs can create a difficult barrier for many. For example, Catholicism does not condone the use of contraceptives, including emergency hormonal contraception (so-called 'abortion pills'), while several religions, including Hinduism, Judaism and Islam, prohibit the consumption of swine and bovine products; this is important as more than 1000 medications contain inactive ingredients derived from these sources [38]. Since patients have the right to make informed decisions about their drug treatment but are often unaware of the ingredients in their medicines, health professionals should be proactive and not leave it up to them to broach the subject [39]. The interpretation of religious laws and guidance is another factor affecting drug use. For example, a study of patients with type 2 diabetes from a Muslim background revealed changes in medicine use during Ramadan that were not always discussed with health care professionals. Many Muslim patients found that fasting during Ramadan was beneficial to their well being and therefore chose to fast despite the Islamic rule of exemption [40].

Cultural and health beliefs about different ways of managing illness can also result in variation in the use of complementary and alternative medicines among different racial/ethnic groups, as seen in the United States [41].

Although these religious and cultural factors have been observed and reported for decades, their implications for the use of medicines are rarely considered in drug utilization research studies.

Actual use of medicines

For prescribed medicines, once a health professional has provided a prescription, the patient may decide to have it dispensed or not, and subsequently they may or may not take the medicine as prescribed (see

Section F). Even when patients have chosen to use a medicine that has been prescribed for them, they may use it in different ways. On the basis of a synthesis of qualitative studies of lay perspectives, there is considerable evidence for the different ways in which patients test their medicines [42]: by using the occurrence of symptoms or side effects to evaluate changes in dosing or timing; by assessing impact on everyday life; by stopping the medication; by taking 'drug holidays' to see what happens; by observing others or obtaining information from others; and by using subjective rather than objective indicators. Pound et al. [42] produced a model of medicine use that distinguished four types of medicine-takers: passive accepters, active accepters, active modifiers and rejecters. These groups are not necessarily static, as patients may take different approaches to using medicines in different contexts and at different times [43]. Those who accept medicine-taking without necessarily giving it a great deal of thought may be characterized as passive accepters. They are content to trust their doctor and do whatever the doctor asks them to do. In contrast, active accepters are those who think about their medicine-taking; although they may test them, they take their medicines as prescribed. Active modifiers are those who test their medicines and then modify their regimens [44]. Rejecters are those who reject their medicines, whether after a period of testing or not. Rejecters may be willing to tolerate their symptoms or risk factors or may prefer to use complementary and alternative therapies to prescribed medicines. Pound et al. [42] concluded that widespread reluctance can be characterized as resistance to medicine-taking, as it captures the ways in which people take medicines while at the same time attempting to minimize their intake.

People with chronic illness normally have to take medicines for the rest of their lives. Some medicines will provide symptom relief and some will be taken for prophylactic purposes. Patients face numerous challenges in everyday medication management; the main one is to develop, maintain and adjust daily routines of medicine-taking. Haslbeck & Schaeffer [43] argue that a trajectory perspective is required to understand the different challenges at different points in an illness and in the medication experience. When patients are first diagnosed with a chronic illness, they may be highly motivated to take medicines as prescribed in the hope of leading a 'normal life'. Later in the illness trajectory, they may try to deescalate the increasingly complex problems of medication management. Chronic illness often requires constant self-monitoring. Patients taking multiple medicines illustrate how living with medicines can be just as difficult as living with symptoms. At one time or another, many such patients seek to substitute conventional medicines with nonpharmacological methods of treatment, before reluctantly returning to conventional medicine treatment [45]. Some adopt a 'minimax' strategy: minimal (thus, 'responsible') use of drugs and maximum use of other strategies, such as going to bed or avoiding certain activities, in order to restrict the amount of medication they need [46]. Long-term use of medicines has an impact on people's daily lives, from the processes of obtaining and maintaining supplies through to effects on relationships, social life and work-related activities, most of which is barely recognized by health professionals [47]. Health professionals are usually unaware of all the overwhelming barriers people with chronic conditions have to face when developing routines for managing their medications, as well as of the emotional pressure to take medicines [43]. Haslbeck & Schaeffer [43] propose the notion of 'stressed adherence' to convey the neglected affective component of medicine-taking.

For many patients, the cost of medications leads to underuse. A nationwide survey of over 2000 chronically ill adults in the United States found that 23% reported forgoing medication in the previous year due to cost. This was more likely for symptom relief medications than for primarily preventive medications [48].

The problem of nonadherence has been extensively discussed and researched in the professional literature for several decades, although few clear solutions have emerged. Stimson [49] pointed out 40 years ago that the notion of compliance requires patients to be 'passive, obedient and unquestioning': requirements that are increasingly anachronistic. Donovan [50] identified a number of assumptions inherent in the concept of 'compliance': that doctors know what is best for their patients; that they are able to impart medical information clearly and neutrally; that they prescribe effective treatments rationally; and that they are the main contributors to decisions about medicines. These assumptions are questionable. Much of the research on nonadherence ignores the patient perspective, despite the fact that much is now known about patients' perceptions and use of medicines, as well as what professionals can do to better support them (see Section F).

Use of information about medicines

People's use of medicines is influenced by information – both about medicines themselves and about health conditions. The availability of information about both has become ubiquitous in recent years through a variety of media, including newspapers, magazines, television and the Internet. All are easily accessible and relatively uncontrolled in the extent to which the information they put out is accurate and reliable. As already mentioned, the Internet also allows products to be purchased directly for a range of conditions, frequently self-diagnosed using the same information sources. Use is increased in some countries by DTCA (see Chapter 31).

The desire for information about medicines among patients has for many years been greater than its provision by health professionals [14,51], who may be unwilling to provide what patients want. Studies suggest that health professionals view written information in particular as being mainly designed to improve adherence and think that it should therefore be brief and simple, with only partial disclosure of side effects [52]. Some may believe that warning patients about side effects will lead them to believe they are experiencing them, but studies show that providing information about side effects does not result in their being experienced [53,54].

Nowadays, many people in high-income countries are provided with written information about prescribed or purchased medicines in the form of patient information leaflets (PILs) or inserts within the original packs of medicines supplied by the manufacturers. PILs are a legal requirement in EU countries, and their content is closely controlled, but many patients will seek further information from a range of sources, notably the Internet. In a number of countries, these leaflets are made freely available online. This contrasts to the situation in the United States and Canada, where only 'high-risk' medicines have mandated leaflets, for which the manufacturer must make a medication guide or 'MedGuide' available. US Food and Drug Administration (FDA) package insert guidelines require a section summarizing the most important information on benefits and risks. In practice, PILs may not reach the patient, as most medicines are not supplied in their original packs.

Well-controlled and accurate information sources are not available everywhere. In Thailand, for example, information leaflets for medicines have been introduced only relatively recently and their availability is highly variable. They are frequently written in English and designed for health professionals, not patients/the public (N. Jarernsiripornkul, pers. comm.).

To ensure they are useful and relevant, usability testing of PILs is now a requirement in many high-income countries, having been pioneered in Australia in the early 1990s. Information about side effects may nonetheless not be provided in a format that is easily understood [55].

Any individual patient's understanding of the information provided is of course dependent on their health literacy, defined by the US National Institutes for Health (NIH) as 'the degree to which individuals have the capacity to obtain, process and understand basic health information and services needed to make appropriate healthcare decisions' [56]. Research into health literacy has expanded considerably in recent years, primarily in the United States and Canada, where poor health literacy has been associated with reduced adherence to medicines (e.g. [57]). Studies have also shown that the ability of the public to correctly interpret even simple instructions on medicine labels is worryingly poor [58]. The practice of providing medicines in paper screws with no written instructions at all or in preprinted plastic bags with little information is still the norm in some low- and middle-income countries, where there is thus a need for verbal information.

Verbal information should, of course, be readily available from the medicine providers, but this is dependent on many factors. If medicines are purchased from licensed medicine sellers, the likelihood of receiving comprehensive, up-to-date, accurate information is much less than if they are obtained from a pharmacist. While good pharmacy practice includes the provision of verbal information about all medicines [59], this is still not the norm everywhere. Not all countries require that a pharmacy has a pharmacist on the premises at all times, and medicines can be sold by other pharmacy staff, who may or may not have been required to undergo training. Time may also be a limitation. Doctors are the preferred source of information about medicines (particularly prescribed medicines) for many patients, but their consultations with patients do not always ensure clarity of information [60,61]. The language used by health professionals is obviously important, as is timing: excessive information on medicine use at the time of a new diagnosis may not be absorbed or understood, and the need for information about medicines can change over time.

In order to make decisions about whether to take the medicines prescribed or recommended for them, patients must be able to weigh up the risks and benefits each provides. The way in which this information is provided is crucial, but as yet no ideal method has been devised. Health professionals and the industry extol the virtues of medicines, the professions in particular being encouraged to promote prophylactic measures for reducing risk of cardiovascular and other diseases, using evidence-based findings of population benefit. However, patients may – not unreasonably – see the benefits of reducing population risk, as opposed to their own risk, less positively.

The negative aspects of medicine use are frequently omitted from consultations, leaving patients to make their own judgements, through learning about risks from PILs and other sources. Since patient perceptions of risk and benefit are key to their decision on whether to use a medicine recommended or prescribed to them, patients have the right to information about both risks and benefits. While methods of providing information about risks have been closely studied, less attention has been paid to information about benefits. Some work suggests that adding 'benefit' statements to PILs, describing the anticipated effects of the drug, can change patient perceptions of the risk–benefit balance in favour of benefit [62]. Recent research is exploring the value from the patient perspective of adding information about the 'chance of benefit' for medicines used prophylactically [63].

Determining the patient perspective on medicines

Researching the patient perspective is no easy task, but is essential to a complete understanding of medicine use. Differences exist between the perspectives of patients and prescribers, but attempts to gain the patient perspective in studies of appropriate prescribing are few in number [64,65]. This often sets the stage for misunderstanding, as the researcher's approach – the questions they want the patient to answer – is frequently set before the study starts, placing restrictions on the types of answer they expect. Whoever defines the 'problem' sets boundaries for its 'solution'. Furthermore, patient perspectives are complex and often difficult to discover; they are not always verbalized or made accessible to researchers or health professionals, because people want to please, and so make themselves appear more positive than they really are. Patient perspectives also differ fundamentally from those of health researchers in that the vocabulary is different (for example, using feelings and emotions to describe physical states), leading researchers researchers to dismiss or discredit patient perspectives because they are difficult to measure – they differ from what many scientists would call 'systematic, rational thinking'.

These differences in perspective create several problems. If a patient knows what they are 'supposed' to be doing and fears reprisal for not doing it, they may not wish to seem disobedient. If they do not agree with, or trust, the doctor's advice, they may say nothing. The doctor may think that the consultation has gone well, when in fact the patient is making their own decision about whether or how to take their medicines. The fear of reprisal is a major impediment to open communication about medicines for those who are modifying their medication regimes [66]. It also makes it difficult for professionals to determine whether their care is effective. Other situations in which the difference in perspective is problematic include when DTCA causes patients to self-diagnose and ask for inappropriate treatments [67].

There is a plethora of instruments specifically designed to gather the views, attitudes and beliefs of patients about medicines, many developed with little patient involvement. Nonetheless, their use is widespread and highly relevant to how medicines are used. There are scales by which to measure patient beliefs about medicines and patient satisfaction with information on medicines, with medicines themselves and with their own ability to manage medicines [68–71]. Development of an instrument by which to measure the impact of medicine use from the patient perspective is underway [72]. Drug utilization research studies evaluating interventions designed to improve prescribing and use of medicines or to reduce costs need to involve the end user. Although the quantitative methods listed here have limitations, they can provide valuable insight into the reasons for variations in use.

In order to understand how people perceive and use medicines within the contexts and constraints of their everyday lives, it is necessary to use qualitative methods (see Chapter 13). This will necessarily involve the inclusion of researchers from other disciplines, who bring with them experience in studying the patient perspective and a wealth of expertise in areas not often used in current drug utilization research. Many randomized controlled trials (RCTs) now include embedded qualitative process evaluations to investigate the acceptability of new interventions (drugs) to patients, among other things. This combination of methods and disciplines is likely to make a productive contribution to drug utilization research in the future.

Involving patients in drug development and monitoring

Patients and the public are increasingly becoming involved in decisions about the recommended use of medicines. In the United Kingdom, for example, the National Institute for Health and Care Excellence (NICE) encourages patients to submit topics and help develop guidance, and its Public Involvement Programme informs, trains and supports lay people to contribute to (lay versions of) guidelines. Patients contribute to pharmacovigilance in many countries, where their reports of adverse drug reactions (ADRs) are perceived as adding valuable data to those of health professionals [73]. However, they are not usually involved directly in decisions about the licensing of medicines, although their representatives can become vociferous in demands for changes to licensing, such as allowing the use of drugs in serious conditions where regulators have deemed them too dangerous [74]. Eichler et al. [75] are of the view that the patient contribution to decision-making at this level is overdue. An exploratory study has already been carried out, which suggests that, with the right support, patients can make a useful and distinctive contribution to drug licensing decisions. It has also been argued that the patient voice is not heard in drug development (e.g. in phase 2 trials), where it might make a valuable contribution [76].

Conclusion

In conclusion, we propose that the future success of drug utilization research depends on the broadening of the existing multidisciplinary collaboration between epidemiologists, clinicians, clinical pharmacologists and pharmacists to include researchers from the social sciences and humanities. Broader collaborations will enable the pursuit of a wider range of research questions, using both qualitative and quantitative research methods, and promises to deepen our collective understanding of the ultimate end user of all drugs: the patient.

CHAPTER 34
An introduction to adherence research

Bernard Vrijens
WestRock Healthcare & University of Liège, Belgium

KEY POINTS

- Medication adherence is the process by which patients take their medications as prescribed. It is a dynamic process, comprising three elements: initiation of therapy, implementation of the dosing regimen and persistence with treatment.
- Medication adherence can be measured using different methods, including pill counts, self-report, therapeutic drug monitoring, electronic prescription/refill databases and automatic/electronic compilation of dosing history data.
- Electronic detection of package entry is considered the current gold standard for automatically compiling drug dosing history data.
- Interventions intended to improve medication adherence need to address the three elements of the process, as well as the changes required in the health care system.

Definition and taxonomy

During the 4 decades of adherence research to date, and drawn from a variety of perspectives and academic disciplines, a diverse and sometimes conflicting terminology has been generated [1]. With the growing interest in adherence-related sciences, there is now a need for consistent, transparent taxonomy and definitions. As a part of the Ascertaining Barriers to Compliance (ABC) project, Vrijens et al. [1] proposed a new taxonomy for behaviours related to taking medication. ***Adherence to medication*** (or ***medication adherence***) is defined as the process by which patients take their medications as prescribed. This process starts with ***initiation*** of the treatment, which occurs when the patient takes the first dose, and continues with the ***implementation*** of the dosing regimen, represented by the extent to which a patient's actual dosing corresponds to the prescribed dosing regimen from the first to the last dose. The quantification of implementation requires the comparison of two time series: the prescribed drug dosing regimen and the patient's actual drug dosing history. ***Discontinuation*** of therapy happens when the patient stops taking the prescribed medication. ***Persistence*** is defined as the length of time between initiation and discontinuation of therapy. In clinical studies, the first dose is typically administered on-site, so it is often assumed that initiation is implicit for all included patients. In such a case, persistence is defined as the time from inclusion until discontinuation.

Management of adherence is the process of monitoring and supporting a patient's adherence to medication, carried out by health care systems, providers, patients and their social networks; its goal is to help patients follow appropriately prescribed drug dosing regimens in order to maximize their effects and minimize their harms (Figure 34.1). ***Adherence-related sciences*** close the loop between medication adherence and adherence management, and comprise those disciplines that seek understanding of the causes or consequences of

Drug Utilization Research: Methods and Applications, First Edition. Edited by M. Elseviers et al.
Published 2016 by John Wiley & Sons, Ltd.

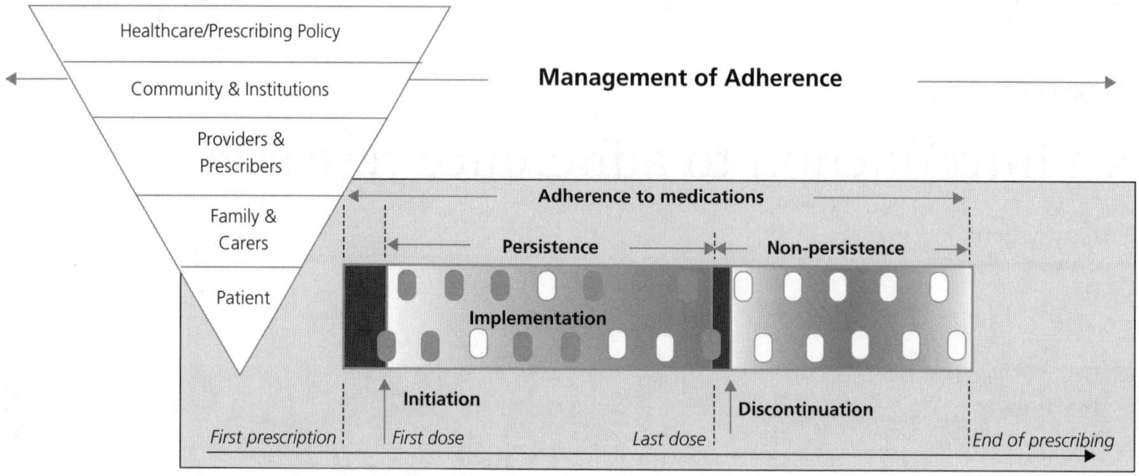

Figure 34.1 Adherence to medication and management of adherence.

Source: Vrijens et al. 2012 [1]. Reproduced with permission from John Wiley and Sons.

differences between prescribed and actual exposures to medicines. These sciences cross the boundaries between many fields, including (but not limited to) medicine, pharmacy, nursing, behavioural science, sociology, pharmacometrics, statistics and economics.

The importance of patient adherence to medications

Medication adherence is now recognized as a global issue of major public health concern [2]. It is also a major economic burden, because it undermines the effectiveness and may compromise the safety of certain prescription medicines that are subject to hazardous rebound effects during periods of interrupted dosing or to recurring first-dose effects as dosing resumes after periods of interruption [3]. At the Health Ministers' Summit held in Amsterdam on 3 October 2012, it was claimed that a USD474 billion avoidable cost opportunity, or 8% of the world's total health expenditure, exists in the area of medication adherence. The most expensive medication is the one that is paid for but never taken.

For many years, medication adherence has been considered solely a patient problem, and has received too little attention. Today, we know that we can provide effective adherence management that enhances medication adherence and achieves continuity of patients' exposure to – and thus continuity of the therapeutic actions of – prescribed drugs. There is, however, no single 'fix' by which to achieve this objective. Interventions intended to improve patient adherence need to address the three elements of the process, as well as the changes required in the health care system that will enable successful management of patient adherence to medication. The solution must be based on reliable quantification of the dosing errors incurred by patients. It must not be limited to simple quantities of doses missed, but should include reliable data on when lapses in dosing occur and for how long, as well as on the dosing patterns that prevail as patients resume dosing (which may or may not be correctly timed; for different patterns of dosing errors, see Figure 34.2). Such data are the logical foundations for new models of integrated care. Thus, reliable measurement of patients' dosing patterns (i.e. the proper measurement of adherence) is the foundation for effective and efficient corrective action [4].

Measurement of adherence

Besides a transparent and well-defined taxonomy, it is critical to appropriately quantify the three elements of medication adherence. Appropriate quantification should provide researchers, clinicians and patients with meaningful metrics by which (i) to describe different experimental investigations, (ii) to assess quality of care and (iii) to demonstrate achieved performance. Such

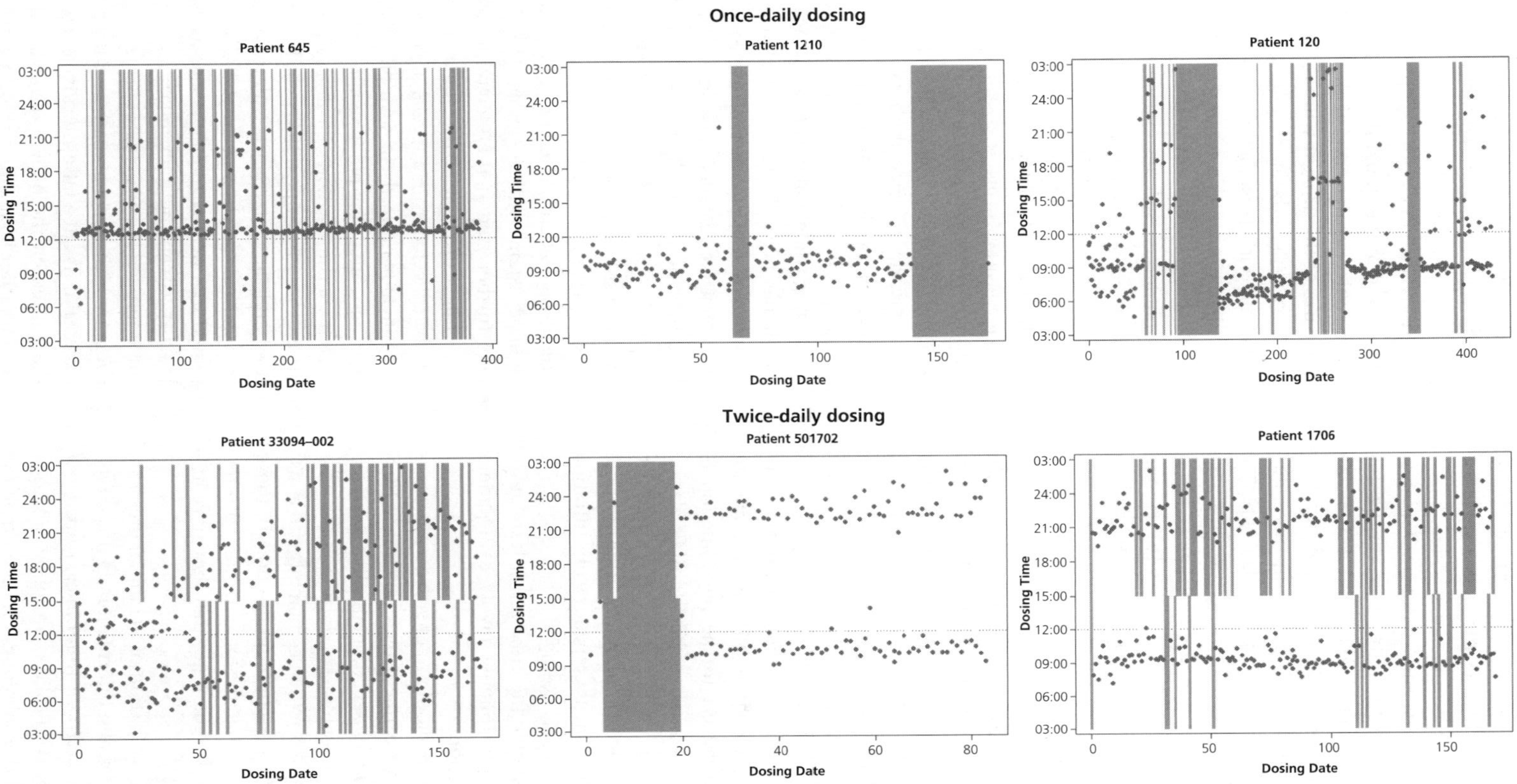

Figure 34.2 Electronically compiled drug dosing histories of 22 patients, each of whom took 81% of their prescribed dose during the observation period. The dots represent electronically captured dosing times and the vertical bars show omitted doses. This is an abridged version of the figure. For the complete, large version, please refer to the companion website: www.wiley.com/go/elseviers/drug_utilization_research.

adherence metrics should be reliable, trackable over time, coherent with the three elements of medication adherence and implementable on a large scale.

Methods that rely on patients' recall and/or allow patients to censor information on their dosing histories have repeatedly been discredited, as they are strongly biased toward overestimation of drug exposure. Attempts to use such data are not only misleading but typically add burden to the patient's daily life. The counting of returned, untaken doses ('pill counts') has been repeatedly discredited since the first reliable test of their validity by chemical marker methods [5]. Despite virtual uniformity of repetition of the 1989 work of Pullar et al. [5], clinical researchers continue to report pill-count data as if no one had ever questioned their reliability.

Clearly and self-evidently, anything depending on the recall of patients is doomed from the outset, because who can recall what they took last Tuesday? Beside recall bias, patient self-report is affected by desirability bias and is easily censored by the patient, resulting in misleading sky-high adherence levels (for more detailed discussion of this, see Chapter 35).

Methods that are based on sampling performed during a clinical visit (e.g. blood sampling for therapeutic drug monitoring) are subject to the phenomenon of 'white-coat adherence', which is a short-term escalation in adherence during the few days prior to a scheduled visit to the clinic or laboratory [6]. Many drugs (but not all) can be restored to their therapeutic concentration ranges by 1–3 days of correct dosing.

Apt quantification should therefore result from automatic compilation of the routines involved in patient adherence to a medication.

- The first act of the medication adherence process is the prescription of a treatment by a physician. ***Electronic prescription databases*** automatically track each prescription issued by a physician, including the time at which they are issued. When combined with a dispensing record of the prescription (also timed), these provide confirmation that the patient has acquired the medication – but no guarantee that they have initiated the treatment.
- The second act is the collection of the initial prescription and subsequent refills. Information on this is typically available from ***electronic (pharmacy) dispensing databases***. A patient who collects an initial prescription but fails to collect a subsequent refill on time (or at all) may be regarded as having not satisfactorily adhered to the prescribed medicine, although it will be unclear how much drug they have taken, or when they took it, simply from the time elapsed between the dispensing of the initial prescription and the request for a refill. Furthermore, if the patient discontinues their use of the drug, it will take a minimum of two refill intervals without evidence of use before one can conclude with reasonable certainty that the patient has discontinued the treatment altogether. The use of dispensing databases is thus a vague indicator of an ambulatory patient's exposure to a drug, with the added problem that the information is so late in coming as to be of very limited utility in the management of the patient's medications.
- The third act is the activation of the package to remove the medication. This step can easily be monitored through ***electronic detection of medication package entry*** by the patient (***Smart Package***). This method has been extended to detect the activation of a pump [7] or an injection [8]. It can also capture the time of disposal of syringes [9]. It is, of course, an indirect method of estimating when and how much drug is administered, but it has been shown to correlate well with drug concentration in plasma [10,11]. This approach delivers a reliable, detailed assessment of dosing history data over time (see Figure 34.2). Feeding this information back to the patient constitutes the cornerstone of a focused discussion between patient and health care provider, which has been proven successful in enhancing patient adherence and maintaining long-term persistence with treatment [12].
- One further step is the electronic detection of the appearance of a tablet in the stomach. This information can be collected from a special microcircuit on a small chip included directly in each pill (***Smart Pill***). Once the chip-containing pill is swallowed, a signal is generated via the creation of a short-lived voltage difference caused by ionic differences between the gastric fluid and the chip, which is detected by an antenna in a dermal 'patch' and amplified so as to be transmitted to a nearby mobile device and on to a server [13,14]. Given the high reliability of package entry, this approach is probably not justified, given its drawbacks, which include patient intrusiveness, safety issues, the risk of a false-negative event detection and the burden on the patient of having to continuously wear a rather large adhesive skin patch [11].

In ***prospective clinical trials***, electronic detection of package entry enables a thorough characterization of adherence, with clear distinctions between initiation, implementation and discontinuation. It is the current gold standard for automatically compiling drug dosing history in trial settings and has been recommended by the US Food and Drug Administration (FDA) draft guidance enrichment methods for drug development [15].

In ***medical practice***, the use of electronic detection of package entry is the simplest and least demanding method by which to monitor and manage therapies, especially those with a narrow therapeutic window that require strict implementation of the prescribed dosing regimen. Since acquisition of prescribed medication typically precedes the use of electronic monitoring, the use of electronic prescription databases is probably the most efficient approach to measuring treatment initiation. Moreover, patients who discontinue their treatment are often not motivated to return their electronic monitoring device, meaning that their adherence cannot be assessed. Therefore, in medical practice, the best estimation of persistence with a specific treatment, a class of treatment or switches between treatments is provided by pharmacy dispensing databases, if they are available and well designed. This information can be used upfront to identify patients who are at risk of treatment discontinuation based on previous data, but it typically comes too late to be useful in the effective management of a patient's use of current medications.

In medical practice, there is thus probably no single gold standard, as information from different sources must be combined in order to best estimate the three elements of medication adherence.

Considerations for future research

While medication adherence is a blanket qualitative term that describes the process of taking prescribed medications, it is critical for future research that the three elements of initiation, implementation and persistence with treatment are properly distinguished. Besides these elements, medication adherence has multiple other dimensions, many of which still need to be discovered and studied. A nice parallel is surgery, which moved from a general discipline towards specialization, not only by body parts (cardiac, gastrointestinal, orthopaedic, etc.), but also based on timing (elective versus emergency), purpose (exploratory versus therapeutic) and equipment (laser, scalpel, robotic).

The multidimensional aspect of patient adherence to medications is a real challenge for future research, which needs to specialize and to specify precise objectives. In this context, the matrix presentation of Table 34.1 may be a useful guide, as illustrated in the following examples:

- The concept of drug forgiveness, defined as the post-dose duration of therapeutically effective drug action [11,16], is mainly related to cell 2.2. When a treatment is not initiated or is discontinued too early, no efficacy should be expected. In the presence of variable drug exposure due to suboptimal patient implementation of a dosing regimen, to guarantee continuity of drug action it is essential to understand the degree of the drug's forgiveness and to support the patient's implementation in order to avoid critical deviations.
- The assessment of a patient's beliefs and/or concerns [17] over the prescription of a new treatment

Table 34.1 Matrix for characterization of medication adherence research into its three elements: initiation, implementation and discontinuation.

	Medication adherence		
	Initiation of treatment	*Implementation* of the dosing regimen	*Discontinuation* of treatment (nonpersistence)
Determinants	1.1	1.2	1.3
Consequences	2.1	2.2	2.3
Costs	3.1	3.2	3.3
Measures	4.1	4.2	4.3
Interventions	5.1	5.2	5.3
Benefits of intervention (clinical and economical)	6.1	6.2	6.3
Other topics of interest	7.1	7.2	7.3

is related to cell 1.1, the determinants of treatment initiation, and to a lesser degree to cell 1.3, short-term discontinuation. In fact, a patient's beliefs and/or concerns may change over time and are often influenced by the patient's own experience with treatment (side effects or efficacy), which limits the explanatory power of such assessment at baseline.

- The development of interventions to enhance patient adherence should clearly identify which of their components address each of the three elements: How can we initiate more patients? (cell 5.1); How can we support patients to implement the prescribed dosing regimen and so deliver continuity of drug action? (cell 5.2); How can we maintain long-term persistence and avoid treatment discontinuation? (cell 5.3).

To conclude, adherence-related sciences have a promising future in a wide variety of disciplines, including medicine, nursing, pharmacy, psychology, statistics and economics. Patient adherence to prescribed medications is a complex problem with multidimensional interacting components. It is therefore unsatisfactory, misleading and unacceptable to summarize patient adherence in a single number, such as proportion of prescribed doses taken (PDT), or, even worse, to dichotomize a patient as being adherent if their PDT exceeds 80%.

To progress in adherence research, it will become critical that the multidimensional aspects of patient adherence to treatment be better addressed and more precisely described in the literature. Special consideration should focus on:

1 The identification of the three components of medication adherence: initiation, implementation and discontinuation.
2 The use of the most appropriate measure for the given clinical situation (trial, research and medical practice) and specific component of adherence.
3 The type of research interest, as listed in the first column of Table 34.1 (determinants, consequences, costs, interventions, etc.).
4 For interventions: a precise description of the behavioural components, using a consistent taxonomy, as proposed by Michie et al. [18]; specification of the standard of care used for comparison [19]; and clear identification of the changes required of the health care system and of the person responsible for delivering the intervention.

CHAPTER 35

Assessment of medication adherence in field research

Monique Elseviers[1] & Bernard Vrijens[2]

[1]*Centre for Research and Innovation in Care, Faculty of Medicine and Health Sciences, University of Antwerp, Belgium*

[2]*WestRock Healthcare & University of Liège, Belgium*

KEY POINTS

- Medication adherence is the process by which patients take their medications as prescribed. It constitutes three elements: initiation, implementation and discontinuation.
- Given the different natures of the three elements, medication adherence cannot appropriately be summarized using an average rate of prescribed doses taken over a defined period of time.
- The choice of adherence measures largely depends on the purpose of use, be it routine clinical practice or more research-oriented.

Introduction

In recent years, the clinical problem of nonadherence by individual patients has gained in interest. Clinicians realize that nonadherence may be the most plausible explanation for the lack of therapeutic efficacy of a prescribed drug. A reliable assessment of the medication-taking behaviour of a patient remains a serious obstacle to distinguishing between treatment resistance and medication nonadherence, however.

While there is an increased focus on adherence-related sciences, drug utilization research and the broader field of pharmacoepidemiology seldom address the specific problem of medication nonadherence. Drug utilization researchers use pharmacy refill or claims databases to express drug exposure as the amount of medication prescribed or dispensed over a defined period of time, without any adjustment for medications that are delivered but not consumed. Related estimations of the clinical and economic consequences of nonadherence are hard to firmly establish. Additionally, a systematic review of randomized controlled trials (RCTs) focusing on medications intended for long-term use in adults reveals that in this specific research area, the reporting of adherence is poor and the methodology inconsistent, making comparison between studies hard to interpret [1] (see also Chapter 34).

Assessment of adherence

The assessment of medication adherence remains a challenging problem. A reliable assessment tool needs to be capable of distinguishing between the three elements of adherence: initiation of therapy, implementation of the dosing regimen and discontinuation of therapy. ***Initiation of therapy*** occurs when a patient takes the first dose of a medicine and continues with the implementation of the dosing regimen, represented by the extent to which a patient's actual dosing corresponds to the prescribed dosing regimen from the first to the last dose. The quantification of ***implementation*** requires two time series to be compared: the prescribed drug dosing regimen and the patient's actual drug dosing history. ***Discontinuation of therapy*** happens when a patient stops taking the prescribed medication [2] (see also Chapter 34).

Drug Utilization Research: Methods and Applications, First Edition. Edited by M. Elseviers et al.
Published 2016 by John Wiley & Sons, Ltd.

In field research, medication-taking behaviour can be approached by objective and direct methods (e.g. by measuring drug concentrations in the blood) or by more subjective and indirect ones (e.g. by interviewing the patient about their medication intake pattern). The most reliable tool by which to measure adherence is electronic detection of package entry. Electronic monitoring can be considered the gold standard assessment of adherence in clinical trials [3].

Apart from clinical trials, prescription and dispensing databases are commonly used for the global and individual assessment of adherence, based on existing and available data sources (see Chapter 36).

Reporting adherence estimates

Estimates of adherence are usually reported as the percentage of the prescribed dose of a medication taken by a patient over a specified period of time. Such rates are misleading as they do not distinguish between the three elements of adherence. For example, an adherence rate of 50% does not allow a patient who stops treatment halfway through the observational period to be distinguished from one who persists with treatment but takes the dose only every other day.

There is no accepted standard for what constitutes adequate adherence [4]. The confusion between the three elements of medication adherence when reported as a rate over a period of time has led to the very misleading threshold of 80% being used to judge whether or not a patient can be classified as adherent. This threshold does not make any pharmacological sense, given that the many different treatments used across many different therapeutic areas have very different half-lives and durations of action. In recent years, increasing insight into medication-taking behaviour has revealed that a single standard for all patients, for all kinds of medication and for all intake patterns (ranging from missing part of one's intake every day to taking real drug holidays for several days) is senseless.

Consensus is growing that all reporting on adherence should start from the distinction between the three dimensions of adherence, with separate sections devoted to the initiation and discontinuation of therapy. Initiation has to be reported as a dichotomous outcome (yes/no), implementation as a longitudinal set of data (time series data) and discontinuation as a time to event [4]. In order to determine a standard of adequate adherence, one must take into account the pharmaceutical properties of the medication, the therapeutic goals in relation to the specific disease and the individual characteristics of the patient [4]. Rather than a general standard, deciding upon adequate adherence will evolve in the direction of a patient-oriented approach.

Additionally, assessment tools capable of distinguishing between intentional and unintentional nonadherence are gaining in attention. Unintentional nonadherence is merely a result of forgetfulness [5]. The distinction between the two is of particular interest in the development of interventions (see Chapter 37).

Reported adherence estimates are typically higher among patients with acute conditions than those with chronic conditions [6]. Simple dosing regimens (once daily) lead to better regimen implementation compared to more complicated dose regimens, but this slight improvement in adherence does not necessarily translate into better clinical outcomes [3,7,8]. In particular, noninitiation and early discontinuation differ considerably across different clinical conditions (see Figure 35.1). Greater adherence is also reported in clinical trials than in medical practice, primarly driven by better initiation and lower compliance [9]. Moreover, large differences in adherence rates are observed in comparative studies in which different methods of assessing adherence are used simultaneously in the same patient [10,11].

Measuring adherence using electronic monitoring

Automatic compilation of drug dosing histories can be realized by incorporating microcircuitry into pharmaceutical packages of various designs, such that the manoeuvres needed to remove a dose of drug are detected, time-stamped, analysed, stored and communicated to the appropriate caregiver(s) and/or the researcher(s). While electronic detection of package entry is an indirect method of estimating when a drug is administered and how much is used, it can accurately project the time-course of drug concentrations in the plasma [12].

A medication event monitoring system (MEMS) is a smart package in the form of a pill bottle cap containing an electronic chip that registers the time and date of every opening. It has been widely used in clinical trials, as illustrated by almost 700 peer-reviewed publications (www.iAdherence.org). Smart packages are

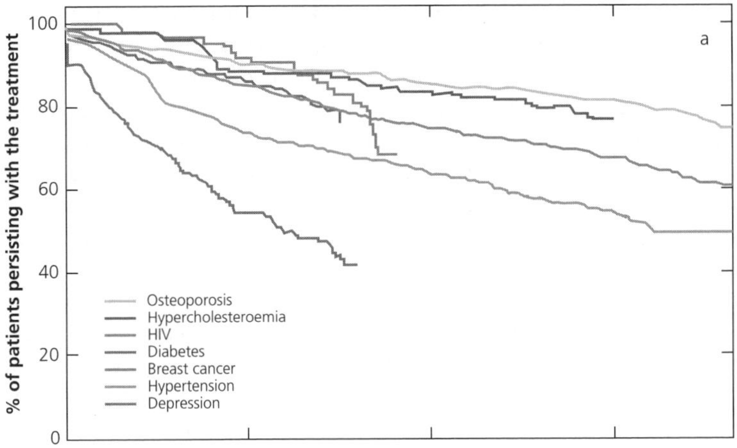

Figure 35.1 Differences in adherence according to different disease conditions, showing noninitiation and short persistence in seven disease conditions based on Kaplan–Meier persistence curves across different therapeutic areas. Note the between-disease differences in the percentage of patients who initiated the prescribed treatment. For colour details, please refer to the colour plates section.

Source: Adapted from Blaeschke et al. 2012 [4].

safe, unintrusive and easy to use, have long-lasting battery times and can easily be adapted to any form factor, including blister packs, inhalers, injectables and polymedication. The resulting adherence data are reliable and detailed, allowing the problems of nonadherence to be entangled with noninitiation, poor implementation and early discontinuation (Figure 35.2).

In clinical trials, smart packages constitute the gold standard of measurement of the three elements of medication adherence. It provides information on when

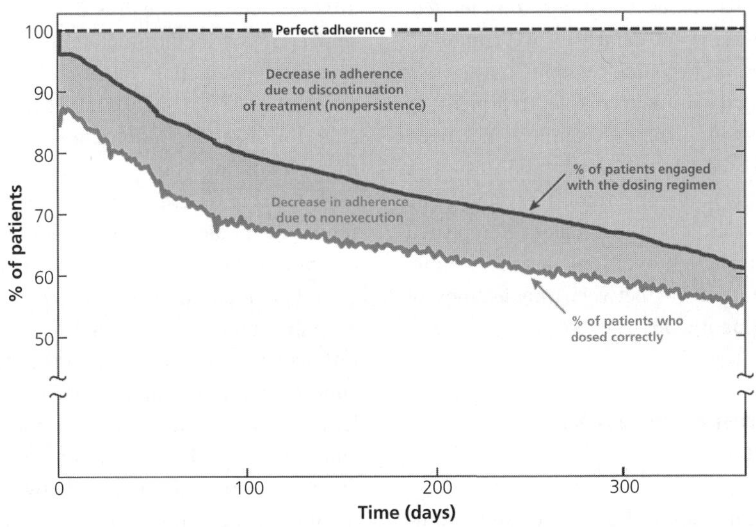

Figure 35.2 Kaplan-Meier plots of the time course of adherence parameters of 16 907 patients prescribed oral medications for one of a variety of medical conditions in 95 studies, during the first year of electronic compilation of the patients' dosing histories. The horizontal dashed line illustrates how perfect adherence by all patients would be depicted. The top line shows the percentage of patients still engaged with their dosing regimen as time passes following the start of treatment. The abrupt drop at zero time reflects noninitiation of treatment by approximately 4% of the patients. Thereafter, the decline indicates patients' permanent discontinuation of their engagement with the dosing regimen, which occurs at a somewhat higher rate during the first 100 days than thereafter. The bottom line shows the percentage of patients who dosed correctly on each day after the start of the observation period. Thus, it wobbles slightly from day to day. The area between the top and bottom lines indicates the shortfall in drug exposure arising from missed doses. The area above the top line indicates the shortfall in drug exposure arising from noninitiation by approximately 4% of patients and subsequently from short persistence with the prescribed dosing regimen by approximately 35% of patients.

Source: Adapted from Blaeschke et al. 2012 [4].

a participant initiates treatment. It delivers a reliable and detailed assessment of the implementation of a dosing regimen over time, allowing the identification of different patterns of adherence (see Figure 35.2). Finally, it allows one to determine precisely when a participant discontinues treatment.

In medical practice, the use of smart packages is most cost-effective with therapies that have a narrow therapeutic index and require precise implementation of the prescribed dosing regimen. Strategic time points for the use of electronic monitoring are at treatment initiation, to support the habit of medication taking [13], and at treatment failure, to avoid unnecessary dose increases or changes in treatment.

Electronic monitoring of adherence focuses particularly on the implementation of the dosing regimen, offering detailed information on intake frequencies and timing. Outside clinical trial settings, electronic monitoring requires patient activation and buy-in to the system. Therefore, in order to gain accurate information on noninitiation and long-term persistence with therapy, the use of electronic databases is highly recommended. When electronic prescription databases are combined with refill databases, it becomes feasible to precisely identify which patients do not initiate treatment or delay initiation. Assuming that a treatment has been initiated, refill databases – based on gap analysis – can detect when a patient is discontinuing treatment. The strength of this approach is that it can identify repeated sequences of discontinuation over long periods of time, taking into account switches between medications of the same class (see Chapter 36).

Measuring adherence using questionnaires

Although a large bibliography shows electronic monitoring to be the most accurate and best validated tool for adherence research purposes, its use in clinical practice is still limited. Many other assessment tools are used in clinical practice (as well as in field research), showing different degrees of consistency, validity and responsiveness [14]. Examples of field research using different assessment tools are summarized in Table 35.1.

There is a great need among clinicians and researchers for an adherence assessment tool that is cost-effective, easy to administer and accurate in measuring a patient's medication-taking behaviour. A large number of ***self-report questionnaires*** have been proposed for this purpose. Self-reports can focus on a particular patient population or may be suitable for use in different populations, diseases and types of medication. They examine implementation of dosing regimens, focusing particularly on repeated dose omissions and drug holidays. Initiation and discontinuation are seldom examined. In most self-reports, patients have to describe their own medication-taking behaviour by answering several questions using dichotomous (yes/no) or Likert-like answer categories. Some use a visual analogue scale (VAS) to quantify the amount of medication taken. Apart from questioning concrete medication-taking behaviour, most self-reports also contain questions on barriers to adherence and beliefs about medicines, aiming to indirectly identify patients at risk for nonadherence.

In recent years, several ***systematic reviews*** evaluating the suitability of different assessment tools for routine clinical use have been published [14–18]. These reviews are useful for all those in search of a suitable and reliable self-report of medication adherence (see Table 35.2). The number of tools included in such reviews ranges from 20 to 58. Dobbels et al. [14] looked at scales suitable for assessing adherence to immunosuppressive therapy among transplant patients. They focused on tools capable of assessing both medication use and the timing of medication use. Alghurair et al. [16] offered an overview of observed barriers to adherence. Ramsey et al. [17] focused on adherence in patients with headache and used broad criteria to select assessment tools for inclusion. Nguyen et al. [18] included 43 self-report adherence questionnaires that were correlated with at least one comparator of medication-taking behaviour. Only in this review was attention given to the ability of self-reports to distinguish between initiation, implementation and discontinuation. All scales assessed implementation, but only 14/43 handled discontinuation and only one also included initiation (Table 35.2). Garfield et al. [15] offered the best overview of assessment tools that directly focus on reporting adherence patterns, using 1–21 items with either dichotomous or Likert-like answer categories. Four questionnaires handled the distinction between intentional and unintentional nonadherence.

In research settings, most of these self-reports are validated using other assessment tools to compare for

Table 35.1 Examples of different assessment tools used in field research

Reference	Population	Details	Validation tools
Determination of drug levels			
Strauch et al. 2013 [27]	339 patients with resistant hypertension	Determination of antihypertensive medication in a blood sample	None
Mkopi et al. 2014 [30]	651 patients with tuberculosis in Tanzania	Determination of antituberculosis medication in a urine sample	Recall interview Self-report (MMAS) Pill count
Pill count			
Brain et al. 2013 [25]	117 patients with schizophrenia	Pill count	Electronic monitoring Recall interview Plasma levels
Bosman et al. 2014 [10]	41 pregnant women with depression	Pill count	Electronic monitoring Self-report Plasma levels
Self-report by scale			
Fernandez et al. 2008 [31]	168 African Americans with hypertension	MASES	Electronic monitoring
Gialamas et al. 2009 [32]	4968 diabetic patients	MARS-5	Clinical outcome
Kalichman et al. 2009 [11]	298 HIV patients	VAS 100-point scale with three marked points (0, 50, 100%)	Pill count Recall interview
Jonsdottir et al. 2010 [33]	280 patients with severe mental disorders	VAS 100-point scale with five marked points (0, 25, 50, 75, 100%)	Plasma levels Self-report MARS-5 Provider report
Tommelein et al. 2014 [34]	734 COPD patients	MARS-5	Medication refill
Almeida et al. 2014 [35]	135 patients with malaria	Five-item self-report adapted from MMAS	Pill count
Self-report by diary			
Bruce et al. 2010 [19]	67 patients with MS	Written medication diary	Electronic monitoring (sharps container) Recall interview
Mutschler et al. 2012 [36]	18 patients with schizophrenia and bipolar disorders	Electronic medication diary combined with reminder and symptom report	None
Gordon et al. 2013 [20]	1500 chronic hepatitis C patients	Electronic dosing diary	Pill count Virological response
Recall interviews and caregiver report			
Khanam et al. 2014 [21]	4097 hypertensive patients in Bangladesh	Structured questionnaire with one question on discontinuation of therapy after diagnosis	None
Gelaw et al. 2014 [22]	270 diabetic patients in Ethiopia	Structured questionnaire with questions on adherence and reasons for nonadherence	None
Vreeman et al. 2015 [24]	191 HIV-infected children	Caregiver report	Electronic monitoring

MMAS, Morisky Medication Adherence Scale; MASES, Medication Adherence Self-Efficacy Scale; MARS-5, Medication Adherence Report Scale 5 item; VAS, visual analogue scale; HIV, human immunodeficiency virus; COPD, chronic obstructive pulmonary disease; MS, multiple sclerosis.

Table 35.2 Systematic reviews of self-reported medication adherence tools.

Reference	Number of selected questionnaires	Inclusion criteria	Exclusion criteria	Number handling initiation (I) or discontinuation (D)	Number handling barriers (Ba) or beliefs (Be)	Validation against other assessment tools
Dobbels et al. 2010 [14]	20	Adults	Specific disease	ND	Ba 5/20	9/20
Garfield et al. 2011 [15]	58	Validated self-reports	Specific disease Beliefs only	ND	Ba 27/58	54/58
Alghurair et al. 2012 [16]	51	Adults Hypertension	Adherence rates only	ND	Ba 51/51	6/51
Nguyen et al. 2013 [18]	43	Validated self-reports	ND	I 1/43 D 14/43	Ba 30/43 Be 7/43	43/43
Ramsey et al. 2014 [17]	32	Headache	ND	ND	Partly handle both	2/32

ND, not determined.

concurrent validity. Garfield et al. [15] and Nguyen et al. [18] compared the results of the self-report scales with electronic monitoring in 30/58 and 12/43 scales, respectively. The comparisons revealed only a positive association in about one-third of the scales. Moreover, only a few scales kept their concurrent validity when used in other settings or other types of medicine [18].

A particular form of self-reporting adherence consists in the daily registration of medication-taking behaviour in a ***patient diary***. Bruce et al. [19] compared adherence reported in a written diary with electronic monitoring in patients with multiple sclerosis (MS) and found high correspondence between the two methods. Electronic recording in a patient diary was used in combination with pill count and virological response to assess adherence in patients with chronic hepatitis [20]. Recently, more sophisticated systems have become available, combining the functions of a diary with a registration of current disease symptoms in a pocket-sized tool [20].

More qualitative methods such as ***recall interviews*** can be used to assess adherence. This is the method of choice in populations with a high degree of illiteracy, as recently demonstrated in hypertensive patients in rural Bangladesh [21] and diabetics in Ethiopia [22]. Promising results have recently been reported in inpatient settings and ambulatory care clinics, where trained pharmacy technicians question patients about their medication history [23].

Health care workers and caregivers can be used to obtain a more indirect assessment of medication-taking behaviour. Although labour-intensive, ***caregiver reports*** are still in use, particularly in children and patients with mental illness [24].

Other as measures of adherence in field research

Pill count (counting the remaining tablets after a period of suspected medication intake) was one of the earliest methods used to assess patient adherence with prescribed therapy. Positive results were reported in the Swedish COAST study, which compared electronic monitoring, pill count, plasma levels, self-report and caregiver reports in measuring adherence to schizophrenia treatment [25]. In a study focusing on adherence to antidepressants during pregnancy, pill count showed good agreement with electronic monitoring, whereas a self-report scale and blood-level monitoring did not [10]. Returned tablet counts show only aggregate consumption, however, and are subject to upward bias through prevalent dumping of untaken dosage forms. Returned tablet counts 'grossly overestimate' what patients have actually taken. Comparisons between electronic monitoring data and returned pill counts are a common feature of studies in which MEMS monitoring is used; gross overestimation by pill counts of what was taken are a regular feature of such comparisons [6].

The ***direct observation of pill intake*** can be considered the most accurate method of ensuring that every patient receives every dose. However, direct observation is labour-intensive, expensive and, thus, seldom used beyond phase I and limited phase II studies. Of note is the successful use of direct observation of therapy for the management of tuberculosis in New York City over the past 2 decades. A reduction in the dosing regimen to three times a week combined with a high density of population and medical care makes it cost-effective to use direct observation of therapy in this particular setting, but it has failed in many other conditions [26].

The ***level of the drug, its metabolite(s) or a biological marker*** related to the drug can objectively be measured in body fluids. In RCTs in particular, the addition of a marker to both the medication and the placebo enables adherence to be measured in both arms of the trial. This approach requires a clinical visit and is costly, sparse and ultimately subject to white-coat adherence, which is a short-term escalation in adherence during the few days prior to a scheduled visit to the clinic or laboratory. The method was successfully used to assess the prevalence of pseudoresistance caused by nonadherence among patients with severe resistant hypertension [27]. Unplanned blood sampling was performed in all patients in order to assess antihypertensive drug concentrations. The observed low adherence in outpatients with resistant hypertension (23% partially and 24% totally noncompliant) led to the conclusion that nonadherence has to be considered and tackled as a primary cause of resistance to hypertensive treatment. In this study, the key was to perform unplanned sampling, which is very intrusive, costly and resource-intensive, making this approach almost inapplicable in practice.

Advantages and disadvantages of different adherence assessment tools

Sources of bias among the different tools currently used to assess adherence are summarized in Table 35.3. In order to evaluate the advantages and disadvantages of these tools, research requirements must be distinguished from needs in daily clinical practice.

In research, there is a need for assessment tools that are reliable and unbiased and which offer measures of adherence that enable accurate identification of subtle differences. Today, electronic monitoring combined with information obtained from refill databases is becoming the gold standard for assessment of adherence. In order to move adherence-related sciences forward, it is essential that future research uses appropriate metrics for the three elements of medication adherence. Reliable and precise measures constitute the cornerstone of study of the determinants and consequences of medication adherence. Understanding of these elements is the basis for a successful intervention to enhance medication adherence and maintain long-term persistence with prescribed therapies.

Clinicians want tools that are cost-effective and easy to assess and to score. The patient who self-reports not taking medication is the most cost-effective identification of nonadherence. While this approach has a high positive predictive value (PPV), its negative predictive value (NPV) is extremely low, due to desirability bias. Self-report tools are still the most common method, despite the major disadvantages of being subjective, unreliable and prone to bias. The reliability of self-reports – but also of pill counts and recall interviews – suffers from white-coat expectations: patients want to give the impression that they handle in accordance with the expectations of the health care provider, and try to deny incomplete medication intake. The reliability of these tools improves in settings where the relationship between patient and health care worker is based on mutual respect and shared decision-making (see Chapter 33).

A critical review of the high number of self-report adherence scales available revealed that most have large methodological shortcomings and limited proofs of validity [14,15,18]. Apart from assessing real medication intake pattern, most self-reports also focus on

Table 35.3 Sources of bias in different adherence assessment tools.

Source: Adapted from Vrijens & Heidbuchel 2015 [3]. Reproduced by permission of Oxford University Press.

	Initiation	Implementation	Discontinuation
Electronic monitoring	Gold standard in clinical trials	Gold standard	Gold standard in clinical trials
Prescription and refill databases	Gold standard	Only aggregate summary	Gold standard
Direct determination in body fluid	Requires sampling after prescription	Sampling is too sparse	Subject to white coat adherence
Self-report	Desirability bias	Recall bias	Desirability bias
Pill counts	Easily censored by patient	Only aggregate summary	Easily censored by patient

barriers and beliefs about medications. In many tools, however, reported adherence estimates are based on a mix of intake patterns, barriers and beliefs. As a result, many are not sufficiently precise to measure subtle changes in individual adherence patterns and are unreliable in comparison with more objective assessment tools [17].

For the accurate measure of the three elements of medication adherence (initiation, implementation and discontinuation), a combination of electronic monitoring and refill databases is desirable. The data produced can then be used to enable a focused discussion between health care providers and the patient. Intentional and nonintentional reasons for nonadherence can be identified and addressed with the patient. This adherence feedback approach has been shown in clinical trials to enhance adherence and maintain long-term persistence with treatment [28,29]. Its implementation in medical practice can largely be improved by a multidisciplinary approach, including not only all health care providers but its implementation in medical practice can largely be improved by a multidisciplinary approach including not only all health care providers but giving a central role to the patient and his informal caregivers.

Conclusion

Medication adherence is the process by which patients take their medications as prescribed. It constitutes three elements: initiation, a dichotomous variable (yes/no); implementation, a dosing history (time series data); and discontinuation, a time to event outcome. Given the different natures of these three elements, medication adherence cannot appropriately be summarized using an average rate of prescribed doses taken over a defined period of time. Choice of adherence measures largely depends on the purpose of use, whether it be routine clinical practice or more research-oriented.

Future field research must focus on the separate assessment of initiation, implementation and discontinuation of therapy, the combination of results deriving from different measurement approaches, the distinction between intentional and nonintentional nonadherence and a more multidisciplinary and patient-centred approach.

CHAPTER 36

Assessment of adherence to drug treatment in database research

Jean-Pierre Grégoire & Jocelyne Moisan
Faculty of Pharmacy, Laval University, Canada
Population Health and Optimal Health Practices Research Unit, CHU de Québec Research Centre, Canada

KEY POINTS

- Prescription and dispensing data can be useful in assessing adherence to treatment in a given population.
- Drug adherence researchers are strongly recommended to provide a good description of the adherence construct being measured, the measure being used (including any treatment reference time window or any permissible gap period) and the results of their sensitivity analyses.
- If used judiciously, administrative data can provide adequate measures of drug treatment initiation, persistence and compliance.

Introduction

In a report published by the World Health Organization (WHO) in 2003, adherence is defined as 'the extent to which a person's behaviour – taking medication, following a diet, and/or executing lifestyle changes, corresponds with agreed recommendations from a health care provider' [1]. Adherence is an umbrella term made up of three main constructs: initiation (or primary adherence), persistence and compliance (or implementation) [2,3] (see Box 36.1). Initiation entails the patient's acceptance of the treatment. Persistence involves the patient maintaining the treatment for the prescribed duration. Compliance involves the patient taking the recommended number of doses and following the recommended schedule.

Box 36.1 Adherence to treatment.

Adherence is a broad term defined as the extent to which a person's drug-taking behaviour corresponds with agreed recommendations from a health care provider.

Adherence constructs

- Initiation: the extent to which a newly prescribed drug treatment is undertaken.
- Persistence: the extent to which the treatment is taken for the recommended duration (this applies to medium- or long-term treatments, not to single courses).
- Compliance: the extent to which the drug is taken at the recommended doses and following the recommended schedule (this does not apply to 'as needed' drug treatments).

Adherence to drug treatment can be assessed in a number of contexts. In clinical trials and comparative effectiveness and safety studies, adherence is generally measured to provide an estimate of the intensity of drug exposure (see [4]). In the context of drug utilization research, adherence can be used to describe patients' adherence behaviours, identify the determinants of those behaviours and develop and test interventions to optimize drug use. This will be our focus in this chapter. We will present some methods for the assessment of the three adherence constructs in administrative database drug utilization research and will discuss some of the issues surrounding this assessment.

Drug Utilization Research: Methods and Applications, First Edition. Edited by M. Elseviers et al.
Published 2016 by John Wiley & Sons, Ltd.

Measuring adherence: prescription versus dispensing administrative data

Prescription and dispensing data drawn from medical record databases or health programmes can be useful in assessing adherence to treatment (see Table 36.1). The Clinical Practice Research Datalink (CPRD) and The Health Improvement Network (THIN) both contain prescription data, for example [5]. These data can be used to assess adherence, but a number of assumptions must be made in order to do so, the validity of which is difficult to check. For example, when assessing persistence with treatment using prescription data, one needs to assume that prescriptions are being filled by patients on the same day as they are issued and that treatments are taken as prescribed. One has also to assume that, as long as a physician is prescribing a drug, the patient is taking it.

Dispensing data provide information on prescribed drugs in a patient's possession. If the research focus is on quality of prescribing, dispensing data are less informative than prescription data. For example, errors of omission by physicians (e.g. not prescribing a required drug) are likely to be overestimated by dispensing data, as an unknown proportion of prescriptions are issued but not filled by patients. However, dispensing data are particularly useful for measuring adherence to treatment, if the administrative database provides information on number of days supplied. Although one must assume that a drug that is purchased is taken, in order to be taken, a drug needs first to be in the patient's possession. Dispensing data have their limitations, however. First, they do not contain information on whether a drug is still being prescribed. Therefore, patients whose drug has been discontinued may wrongly be considered nonpersistent if they stop filling it. Second, they are sensitive to reimbursement and to administrative rules. For example, if a drug is not (or is no longer) covered by a drug plan, a patient may be considered nonpersistent even if they continue to take it by paying out of pocket (a majority of administrative databases do not capture out-of-pocket transactions). Researchers must therefore be aware of the reimbursement and administrative rules that apply to any administrative data they use to measure adherence.

Table 36.1 Sources of administrative data used to measure adherence.

Source	Construct	Advantages	Limitations
Prescription data	Initiation	Allows initiation to be measured, if linked with dispensing data	Initiation cannot be measured unless linked with dispensing data
	Persistence	Confirms the drug is still being prescribed	Requires one to assume that the prescription is filled the same day it is issued and that patients fill all prescribed renewals
	Compliance		Requires one to assume that the prescription is filled the same day it is issued, that patients fill all prescribed renewals and that the drug is taken according to the prescribed dosage regimen
Dispensing data	Initiation	Allows initiation to be measured, if linked with prescribing data	Initiation cannot be measured unless linked with prescribing data Sensitive to reimbursement rules[a]
	Persistence	Provides information on drug possession	Requires one to assume that drugs in a patient's possession will be taken and that the patient is still on treatment with all such drugs Sensitive to reimbursement rules[a]
	Compliance	Informs on the possession of the drug	Requires one to assume that drugs in a patient's possession will be taken and that such drugs are still being prescribed Cannot measure the adequacy of the drug schedule Sensitive to reimbursement rules[a]

[a]For example, the dispensing of drugs that are not reimbursed may not be recorded in the database.

Table 36.2 Measures of adherence constructs using administrative data.

Adherence construct	Measure	Type of administrative data
Initiation (acceptance or primary adherence)	Drug is filled within an acceptable period after the prescription is issued (yes/no)	Prescription and dispensing
Persistence (discontinuation)	1. Time between filling of first prescription and discontinuation 2. Initiated drug is refilled: • within the no. of days of supply (plus a permissible gap) (yes/no) • sufficiently close to a given initiation anniversary date (based on no. of days of supply plus permissible gap) (yes/no)	Dispensing
Compliance (implementation)	1. Proportion of days covered (PDC) 2. Proportion of prescribed doses taken 3. Calculated proportion is higher than a predetermined threshold value (yes/no)	Dispensing

Measurement selection

There is no gold standard of adherence measurement using administrative data. All methods have their limitations, but some are more suitable than others for use with a particular construct. Measurement selection should therefore primarily be guided by the construct of interest. For example, if a study aims to describe the dynamics of patients' treatment discontinuation (nonpersistence) and return to therapy, the focus should be on measuring nonpersistence. A measurement based on gaps in refilling a prescription will then be more appropriate than one based on the proportion of days potentially covered by filled prescriptions. Table 36.2 summarizes some methods that can be used to measure adherence, according to the construct of interest.

Measuring initiation

Until recently, little was known about the extent to which patients filled drug prescriptions issued by their physicians. Early studies on this topic were small in size [6] and limited to single practice settings [6,7]. Dispensed data had to be compared with hand-written paper copies of prescriptions issued. The availability of electronic prescribing data that can be linked with pharmacy claims data [8] and of prescription data entered by physicians in their electronic health records (EHR) [9] has made it easier to estimate drug treatment initiation.

Although measuring initiation may at first look easy, there are two major issues: (i) Should initiation be measured using new prescriptions only? and (ii) What should be considered an allowable time window between when a prescription is issued and when it is filled?

New versus repeat prescription or dispensing

Should we measure initiation using repeat prescriptions or just first issues? Based on the definition of initiation ('when the patient takes the first dose' [3]), it looks as though only new prescriptions should be considered. However, some might interpret this definition in a broader sense as 'when the patient takes the first dose of the latest prescription issued'. In such a situation, one might consider mixing prescriptions issued to patients who have already initiated their treatment with prescriptions issued to drug-naïve patients, but this would make the interpretation of results problematic. Indeed, since time on treatment is a strong predictor of treatment continuation, it is likely also to be a strong predictor of whether a reissued prescription is filled. The proportion of filled prescriptions is therefore expected to be higher among 'ongoing users' than among 'potential new users'. This is illustrated in a study conducted in the United States linking electronic prescribing data issued between 1 April 2004 and 31 March 2005 with pharmacy claims data [8] (see Box 36.2). This study found that 78.1% of all prescriptions of antidiabetic medicines were filled, but when only new prescriptions were considered, the

Box 36.2 Primary medication nonadherence: analysis of 195 930 electronic prescriptions.

Main objective

- To evaluate primary nonadherence (noninitiation) across different classes of drugs.

Population

- Patients (n = 75 589) issued one or more electronic (e) prescriptions by a community-based physician as part of the eRx Collaborative in Massachusetts between 1 April 2004 and 31 March 2005.

Data sources for adherence measurement

- e-prescribing transactions linked with pharmacy claims files.

Adherence

- Construct measured: noninitiation (or primary nonadherence).
- Measure: a prescription was considered filled if there was a corresponding claim in the pharmacy file at any time between the date the prescription was issued and the end of the study.

Main results

- Out of 195 930 prescriptions issued, 78% were filled. This proportion was 72% for new prescriptions.
- Among patients aged 19 and over, the proportion of primary nonadherence (never-filled new prescriptions) varied between 25% for antianxiety drugs and 55% for pain drugs.

Issue

- Results were difficult to interpret, as the available time window in which to assess whether issued prescriptions were filled varied from 0 to 365 days.

Source: Fischer et al. [8].

proportion was 9.5% lower. The gap was as high as 20% for prescriptions issued for pain drugs.

If the focus is on new prescriptions only, defining what is a new prescription could be challenging using administrative data. The best approach is to look back through the pharmacy claims data to check whether a prescription for the same drug was filled in a prespecified period of time before the 'index' prescription being considered. How long this washout period should be depends on the study objective and on the population and target drugs. For example, if the research objective is to assess 'initiation of a new antidepressive treatment', one might want to consider new episodes of treatment, irrespective of prior treatments. Then, a washout period of 3 months might be considered acceptable to define the prescription as being for a new episode. On the other hand, the concept of 'new episodes' may not apply for the treatment of diseases such as hypertension, diabetes or dyslipidemia. The duration of the washout period will then be mainly determined by the extent to which specificity has to be maximized. For example, if it is important to consider only lifetime drug-naïve individuals, the longer the washout period, the higher the specificity. This comes at the expense of a lost in efficiency, however, since gains in specificity will eventually reach a plateau. Besides, historical data may simply not be available. Determining a relevant washout period also depends on the characteristics of the administrative data. In some drug plans, prescriptions are dispensed for 30-day periods, while in others they are dispensed for longer (90 days or more). This type of administrative rule has to be taken into consideration when defining the washout period.

Time window between prescription and dispensing

Determining the appropriate time window within which a prescription issued should be filled is another important issue to consider when measuring initiation. Specifically, what is the maximum appropriate time between when a prescription is issued and when it is filled? There is no easy answer to this question. The duration selected will have an influence on the calculated proportion of individuals initiating a drug treatment: the longer the duration, the higher the proportion is likely to be.

In past research on this topic, either no time window was defined [7,8] or it was defined arbitrarily. In the study by Fischer et al. [8], in order to be considered to have initiated a prescribed treatment, patients had to fill the prescription at any time before the end of the study (i.e. 31 March 2005). The time window was thus variable, and depended on the date on which the prescription was issued. It went from 0 days for electronic prescriptions issued on 31 March 2005 to 365 days for those issued on 1 April 2004. Results are therefore difficult to interpret, as it is unknown to what extent they would have been different if the time window had been the same for all prescriptions issued. On the other hand, a time window of 30 days has been used in two studies [9,10]. In Raebel et al. [9], patients were considered 'primary nonadherent' if a prescription for an antihypertensive, an antidiabetic or a lipid-lowering oral drug was not filled within 30 days of issue.

Clearly, the duration of the time window should be fixed and should take into account the period of legal validity of prescriptions in a given jurisdiction. The time window should also be determined according to the clinical situation for which a drug is being prescribed.

Finally, it is recommended that sensitivity analyses be conducted to check whether initiation results are robust to changes in the duration of the drug-naïve washout period and in the duration of the time window within which an issued prescription should be filled.

Measuring persistence/ discontinuation

Persistence with treatment and discontinuation are two related constructs. Both persistence and discontinuation can easily be measured using administrative data, provided the following dispensing information can be retrieved: name of drugs dispensed and number of days of supply (or, alternatively, the quantity dispensed and the prescribed dose). There are two main assumptions being made here: (i) to be taken, a drug needs to be in the patient's possession; and (ii) once dispensed, a drug will be taken by the patient.

Prescribing data can also be used in place of dispensing data. An example is studies relying on medical record data [11,12]. Persistence is then likely to be overestimated compared with pharmacy-based estimates. Even if a physician keeps issuing prescriptions, their patients may never initiate treatment, or if they do, they may later stop refilling their prescription. Such patients will be misclassified as persistent.

Persistence can be measured using either of two principal methods: the refill-gap method and the treatment anniversary method.

Refill-gap method

With the refill-gap method, a patient can be considered persistent on a drug treatment as long as they keep refilling the drug within a pre-specified period of time. This period is specified according to the dispensed number of days of supply. A patient is then expected to refill the prescription before or on the date on which they will run out of drugs. Otherwise, they will no longer be considered persistent. A permissible gap can be added to the expected date of refill. This allows the fact that a patient may indeed be persistent with a treatment even though they are not taking all prescribed doses to be taken into account. In other words, the patient may be persistent but not compliant (or may show suboptimal implementation). This permissible gap needs to take into account periods during which the patient is hospitalised, particular if the in-hospital use of drug is not captured in the administrative database. When a patient is considered nonpersistent, it can be useful to define the date of discontinuation. This is often arbitrarily set as the date on which the patient was expected to refill the prescription, or in other words, the date they would have run out of supply if they had been compliant. Notably, this can be done so long as the prescribed daily doses (PDDs) or number of days of supply are available. It should not be done based on defined daily doses (DDDs) only, as this entails the problematic assumption that DDD equals PDD.

The refill-gap method can be applied for as long as a patient is followed up, since the patient will be censored at the date of discontinuation, loss of drug coverage (e.g. due to hospitalization or migration) or death, whichever comes first.

In order to illustrate the refill-gap method, we will refer to the hypothetical case of a patient who initiates a treatment prescribed for a long period (see Figure 36.1). Measurements are based on outpatient administrative data. All prescriptions are dispensed for 30 days. The patient gets the first two refills (D2 and D3) on days 30 and 60, as expected. The next refill (D4) seems to be late at day 110. However, as the patient has been hospitalized for 20 days, the treatment is still being refilled within the expected period (day 90 + 20 days = day 110). Considering this last refill was at day 110, the

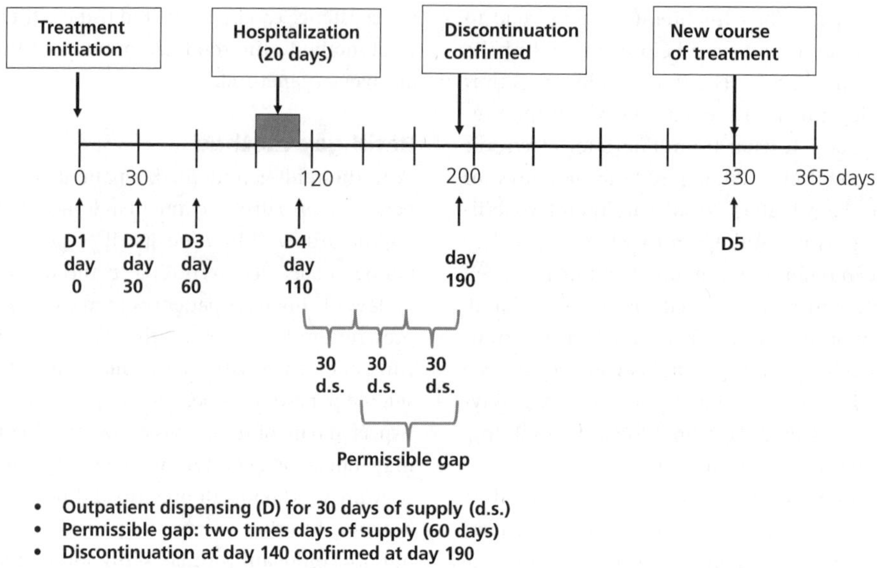

Figure 36.1 Measuring persistence: the refill-gap method.

patient is then expected to refill again before or at day 140. Given a permissible gap of two times the days of supply (i.e. 60 days), the patient would still be considered persistent with the treatment if the prescription was refilled before or at day 200 (day 110 + 30 days of supply + (2 × days of supply = 60) days of supply = day 200). The patient fails to refill their prescription by day 200, however, so is no longer persistent. Discontinuation is confirmed at day 190. The patient is considered to have discontinued the treatment at day 140; that is, at the end of the most recent 30-day supply. The patient eventually refills the treatment (D5) at day 330. This is considered a new course of treatment.

The refill-gap method is particularly useful when the focus of a study is on persistence or discontinuation patterns. In order to develop interventions aimed at preventing discontinuation, it is important to describe these patterns in terms of occurrence and timing. The timing of occurrence can be estimated by measuring the time from initiation to a first discontinuation, or the time from a new course of treatment to a second discontinuation, using Kaplan–Meier survival curves. This approach has been used to describe persistence patterns in the treatment of hypertension [13], dyslipidaemia [14] and type 2 diabetes [15] (see Box 36.3). It can help identify some determinants of a first or second discontinuation, upon which an intervention can be built.

The refill-gap method has some limitations. First, persistence estimates are sensitive to the permissible gap definition. It is therefore suggested that sensitivity analyses be conducted in order to verify whether different definitions of permissible gap affect the robustness of results. Second, not taking into account stockpiling from previous supplies can overestimate discontinuation, as patients may be late to refill because they are taking their accumulated supplies [16]. The shorter the permissible gap, the higher the risk of overestimating discontinuation. Third, in assessing persistence with treatment at a pre-specified point in time after treatment initiation (e.g. 1 year after initiation), the refill-gap method will provide an underestimate if patients are censored at the first discontinuation on the assumption that they will never return to treatment. Research has shown that this assumption does not hold [13–15]. This limitation can be avoided by using another approach: the treatment anniversary method.

Treatment anniversary method

This method consists in assessing whether or not patients are still taking a treatment a given period of time after treatment initiation. It can be applied for as long as a patient remains followed up, until the anniversary date (e.g. the 6, 12 or 24-month anniversary). It is illustrated in Figure 36.2, using the same hypothetical

Box 36.3 Patterns of persistence with oral antidiabetic drug (OAD) treatment in newly treated patients – a population-based study.

Main objective

- To evaluate persistence patterns in new users of metformin and insulin secretagogues sulfonylureas.

Population

- Individuals aged 18 years and older covered by the Quebec public drug plan who had a first claim (wash-out period of 1 year) of metformin or of insulin secretagogues sulfonylurea between 1 January 1998 and 31 December 2003 (n = 98 940).

Data sources for adherence measurement

- *Régie de l'assurance-maladie du Québec* pharmacy claims files.

Adherence

- Constructs measured:
  - Persistence with OADs.
  - Reinitiation.
- Measures:
  - Persistence with initial OADs, defined as continuously refilling within three times the number of days of supply of the preceding claim, regardless of add-on OADs or insulin (excluding hospital days).
  - Reinitiation, defined as treatment initiation with any OAD after a first treatment discontinuation.

Main results

Based on Kaplan–Meier curves:

- The probability of persisting with initial OADs went from a high of 65% after 1 year to a low of 28% after 6 years.
- Among those who discontinued their initial OADs, the probability of initiating a new course of treatment was around 60% in the first year after discontinuation, reaching over 80% after 6 years.

Issue

- Since the refill-gap method was used to measure persistence, compliance is hard to measure.

Source: Gregoire et al. [15].

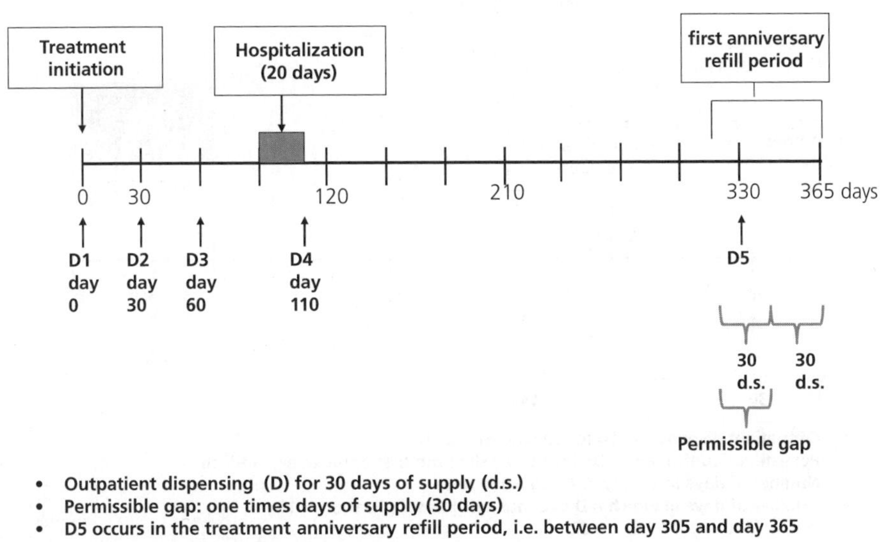

Figure 36.2 Measuring persistence: the treatment anniversary approach.

case of a patient who initiates a treatment prescribed for a long period of time and dispensed for 30 days. The objective here, however, is to determine persistence with treatment specifically at the 1-year anniversary of treatment initiation. This involves assessing whether the patient is taking the treatment at day 365. Here, the challenge involves defining an appropriate anniversary refill period. At the minimum, this period should be equal to the number of days supplied at the most recent dispensing before or at the anniversary date. If compliant, the patient will then be in possession of enough units of drug to take it at the anniversary date. However, as already mentioned, persistence and compliance are different constructs. A patient can therefore be persistent yet noncompliant.

As in the refill-gap method, it may be appropriate to add a permissible gap when defining the anniversary refill period. In our example, the permissible gap is defined as one times days of supply (i.e. 30 days). The first anniversary refill period zone goes from day 305 ((365 − 30 days of supply) − (1 × days of supply = 30) days)) to day 365. In this example, as the patient is dispensed a prescription (D5) at day 330, which is within the first anniversary refill period, she/he is considered to be persistent with the treatment.

This method has its limitations and strengths. On one hand, it is insensitive to discontinuation periods that occur before the treatment initiation anniversary. Indeed, in the example presented in Figure 36.2, it does not capture the fact that the patient has been off treatment for 89 days (i.e. from day 140 until day 330, excluded). On the other hand, it is easy to compute. It also has the advantage that it can be coupled with a compliance measure (see Figure 36.3). This makes it possible to characterize two different adherence constructs in a single person: persistence and compliance.

Persistence with initial drug versus persistence with therapy

The focus of a persistence study can be either the initial drug/drug class or any drug taken to treat a condition (therapy persistence). The focus of early studies in the field of hypertension was on the initial drug prescribed [11] or dispensed [17]. Focusing on the initial drug may be relevant if one wants to describe patterns of newly used drugs. In addition, it is sometimes used as a measure of treatment effectiveness (e.g. in schizophrenia [18]). On the other hand, if the purpose of a study is to assess whether patients are still being treated for their condition, then the focus of the persistence

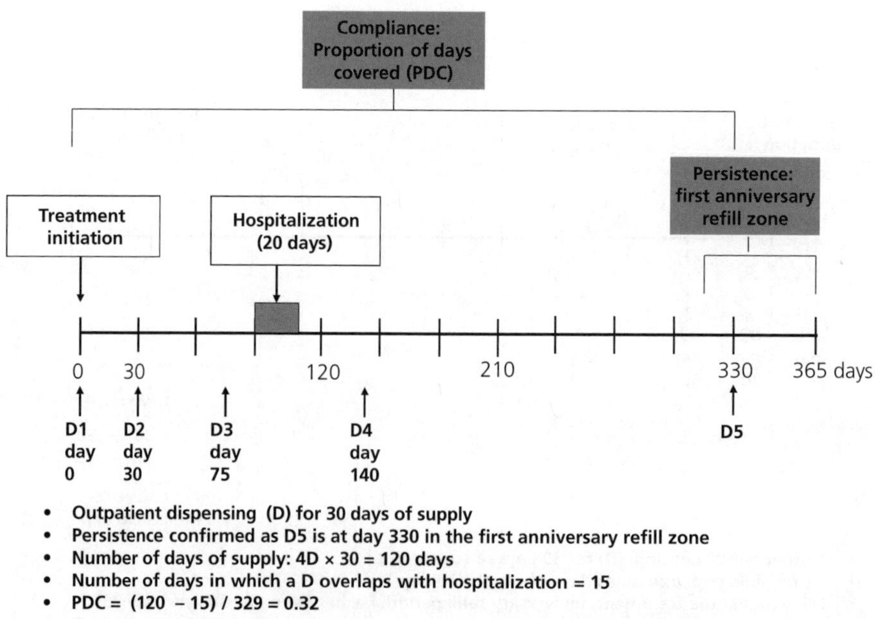

Figure 36.3 Measuring compliance in those who are persistent.

measure should not be restricted to the initial drug but rather should include any treatment recommended for that condition. This is particularly relevant in chronic disease areas for which clinical guidelines recommend multiple-line drugs. For examples of studies of persistence with any treatment, see Qvarnström et al. [19] (hypertension), Cooper et al. [20] (schizophrenia) and Grégoire et al. [15] (diabetes).

Measuring compliance (implementation)

Once a treatment has been initiated, compliance can be measured using administrative data, provided the following information can be retrieved: the identity of the drugs dispensed and the number of days of supply (or, alternatively, the quantity dispensed and the prescribed dose). This information generally comes from pharmacy claims data. The compliance measure is based on the quantity of drug available to the patient during a given period of time. As for the measure of persistence, assessment is made under the following assumptions: (i) in order to take a drug, a patient needs to have it in their his/her possession; and (ii) drugs acquired at the pharmacy will be used.

Metrics based on drug gaps have been proposed for the measurement of compliance [21], but they are not often used. A series of metrics based on drug possession [22] are more popular. Among them, the proportion of days covered (PDC) is the most widely used. The PDC is the total number of days of supply dispensed during a specified period of time divided by the length (in days) of that period. The period starts at the date of treatment initiation (date of first fill or day 0) and ends according to the research objective. If the objective is to measure compliance over a 1-year period, for example, the period might end at day 365. It might also end at the date of the most recent fill (prior to day 365) or at any other date specified by the researchers. If, over the observation period, a patient fills more units than the prescribed number, the total number of days of supply will then exceed the number of days in the observation period and the PDC will then be greater than 1. Most researchers choose to cap the PDC at 1. Exceptions may be made in situations for which it is relevant to capture a potential drug overconsumption or abuse. An efficient approach consists in programming the PDC calculation in such a way that drug possession is assessed for each day of the observation period, based on the number of days of supply of drug previously dispensed. As for the measure of persistence, one may consider excluding hospital stays from the calculation. The 'medication possession ratio' and the 'continuous measure of drug availability' are two other popular measures of drug possession that are similar to the PDC.

An example of the calculation of PDC is given in Figure 36.3. The observation period goes from day 0 (date of initiation) until day 330 (date of last dispensation). Since the patient has the prescription dispensed four times during that period, the number of days covered by the drug is 110 (i.e. 4 dispensings × 30 days), minus the 10 days for which a dispensation overlaps with hospitalization. The percentage of days covered with the drug is 32% (i.e. 110 out of 329 days). If the observation had gone from day 0 until day 365, the number of days covered would then be 150 days (5 dispensings × 30) minus 10 days of hospitalization overlap, for a PDC of 0.38.

A first challenge is to determine the treatment period in reference to which the PDC should be calculated. Let's assume a patient initiates the treatment with a dispensing for 30 days. If the patient discontinues the treatment at any time during this 30-day period, there will be no other recorded dispensation in the database. If we calculate the PDC in reference to a treatment period duration of 60 days then the PDC will equal 0.5 (30 days supply/60 days). As the drug has not been refilled following the initial dispensation, one has to assume the patient is still taking it at day 60. In this example, given that the patient has discontinued the treatment after the initial dispensation, the PDC measure decreases inversely with an increase in the duration of the PDC measurement reference period. For instance, for a reference period of 90 days after treatment initiation, the PDC will be 0.3 (30 days of supply/90 days). For a 365-day reference period, the calculated PDC will be 0.08 (30 days of supply/365 days). In a compliance study, given the sensitivity of the PDC calculation to the duration of the treatment reference period, it is very important that the duration be the same for all patients.

As we have just seen, a major limitation of the PDC is its inability to capture periods of nonpersistence. Indeed, with the PDC, it is difficult to distinguish patients with a low compliance who persist with treatment from those who have discontinued their treatment early. The example in Figure 36.3 helps to illustrate this limitation. The patient has a low PDC of 0.32 but is still using the drug treatment 1 year after initiation, yet a patient who was fully compliant with the treatment for the first 4 months but who discontinued it thereafter would have a similar PDC.

The PDC may not provide an accurate measurement of compliance in patients who have initiated treatment but not persisted with it. Persistence therefore has to be measured first, using the treatment anniversary approach (see Figure 36.3). Compliance with treatment can then be assessed for patients who persist at treatment anniversary, by calculating the PDC for the prescribed drug over the observation period. In Figure 36.3, the patient is persistent with the treatment 1 year after initiation, allowing the PDC to be calculated (= 0.32). If the last dispensation (D5) had occurred at day 210 rather than at day 330, this patient would not be persistent. It would then not be relevant to calculate the PDC, as they would no longer be taking the drug.

For an example of this approach, we will refer to a health administrative database study conducted to assess the determinants of persistence and compliance among 6662 new users of an antipsychotic for the treatment of schizophrenia [20] (see Box 36.4). A total of 4495 patients (67.5%) were persistent with the treatment 1 year after initiation; among them, 3534 (78.6%) had an antipsychotic in their possession for at least 80% of the first year and were therefore considered compliant. This approach has also been used in a study assessing the determinants of persistence and compliance among 151 173 new users of oral antidiabetic drugs (OADs). Among them, 119 832 (79.3%) were persistent 1 year after treatment initiation, and 93 418 (78.0%) of those had an antidiabetes drug in their possession for at least 80% of the time [23].

In general, the PDC calculation does not take into account stockpiling from previous supplies. This is

Box 36.4 Adherence to atypical antipsychotic treatment among newly treated patients: a population-based study in schizophrenia.

Main objectives

- To measure the proportion of atypical antipsychotic users still on antipsychotic treatment 1 year after initiation.
- To measure the proportion of compliant users among persistent users.

Population

- Outpatient individuals suffering from schizophrenia who had a first claim (wash-out period of 6 months) of an atypical antipsychotic between 1 January 1997 and 31 August 1999. They had to be covered by the Quebec public drug plan for a minimum of 1 year after treatment initiation (n = 6662).

Data sources for measurement of adherence

- *Régie de l'assurance-maladie du Québec* pharmacy claims files.

Adherence

- Constructs measured:
  - Persistence with any antipsychotic drug (therapy persistence).
  - Compliance.
- Measures:
  - Therapy persistence, defined as refilling any atypical antipsychotic in the 45 days before the 1-year anniversary of treatment initiation.
  - Coverage by an atypical antipsychotic for ≥80% of the days of study (hospital days excluded). The sensitivity of the 80% cut-off point to compliance results was tested.

Main results

- 4495 individuals (67.5%) were persistent with the atypical antipsychotic treatment 1 year after initiation.
- Of those who persisted, 3534 (78.6%) were compliant.
- Overall, 53% of individuals were both persistent and compliant.

Issue

- Since persistence was measured using the treatment anniversary method, episodes of discontinuation outside the treatment anniversary period were not captured. They were, however, reflected in the compliance measure.

Source: Cooper et al. [20].

another limitation, as the PDC is likely to be underestimated for patients who are taking accumulated drugs from previous supplies. In addition, calculating the PDC for patients taking more than one drug is challenging. This situation occurs when a new drug is added to an existing one. The two drugs should then be taken concurrently. By contrast, it can also occur when the initial drug is stopped and the patient is switched to another one, but some of the days of supply of the two drugs overlap. It is difficult to disentangle the latter situation from the former. If the new prescribed drug is from the same therapeutic class as the previous one, one option is to assess whether the patient has at least one drug in their possession on each of the days of the observation period. However, if the patient is indeed prescribed both drugs, the PDC may overestimate compliance, since, to be considered compliant, a patient needs only to be in possession of one of the two drugs. Similarly, if the patient has been switched to a new drug, compliance may be overestimated in the period during which both the withdrawn and the newly prescribed drug are in the patient's possession. On the other hand, if the new prescribed drug is clearly for the treatment of a condition other than the one for which the initial treatment was prescribed, then one could opt to calculate the PDC for each prescribed drug. Assessing compliance with multiple treatments remains a challenge that requires further methodological research.

Limitations of administrative data

The measurement of adherence with administrative data has some limitations (Table 36.3). First, as we have already seen, adherence measures are based on the assumption that a prescribed or filled prescription will be taken. Many pharmacists conducting medication home reviews have seen patients stocking filled prescriptions without actually taking the drug. If this situation occurs, the PDC will overestimate compliance. Second, drug samples given by physicians to patients are generally not recorded in administrative databases. This can lead to underestimation of initiation, since patients provided with samples will be misclassified as noninitiators if they do not need to fill their prescription within the designated time window. Drug samples are less likely to affect persistence and compliance estimates, unless samples are given on a frequent basis (e.g. to low-income patients). In this situation, some patients may decide not to refill their prescriptions and so be misclassified as nonpersistent or noncompliant.

Third, some drug acquisition transactions are not captured in administrative databases. This is generally the case with drugs not listed on a drug plan formulary. It can lead to substantial underestimation of drug exposure [24], and therefore of drug adherence. For example, patients already treated with an antidiabetic drug might be switched to a newly marketed drug; even if those patients fill their prescriptions and use the drug, this transaction might never be recorded in the administrative database if the drug is not reimbursed by their drug plan. Such patients will be misclassified as noninitiators, nonpersistent or noncompliant. This could also be the case for patients using drugs that do not require a prescription. Even if a drug is covered by a patient's drug plan, they might still buy it over the counter. For example, patients who initiate an antiplatelet treatment with acetyl-salicylic acid, a nonprescription drug, may be misclassified as noninitiators if they buy it over the counter. Alternatively, if they get their first prescription

Table 36.3 Limitations resulting from the assumptions made when measuring adherence with administrative data.

Assumption	Limitation	Effect on adherence measure
A drug prescription that is issued will be taken	The drug prescription may not be filled	Persistence and compliance will be overestimated
A drug prescription that is filled will be taken	The filled prescription may not be taken	Initiation, persistence and compliance will be overestimated
The only drugs used are those recorded in the database	Drug samples may be given	Initiation, and to a lesser extent persistence and compliance, will be underestimated
	Prescribed drugs bought over the counter may not be recorded	Initiation, persistence and compliance will be underestimated
	Nonreimbursed drugs may be bought but not recorded	Initiation, persistence and compliance will be underestimated

filled at the pharmacy but stop refilling it because they prefer to buy it over the counter then the administrative data will provide underestimates of persistence and compliance.

Conclusion

Prescription and dispensing administrative data can be useful in assessing adherence to treatment. It is no surprise that administrative data have been increasingly used over the years to assess patients' adherence behaviours and to identify determinants of those behaviours. This has produced findings that are sometimes difficult to interpret and to compare across studies, mainly due to variations between studies in the way adherence is defined and measured and to the fact that too often researchers do not provide a good description of their measures of adherence. Consequently, we strongly recommend that drug adherence researchers provide a good description of the adherence construct being measured, the measure being used (including any treatment reference time window) and any permissible gap period.

Since time windows and permissible gap periods are often arbitrarily determined, we also recommend researchers conduct sensitivity analyses in order to determine to what extent initiation or persistence results are robust to changes in the duration of those periods. In addition, when there is a need to dichotomize compliance based on the PDC, it is also recommended that sensitivity analyses be conducted using different cut-off points for the PDC.

We have highlighted in this chapter the importance of pre-determining which of the adherence constructs will be the focus of an assessment, as measurement methods will differ accordingly. Being conscious that other methods exist, we have presented those that are most commonly used and discussed under what circumstances they can best be applied to the measurement of initiation, persistence and compliance.

It is important to remember that the characteristics of administrative data are likely to vary from one jurisdiction to the next and from one drug plan to another. Researchers have to be aware of prescribing and dispensing regulations, as this may help them better design their assessment approach. The same is true of reimbursement rules.

We suggest the reader keep up to date with future methodological work. New methods are likely to provide new insights into adherence behaviours. For example, the recently proposed group-based trajectory models may help better characterize long-term compliance patterns [25].

The ultimate goal of adherence research is to develop and propose efficient means of helping patients better manage their drug treatments so that they obtain optimal health outcomes. Adequate measurement is a prerequisite for the development of sound interventions. If used judiciously, administrative data can provide adequate measures of drug treatment initiation, persistence and compliance.

CHAPTER 37

Interventions to improve adherence to drug treatment

Marie-Paule Schneider[1,2], Jennifer Celio[1,2], Yoleen van Camp[3] & Matthias Cavassini[4]

[1]*Community Pharmacy, School of Pharmaceutical Sciences, Universities of Geneva, University of Lausanne, Switzerland*

[2]*Community Pharmacy, Department of Ambulatory Care & Community Medicine, University of Lausanne, Switzerland*

[3]*Centre for Research and Innovation in Care (CRIC), Faculty of Medicine and Health Care, University of Antwerp, Belgium*

[4]*Service of Infectious Disease, Centre hospitalier universitaire vaudois and University of Lausanne, Switzerland*

KEY POINTS

- Medication adherence, determining population drug exposure and patterns of use over time, is a complex and dynamic behaviour; it is shaped by many determinants – intentional and unintentional, modifiable or unmodifiable. This behaviour influences medication initiation, implementation and persistence.
- The effectiveness of medication adherence interventions is a difficult field of research and the evidence across randomized clinical trials is inconclusive. No consensus about effective interventions can be provided. However, most effective interventions are usually complex, echoing the complex nature of adherence.
- Long-term medication adherence interventions should: (i) be embedded in a theoretical framework; (ii) address patients' perceptions of barriers and facilitators; and (iii) be tailored to patients' needs and adherence subproblems. Patients should be supported in putting forward solutions that might work for them.
- There are several levels of medication adherence in routine care: patient, professional, institution and system. Addressing more than one at a time facilitates uptake and sustainability.
- Overcoming the problem of suboptimal adherence requires that physicians, pharmacists and nurses collaborate across disciplines by identifying each professional's expertise and articulating it in a structured programme to support patients' adherence and care.

Introduction

Medication nonadherence is a widespread behaviour, encountered in many patients, which is deleterious from the perspectives of clinical outcomes and health hazards. It leads to increased morbidity, mortality and avoidable health care costs in chronic care [1,2]. Research on medication nonadherence describes patients' behaviours, drug exposure and patterns of use over time and analyses their determinants and their effect on clinical outcomes, quality of life, morbidity and mortality. As drug utilization-oriented research, it also aims at improving quality of drug use through educational and behavioural interventions [3].

The literature increasingly provides insight into patients' needs, attitudes and perspectives in terms of disease and treatment management. Ways of measuring adherence have also progressively developed, as well have interventions to improve adherence [4–6]. Still, the gap between the literature and routine clinical care remains substantial [7].

Efforts to increase and support medication adherence aim at achieving planned clinical outcomes while preserving patients' quality of life and autonomy. As prerequisite to any adherence intervention programme, medicines need to be prescribed and dispensed appropriately in order to ensure their safe, effective and adequate use [8]. This involves all stakeholders,

Drug Utilization Research: Methods and Applications, First Edition. Edited by M. Elseviers et al.
Published 2016 by John Wiley & Sons, Ltd.

including physicians, pharmacists and nurses. Moreover, patients have a central and active position in this framework, collaborating with each stakeholder [9].

This chapter will discuss medication adherence interventions and their effectiveness and make recommendations for the transfer of interdisciplinary, multilevel interventions.

Determinants of medication adherence

Medication adherence is a dynamic behaviour that is shaped by many determinants. The World Health Organization (WHO) classifies these determinants according to five related dimensions (see Figure 37.1): patient-related (e.g. no belief in the effectiveness of the medication), disease-related (e.g. depression, which may negatively impact a patient's motivation to adhere to any chronic treatment), treatment-related (e.g. a complex medication scheme), socioeconomic-related (e.g. shame around taking medication) and health systems-related (e.g. appointments only possible during working hours) [2]. Some determinants are disease-specific (e.g. shame and the need for confidentiality in human immunodeficiency virus (HIV) disease), while many are present across diseases. This explains why many intervention components are effective across diseases (e.g. social support), while others only work in one specific disease or setting (e.g. financial support in developing countries).

Kardas et al. [10] identified over 700 medication adherence determinants (see Table 37.1). Most influence medication implementation (defined as the extent to which a patient's actual dosing corresponds to the prescribed dosing regimen), but a few also influence initiation (defined as taking the first dose of a prescribed medication) and persistence (defined as the length of time between initiation and the last dose, which immediately precedes discontinuation) [11]. For instance, patient's readiness to start treatment influences initiation, while high drug costs, poor provider follow-up and regimen complexity influence persistence [11].

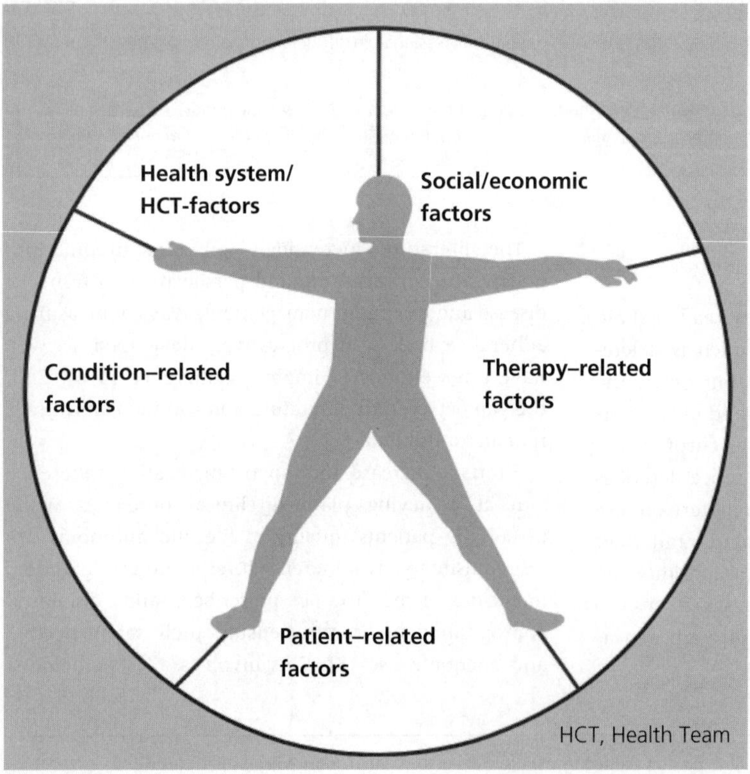

Figure 37.1 The five dimensions of adherence.

Source: Sabate E. 2003 [2]. Reproduced with permission from World Health Organization.

Table 37.1 Determinants affecting adherence. Source: Adapted from Kardas et al. 2013 [10]. Copyright © 2013 Kardas, Lewek and Matyjaszczyk.

Therapy-related factors affecting adherence	Adverse effects Pill burden Drug effectiveness Duration of treatment Alignment between treatment and patient's lifestyle
Condition-related factors affecting adherence	Disease severity Presence of symptoms Disease duration Depression/anxiety Social stigma Presence/absence of clinical improvement
Health care team- and system-related factors affecting adherence	Health care provider–patient communication and relationship Health care follow-up and continuity in care (e.g. type, frequency, reminders) Information about drug use and administration Barriers to health care (environmental and economic) Treatment availability
Socioeconomic factors affecting adherence	Social support (family, significant others, peers) Socioeconomic status Costs of drugs and treatment Health insurance and prescription coverage

Determinants can be further classified as intentional (e.g. deliberately not taking medication to avoid side effects) or unintentional (i.e. forgetfulness) and as modifiable (e.g. pill burden) or nonmodifiable (e.g. patient's personality traits). Determinants can be either facilitators of (e.g. positive beliefs, absence of side effects) or barriers to (e.g. negative attitudes, difficulties in finding appointments with doctors) drug intake.

Research on medication adherence-enhancing interventions

From simple to multifaceted interventions

Interventions to improve patients' adherence can either be simple (e.g. one-time intervention) or complex (e.g. multifaceted). During the first decades of adherence research, simple interventions were studied most often [12], with research tackling a single component (e.g. giving education). Nowadays, adherence is acknowledged as a complex behaviour, as illustrated in the preceding section, and the limitations of simple interventions have become clear [5]. For instance, sending patients reminders to take their dose might work if they are unintentionally forgetting but has no effect if they are intentionally skipping doses because they have experienced side effects. Multifaceted interventions are needed, which combine two or more successful intervention components. For example, patient education combined with pharmacist-led medication reconciliation, medication tailoring, collaborative care between pharmacist and physician and voice messaging increased adherence to medication regimens in the year after acute coronary syndrome hospital discharge [13]. In 2014, the Cochrane collaboration published an updated review of interventions aimed at enhancing medication adherence [5]. The review identified 17 (out of 182) randomized controlled trials (RCTs) with a minimum risk of bias for both the study design and the primary clinical outcome. In these studies, different approaches were proposed to enhance medication adherence, most of them involving complex interventions: counselling (e.g. motivational interviewing or cognitive behavioural therapy (CBT)) and/or daily treatment support (alarms, text messages, written or visual educational material), interventions provided by allied professionals and programmes involving families or peers. Nine RCTs showed a positive effect on adherence, but only five reported improvements in both adherence and clinical outcomes. Table 37.2 summarizes the principal characteristics of these five studies. They were heterogeneous, and no common intervention characteristics were identified. Such heterogeneity (in intervention designs, medication adherence and clinical outcome measurements) represents a main concern in medication adherence interventions, according to most systematic reviews. For example, Viswanathan et al. [6] described heterogeneity in

Table 37.2 Cochrane collaboration review of interventions aimed at enhancing medication adherence: characteristics of five randomized controlled trials (RCTs) reporting improvements in medication adherence and clinical outcomes [5].

Study	Setting and number of patients (Ig/Cg)	Pathology	Duration	Types of intervention	Outcomes	Adherence measure instrument	Main results
Farooq et al. [15]	Lady Reading Hospital (Pakistan) (55/55)	Schizophrenia	12 months	Specific education was provided to the key care supervisor (a family member living with the individual for at least 6 months), providing support for the treatment	1. Medication adherence 2. Symptoms and functioning (GAF and PANSS)	Questionnaire: five-item self-report scale	1. Percentage of patients with perfect adherence – was higher at 3 and 12 months in the Ig (but not at 6 months) 3 months: 69.1% (Ig) versus 28.0% (Cg), ($p = 0.05$) 12 months: 67.3% (Ig) versus 45.5% (Cg) ($p < 0.02$, RR 1.59, 95% CI 1.03–2.53) 2. The participants in the Ig showed significantly greater improvement in symptoms and functioning
Gray et al. [16]	Manchester Royal Eye Hospital (MREH) clinics (United Kingdom) (64/63)	Ocular HBP or open-angle glaucoma	12 months	Individual assessment of health care needs and beliefs (provided by a nurse) Follow-up including education, support and training (approximately five 15-minute face-to-face or telephone consultations per year)	1. Medication adherence 2. Glaucoma knowledge, beliefs about illness and medicines, quality of care, IOP fluctuation, changes in clinical management (change or addition of eye drops and/or surgical intervention)	Refill and self-report (GAQ-R)	1. 12-month refill adherence significantly better in the Ig (70 vs 43%, $\chi^2 = 9.75$, df = 1, $p = 0.002$). Ig collected significantly more prescriptions than Cg (Mann-Whitney $Z = -3.56$, $p < 0.001$) Self-report adherence was better in Ig for patients who intentionally (Mann-Whitney $Z = -6.22$, $p < 0.001$) and unintentionally (Mann-Whitney $Z = -6.68$, $p < 0.001$) missed drops 2. At 24 months (1 year after intervention stop), Cg had more IOP fluctuations (2.7, SD 1.5 vs 3.4, SD 1.5 mmHg; $t = -2.53$, df = 119, $p = 0.013$) and more changes in clinical management ($\chi^2 = 4.39$, df = 1, $p = 0.036$)

Lester et al. [17]	Three HIV clinics in Kenya (273/265)	HIV	12 months	Mobile phone SMS intervention. Patients in the intervention group received weekly SMS messages from a clinic nurse and were required to respond within 48 hours	1. Medication adherence 2. Plasma HIV-1 viral RNA load suppression	Self-report (number of pills missed in the last 30 days)	1. Medication adherence was reported in 168/273 (Ig) and 132/265 (Cg) patients (RR for nonadherence = 0.81, 95% CI 0.69–0.94, $p = 0.006$) 2. Suppressed viral loads were reported in 156/273 (Ig) and 128/265 (Cg) patients (RR for virologic failure = 0.82, 95% CI 0.71–0.99, $p = 0.04$)
Morgado et al. [18]	Secondary care hypertension/ dyslipidaemia outpatient clinic (Cova da Beira Hospital Centre, Covilhã, Portugal) (98/99)	HBP	9 months	Quarterly follow-up by a hospital pharmacist Pharmacists interviewed and educated patients, identified problems and communicated with physicians	1. Medication adherence 2. SBP, DBP	Five-item questionnaire (derived from the Morisky four-item scale)	1. Medication adherence was higher in the Ig (74.5 vs 57.6%, $p = 0.012$) 2. BP control was higher in the Ig (63.3 vs 43.4%, OR 2.2; 95% CI 1.3–4.0, $p = 0.005$). SBP and DBP were significantly lower in the Ig (SBP: −7.4 (Ig) vs −0.9 (Cg) mmHg, $p = 0.006$; DBP: −2.7 (Ig) vs −1.0 (Cg) mmHg, $p = 0.020$)
Wu et al. [19]	Prince of Wales Hospital (Hong Kong) (223/219)	Polypharmacy	24 months	Six to eight 10–15-minute telephone calls between a pharmacist and the patient to discuss issues related to the treatment, provide information about side effects, promote medication adherence and supervise medical follow-up	1. Medication adherence 2. Time from randomization to death from any cause	Questionnaire (developed for the purpose of the study)	1. Ig had fewer baseline nonadherent patients who remained nonadherent (7 vs 18%, $p < 0.001$) and more baseline adherent patients who remained adherent (81 vs 58%, $p = 0.038$) Adjusted RR for death: 1.61 (1.05–2.48; $p = 0.029$) and 2.87 (1.80–2.56) in patients with adherence scores of 34–66% and 0–33%, compared with those with adherence scores of 67% or more 2. After adjustment for confounders, telephone counselling was associated with a 41% reduction in the risk of death (RR 0.59, 95% CI 0.35–0.97, $p = 0.039$)

Ig, Intervention group; Cg, control group; GAF, Global Assessment of Functioning Scale; PANSS, Positive and Negative Syndrome Scale; HBP: high blood pressure; IOP, intraocular pressure; GAQ-R, Revised Glaucoma Adherence Questionnaire; HIV, human immunodeficiency virus; SMS, short message service; SBP, systolic blood pressure; DBP, diastolic blood pressure; BP, blood pressure.

both simple (e.g. one-time mailings) and multifaceted (e.g. collaborative care) interventions. Hence, no present consensus on effective interventions can be provided. In addition, Oberjé et al. [14] identified 14 RCTs examining the cost-effectiveness of adherence interventions. Some studies showed favourable cost-effectiveness ratios, but heterogeneity and methodological weaknesses impeded any conclusion.

Behavioural skills, knowledge and social support

Based on the literature best evidence, the factors most likely to act as prerequisites for adherence include knowledge, social support and behavioural skills. These might be established by giving education, involving a caregiver and providing skills training (e.g. cue-dose training: linking the intake of medication to a habit, such as brushing teeth).

One-time interventions may not ensure adherence, but rather provide an educational prerequisite to ensure that patients understand the purpose and correct dosing of their medication. Failure to understand the purpose of medication may be associated with nonadherence.

In the literature, the importance of knowledge and social support is still controversial: in many studies, they appear to be determining factors of medication adherence, but in some they do not [20]. For example, fully knowledgeable patients may still be nonadherent: they can experience side effects that 'overpower' their awareness of the importance of the medication or else fear potential long-term side effects [21].

Several theoretical frameworks model patients' behaviour and behavioural changes. These include ***social cognitive theory***, ***theory of planned behaviour*** and ***self-regulation theories*** [22]. Behavioural theory helps strengthen the design of medication adherence-enhancing interventions [22]. For example, in their behavioural model for medication adherence, de Bruin et al. [23] postulate that a key concept in medication interventions is the intention of the patient to adhere, which is modulated by many determinants, including personality traits, facilitators and barriers and the patient's cognitive and emotional evaluation of the situation. In sum, these theories assist researchers and health care givers in the design of behaviour change interventions by explaining the patient's behaviour and its determinants.

Electronic monitoring and new technologies

Innovative technology is increasingly applied in the field of adherence management (e.g. electronic pill bottles or blister packs and smartphones (text messages, reminders, apps, etc.)) [24–27]. Demonceau et al. [28] found electronic feedback to patients (through a digital report on their recent drug dosing history) to be one of the most successful intervention components. Vervloet et al. [29] reviewed the effects of electronic reminders on adherence and found them to be significant. Internet-based interventions are increasingly common. They have the advantage of being able to tailor interventions to the patient's needs and can reinforce the alliance between health care providers and patients by filling time gaps between visits and allowing patients to share material [25,30]. However, the effectiveness of Internet-based interventions still needs to be established.

Tailored medication adherence interventions and patient-centred care

The complexity of addressing nonadherence might explain the success of one-on-one interviews in which intake behaviour is discussed from a psychosocial viewpoint [24]. When discussing adherence, it is extremely important to have a nonjudgemental approach [2]. Patients who do not feel supported or understood will be less likely to 'admit' to difficulties in taking doses as prescribed. Further, the importance of self-efficacy and empowerment is increasingly acknowledged. Rather than just offering solutions, patients should be supported to identify possible adherence barriers themselves and to put forward solutions that might work for them. Presently, emphasis is put on tailoring interventions: customizing them to the unique characteristics of the individual patient. Tailored interventions based on types and causes of nonadherence and on patients' needs have a greater impact than generic interventions [31,32].

Future directions for research

In sum, adherence-improving interventions follow the evolution of research into this complex behaviour and its determining factors. Early research was narrowed to mainly medical, pharmacological and demographic factors. Hence, interventions were single and were aimed at increasing knowledge. Decades of research have led to a better understanding of adherence as a complex behaviour, requiring a nonjudgemental, tailored and long-term approach. However, which multifaceted, tailored interventions over what period of time will most (cost-)effectively improve adherence remains unclear.

Qualitative research is needed to map the exact needs of specific populations (e.g. HIV patients might benefit from interventions aimed at addressing shame, which might be less of an issue in another population). Such qualitative insights are crucial to understanding what adherence really means from the patients' point of view and what drives such behaviour. Indeed, the discrepancy between the perceptions of patients and of health care providers has long been underestimated. For instance, health care providers often correlate nonadherence to patient incompetence, and so focus their efforts on education in an attempt to increase patient knowledge.

Transfer of intervention programmes in routine care

There are several levels of medication adherence in routine care: patient, professional, institution and system (Table 37.3). Addressing more than one at a time facilitates uptake and sustainability.

Table 37.3 Levels of medication adherence interventions in routine care.

Patient-level	Health care professional-level	Health care institution-level	Health care system-level
Provide a person- and patient-centred intervention Invite the patient to become an active and consenting partner Evaluate the patient's perceptions of personal barriers and facilitators: what are their priorities, perspectives, attitudes and beliefs? What are the patient's needs in terms of education, motivation and medication management skills? These will determine the level of the intervention: low, medium or high What stage is the patient in, in terms of initiation, implementation and persistence (e.g. long-term pill fatigue, pill burden, side effects)? What about the patient's social support, affective life and affective disorders? What about the patient's comorbidities and co-treatments? How do these affect the patient's adherence? What material and technologies might be helpful (e.g. pill boxes, brochures, text messages, written information, websites)?	Provide education (pre- and postgraduate): • medication adherence • adherence intervention programmes Practice motivational interviewing (e.g. empathy, active listening, identification of patients' fears and needs, rolling with resistance, avoiding argumentation) Develop and endorse a semistructured programme manual Ensure continuity of care	Ensure leadership Organize teamwork (time, human resources, adequate facilities) Ensure team competencies and satisfaction Link research with practice Develop interdisciplinarity Implement a quality process manual Disseminate new skills Structure activity within the workflow	Reimburse medication adherence programmes Advocate through national and international institutions (e.g. WHO)

Patient-level interventions

In routine care, the objective of intervention by health care providers is to support patients in improving and sustaining their drug intake behaviour according to their ability and willingness, while respecting their integrity and striving for the best possible quality of life. A patient's resistance to adherence with an evidence-based treatment is informative and can be useful in guiding the intervention. Particular steps to monitor are: (i) informed decision process at initiation (shared decision-making) [33]; (ii) patient readiness to treatment [34]; (iii) implementation and persistence; and (iv) prevention and management of discontinuation. Setting realistic goals, planning self-management, acquiring a sufficient level of knowledge and identifying ways of reinforcing self-efficacy or adjusting social support all aid in promoting adherence (see also Chapter 33).

A main issue is to increase retention in the care of intentionally nonadherent patients and patients not ready to start treatment, who are at high risk of being lost from follow-up (pre-contemplative patients, according to Prochaska's definition) [35]. The main goal in this situation is to preserve the relationship between the patient and the provider, without pressuring the patient to accept a prescription if they are not ready to start or resume treatment. Other resources can be reinforced in parallel (e.g. patient support groups).

Health care professional-level interventions

Interventions to support medication adherence entail several health care professional competencies: (i) rational prescribing and dispensing, to ensure treatment effectiveness and patient safety; (ii) pre- and postgraduate education in nonadherence monitoring and management [2]; and (iii) training in communication skills [36,37] (Table 37.3).

Health care institution-level interventions

Adequate human resources, leadership, facilities and quality processes are prerequisites for implementing and sustaining an effective medication adherence programme in both public and private routine care settings [38,39] (Table 37.3).

For example, missed appointments with health care providers are one of the first red flags for nonadherence to medical follow-up, and probably to medication [40]. Appointment reminders and follow-ups with patients who did not show up are easy to implement.

Health care system-level interventions

As part of the shift from acute to chronic health care and the development of new care models, effective medication adherence interventions should be considered for reimbursement by public health funds [41] (Table 37.3). This will require more robust effectiveness and cost-effectiveness data for medication adherence interventions [14].

Interdisciplinary approaches

A patient goes through a continuum of care, provided by a number of professionals. Rather than focusing on a single profession, there is a strong need for studies aimed at interprofessional approaches to addressing medication adherence. An interdisciplinary collaboration is characterized by the acknowledgement and integration of the unique knowledge and expertise of different professionals [42,43]. The involvement and expertise of different professionals have become essential to improving care and health outcomes [42,44,45].

In 2013, the ***World Health Professions Alliance (WHPA)*** issued a major new statement on collaborative practice [46]. Effective collaborations were associated with increased patient and health professional satisfaction, with the possibility of patients taking part in medical decisions, with a reduction in morbidity and mortality and with an increased quality of care (and quality of life). Interdisciplinary collaborations allow a better use of resources, can reduce health costs and improve quality at work [44,46–48].

Furthermore, multidisciplinary and interdisciplinary collaborations may have a positive impact on medication adherence and various treatment goals, although the evidence to support this is still limited [49].

Collaboration from diagnosis to long-term follow-up

Diagnosis and drug prescription

Physicians are in the position to stress the importance of medication adherence when they prescribe a treatment during medical consultations [50,51]. Additionally, they are in the position to confirm/question adherence results and foresee adherence problems by assessing clinical outcomes. Physicians and nurses can provide complete and individualized information about a diagnosis and disease to a patient [52]. Physicians can also clarify treatment options with patients (shared decision-making, readiness for treatment and self-efficacy) [33,50,53] (see Figure 37.2). For example, decreasing the number of daily doses and lowering pill burden help promote medication adherence [54]. During follow-up, physicians and pharmacists can identify treatment-related problems and manage drug side effects and interactions [50,55].

Screening for risks of nonadherence

Physicians, pharmacists and nurses have a fundamental yet challenging responsibility to screen and identify patients with suboptimal adherence [57]. This task has been described as highly difficult, due to the diversity and complexity of determinants and the absence of a comprehensive screening approach. However, integrative, interdisciplinary collaborations can help increase

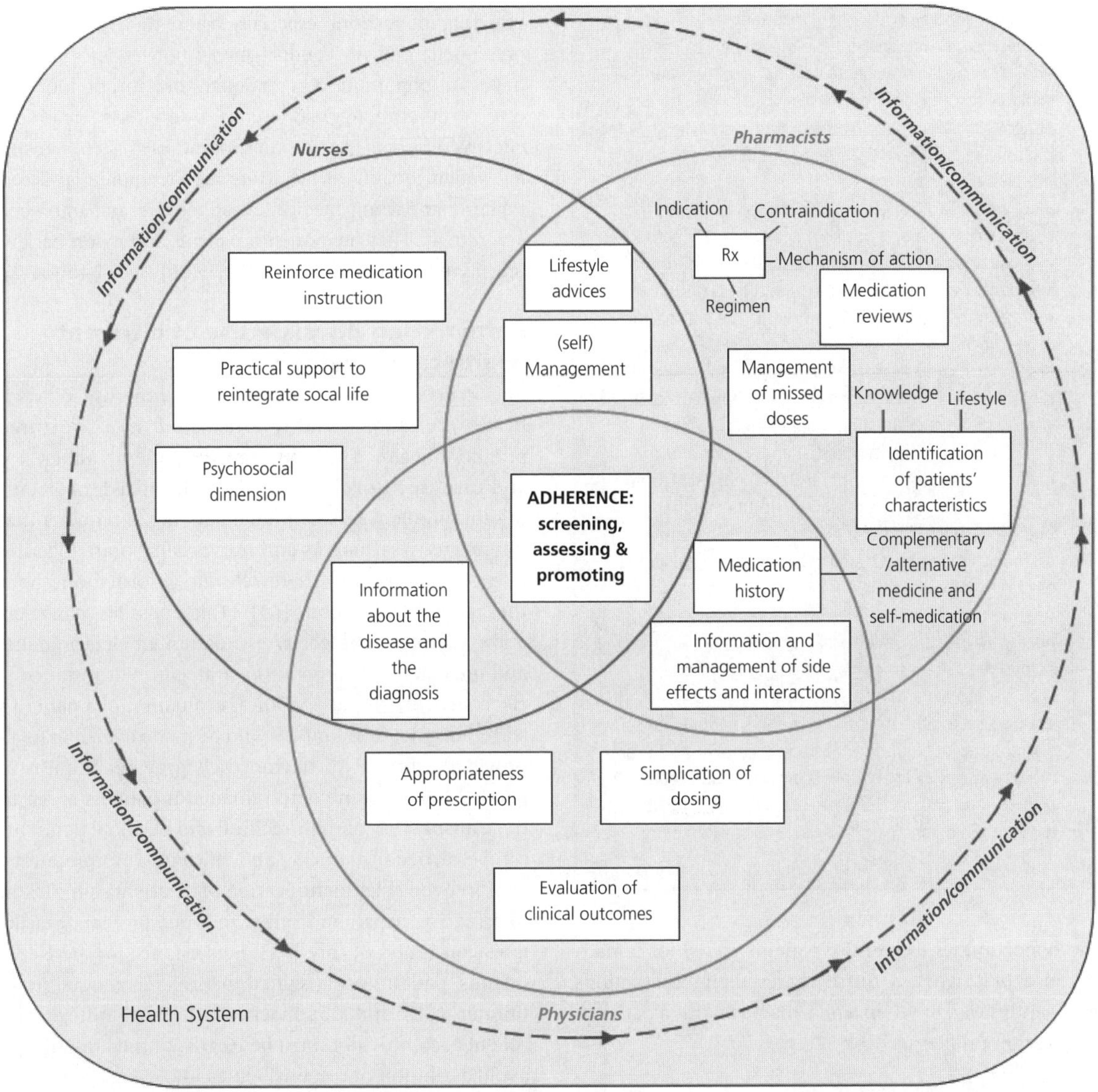

Figure 37.2 Interdisciplinarity in medication adherence-enhancing programmes: expertise of physicians, pharmacists and nurses.

Source: Adapted from.Celio et al. 2014 [56]. Reproduced by permission of the author.

Box 37.1 Interdisciplinary collaboration around an HIV+ woman [61].

In 2006, a young Caucasian teenage woman with congenital HIV is referred by her doctor to a pharmacist-led interdisciplinary adherence programme, consisting in a multifactorial intervention combined with electronic drug monitoring (EDM). During semistructured motivational interviews, the pharmacist: (i) explores the patient's motivation for treatment; (ii) discusses her daily treatment management, based on the EDM feedback and side effects (e.g. management of missed doses, the time required for the medication to have an effect, the patient's ability to self-manage treatment); (iii) explores the need for information; and (iv) evaluates the patient's social support. At the end of each interview, the pharmacist provides a medication adherence report to the physician and nurse.

During the 8-year follow-up within this programme, the patient's clinical outcomes and medication adherence improve and her alliance with medical staff strengthens. The patient accepts the diagnosis and feels progressively more comfortable with the treatment. The contribution of each health professional was crucial to this success. Physicians recommend that the patient enter the medication adherence-enhancing programme, monitored viral load and relevant clinical parameters, adapted the prescription according to the patient's needs and the medication adherence report and, in the most critical periods, established directly observed therapy (DOT) under the supervision of a pharmacist. Pharmacists monitored the patient's medication adherence using electronic pill containers, supported the patient in treatment and in pocket-dosing management and, when necessary, met the patient daily. Psychosocial nurses helped the patient to manage a difficult relationship with her mother and to accept her congenital HIV status, the disease and the treatment. They also addressed safe sex, contraception and gynaecological problems. Several medical interdisciplinary networks were organized – often on the patient's request – to discuss the most relevant clinical and psychosocial problems affecting adherence to HIV drugs.

the opportunities to identify patients at risk of nonadherence (e.g. when a nurse shares their observations with a physician or when a pharmacist shares a patient's medication profile; see Box 37.1).

Supporting and promoting medication adherence

Pharmacists' usual role is to dispense effective, safe and economic medication, using information from medication refills among other things. They endorse responsibilities in evaluating, promoting and supporting medication adherence through tailored cognitive and behavioural pharmaceutical services (e.g. medication therapy management) [50,55,58] (see Figure 37.2). Pharmacists: (i) identify patients' characteristics, perspectives and particular needs; (ii) provide patient-centred information about a treatment: its aims, risks, benefits and proper use; (iii) support development of medication self-management skills (including side effects and missed doses); (iv) supervise drug interactions, especially where there are multiple prescribers; and (v) conduct medication reviews. Nurses have an important observational role throughout the care continuum (e.g. adherence, side effects, treatment effectiveness, emerging problems at each step), ensuring patient quality of life. They monitor potential determinants impacting medication adherence and intervene accordingly. They advocate for patients and report back to practitioners and pharmacists [50,59,60] (see Figure 37.2).

Harmonizing the expertise of different health care providers

It is crucial to clearly identify the expertise of each health professional and to articulate it in a structured programme aimed at supporting the patient's adherence and care (see Boxes 37.1 and 37.2). Indeed, overcoming the problem of suboptimal adherence requires that physicians, pharmacists and nurses collaborate together in a continuum and share relevant information about the patient's situation [63]. This includes consideration of treatment goals, evaluation of determinants and provision of intervention strategies. For instance, a clear, structured and periodical evaluation of a patient's adherence determinants should be made available to all providers, instead of having each provider inquire in parallel for the same determinants. If patients agree to the transmission of their medical and personal data, this can be carried out quickly and efficiently by computer.

Moreover, clear identification of a patient's physician, pharmacist, nurse and other relevant providers facilitates continuity of care [51]. For instance, in the Netherlands, patients are assigned to a referee general practitioner (GP) and pharmacist [64]. Furthermore, the role of each provider must be clearly defined in order to avoid a dilution of responsibilities [47].

Finally, to promote adherence and patient self-efficacy, all information transmitted to the patient should be clear, coherent and unanimous (reflecting the common

Box 37.2 A multidisciplinary intervention programme in Alberta, Canada [62].

Farris et al. [57] describe a multidisciplinary intervention programme involving six health care teams, consisting of a family physician, a family physician's office nurse, a pharmacist and a home care nurse case manager. During the pre-implementation period, the teams decided how to organize and share responsibilities. Between September 1999 and April 2000, they met for an hour and a half once a week to discuss different patients' situations and related difficulties. The pharmacist's role consisted in the presentation of the patient medication histories during the meeting and the conduct of medication reviews during home visits. Home care nurses were responsible for patient care, while office nurses had an important role in patient screening. Medication and health issues were identified by the team, which then decided how to proceed. Patient follow-up was conducted by telephone or in person by the most suitable health professional, who then shared the information with the team. Results showed that medication adherence improved at 3 and 6 months, and that patients required fewer doctors and emergency consultations. Health professionals were generally satisfied with the programme and felt they better understood each professional's role in the team.

objectives of the professional team; regular team meetings help define common objectives, as well as quality procedures).

Conclusion

Medication adherence and patient self-care are determining issues in chronic care, where tension between resources and expenses is at a culmination point. The number of chronic patients continues to increase, and treatments are targeted, high-technology, long-term and hence expensive.

Patients should not be blamed and stigmatized for nonadherence as they share the responsibility with providers and health care systems. Nonadherence is common and deleterious, and needs to be addressed empathically through effective, collaborative and interdisciplinary patient-centred care programmes. Such programmes increase patient and health professional satisfaction, allow patients to take part in medical decision-making, reduce morbidity and mortality and increase quality of care and patient quality of life [44,46,47].

Research in this area must be disseminated in clinical care through feasible and scalable interventions, both generic and targeted. Much has to be done to dismantle clinical inertia, and a close collaboration between academia and practice is needed to shape the person-centred health care system of this century. Medication adherence interventions demand an interdisciplinary approach, tailored to the specific needs of the population or individual patient and to the particular adherence subproblem (noninitiation, poor medication implementation, discontinuation) and barrier (e.g. shame, knowledge deficit, side effects).

Most importantly, it is time to investigate the impact of interventions on the pattern of use of drugs at the societal level. Drug utilization research is needed to inform national and international drug policy and so help prevent avoidable and deleterious medication nonadherence.

SECTION G The role of drug utilization within the field of pharmacoepidemiology

CHAPTER 38

Drug utilization research and risk management

Giampiero Mazzaglia[1] & Peter Mol[2]

[1]*Scientific and Regulatory Management Department, Human Medicines Evaluation Division European Medicines Agency, United Kingdom*

[2]*Department of Clinical Pharmacy and Pharmacology, University Medical Centre Groningen, University of Groningen, The Netherlands.*

KEY POINTS

- Good risk management requires continuous evaluation and improvement of planned activities.
- The evaluation impact of risk management activities requires robust study designs and carefully selected outcome measures.
- Key learnings and caveats from drug utilization research should be applied to the field of risk management plan (RMP) impact assessment (e.g. shortcomings of ecological studies, data collection, cross-country comparisons).

Introduction

Knowledge of the full risk–benefit balance of a medicinal product is limited at the time of licensing and can change after approval, when serious safety issues may emerge [1]. This is a consequence of the inherent limitations of preregistration trials, which often include a relatively homogenous population in order to achieve internal validity and maximize the discriminatory power of drug effects. Additional studies may be performed to support new drug indications or population subgroups underrepresented in the preauthorization phase; however, drugs will be used in clinical practice as such before these studies are finalized and formally evaluated. Therefore, the risk–benefit balance requires continuous assessment and evaluation throughout the product life cycle (i.e. in both the pre- and the post-authorization phases) [2].

Proactive pharmacovigilance is part of the life cycle approach aimed at early detection and minimization of risks, as stated in the strategic plans of the European Medicines Agency (EMA) and the US Food and Drug Administration (FDA) [3]. For this purpose, a risk management plan (RMP) has been implemented in the European Union since 2005; the new EU pharmacovigilance legislation that came into force in July 2012 further embeds the RMP as a key tool in proactive pharmacovigilance [4–5].

An RMP consists of a set of activities and interventions that are designed to identify, characterize, prevent or minimize risks during the life cycle of a drug. It aims to ensure that the benefits of a medicinal product exceed its risks to the largest possible extent, both at the individual and at the population level [6].

However, the final purpose of risk identification and characterization is to allow for risk minimization or

Drug Utilization Research: Methods and Applications, First Edition. Edited by M. Elseviers et al.
Published 2016 by John Wiley & Sons, Ltd.

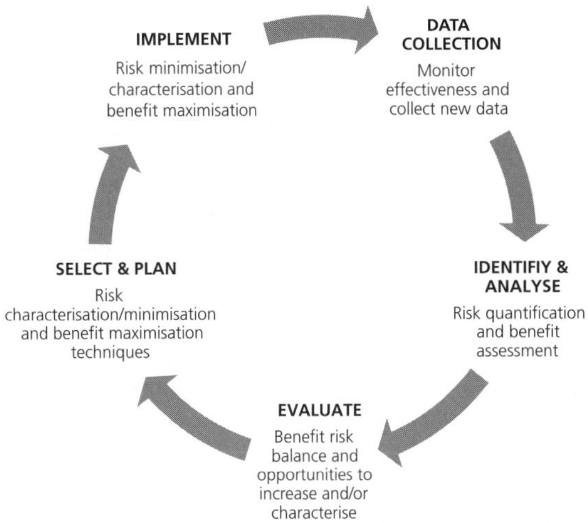

Figure 38.1 The risk management cycle as reported in the Guideline on Good Pharmacovigilance Practices (Module V) of the European Medicines Agency (EMA).

Source: European Medicine Agency 2012 [6]. © European Medicines Agency and Heads of Medicines Agencies, 2014.

mitigation wherever possible (Figure 38.1). Therefore, risk management has three stages, which are interrelated and reiterative:

1 Identification of the safety profile of the medicinal product.
2 Planning of pharmacovigilance activities to characterize known risks, identify new risks and increase knowledge in general about the safety profile of the medicinal product.
3 Planning and implementation of risk minimization or mitigation and assessment of the effectiveness of these activities.

Drug utilization research and risk assessment

Risk identification and characterization

The Guideline on Good Pharmacovigilance Practices on the RMP (GVP-RMP), issued by the EMA in 2012 [6], asks pharmaceutical companies to provide cumulative data on post-marketing drug exposure, including user characteristics, dose, duration and concomitant medication use. Such information can form an important part of a product-related RMP and allows off-label use to be captured from real-life clinical practice, enabling identification of targeted scenarios requiring close post-marketing surveillance.

Ecological studies

Correlating a drug's risk, as assessed using spontaneous reporting systems or the results of pharmacoepidemiological studies, to population exposure may help regulators in: (i) measuring the public health impact of adverse drug reactions (ADRs) (i.e. mapping the risk of a given drug either by country or across different population subgroups); (ii) interpreting pharmacovigilance data; and (iii) calculating reporting rates (i.e. raw risk estimates, following a causality assessment on cases obtained from efficient pharmacovigilance systems only).

For example, an ecological study combined information from the FDA Adverse Event Reporting System (FAERS) (characterizing the torsadogenic profile of antipsychotics) with drug utilization data from 12 European countries to assess population-based antipsychotic exposure over the years 2005–10 [7]. Although the validity of this strategy may be questioned due to the inherent limitations of spontaneous reporting systems and the lack of linkage between drug exposure and adverse events, its potential applicability in ranking signals for prioritization should be acknowledged. In fact, this parallel approach has identified drug and country-specific scenarios requiring potential regulatory action, including levomepromazine in Serbia, fluphenazine in Slovenia and cyamemazine in France.

A study conducted in the United States evaluated the impact of an extended-release oxycodone (ERO), reformulated to deter abuse, on reports of fatalities submitted to a pharmacovigilance database [8]. ERO fatality reports were combined with prescription data to calculate reporting rates, demonstrating a 5, 58 and 80% decrease at the first, second and third years, respectively, after reformulation. Nevertheless, this study suffered from the same limitations as other ecological studies.

Prescription event monitoring

Drug utilization data from electronic prescription databases or automated health insurance claims may also be used to identify cohorts of patients exposed to new medicinal products. A follow-up questionnaire can then be sent to each prescribing physician or patient at pre-specified intervals to obtain outcome information. Information on patient demographics, indication for treatment, dose, duration of therapy, clinical events and reasons for discontinuation can be included in the questionnaire.

This noninterventional cohort pharmacovigilance activity, commonly termed prescription event monitoring (PEM) [9], provides valuable drug utilization information for new medicines, as well as estimates of incidence rates for events reported in the exposed cohort. It also provides the opportunity for further clinical evaluation of selected events of interest using bespoke follow-up questionnaires.

PEM has disadvantages and limitations too, however. First, data collection entails a high workload for primary care physicians, with the potential for low response rates, which might bias the incidence of reported events. Second, no information on drug use is provided for those who are not exposed, limiting these studies to use in pharmacovigilance hypothesis generation. Third, hospital prescriptions are generally not included in PEM studies. Therefore, for drugs started in hospital or used only in hospital settings, PEM is unlikely to provide reliable results.

However, in recent years a number of enhancements have been made in order to facilitate more targeted safety surveillance. This has led to the evolution of the 'Modified PEM' (M-PEM). The customized questionnaires used in M-PEM studies are designed to collect relevant additional information in order to allow more detailed exploration of specific safety issues. The underlying process remains the same as in conventional PEM, but M-PEM attempts to overcome some of its limitations, particularly by providing reimbursement to primary care physicians in order to increase response rates.

PEM and M-PEM are extensively used in several countries, where a number of important safety issues have been studied, including serious cardiovascular events with erectile dysfunction drugs, deep vein thrombosis (DVT) with oral contraceptives and serious skin reactions with selective cyclooxygenase 2 inhibitors. Therefore, PEM and M-PEM may be considered valuable tools in the development of RMPs for the evaluation of medicinal product safety profiles.

Off-label use

Off-label use relates to situations where a medicinal product is intentionally used for a medical purpose not in accordance with the authorized product information. This is particularly relevant when a medicinal product has an indication restricted to a subset of the population within a disease area or when it must not be given for safety reasons. It also occurs when a drug is given for indications for which there is a weak evidence of clinical benefit.

The GVP-RMP [6] specifically requests that pharmaceutical companies provide information from drug utilization studies in order to quantify the off-label use of an authorized product. In fact, studies of drug utilization in daily practice have consistently shown that drugs are frequently prescribed or taken for nonapproved conditions or otherwise not in accordance with the label, as real-life treatment scenarios are characterized by even wider variability than 'on-label' use. Box 38.1 presents the marketing history of rimonabant as an example of the importance of drug utilization studies in evaluating off-label use and actual risk–benefit profiles.

Box 38.1 Rimonabant marketing history.

Rimonabant was licensed in the European Union in 2006 as an adjunct to diet and exercise for the treatment of obese or overweight patients with associated risk factors such as type 2 diabetes mellitus or dyslipidemia. At that time, EU regulators concluded that in the clinical trials presented for approval, the weight-reducing effect was moderate and of clinical relevance for 20–30% of treated patients when they were treated for more than 1 year. There were also safety questions, since increased rates of depressive disorders and suicidal and aggressive behaviour were reported, although, based on the incidences observed in the trials, these adverse effects were considered less significant than the benefits [10].

In the post-marketing stage, however, drug utilization data [11] indicated that only 33% of rimonabant users remained on treatment after 1 year and that 30% were neither obese nor overweight, with consequent reduced beneficial effects on their body weight.

At the same time, safety also became an issue. A prescription survey revealed that among all rimonabant users, only 70% were diagnosed with diabetes or dyslipidemia and that 58% had psychiatric conditions at the time of their first prescription. It became apparent therefore that in the real-life setting, the combination of poor patient persistence (which reduced the effect size), off-label prescribing by physicians and increased susceptibility to adverse effects as a result of a preexisting comorbidity entailed a shift in the risk–benefit profile such that adverse mental effects could outweigh the benefits of weight loss. Based on these data, rimonabant was taken off the market in the European Union in 2009.

Drug utilization research and risk minimization

Rationale

Drug approval in Europe involves an assessment of the need for additional activities to ensure the risk–benefit balance remains optimal when a drug is used in clinical practice. The specific indication, dosage recommendations, contraindications and warnings are given in the summary of product characteristics (SmPC) and the package leaflet. These represent the mainstay tools of risk minimization, as they constitute a controlled and standardized format for informing health care professionals and patients about a given medicinal product [12]. Although not all health care professionals will have detailed knowledge of an SmPC, the document serves as a source for textbooks and electronic prescribing systems; it also sets the limits for drug advertising by pharmaceutical companies.

In addition, product-related RMPs may include a set of additional risk minimization measures (RMMs; see Box 38.2), aimed at reducing the probability or severity of identified or potential adverse effects [13]. These measures are intended for use with drugs for which routine risk management activities are not considered sufficient, whether due to concerns over the risk–benefit balance in daily practice or to anticipated problems with adherence to special recommendations/warnings given in the SmPC.

The impact of RMMs in health care systems requires assessment to ensure that their objectives are fulfilled and that the measures in place are proportionate, taking into account the risk–benefit profile of the product and the efforts required by health care professionals and patients to implement them. Successful implementation of RMMs is in fact not straightforward, as it requires contributions from all involved stakeholders, including pharmaceutical companies, patients and health care professionals.

The increasing number of safety issues being addressed [14] and the increasing risk awareness of the public, media and regulators [15] are among the key factors which might contribute to confusion among prescribing physicians and ultimately reduce the effectiveness of RMMs [16].

Methodological issues

Quality indicators

Prieto et al. [17], in describing the approach required to evaluate the effectiveness of RMMs, stressed the importance of building an assessment on two distinct levels of evidence: (i) process quality indicators (i.e. drug

Box 38.2 Risk minimization measures (RMMs) [13].

- Educational programmes (targeted communication to supplement the information in the SmPC and package leaflet):
  - educational tools targeting health care professionals (specific recommendations on what to do/what not to do/how to manage adverse reactions associated with a certain drug);
  - patient checklists, brochures, posters and so on;
  - educational tools targeting patients and/or caregivers (these enhance the awareness of patients or their caregivers about the signs and symptoms relevant to the early recognition of specific adverse reactions);
  - patient alert cards (these ensure that special information regarding a patient's current therapy and its risks is held by the patient at all times and reaches all relevant health care professionals).
- Controlled access programmes (interventions seeking to control access to a certain drug):
  - patient screening (to ensure compliance with strictly defined clinical criteria);
  - prescriber, dispenser and/or patient documentation of their receipt and understanding of information on the serious risks of the product;
  - systematic patient follow-up, through enrolment in a specific data collection system;
  - select pharmacies (registered and approved to dispense the product).
- Other measures:
  - pregnancy prevention programmes (aimed at minimizing pregnancy exposure during treatment using drugs with known or potential teratogenic effect);
  - direct health care professional communication (information delivered to health care professionals to inform them of the need to take certain action in order to minimize the risk of the product).

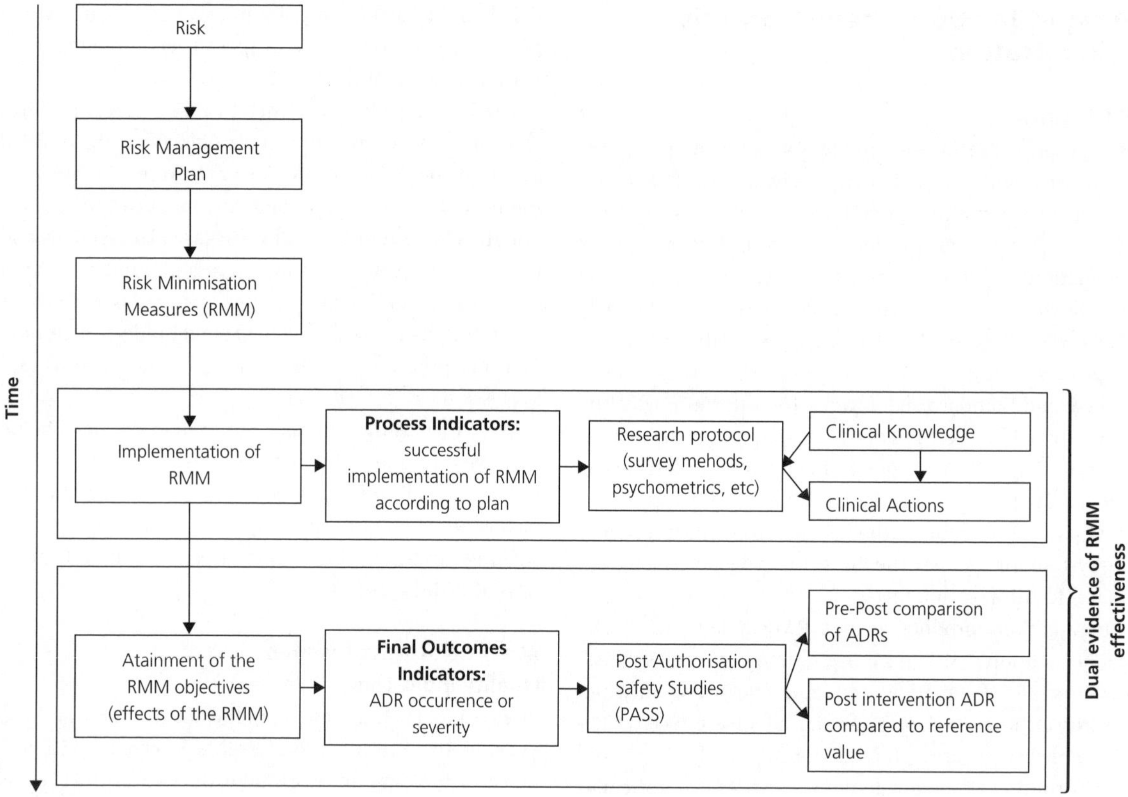

Figure 38.2 Dual evaluation of the effectiveness of risk minimization measures (RMMs).

Source: Prieto et al. 2012 [17]. Reproduced with permission from John Wiley and Sons.

use, contraindicated use, etc.), to measure the actual implementation; and (ii) outcome quality indicators, to determine the attainment of the final objective(s) (i.e. (reduced) occurrence of safety events) (Figure 38.2).

Measurement of the implementation of RMMs can be further subdivided into two levels of evaluation: (i) the assessment of clinical knowledge, usually employed through tailored cross-sectional surveys, where appropriate consideration of representativeness and sample size, choice of measurement instruments and operational definitions of independent/dependent variables are taken into account; and (ii) the assessment of clinical actions, generally requiring the establishment of prescribing measures and indicators, together with the use of available electronic health care/claims databases.

The structure of the health care system should also be considered – particularly how the system is organized, how the quality of RMMs is ensured and how logistics are organized and monitored (i.e. structure indicators).

This conceptual model of structure–process–outcome was first proposed by Donabedian [18] in 1988, and formed the basis for the recommendations issued at the European expert meeting on indicators of prescribing quality in drug utilization research [19]. The assumptions of such models are challenged, however, by a systematic review published in 2012, which showed that for many widely used quality indicators (structure or process), there is insufficient evidence demonstrating that they are predictive of better patient outcomes [20].

It is therefore important to carefully check how quality indicators are employed to measure the implementation of RMMs. On one hand, evaluating what proportion of targeted health care professionals have received a certain risk communication message may be considered part of the assessment of risk minimization activities, as there are several barriers across health care systems which might influence the practical implementation of regulatory measures. For example, in a study conducted in the Netherlands [21], it was found that 16% of health care professionals (ranging from 5% of hospital pharmacists to 28% of general practitioners) did not know what a direct health care professional communication (DHPC) was and could not recollect ever having received one.

On the other hand, specific attention should be given to employing appropriate process indicators, particularly if detailed information on drugs (dose, duration, clinical indication) and patients (comorbidity, clinical values) is required for their assessment. For example, in a study conducted in the United Kingdom [22] to measure the impact of regulatory warnings issued between May 2007 and January 2008 concerning the cardiovascular safety of thiazolidinediones (TZDs), patient-level information on TZD use was linked with cardiovascular morbidity. It was therefore possible to define measurable process indicators in order to demonstrate a significant decrease in the proportion of new users of TZD with contraindicated history of heart failure, myocardial infarction, cerebrovascular disorders and angina, resulting from the FDA and EMA warnings.

It is also important to ensure that the established process measures are comparable across the different countries where the study is conducted and that the study results are reliable enough to be generalizable to those countries where routinely collected health care information is not available.

Hospital-based data are even more difficult to obtain, suggesting that tailored field studies are sometimes needed to evaluate the impact of risk minimization activities in hospital settings. Initiatives such as the European Network of Centres for Pharmacoepidemiology and Pharmacovigilance (ENCePP) database of research resources [23] and the Pharmacoepidemiological Research on Outcome of Therapeutics by a European Consortium (PROTECT; see Chapter 14) inventory of drug consumption databases [24] may help drug utilization researchers in retrieving the most feasible data source for measuring the impact of regulatory measures.

Study design

Two recent systematic reviews [25,26] outlined the need to employ more rigorous criteria in investigating the impact of safety-related regulatory actions. Overall, the authors concluded that: (i) when regulatory actions were evaluated, a significant percentage of studies showed inadequate methodological standards, which might have resulted in an overestimation of the impact of RMMs; and (ii) generally, studies tended to examine only changes in the use of the targeted medical product (i.e. intended impact), without assessing either the unintended impact of the RMMs (i.e. increases in the use of substitute product or services) or outcome measures directly related to patient health and adverse effects. For example, the safety warnings for selective serotonin reuptake inhibitors (SSRIs) resulted in intended reduced prescription in the population at risk following identification of an increased risk of suicidality and suicidal thoughts in children and adolescents, but also resulted in decreased prescription in adults, thus potentially increasing the risk of suicidality in the general population [27].

As a consequence, a consensus panel has identified seven research design and analytic methods suitable for the evaluation of regulatory actions [25]. Among them, two – the interrupted time series (ITS; see Chapter 2) and the regression discontinuity (RD) design – are relatively easy to conduct and have been proven to offer strong methodological advantages in their ability to control for many potential time-varying threats to internal validity.

In the case of ITS, data are collected at multiple instances in time before and after a regulatory measure (interruption) is introduced to detect whether the intervention has an effect significantly greater than the underlying secular trend [28]. An advantage of an ITS design is that it allows for the statistical investigation of potential biases (i.e. secular trends, seasonal effects, duration, random fluctuations and autocorrelations) in the estimation of the effect of the intervention. It can also be performed using aggregate-level longitudinal data and it does not require a control group.

The RD design is most appropriate for assessing the impact of regulatory measures applied to a subgroup population defined by a continuous measure with a fixed threshold (i.e. contraindication in patients aged ≥65 years). It is characterized by its method of assigning subjects, which employs a cut-off score on an assignment measure. All subjects who score on one side of the cut-off (e.g. age ≥65 years) are assigned to the intervention group, while those scoring on the other side are assigned to the control group. Based on the control group's regression equation pre- and post-intervention, one can predict what the intervention group's values would have been if the programme had had no effect [29]. The RD design is a reasonably robust quasi-experimental design and may be especially useful when pre-intervention data are limited, although it requires individual-level data and it has rarely been used in medical research. Experience with this design is more limited than that with ITS designs.

Conclusion

Drug utilization studies describe the prescription, dispensing and use of medicines in defined populations. They can be used to track off-label use of drugs and can form the basis for evaluating the safe and effective use of medicines. The ability of these studies to identify prescribing patterns, to provide denominator data for the calculation of reporting rates in special populations, to characterize baseline risk profile in patients, to estimate potential drug abuse and to assess the effectiveness of risk minimization activities are only some of their potential applications in risk management.

The new EU pharmacovigilance legislation strengthens the role of the RMP as a key tool in proactive pharmacovigilance and highlights the need to measure the impact of risk minimization activities to ensure that the effectiveness of regulatory actions is demonstrated. Therefore, this new framework represents a relevant opportunity for drug utilization researchers to identify the most rigorous criteria for ascertaining prescribing quality and for conducting well-designed studies to measure the impact of risk minimization activities.

Disclaimer

The views expressed in this chapter are the personal views of the author(s) and may not be understood or quoted as being made on behalf of or reflecting the position of the EMA or one of its committees or working parties.

CHAPTER 39
Drug utilization research and pharmacovigilance

Emanuel Raschi & Fabrizio De Ponti
Pharmacology Unit, Department of Medical and Surgical Sciences, University of Bologna, Italy

KEY POINTS

- Drug utilization data have rarely been combined with spontaneous reporting system (SRS) data, despite the fact that they add a population (country-level) perspective to SRS (individual-level): a crucial dimension perfectly in line with new European legislation.
- Combining drug utilization data with SRS requires a comprehensive knowledge of the strengths, pitfalls and technicalities of each approach.
- There are three main goals when combining drug utilization data with SRS: (i) to calculate the reporting rate, which complements disproportionality techniques by highlighting possible risk differences among medicines (especially for vaccines and designated medical events (DMEs)); (ii) to weigh the drug risk at the population level (and assess the public health impact of adverse drug reactions (ADRs)); and (iii) to prioritize safety signals emerging from traditional disproportionality approaches.

The new era of pharmacovigilance in Europe

The need for transparency has changed the approach to pharmacovigilance, which has become a multifaceted field in which all stakeholders (pharmaceutical industry, regulators, academia, the public, media) are starting to share a common multidisciplinary environment [1]. Indeed, the new European pharmacovigilance legislation, in force since July 2012, attempts to rationalize and strengthen the role of the post-marketing phase, which is now explicitly intended to 'promote and protect public health by reducing burden of adverse drug reactions (ADRs) and optimizing the use of medicines' [2,3]. A number of tools can help in this, including the so-called post-authorization safety and efficacy studies (PASS and PAES, respectively; see also Chapters 38 and 40). Thus, pharmacovigilance is becoming a holistic proactive discipline, moving beyond the generation of simple alerts towards an overall risk–benefit assessment at both the individual patient level and the population level (epidemiological perspective). The main future challenge for pharmacovigilance is to integrate all the different heterogeneous pieces of evidence into a unified indicator through innovative and easily replicable technologies.

The recent exponential increase in the number of spontaneous ADR reports has prompted regulators and researchers to develop automated data-mining approaches that can deal with large spontaneous reporting systems (SRSs) recording millions of reports. Data-mining algorithms (DMAs) were developed as quantitative measures by which to assess, from a statistical standpoint, the association between a particular drug and a given clinical event [4]. DMAs are now routinely adopted by regulators investigating large volumes of data, in order to focus on issues of importance to public health. The remarkable trends in DMA-related publications demonstrate an active field of research, with a number of novel approaches under development and refinement [5] (see Box 39.1).

Drug Utilization Research: Methods and Applications, First Edition. Edited by M. Elseviers et al.
Published 2016 by John Wiley & Sons, Ltd.

Box 39.1 Development of spontaneous reporting system (SRS) databases.

From a methodological standpoint, the most important step in data mining relates to the *a priori* management of a database before the application of data-mining algorithms (DMAs) (i.e. the definition and processing of the initial raw dataset) [9]. This aspect is of great importance, especially as commercial tools become publicly available, as health care workers and the general public are usually unaware of all the technical issues surrounding these types of analysis. Several aspects must be carefully considered (these may differ between SRSs):

- **Drug and event codification (data mapping):** In the public version of the US Food and Drug Administration Adverse Event Reporting System (FAERS), drugs are reported in the 'DRUGNAME' field as free text: either the brand or the generic name can be reported, but so can a combination of both, and misspellings are relatively frequent. Thus, a significant amount of time is spent in the *ad hoc* creation of a drug name archive using a number of available drug dictionaries. For instance, in Vigibase, drugs are coded according to the World Health Organization (WHO) Drug Dictionary, which is maintained by the Uppsala Monitoring Centre (UMC). It is also recommended that codified active substances be indexed according to Anatomical Therapeutic Chemical (ATC) classification. As regards event codification, MedDRA and WHO-ART are the key medical terminologies used in the analysis of SRSs. Notably, these terminologies are not regularly updated with new terms, and even where new terms appear, symptoms may continue to be recorded using a more general one for some time. This causes problems with retrospective analysis (reports are 'hidden'), which can be very resource-intensive.
- **Data counting:** Usually, each report may contain several different adverse reactions, and each reaction term belongs to a body system organ class (SOC). When analysing counts of reactions, it is important to keep in mind that 'number of reactions' is not the same as 'number of reports'. For instance, if a report mentions two reactions and the count is made on the reaction level, this will result in two counts for this report. Where a report mentions several different reactions, two or more of which belong to the same SOC, the count can be conducted in two different ways: a report of rash (SOC Skin), urticaria (SOC Skin) and hepatitis (SOC Liver) can be counted as one occurrence of 'Skin' and one of 'Liver' or as two occurrences of 'Skin' and one of 'Liver'. The first method assigns equal weight to the two SOCs, irrespective of the number of terms reported for each, while the second puts more emphasis on the individual terms. Whenever an adverse reaction profile that involves SOC counts is produced, it is important that it states how the count was made.
- **Missing data:** The extent of missing data has not been systematically quantified in all SRSs, and it may vary depending on the field under study. Key information that is usually missing in more than 50% of reports in large international databases includes treatment dates, indication and dosage. Very recently, UMC developed the VigiGrade completeness score to measure amounts of clinically relevant information in a structured format. The overall quality is low (median completeness 41%), with the highest rate of well-documented reports occurring in Italy (65%) [10]. Single or multiple imputation strategies can be applied to deal with missing data.
- **Duplicates:** The presence of duplicates reporting the same individual event is a well-known phenomenon, especially in international SRSs. In addition, multiple records can be found when follow-up was submitted for an already reported event. All SRSs implement automatic 'data-cleaning' techniques to routinely remove duplicates and multiple records.

In parallel, the increasing availability and quality of health care databases (HCDs) based on administrative and claims data has boosted interest in the integration of evidence from multiple heterogeneous sources as a pharmacoepidemiological tool by which to evaluate drug safety [6,7] (see Chapter 41). The complementarity between SRSs and HCDs is a driving force behind several international multidisciplinary projects (US and European consortia, some of which are currently ongoing), often relying on a combination of different databases for signal detection (Table 39.1).

However, when aiming at early signal detection, SRSs remain the primary source for drug safety information, especially when exploring the risk profile of new drugs or investigating rare events with high drug-attributable risks, such as torsades de pointes and pancreatitis, known in pharmacovigilance as designated medical events (DMEs). The use of individual spontaneous reports represents a ready-to-use source of clinical data that can be mined successfully in a reasonable period of time and, through the evaluation of patient-related risk factors (demographic characteristics, concomitant disorders or medications, past medical history), show foci of lack of appropriateness in the use of specific drugs included in adverse event reports.

Table 39.1 Recent international drug safety initiatives using spontaneous reporting systems (SRSs) as key sources of signal detection.

Project	Funding	Timeframe	Partners	Drugs under investigation	Outcomes under investigation	Data sources
ARITMO, Arrhythmogenic Potential of Drugs (http://cordis.europa.eu/project/rcn/94061_en.html)	FP7	January 2010–June 2013	19 (academia and AstraZeneca)	Antipsychotics, antiinfectives, antihistamines	Arrhythmias	International (FAERS, EudraVigilance, Vigibase) and national (Italy, France, Germany, United Kingdom) SRSs HCDs Administrative claims
SAFEGUARD, Safety Evaluation of Adverse Reactions in Diabetes (http://www.safeguard-diabetes.org/)	FP7	October 2011–September 2014	14 (academia, including US university/research organizations)	Antidiabetics	Cardio/cerebrovascular and pancreatic safety	International (FAERS, EudraVigilance) and national (Germany, United Kingdom) SRSs HCDs Administrative claims
GRIP, Global Research In Pediatrics (http://www.grip-network.org/index.php/cms/en/home)	FP7	January 2011–December 2015	21 research institutions, including the WHO and EMA	Vaccines	Paediatric pharmacoepidemiological studies	12 HCDs, 3 SRSs (FAERS, VAERS and Vigibase)
PROTECT, Pharmacoepidemiological Research on Outcomes of Therapeutics by a European Consortium (http://www.imi-protect.eu/)	IMI	September 2009–September 2014	34 (public and private institutions coordinated by the EMA)	All drugs in the network	Methodological aspects unrelated to a pre-specified outcome (in some cases, specific drugs and outcomes have been used, such as antibiotics and liver injury)	SRSs (EudraVigilance, Vigibase and databases from drug companies) and HCDs
OMOP, Observational Medical Outcomes Partnership (http://www. omop.org/)	United States	Late 2008–December 2014	More than 10 (FDA, foundations, PhRMA)	ACE inhibitors, amphotericin B, antibiotics, antiepileptics, benzodiazepines, beta-blockers, tricyclic antidepressants, second-generation antipsychotics, warfarin	Bleeding, aplastic anaemia, angioedema, acute liver injury, gastrointestinal ulcer hospitalization, myocardial infarction, mortality after infarction, renal failure, hospitalization and other outcomes recorded in databases	Network of electronic medical records and claim databases International SRSs, such as FAERS

FP7, 7th Framework Programme; FAERS, US Food and Drug Administration Adverse Event Reporting System; HCD, health care database; WHO, World Health Organization; EMA, European Medicines Agency; VAERS, Vaccine Adverse Event Reporting System; IMI, Innovative Medicines Initiative; FDA, US Food and Drug Administration; PhRMA, Pharmaceutical Research Manufacturers of America; ACE, angiotensin-converting enzyme.

Getting the most out of current SRSs

Each European country collects its own reports in a national spontaneous reporting database, but international SRSs also gather reports, both from direct reporter submission and via systematic flows from the national databases. Collecting information from all these accessible sources is the mainstay of pharmacovigilance. Each source has its specific characteristics and limitations that must be considered when planning a drug safety analysis (e.g. completeness of data, options for database interrogation).

Major international SRSs [e.g. the EudraVigilance database (held by the European Medicines Agency - EMA), Vigibase (maintained by the Uppsala Monitoring Centre - UMC) and the US Food and Drug Administration Adverse Event Reporting System - FAERS] offer great opportunities for early and timely detection of signals of risk for rare events, by virtue of their large catchment areas (Table 39.2). The analysis of multiple international databases has the advantage that it covers a very large population and heterogeneous patterns of reporting for ADRs.

In the recent past, efforts were made to increase overall transparency in data analysis by providing public access to several databases. For instance, EudraVigilance data are available for research upon request, based on the EMA data access policy. Vigibase can be accessed and mined through specific Web-based tools: Vigisearch and Vigimine (formal requests to access full data can also be made). FAERS has provided public access to data since 2004 (both US and rare/serious European events), with full access to previous reports obtained through *ad hoc* requests. Notably, the US Food and Drug Administration (FDA) has launched the openFDA initiative (open.fda.gov), a beta research project aiming to provide open access to large health datasets collected by the agency.

Conversely, a single national SRS, as compared to international databases, is often insufficient to address the entire spectrum of drug safety (especially for rare events), mainly because of its limited population coverage. Nonetheless, national databases have the advantage of providing the local picture of a risk (which depends on local drug use) and offering access to patient medical histories (the so-called 'narratives'), thus potentially increasing the sensitivity of signal detection when performing a case-by-case analysis.

Ideally, the most accurate analysis should be based on the overall case listing, derived from a combination of all available SRSs, with the aim of creating a single database comprising pooled/aggregated data on ADRs worldwide. This theoretical scenario, unfortunately, is still unfeasible when performing drug safety studies, for several technical reasons. Apart from differences among various databases in terms of the terminologies and coding systems used to record both events and drugs, overlaps are likely to exist among national and international SRSs, mainly because reports submitted to national SRSs are sent on to international databases (especially those recorded as serious). In addition, a non-negligible but unmeasured proportion of reports recorded in national databases remains undetected in international SRSs (Figure 39.1). Redundancy among databases should be distinguished from intradatabase duplicates (i.e. duplicate reports caused by submissions from different reporters of the same individual event; see Box 39.1). No formal quantification of the actual extent has been attempted to date, making this an area for further research. It may vary with the ADR under investigation.

In summary, exploitation of different databases is important to covering all safety aspects and gaining the highest statistical power in signal detection (increased sensitivity) [8]. We believe that this modern view of pharmacovigilance – embraced, for instance, in the ARITMO project (http://cordis.europa.eu/project/rcn/94061_en.html) – will be of benefit to future research on drug safety.

Combining drug utilization data with spontaneous reports

The link between drug utilization data and spontaneous reports is not straightforward. In most cases, adverse events track the magnitude of utilization, meaning that the volume of spontaneous reports largely mirrors the exposure trend. However, drug utilization data can have an important role in approaching pharmacovigilance data from a population risk perspective, rather than the classical single patient perspective. These correlational studies refer to populations rather than individuals, so it is not possible to link exposure to occurrence of an outcome in a single person. Moreover, it should be kept in mind that results derived from a combination of both data sources must be interpreted very cautiously because they come from different databases, affected by different

Table 39.2 Overview of international spontaneous reporting systems (SRSs) from a research perspective: differences and similarities.

Database (public access)	Access	Timeframe	Drugs	Source of reports	Content of reports	Current number of reports available	Origin of submitted reports
FAERS (http://www.fda.gov/Drugs/GuidanceCompliance RegulatoryInformation/Surveillance/AdverseDrug Effects/default.htm)	Free only for data since 2004 Fredom of Information Act can be requested	1969–present (FAERS)	All drugs and biologics globally that provide a report of ADRs	Health care professionals, pharmaceutical companies, patients/consumers	Mandatory postmarketing report of serious and unexpected ADRs from drug companies Voluntary report (via MedWatch) from health care professionals/the public on ADRs with drugs	>8 million (as of December 2014); approximately 500 000 per year (2009–12)	Mostly the United States, but also serious/unexpected reports from the European Union, Japan and other non-US countries
Vigibase (WHO Global ICSR database) (http://www.vigiaccess.org/)	Web-based interface (VigiLize, VigiFlow, VigiMine applications[a]	1968–present	All drugs and biologics globally that provide a report of ADRs	National and regional pharmacovigilance centres (which may receive reports from patients, health care professionals or drug companies)	Individual case safety reports of suspected ADRs, case reports from studies and special monitoring	>12 million (as of January 2014); 200 000 per year	Global (107 official members and 33 associate members), but the majority come from the European Union and United States
EudraVigilance http://www.adrreports.eu/	Web-based interface (different access policies[b]	2001–present	All drugs and biologics authorized in the European Economic Area	National and regional pharmacovigilance centres (which may receive reports from patients, health care professionals or drug companies)	Individual case safety reports of suspect ADRs associated with medicinal products authorized in Europe Suspected unexpected serious reports from clinical trials	>8 million ADR reports received (as of December 2014)	European Economic Area
Canada Vigilance Adverse Reaction Online Database (http://www.hc-sc.gc.ca/dhp-mps/medeff/databasdon/index-eng.php)	Web-based interface	1965–present	Medicines and vaccines (since 2011) marketed in Canada or reported to Health Canada	Health care professionals and consumers, pharmaceutical companies, marketing authorization holders	Mandatory report from drug companies of marketing authorization holders Voluntary report from health care professionals and patients	No public data provided	Canada
DAEN TGA (https://www.tga.gov.au/database-adverse-event-notifications-daen	Web-based interface (free access to drug summary and list of reports)	1971–present	Medicines, vaccines and devices used in Australia	Health care professionals and patients	Voluntary report from health care professionals and patients	No public data provided	Australia

[a] Freely available to all members of the WHO Program for International Drug Monitoring.

[b] Specific access policies are described according to stakeholder groups. For details, see http://www.ema.europa.eu/docs/en_GB/document_library/Other/2015/12/WC500199048.pdf (last accessed).

FAERS, US Food and Drug Administration Adverse Event Reporting System; ADR, adverse drug reaction; WHO, World Health Organization; ICSR, Individual Case Safety Reports; DAEN TGA, Database of Adverse Event Notifications – the Therapeutic Goods Administration.

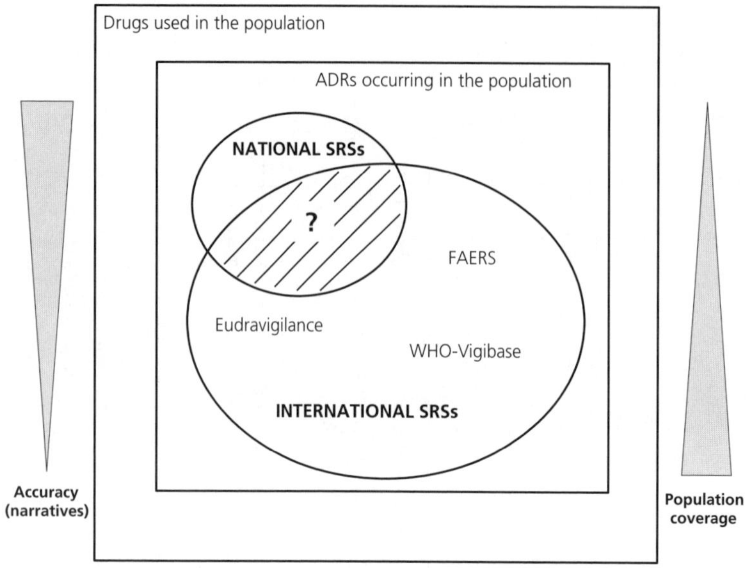

Figure 39.1 Issues to consider when planning an analysis using spontaneous reporting systems (SRSs): (i) relationships among the different databases (overlaps); (ii) their differences in terms of population coverage (sensitivity as a direct consequence of the catchment area) and accuracy in case selection (automated versus free text search strategy); (iii) relationships among patients exposed to drugs and experiencing adverse drug reactions (ADRs) and actual reporting (used to calculate disproportionality). Areas of circles do not necessarily reflect the precise proportions and relationships existing among them.

bias (e.g. under-reporting for SRSs, discrepancies with actual drug administration for prescription data).

Currently, only a few projects have attempted to address the combination of drug utilization data and data from SRSs. Apart from the ARITMO project, discussed later, the PROTECT project (http://www.imi-protect.eu/; see also Chapter 14) recently addressed the possible role of drug utilization data in drug safety studies, by reviewing, compiling and updating current knowledge of European sources of data on drug utilization in the out- and inpatient health care settings [11,12]. These documents are publicly available, in order to provide an accurate inventory of the sources available for use in planning clinical research. In addition, a database was created by the EMA and other PROTECT partners, using a stepwise approach (automated mapping of ADR terms listed in section 4.8 of the Summary of Product Characteristics to the MedDRA terminology, fuzzy text matching and expert review). The first project aimed at combining numerator data (from VigiBase) with denominator data (from the IMS Health drug utilization database) started in 1995: the ADR Signal Analysis Project (ASAP), funded by the European Union (BIOMED grant BMH1-CT94-1301). The strategic importance of the ASAP approach lies in the gap between when an early signal with possible important clinical and public health implications is found and when expensive case control or cohort studies can be performed. The key topics of published studies are as follows:

- Digoxin [quantitative and qualitative differences were found among countries (a higher reporting of suspected reactions from Australia and a later peak of occurrence with age in France) strengthening the importance of monitoring old drugs, and not just those recently marketed] [13].
- Omeprazole and visual disorders (the signal raised in Germany could not be confirmed by international data, suggesting a peculiar country-related phenomenon to be managed locally) [14].
- Selective serotonin reuptake inhibitors (SSRIs) and withdrawal syndrome (possible qualitative differences were found between the different compounds with respect to the nature of the withdrawal syndrome) [15].
- Tiaprofenic acid plus other antiinflammatory drugs and cystitis (the safety issue is specific to tiaprofenic acid and cannot be accounted for by changes in reporting patterns in certain countries or years) [16].
- Antihistamines and ventricular arrhythmia (some of the alternatives to terfenadine, withdrawn over cardiac risk, may have similar problems, suggesting that comparative risk–benefit assessment is needed) [17].

In research, drug utilization data may be connected (directly and indirectly) with case reports in order to: (i) calculate reporting rates; (ii) assign a given risk to the population; and (iii) prioritize safety signals emerging from the traditional disproportionality approach (Table 39.3).

The ***reporting rate*** is basically the ratio between the number of ADR cases extracted from a given spontaneous reporting database (the numerator) and the extent of drug use (the denominator, which may be expressed in terms of sales, prescription or dispensed data).

Only when the number of recorded cases approximates the number of actual cases (i.e. if under-reporting does not exist) may the reporting rate be viewed as an indicator of incidence. In this theoretical scenario, the critical aspect is in the precise selection of cases, which should be manually validated for plausibility and causality (e.g. by checking concomitant drugs that may play a causative role in the occurrence of ADRs) in order to distinguish correlation from actual causation [18]. The reporting rate is particularly suitable for drug–reaction pairs with the following characteristics: (i) the reactions are known as DMEs; and (ii) the drugs have been on the market for a number of years [5–10]. The former criterion means that reactions have a high drug-induced component; therefore, under-reporting is supposed to be negligible, as clinicians should be aware of the drug-attributable nature. The latter refers to old drugs, which should be associated with a relatively stable reporting pattern over time, because all emerging safety aspects should have been theoretically recognized, provided that therapeutic indications are not expected to change substantially in the near future. Whatever its magnitude, under-reporting does not affect the validity of conclusions if it is assumed that this is more or less identical across drugs belonging to the same therapeutic class, having the same indication and marketed in the same country during the same period of time. Under these circumstances, differences in terms of reporting rate should reflect differences in actual risk. Although this basic assumption was demonstrated 15 years ago [19], there are only a few examples in the literature attempting to calculate a reporting rate for risk estimation and safety comparative assessment [20]. For instance, in Italy, calculation of the reporting rate showed a remarkably higher rate of serious hepatic reactions associated with amoxicillin/clavulanic acid as compared to amoxicillin alone: a difference that was not detected by the traditional disproportionality approach [21].

Table 39.3 Main objectives of using drug utilization data in conjunction with spontaneous reporting systems (SRSs).

Objectives	Achievable goals
Calculation of reporting rate	To provide incidence estimate of the ADR associated with the drug under investigation
	To identify differences in reporting patterns between drugs, between countries and over time
	To identify emerging issues for old drugs
	To elucidate reasons for country differences (e.g. differences in drug use or publication bias influencing reporting)
Weighing drug risk at the population level (pharmacoepidemiological perspective)	To calculate trends of drug utilization over time and examine the impact of a regulatory decision
	To plan additional analytical study in a specific population that may be more susceptible to ADR occurrence
	To estimate the expected number of cases of a medical event in a defined population and period of time (to be compared with the observed number of cases)
	To measure the potential public health impact of ADRs
	To provide background data for the comparison of the safety profiles of several drugs
	To estimate the utilization of drugs withdrawn from the market and identify alternative drugs for the same indication
Prioritization of safety signals	To check the relationship between a detected disproportionality signal and magnitude of use
	To plan additional risk-minimization activities
	To prompt dedicated pharmacoepidemiological studies for risk quantification
	To assign a degree of uncertainty to safety signals

ADR, adverse drug reaction.

As previously emphasized, the merging of the two datasets requires in-depth knowledge of their structures and definitions and the way in which data are recorded. Concerning drug utilization data, it is important to identify the most appropriate source, keeping in mind the characteristics of the drugs under investigation (e.g. reimbursed, sold over the counter (OTC), mainly administered in hospitals). The reimbursement status is a key technical aspect, requiring careful evaluation, especially when investigating recently marketed drugs, for which local drug policies may influence dispensation.

If a given drug safety signal arises from SRSs, or when the accrual of scientific evidence allows better quantification of risk, drug utilization data can provide the ***population perspective*** by weighing the risk according to the magnitude of use, both in terms of aggregate mean use over a given period of time and in terms of secular trends, which may be particularly useful for recently marketed drugs.

For instance, collection and publication of antibiotics data by the European Surveillance of Antimicrobial Consumption (ESAC) project formed the basis for important ecological studies, especially on the relationship between antibiotic use and resistance [22]. The case of nimesulide exemplifies how different drug reporting patterns may strongly influence local regulatory decisions. Following identification of a signal of serious hepatic reactions, nimesulide (used only negligibly in several countries) was withdrawn from many European markets. In Italy, given that (i) it was the most frequently prescribed drug among antinflammatory agents, (ii) the reporting rate for serious hepatic reactions was very low and the overall risk of hospitalization for hepatotoxicity among antinflammatory drugs was low and (iii) it was well tolerated in terms of gastrointestinal risk, nimesulide was not withdrawn, but its supply status was changed from 'renewable' to 'not renewable' prescription, as a measure to reduce its potential inappropriate use and avoid possible switching to other drugs with higher gastrointestinal risk, such as ketoprofen or diclofenac.

In the ARITMO project, a number of European Drug Utilisation Research Group (EuroDURG) researchers were involved in the collection of drug utilization data on antipsychotics, antihistamines and antiinfectives (with ESAC group collaboration) from 19 European countries. Drug utilization data were used within ARITMO to give a population perspective to results on the arrhythmogenic potential of drugs belonging to these therapeutic classes.

Different methodological approaches can be taken to the interpretation of drug utilization data in conjunction with results on arrhythmogenic risk, with important public health implications. In this context, preliminary approaches are under discussion with the EMA, and initial results have recently been published on antipsychotics and antihistamines. Some specific scenarios were identified for particular countries: cyamemazine in France, prothipendyl in Austria and cetirizine in Norway [23–25]. This joint analysis, although preliminary, shows the synergy between drug utilization and adverse event databases in alerting health policy personnel to potential future activities by which to reduce ADRs, especially for drugs associated with a very strong torsadogenic signal.

Some more general indications from the ARITMO project are as follows:

- Large inter- and intraclass differences in drug use are found among countries; as expected from previous studies, Southern European countries are increasingly and remarkably exposed to antibiotics, whereas Northern European countries are typically characterized by large consumption of antihistamines. Antipsychotics are widely used across Europe, with a trend towards newer second-generation agents.
- If a country shows new exposure to a given class or certain drug known for its arrhythmogenic potential on the basis of any drug safety study, the national medicine agency should check with prescribers for potential areas of inappropriate use.
- If a specific high-risk agent within a class generates concern (e.g. due to magnitude of consumption or a remarkable recent trend), the reasons for this should be investigated and a switch towards safer analogues may be considered and possibly promoted, where genuinely safer options are available.
- Drugs with relatively low use should not be ignored or overlooked: both recently marketed drugs (which quickly penetrate the market with increasing consumption) and drugs with peculiar use in a few countries call for *ad hoc* continuing surveillance.
- The three ARITMO drug classes are very heterogeneous in terms of rules of dispensation (some agents in each class are administered in hospital, while some antihistamines are available OTC). This should be taken into account when regulatory decisions are

made at the national level. In this context, hospital use is probably less critical than OTC use from a clinical viewpoint, due to stringent in-hospital patient monitoring, although pharmacokinetic issues (high doses and intravenous administration) and patients' clinical status (disease severity, comorbidities) represent additional risk factors.

Signal prioritization is a term usually adopted by regulators to assign a level of priority to a disproportionality signal identified together with many other signals in an SRS. Typically, different parameters are assessed to prioritize these safety signals: a public health perspective will be strongly considered (e.g. the severity of the event), whereas pharmacological criteria are usually neglected (e.g. the strength of the disproportionality) [26]. In ARITMO, a prioritization tool was developed to highlight signals of arrhythmia through consideration of a number of pharmacological indicators obtained via different data-mining techniques. In addition, efforts were made to assign a qualitative measure to this prioritization tool by calculating a degree of uncertainty (which reflects the confidence in the signal originating from SRSs). In fact, assessment and comparison of drugs based solely on a pharmacological score may be misleading, as several biases compromise the actual ranking through SRSs. Other variables were therefore considered, in particular the time on the market, drug consumption and the consistency of signal among databases. Drugs with a high uncertainty were characterized by recent marketing life and low consumption, both of which reduce the degree of confidence in the value of the score.

A final speculative use of drug utilization data in pharmacovigilance was also hypothesized: the identification of potential low-risk drugs. In our view, at least three criteria must be simultaneously met in order to classify a drug as low-risk: (i) 'negative' pharmacovigilance data (i.e. ideally, no report should be extracted on the event of interest) with a sufficient number of total reports (i.e. such that a safety signal, if it existed, would have emerged); (ii) long time on market (at least 10 years: a reasonable time window in which to fully appreciate the safety profile of a drug); and (iii) detectable use [e.g. at least 0.01 defined daily doses (DDDs) per thousand inhabitants per day (DID)] in a sufficient number of countries (such that a safety issue, if it existed, would have emerged). Notably, based on recently published data, no antipsychotic meets all these criteria; therefore, all antipsychotics appear to carry an inherent torsadogenic risk, and data on use of this class can be considered an indicator of risk in the population [24].

Conclusion

A multidisciplinary, multidimensional environment, encouraged by the new proactive pharmacovigilance legislation, is the main factor in achieving better drug risk–benefit evaluation. In the era of open data, global integration of available evidence is required, from the individual clinical perspective of SRSs to the epidemiological perspective of drug utilization studies.

Current areas of research are struggling with proper merging and combination of (i) the same types of data from different databases (e.g. SRSs and HCDs) and (ii) heterogeneous types of data from disparate sources [e.g. drug utilization data, SRSs (including patient-generated data on the Internet), literature, preclinical data].

Combining drug utilization data with SRSs is a feasible ecological exercise that may help provide insight into public health issues by highlighting additional risk indicators, such as the population-attributable risk and reporting rate for specific drug–reaction pairs. A future challenge will be the integration through record-linkage approaches of information obtained from clinical records with that extracted from SRSs. Of course, ethical issues (protection of patients) will require appropriate management.

Acknowledgements

We would like to acknowledge all persons who in recent years have shared with us ideas and discussions on the topic of this chapter, especially all colleagues involved in pharmacovigilance activities carried out during the ARITMO project (in particular, Elisabetta Poluzzi and Ugo Moretti). In addition, we thank Prof. Marie Lindquist from WHO, who shared important theoretical and technical concepts behind the combination of drug utilization data and spontaneous reporting databases.

CHAPTER 40

Drug utilization research and the regulator's perspective in pharmacovigilance

Xavier Kurz & Kevin Blake
European Medicines Agency, United Kingdom

KEY POINTS

- Drug utilization studies are an increasingly essential component of the risk–benefit monitoring of medicinal products in the postmarketing phase.
- Three important objectives of drug utilization studies are very useful in pharmacovigilance: describing the characteristics of treated patients; estimating the incidence rate or the prevalence rate of drug use; and studying the quality of drug utilization in comparison with a clinical standard.
- Studies recorded in the EU-PAS Register, a publicly accessible resource for the registration of post-authorization studies (PASs), frequently include drug utilization aims.
- Drug utilization studies have acquired an important role in measuring the effectiveness of risk minimization measures and thereby help verify the impact of decisions taken to protect public health.
- Population-attributable risk (PAR) represents a possible approach to the measurement of the public health impact of adverse drug reactions (ADRs): it combines relative risk data with drug utilization data from national or international databases.

Introduction

In the past, decision-making in pharmacovigilance often relied on the results of studies requested to pharmaceutical companies by regulators following the detection of safety signals based on spontaneous adverse drug reaction (ADR) reports. More recently, signal detection and decision-making have been based on complementary sets of data collected by industry, research organizations or public authorities, including data on how drugs are used in populations and how their utilization can be improved [1].

Despite the opening of pharmacovigilance to other types of data, spontaneous ADR reports are still the primary source of information for signal detection. This role still influences the use of absolute numbers of reports and of national sales or prescription data to estimate the risk of occurrence of a drug safety issue in the population and to decide on any protective action. Fundamental problems in this practice have been highlighted [2]. Uncertainties affect both the numerator (i.e. the number of incident cases, due to underreporting and biased reporting) and the denominator (i.e. the number of exposed patients). In many countries where electronic health records (EHRs) are not available at all, have limited coverage or do not contain adequate information, prescription or sales data are used as the primary source of information. In these situations, the estimation of exposure is often complicated by a lack of data on actual consumption (including non compliance), dosage and duration of use (which can vary according to patient groups), as well as the variation over time in the amounts of drugs stored and sold. Any direct comparison of drug safety is therefore impaired by a lack of comparability of the estimates of incident rates for different drugs [3]. These uncertainties have led to recommendations that rates based on spontaneous reports should not be

Drug Utilization Research: Methods and Applications, First Edition. Edited by M. Elseviers et al.
Published 2016 by John Wiley & Sons, Ltd.

used to assign a frequency for an ADR in the product information. For example, in the European Union, the category 'Frequency not Known' should be used in the summary of product characteristics (SmPC) [4].

One approach to addressing these uncertainties is for regulators to require targeted product-specific postmarketing drug utilization studies. This is reflected in EU pharmacovigilance legislation, which provides regulators with a legal basis from which to impose post-authorization safety studies (PASSs) on companies in order to assess patterns of drug utilization (such as indication, dosage, co-medication and medication errors [5]). The conduct of such PASSs has been facilitated by the increasing availability of EHRs containing detailed drug prescription or dispensing data on large populations (see Chapter 38).

Specific objectives of drug utilization studies in pharmacovigilance

Patterns of treatment and characteristics of treated patients differ between clinical trial and postmarketing settings. These differences may have consequences for drug effectiveness and safety [6]. Companies are therefore often requested by regulatory authorities at the time of the initial authorization of a medicinal product, and potentially throughout the post-authorization phase, to conduct studies aimed at determining how the medicinal product is used in routine clinical practice. This might include characterizing who actually uses it and whether specific patterns of use are associated with specific risks. In this context, drug utilization studies have three important objectives in pharmacovigilance (Table 40.1): (i) to describe the characteristics of treated patients, including sociodemographic and clinical characteristics, and their patterns of drug use; (ii) to estimate the incidence rate of drug use (a measure of the number of new users of a specific drug within a given period against the size of the underlying population followed during the same period) or the prevalence rate of drug use (the proportion of a population using a specific drug at a given point in time (point prevalence) or within a given period (period prevalence)); and (iii) to study the quality of drug utilization in comparison with a clinical standard, including persistence (defined here as the continuation of the treatment for the prescribed duration), adherence (the percentage of the prescribed doses of the medication actually taken by the patient over a specified period) and, more generally, compliance (the extent to which a drug is used or prescribed according to the SmPC or clinical guidelines; see Chapter 38).

These objectives allow the pursuit of different achievable goals (Table 40.1). Several objectives are often pursued in the same study, but each objective may require a specific methodological component. Critical to the design of a drug utilization study is the choice of study population, which may be drawn from the general population or may be a sampling of patients with the same disease, treated with the same drug or treated with drugs from the same class. This choice has a profound influence on the goals that can be pursued, the nature of the information that can be collected and the analyses that can be performed.

The collection of scientifically robust data directly from patients or health care professionals may permit a more precise determination of the characteristics of drug users and their patterns of drug use than extraction of data from electronic databases of prescriptions or health records. Primary collection of data may therefore be more appropriate (although it is often also more expensive) when examining adherence and compliance with clinical guidelines and the product information (including an estimation of off-label use) and the factors influencing them. Such information is critical to pharmacovigilance in assessing whether measures taken to minimize the risks associated with a given drug are followed and effective in routine clinical practice. Such measures may include a restriction of indications, new contraindications, new dosage instructions or warnings against certain co-medications [7]. Detailed knowledge of how a drug is used by patients in practice also informs on determinants of the drug's efficacy and safety in terms of actual dosage, treatment schedules and potential confounding factors (such as patient sociodemographic characteristics and concomitant conditions, morbidities and other treatments). A less recognized application is in the estimation of the prevalence of a chronic disease treated with drugs specific to that disease (e.g. antidiabetic therapies). An accurate calculation of this requires data on the total amount of these drugs sold in a given region and on the mean intake of these drugs based on the consumed daily doses estimated from a survey of a representative sample of patients [8].

Where they are available and comprehensive, electronic data sources (e.g. prescription or health care records) may allow a measurement of the incidence or prevalence of drug use in a population. These data are needed for the assessment of drug safety issues based on

Table 40.1 Objectives and achievable goals of drug utilization studies in pharmacovigilance.

Objective	Examples of achievable goals
To describe the characteristics of treated patients and their patterns of drug use	To identify important characteristics of users and utilization patterns that differ between premarketing clinical trials and postmarketing use (e.g. age and sex distribution, comorbidity, dosage)
	To study the distribution of categories of patient-related variables known to be confounders or effect modifiers of drug efficacy or safety in medical practice
	To measure the frequency of prescription of interacting drugs and the resulting risk of ADRs or decreased efficacy
	To determine the effectiveness of risk minimization measures acting on prescription patterns
	To evaluate patients' knowledge and behaviours and the impact of patient information
	To compare the patient profile and utilization patterns of different drugs of the same class or drugs prescribed for the same indication
To estimate the prevalence of a chronic disease treated with specific drugs and to measure the incidence or prevalence of drug use in a defined population	To estimate the prevalence of a chronic disease treated with specific drugs
	To calculate trends of drug utilization over time and examine the impact of a regulatory decision restricting the prescription of or access to a drug
	To plan a pharmacoepidemiological study in the same population (power calculation)
	To estimate the expected number of cases of a medical event in a defined population and a given time period (to be compared with the observed number of cases)
	To measure the potential public health impact of ADRs
	To provide background data for the comparison of the safety profiles of several drugs
	To evaluate switching patterns between drugs and preferential prescribing of new drugs
	To estimate utilization of drugs withdrawn from the market and identify alternative drugs used for the same indication
	To provide data for health services research and planning
To study the quality of drug utilization in comparison to a clinical standard (persistence, adherence, compliance)	To study compliance with clinical guidelines or the product's SmPC in terms of indication, contraindications, dosage (including off-label use, abuse and misuse), co-medication and patient follow-up
	To estimate the success of a treatment and its determinants
	To estimate the quality of therapeutic management
	To compare the public health and economic impacts of different treatments
	To estimate treatment efficacy and safety by level of adherence and compliance

ADR, adverse drug reaction; SmPC, summary of product characteristics.

a comparison of the expected and observed number of cases of a medical event in a treated population. Estimation of incidence and prevalence of drug use may allow an evaluation of discontinuation patterns and switching patterns (e.g. if one drug is no longer available in the market). It may also guide therapeutic strategies by taking into account available alternatives.

Experience of drug utilization studies in the EU PAS Register

The distribution of the three objectives for drug utilization studies has been examined in the EU PAS Register, which is a publicly accessible resource for the registration of post-authorization studies (PASs) (www.encepp.eu). The EU PAS Register does not provide an exhaustive or representative picture of the range of drug utilization studies conducted in the European Union, but among the 202 observational studies registered by 31 December 2013, drug utilization was mentioned in the scope of 78 and was the main scope of 36. Characteristics of these 36 studies were extracted from their methodological description and their protocol, where available, and are given in Table 40.2. Their objectives address the characteristics of drug users or drug use in 15 of 36 cases, the population incidence or prevalence of drug use in 8 and the quality of drug utilization in 25. A total of 24 (66.7%) studies were reported to have been requested by a regulatory authority (the European Medicines Agency - EMA - or a National Competent Authority), and 21 (58.3%) were entirely funded by a pharmaceutical

Table 40.2 Characteristics of studies whose main scope is drug utilization registered in the EU PAS Register by 31 December 2013.

Source: EU Pas Register (www.encepp.eu).

Characteristics	Number of studies (n = 36)
Study objectives (may be more than one in a given study):	
• Characteristics of drug users and drug use	15 (41.7%)
• Incidence or prevalence of drug use in a population	8 (22.2%)
• Quality of drug utilization	25 (69.4%)
• Effectiveness of risk minimization	13 (36.1%)
• Studies requested by a regulatory authority	24 (66.7%)
Source of funding:	
• Industry	21 (58.3%)
• EMA	3 (8.3%)
• EC funding scheme	2 (5.6%)
• Government body	2 (5.6%)
• Research council	1 (2.8%)
• Other	7 (19.4%)
Studies in more than one country:	20 (55.6%)
• 2 countries	3 (8.3%)
• 3 countries	8 (22.2%)
• 4 countries	4 (11.1%)
• >4 countries	5 (13.9%)
Countries involved (may be more than one in a given study):	
• United Kingdom	21 (58.3%)
• Germany	13 (36.1%)
• France	12 (33.3%)
• Italy	9 (25.0%)
• Spain	8 (22.2%)
• The Netherlands	8 (22.2%)
• Denmark	7 (19.4%)
Data collection:	
• Primary	11 (30.6%)
• Secondary	25 (69.4%)
Total number of different established data sources used in secondary data collection	18

EMA, European Medicines Agency; EC, European Commission.

company. Although the EU PAS Register is a public register open to all PASs, these figures reflect the fact that regulatory authorities encourage registration when a study is requested to a marketing authorization holder.

Registering a study and its protocol in a publicly available domain allows the study design and methods to be shared and has been promoted as a means of supporting peer review and study quality [9]. A full protocol was available for 18 of the 36 drug utilization studies registered by the end of 2013, providing a large, readily accessible methodological base to researchers.

The conduct of more than half of the studies in more than one country (with a mode of three countries) shows the feasibility of conducting a drug utilization study on a multinational level. The distribution of countries where drug utilization studies are most frequently conducted may reflect the need for large sample sizes and the availability of electronic health care databases facilitating access to drug utilization data. These aspects are also reflected by the secondary use of data sources in 69% of the registered drug utilization studies.

Measurement of the effectiveness of risk minimization

Drug utilization studies have acquired an important role in pharmacovigilance as a tool by which to measure the effectiveness of risk minimization measures and thereby help verify the impact of decisions taken to protect public health. Such studies are funded not only by industry but also by regulatory authorities and national bodies. Table 40.3 provides information on 13 drug utilization studies registered in the EU PAS Register aimed at measuring the effectiveness of risk minimization measures. The breadth of information in Table 40.3 illustrates the role of drug utilization studies in pharmacovigilance, both in terms of the complexity of the issues they aim to address and the wide range of measures regulators may introduce [7]. Examples include the evaluation of a pregnancy-prevention programme, effects of concomitant drug use, compliance to labelled indications, the impact of educational materials, inappropriate prescribing and compliance to SmPC requirements regarding liver enzyme monitoring, pregnancy testing and contraception methods. While most of the studies are

Table 40.3 Objectives and designs of 13 drug utilization studies registered in the EU PAS Register by 20 December 2013 and aimed at measuring the effectiveness of risk minimization.

Source: EU PAS Register (http://www.encepp.eu/encepp/studySearch.htm).

Lead investigator	Drug or drug class	Objective(s)	Countries	Data sources (actual or estimated number of study subjects for main outcomes)	Study period	Funding	Protocol available in Register	Results available in Register
de Vries C.	Isotretinoin	To measure the effectiveness of the Pregnancy Prevention Programme	United Kingdom, Italy	CPRD (323) Emilia-Romagna GP drug prescription (5882) Emilia-Romagna dermatology clinic (152)	2004–10	EMA	Yes	Yes
Svendsen K.	Cyproterone-ethinylestradiol products, isotretinoin	To measure drug utilization of cyproterone-ethinylestradiol products and co-prescription with isotretinoin	France, Germany, United Kingdom	IMS Disease Analyzer for France (15 141), Germany (43 879) and the United Kingdom (20 322)	2002–11	EMA	Yes	Yes
Sorensen H.T.	Pioglitazone	To measure associations between changes in drug utilization and regulatory decisions To measure alterations in glycaemic control and other objective parameters of disease in patients discontinuing pioglitazone after the Dear Heath Care Professional Communication To measure contraindications and events in patients continuing or starting pioglitazone	Denmark, The Netherlands, United Kingdom	Danish Medical Registries (897) IPCI (667) CPRD (33 308)	2000–12	EMA	Yes	Yes
Sorensen H.T.	Rosiglitazone	To measure trends in the utilization of rosiglitazone-containing preparations over time in response to risk minimization events (switches to and from rosiglitazone-containing preparations) To measure the prevalence of contraindicated and off-label use To measure changes in the objective parameters of disease in medication switchers	Denmark, United Kingdom	Danish Medical Registries (2321) CPRD (25 428)	2000–12	EMA	Yes	Yes
Castellsague J.	Cilostazol	To determine the characteristics of new users of cilostazol according to baseline comorbidity, including conditions listed in the SmPC and the RMP as potential or identified safety concerns and concurrent use of potentially interacting medications	Germany, Spain, Sweden, United Kingdom	IACS (unknown), SIDIAP (3375), GePaRD (4867–9735), THIN (1640), Swedish National Databases (1800–2200)	2002–12	Industry	Yes	No

Actelion Pharmaceuticals	Bosentan	To measure adherence to the SmPC requirements (liver enzymes monitoring, pregnancy testing and contraception methods) and occurrence of specific safety issues	18 countries	Prospective disease registry (5000)	2008–	Industry	No	No
Weatherhall M.	Dexmetedomidine	To measure use in clinical practice and observed compliance with current marketing license	Austria, Finland, Germany, Poland	Patient medical records (2000)	2013–	Industry	Yes	No
Frajzyngier V.	Tigecycline	To measure the effectiveness of risk minimization measures by describing indications for tigecycline use and clinical outcomes among adult patients in the European Union before and after their implementation	Austria, Germany, Greece, Italy, United Kingdom	Medical charts review (600)	2013–14	Industry	Yes	No
Sorensen HT.	Metformine	To measure the prevalence of renal impairment and other characteristics among new and prevalent users of metformin To measure use of metformin in patients with type 2 diabetes according to stage of renal function impairment To assess the safety of metformin regarding renal impairment and lactic acidosis	Denmark, United Kingdom	Danish Medical Registries, CPRD (total 22 000)	2013–14	EMA	No	No
Caetano P.	NSAIDs, PPIs, antiplatelet agents	To determine the superiority of educational outreach visits compared to usual implementation of guidelines regarding the reduction of inappropriate prescribing by family physicians	Portugal	Randomized clinical trial (220)	2013–16	Government (Portuese)	Yes	No
Ataher Q.	Apixaban	To measure utilization patterns and prescriptions within and outside the approved label of apixaban in Sweden	Sweden	Swedish National Healthcare Registries (600)	2012–14	Industry	Yes	No
Gunn S.	Ocriplasmin	To determine the effectiveness of educational material provided to patients prior to injection	Seven countries	Prospective patient-based data collection (600)	2014–18	Industry	No	No
Antinori A.	Tenofovir, emtricitabine, efavirenz, rilpivirine	To quantify prescription errors and identify those that can be avoided by the use of single-tablet regimens	Italy, Portugal, Spain	Routine primary care electronic patient registry, pharmacy dispending records (total 2215)	2014	Industry	No	No

CPRD, Clinical Practice Research Datalink; GP, general practitioner; EMA, European Medicines Agency; SmPC, summary of product characteristics; RMP, risk management plan; IACS, Aragon Institute of Health Sciences (Aragon, Spain); SIDIAP, Information System for the Development of Research in Primary Care (Barcelona, Spain); GePaRD, German Pharmacoepidemiological Research Database; THIN, The Health Improvement Network; NSAID, nonsteroidal antiinflammatory drug; PPI, proton pump inhibitor.

based on electronic health care databases, a large variety of data sources are employed, including prospective disease registries, manual review of medical charts, primary patient-based data collection and randomized clinical trials.

Variability in study design

Drug utilization studies are potentially able to assess a large range of risk minimization factors. However, due to variability in their design, a meaningful comparison and interpretation of results is not always possible. Table 40.4 presents the characteristics of two studies aimed at evaluating the impact of warnings regarding the risks associated with treatment with rosiglitazone. One was performed in the United Kingdom only [10] and the other in both the United Kingdom and Denmark [11]. In the former, the main outcome was incidence and prevalence rates of use of rosiglitazone; in the latter, it was the proportion of rosiglitazone users among users of all oral hypoglycaemic agents (OHAs). Other differences between the two studies concern the terminology used to describe exposures and outcomes, the periods of follow-up, the choice of confounding factors, the definition of prescription duration and the definition of rosiglitazone discontinuation. Although the two studies reached the same general conclusion (a sharp decline in rosiglitazone prescription started in May 2007 following the publication of a meta-analysis [12]), their results cannot be compared or combined at a more granular level of detail. This lack of comparability is not, however, restricted to drug utilization studies [13].

New-user design

When the effectiveness of risk minimization is measured based on patients who continue to use a drug (e.g. a study comparing the occurrence of an adverse reaction before and after the introduction of new recommendations on dosage or patient monitoring), biases may be introduced by the fact that the patients who remain under treatment, and are therefore more likely to be surveyed, are those who use the drug correctly: the so-called 'healthy user effect'. Such an effect depends on time-related factors, including the duration of treatment, patterns of prescription over time and the time period covered by the survey. A new-user design has been proposed to eliminate these biases. This requires the identification of all patients in a defined population (in terms of both people and time period) starting a treatment with the study medication [14]. This is illustrated in a study investigating different regimens of statin therapy for the primary prevention of vascular diseases, where 'first use' of statins is defined by the absence of any recorded prescription of any statin in the time period at least 1 year before the date of the first recorded prescription [15].

Measurement of the public health impact of adverse drug reactions

The measurement of the public health impact of suspected ADRs is an essential regulatory activity that supports the prioritization of actions, the choice of risk management decisions and the evaluation of the effectiveness of those decisions. For European regulators, it is particularly important to collect this information in a comparable manner across several member states, so that findings can be generalized without being affected by local factors. The methodologies by which to do this are not firmly established.

An epidemiological approach to such measurement is illustrated by Khong et al. [16], who estimated the population impact of the use of benzodiazepines on the rate of hip fracture in five large European countries (France, Germany, Italy, Spain and the United Kingdom) and the United States. In the absence of published data comparing consumption of benzodiazepines across multiple countries, they used a sales database to calculate country-specific prevalence rates of benzodiazepine use. They converted sales data to the World Health Organization (WHO)'s defined daily dose (DDD), calculated a consumption of DDDs per 1000 persons per day and estimated the 1-year prevalence of benzodiazepine use; this was done by extrapolating publicly available data containing the total number of DDDs and the number of drug users in three countries (Denmark, the Netherlands, Norway) to the countries under study where such information does not exist. While recognizing the limitations of such extrapolation (the prescribed daily dose may vary from country to country), the authors considered that the method showed the usefulness of sales data for comparisons between countries. Pooled relative risks of the association between benzodiazepine use and hip fractures were combined with exposure data into a population-attributable risk (PAR), which is a measure that estimates how many hip fractures could

Table 40.4 Study design of two studies evaluating the impact of warnings regarding risks associated with rosiglitazone.

	Leal I et al. [10]	Ehrenstein V et al. [11]	
Objective	To analyse the prescription pattern of glucose-lowering drugs (GLDs) in the United Kingdom, with a special focus on the effects of safety warnings about rosiglitazone issued by the FDA and EMA	To study the impact of labelling changes and findings reported in scientific publications on the utilization of rosiglitazone-containing products in Europe and on the glycaemic control of patients discontinuing rosiglitazone	
Country	United Kingdom	United Kingdom	Denmark
Data source	THIN	GPRD	AUPD, LABKA
Study period	1 January 2000–24 November 2009	01 January 2000–31 December 2010	
Study population definition	Patients with type 2 diabetes mellitus with a prescription of at least one GLD during the study period	People who received at least one prescription for any oral hypoglycaemic agent (OHA) during the study period	
Source population (number of subjects in study period)	5 312 567	Not specified	1.8 million
Study population (number of GLD or OHA users in study period)	178 674 (3.4%)	191 276 (-)	67,525 (3.8%)
Main outcome definition	Annual prevalence of use Annual incidence of use Characteristics of new users Switching patterns of GLDs	Proportion of rosiglitazone users among all OHA users Comparison of rosiglitazone users and other OHA users Changes in glycated haemoglobin (HbA_{1c}) and fasting plasma glucose (FPG) levels Switching patterns of OHAs after rosiglitazone discontinuation	
Time periods of interest	Characteristics of new users: • within 6 months prior to FDA warning • between FDA and EMA warnings • within 6 months of EMA warning Switching patterns of GLDs 1 year before and 1 year after FDA alert	Changes in HbA_{1c} and FPG: • 3, 6 and 12 months after rosiglitasone discontinuation during study period Changes in HbA_{1c}: • 3 and 6 months after EMA suspension of rosiglitazone (23 September 2010)	
Definition of			
• loss of glycaemic control		• $HbA_{1c} > 7.5\%$	
• treatment failure		• FPG > 10 mmol/l	
Patient characteristics assessed	Age, sex, concomitant use of insulin, history of heart failure, myocardial infarction or cerebrovascular disorder, primary hypertension, angina, obesity or lipid metabolism disorder	Age, sex, BMI, smoking, Charlston comorbidity index, history of OHA use before baseline,[a] history of hypoglycaemic agent use before baseline, history of other medication use	
Drug identification	Multilex codes	Multilex codes	ATC codes
Definition of prescription length	Total number of units per prescription divided by prescription daily number of these units	Fixed at 130 days[b]	Fixed at 45 days[b]
Definition of rosiglitazone discontinuation	No refill in the year following start of prescription of another GLD (switch)	No refill during period covering at least two prescriptions (260 days)	No refill during period covering at least two prescriptions (90 days)

[a]Baseline date: 1 January 2000 or date of first OHA prescription, whichever came later.

[b]Prescription length based on observed intervals between prescriptions and knowledge about typical prescription practice in Denmark, as well as on prescribing instructions in the British Monthly Index of Medications in the United Kingdom.

FDA, US Food and Drug Administration; EMA, European Medicines Agency; THIN, The Health Improvement Network general practice database; GPRD, General Practice Research Database (currently known as the Clinical Practice Research Datalink, CPRD); AUPD, Aarhus University Prescription Database; LABKA, Laboratory Information Systems of the North and the Central Denmark Regions; BMI, body mass index; ATC, Anatomical Therapeutic Chemical.

Table 40.5 Benzodiazepine use (DDD/1000 persons/day) in five European countries and the United States, calculated using IMS MIDAS drug sales data (2009).

Source: Khong et al. 2012 [16].

Country	Any benzodiazepine	SAB	LAB
France	76.0	64.1	11.9
Germany	18.0	14.0	3.91
Italy	52.4	42.4	10.0
Spain	85.5	67.9	17.6
United Kingdom	19.3	11.6	7.63
United States	82.9	75.9	6.96

DDD, defined daily dose; SAB, short-acting benzodiazepine; LAB, long-acting benzodiazepine.

be prevented if exposure to the risk factor – in this case benzodiazepine use – were eliminated. The results show that there were considerable differences in benzodiazepine use across countries (Table 40.5). The estimated PAR of the use of any benzodiazepine on the risk of hip fractures (Table 40.6) varied between 1.8 and 8.2%. In all countries, this PAR was higher than the separate PARs for short- and long-acting benzodiazepines.

Table 40.6 Estimated population-attributable risk (%) and its 95% confidence interval for hip fractures associated with benzodiazepine use in five European countries and the United States.

Source: Khong et al. 2012 [16].

Country	Any benzodiazepine[a]	SAB[a]	LAB[a]
France	7.4 (4.5–10)	3.7 (1.5–6.1)	1.0 (0.3–1.8)
Germany	1.8 (1.1–2.6)	0.8 (0.3–1.4)	0.3 (0.1–0.6)
Italy	5.2 (3.2–7.3)	2.5 (1.0–4.1)	0.8 (0.3–1.5)
Spain	8.2 (5.1–12)	3.9 (1.6–6.4)	1.5 (0.5–2.6)
United Kingdom	2.0 (1.2–2.8)	0.7 (0.3–1.2)	0.6 (0.2–1.2)
United States	8.0 (4.9–11)	4.3 (1.7–7.1)	0.6 (0.2–1.1)

[a]Percentages of SABs and LABs cannot be combined in order to obtain the percentage of the total group (any benzodiazepine).

SAB, short-acting benzodiazepine; LAB, long-acting benzodiazepine.

This study illustrates the difficulties that are frequently met in multinational drug utilization studies. While a given database may have the advantage of using similar data collection methods across countries, assumptions may still be needed to estimate the number of drug users and the 1-year prevalence rate. Furthermore, data may not allow the estimation of drug use by age and sex groups. In this case, the assumption that benzodiazepine use is equally distributed over the whole population may have underestimated the PAR, since the highest risk of hip fracture is found in the elderly, which is also the group most exposed to benzodiazepines. In addition, results are also dependent on the biases that can affect observational studies used to estimate risks of hip fractures.

Conclusion

Recent experience has shown the ability of drug utilization studies to investigate a large number of different issues (Table 40.1). Despite the limitations of available databases, including EHRs, their increasing sophistication facilitates investigations across several countries and in a short period of time. This increase in versatility may have a price in terms of limited standardization in methods and practices. It is also the case that drug utilization research should not be used for purely marketing or promotional purposes, in line with the requirements for other PASs. Avoiding these potential pitfalls and focusing on the development of a coherent scientific discipline, including making protocols publicly available, will ensure that drug utilization studies become an increasingly essential component of pharmacovigilance activities and, more broadly, of the risk–benefit monitoring of medicinal products in the postmarketing phase.

Disclaimer

The views expressed in this article are the personal views of the authors and may not be understood or quoted as being made on behalf of or reflecting the position of the European Medicines Agency or one of its committees or working parties.

CHAPTER 41

Drug utilization research and outcomes research

Henrik Toft Sørensen[1] & Gianluca Trifirò[2]

[1]*Department of Clinical Epidemiology, Aarhus University Hospital, Denmark*

[2]*Department of Biomedical and Dental Sciences and Morphofunctional Imaging, University of Messina*

KEY POINTS

- Drug utilization research represents a rich pool of strategies for use in drug exposure description and interpretation within outcomes research studies.
- Medications can play a central role in defining exposure groups for comparison, controlling for confounding and measuring outcomes.
- Patient registries, claims databases and general practice databases represent the main sources of data for outcomes research studies.
- Newly developed methodologies that allow multiple health care databases from different countries to be combined further enlarge the scientific opportunities offered by existing data sources.

Introduction

Outcomes research deals with the systematic analysis of the results of health-related actions [1]. Although there is no internationally clear definition of the concept of 'outcomes research', it most often refers to research into outcomes of pharmacological treatment or other clinical interventions in the health care sector, such as diagnostic tests and surgical procedures [2–4]. The outcomes can be hard end points like morbidity and mortality [5] or patient-reported factors like quality of life, adherence and functional status [6]. Given the nature of self-reported data, they will usually be prevalence data, whereas hard end points may be incidence data.

Multiple roles of drug utilization in outcome research

Since outcomes research frequently investigates the health outcomes of drug use (i.e. benefits, adverse effects and economic consequences), valid analysis of drug utilization in the study population should be planned for within the outcomes research design. Drug utilization research provides methods for describing both qualitative and quantitative drug exposure, as well as polypharmacy, adherence to prescribed therapy and differences in exposure among groups of patients. All these data allow us to define exposure groups for comparison and to identify the potency of the study. Drug utilization can also provide an outcome measure per se, such as when starting drug therapy represents a good proxy of outcomes (examples are provided later in the chapter).

In many situations, the concept of comparative effectiveness is also used for health outcomes research, since many elements of routine clinical care are part of a study [1,5,7]. In contrast to randomized clinical trials, which typically focus on one primary end point, such as survival or mortality, outcomes research often focuses on a broad spectrum of health outcomes, including information on economic outcomes (which are often related to use of resources and cost of care for the patient) and clinical quality. Moreover, clinical trials often focus on

Drug Utilization Research: Methods and Applications, First Edition. Edited by M. Elseviers et al.
Published 2016 by John Wiley & Sons, Ltd.

short-term efficacy and safety in a controlled clinical environment among well-educated affluent patients [8]. Furthermore, not all clinical trials take account of co-intervention with therapies given outside the study protocol [9]. All of these issues reduce the reliability of data from randomized clinical trials in informing clinical decision-making in the practice setting.

Observational methods therefore play a major part in health outcomes research. The most commonly used study design is a cohort design, in which one or more treatments or interventions are compared over a broad spectrum of end points (whether clinical end points, patient-related end points (quality of life/satisfaction with care) or health economics) [4].

Since medications are one of the most commonly used clinical interventions, the comparison of various types of treatment plays a major role in health outcomes research. Sometimes, the term 'comparative effectiveness research' is used when two or more treatments are compared [10,11]. In this context, medications are thus the 'exposure' in epidemiological models. However, medications can also play a central part in controlling for confounding or measuring outcomes. Drug utilization research represents a rich pool of strategies for use in drug exposure description and interpretation within outcomes research studies.

A special methodological challenge is the fact that one kind of medication is seldom used alone. Polypharmacy and multimorbidity are more often the rule than the exception [10]. Co-medication is therefore a potential confounding problem in almost all studies. In the remainder of this section, we illustrate the three basic ways of including drug use in outcomes research models.

Drug as exposure

Metformin is a widely used antidiabetic drug with potential antiinflammatory and antithrombotic properties. Despite its potential beneficial effects in critical illness, it is usually avoided due to its potential association with lactic acidosis. In order to examine the effect of early exposure to metformin in critical illness, 7404 intensive care patients with type 2 diabetes were included in a cohort study comparing the impact of preadmission use of metformin on mortality [12]. It was found that preadmission use of metformin was associated with a 20% (adjusted hazard ratio = 0.80, 95% CI 0.69–0.94) reduced 30-day mortality, but former use of metformin was not associated with mortality. As only a few cases developed lactic acidosis, the results challenge the routine discontinuation of metformin upon hospitalization and facilitate interventional studies.

In a case–control study, the risk of developing Alzheimer's disease was examined in individuals with diabetes mellitus treated with metformin or other antidiabetic drugs based on the United Kingdom-based General Practice Research Database [13]. 7,086 individuals with incident Alzheimer's disease identified between 1998 and 2008 and the same number of matched controls without dementia were included. Previous use of metformin or other antidiabetic drugs was compared between cases and controls. Corresponding odds ratios were calculated using conditional logistic regression. Risk estimates were adjusted for potential confounders. As compared with nonusers, long-term users of 60 or more metformin prescriptions were at greater risk of developing Alzheimer's disease (adjusted odds ratio (AOR) 1.71, 95% CI 1.12–2.60), but there was no consistent trend with increasing number of prescriptions. Long-term use of other antidiabetic drugs, such as sulfonylureas (AOR 1.01, 95% CI 0.72–1.42), thiazolidinediones (AOR 0.87, 95% CI 0.31–2.40) and insulin (AOR 1.01, 95% CI 0.58–1.73), was not related to an altered risk of developing Alzheimer's disease. There was a suggestion of a slightly higher risk of Alzheimer's disease in long-term users of metformin.

Drug use as potential confounder

Thomsen et al. [14] examined whether preadmission statin use decreased risk of death based on a cohort study of 29 900 adults hospitalized with pneumonia in Denmark, drawn from administrative databases. Statin use is strongly associated with diabetes, which may confound the results. Therefore, data on the use of antidiabetic drugs as a potential confounding factor were included in a regression model.

Mortality among statin users was lower than among nonusers: 10.3 versus 15.7% after 30 days and 16.8 versus 22.4% after 90 days, corresponding to adjusted 30- and 90-day mortality rate ratios of 0.69 (95% CI 0.58–0.82) and 0.75 (0.65–0.86). The use of statins was thus associated with decreased mortality after hospitalization with pneumonia.

In a cohort study, spironolactone and the risk of incident breast cancer in women older than 55 years was examined using data from the General Practice Research

Database (GPRD) [15]. The study included 1 290 625 female patients aged over 55 years old with no history of breast cancer and drawn from 557 general practices. The exposed cohort included women who received at least two prescriptions of spironolactone after age 55 years, who were followed up from the first prescription (index date). Two unexposed female controls for every exposed patient, matched by practice, year of birth and socioeconomic scores (if available), were selected for a comparison cohort. Potential confounding factors included use of the combined oral contraceptive pill or hormone replacement therapy, use of other drugs that may protect against breast cancer (aspirin, metformin) and use of drugs causing gynaecomastia (digoxin, finasteride, cimetidine, nifedipine). The results showed 29491 new cases of breast cancer in the study population (incidence rate 0.35% per year). The exposed cohort of 28032 patients and comparison cohort of 55961 patients had unadjusted incidence rates of 0.39 and 0.38% per year, respectively, over a mean follow-up of 4.1 years. The study provided no evidence of an increased incidence of breast cancer in patients exposed to spironolactone (hazard ratio 0.99, 95% CI 0.87–1.12).

Drug use as indicator of morbidity

Critically ill patients are exposed to high levels of stress, which may increase the risk of subsequent psychiatric illness. A cohort study included 9921 nonsurgical mechanically ventilated hospital survivors and matched cohorts from other hospitalized patients and the general population. Use of psychoactive drugs was used as a marker for psychiatric illness [16]. Within the first 3 months after discharge, a first-ever prescription for psychoactive medication was filled in 12.7% of mechanically ventilated patients, in 5.0% of hospitalized patients and in 0.7% of the general population. After adjustment for confounders, mechanical ventilation was associated with a 3-fold increased rate of new psychoactive drug prescription compared with hospitalized patients and a 20-fold increased rate compared with the general population.

Knee arthroplasty remains the gold standard in the treatment of severe osteoarthritis. Chronic postoperative pain has been reported with a prevalence ranging from 15 to 47%. In a cohort study of 1939 patients, based on health insurance data, analgesic drug consumption was compared before and after surgery as an indicator of pain after knee surgery [17]. Rate of drug use (all analgesics, antineuropathic drugs, strong opioids) was computed and compared across several periods surrounding the surgery (from 12 months before until 12 months after knee arthroplasty). A multivariate logistic regression model was used to identify factors associated with chronic postoperative pain. An increase in analgesic, antineuropathic and opioid drug consumption was observed in the year after surgery in 47.3, 8.6 and 5.6 of patients, respectively.

Accurate measurement of exposures, confounders and end points is crucial in all types of health outcomes research [18]. Any inaccurate measurements of drug use will lead to bias or residual confounding [19]. The main data sources from which to obtain information about drug use are questionnaires, interviews, medical records and medical databases, but their selection depends on the required data quality, sample size and length and completeness of follow-up. Many administrative data are widely used in outcomes research due to the requirement for high sample size and completeness of follow-up [20].

A health outcomes study needs to be planned with the same stringency as epidemiological studies; that is, with a clearly defined exposure, knowledge of the validity and measure of the exposure, well-defined outcomes and identification of potential confounders.

Most health outcomes research studies are observational, and the point of interest is to quantify an effect for translation into clinical or health care utility terms. Therefore, additive effect measures, such as risk differences, number needed to treat and number needed to harm, are the most informative measures. Relative risk and, in particular, p-values do not play a major part in this type of research.

Advantages and limitations of different sources of drug utilization data in outcomes research studies

Sources of data in outcomes research represent a key component in success of the study. Because of the importance of providing an exhaustive description of exposure, outcomes, risk factors and covariates, high-quality health care databases covering large populations should be identified by considering the specific setting of the clinical question. Since, as already stated, drug utilization can play different roles in outcomes research studies (i.e. drug as exposure, confounder and outcome), the completeness of the drug utilization data in potential sources should be accurately assessed.

Health care databases have been increasingly used for pharmacoepidemiology research in recent decades [20]. Many administrative claims and general practice databases have already individually been extensively used for both safety and effectiveness outcomes research in a growing number of countries [21].

Newly developed methodologies that allow multiple health care databases from different countries to be combined further expand the scientific opportunities offered by existing data sources. Rare outcomes and rare drug exposures can now be better investigated thanks to the ongoing networks of databases covering populations of several million subjects [22]. In a scenario in which large-scale pharmacoepidemiology studies are conducted through database networks, it is essential to recognize both the potentials and the limitations of different data sources (patient registries, claims databases, general practice databases).

Table 41.1 provides information on drug exposure and clinical outcomes from various data sources.

Patient registries

Patient registries are created to evaluate the clinical aspects and management of specific diseases (e.g. diabetes) or special types of health care intervention

Table 41.1 Drug utilization and clinical outcomes from different data sources.

	Drug-based registries	Claims databases	General practice databases
Source of drug information	Prescription	Dispensing	Prescription
Prescribed daily dose	Available	Missing	Available in some databases
Duration of use	Available	Missing Can be estimated based on DDDs and prescribed quantities	Available in some databases as unstructured information Can be estimated based on DDDs and prescribed quantities
Adherence	Not available	Not available Only refilling can be evaluated	Not available Only represcribing can be evaluated
Drugs for which information is available			
• Outpatient drug prescriptions	Only related to the drug that is under registry-based monitoring	Often only for drugs reimbursed by a third-party payer	Complete for drugs reimbursed by a third-party payer, apart from drugs directly dispensed by hospitals Partly available for drugs that are charged to patients (e.g. paracetamol and benzodiazepines in Italy)
• Inpatient drug prescription	Only related to the drug that is under registry-based monitoring	Generally available as aggregated data, but not as individual patient-level data	Not available
• Date of prescription/dispensing	Yes	Yes	Yes
• Dietary supplements	Generally not available	Not available	Not available
• OTCs	Generally not available	Not available	Partly available (no compulsory registration by GP)
Clinical outcomes	Only pre-specified events that are strictly correlated to the drug exposure	All events leading to hospitalization or death (if death registry is available)	All GP-based medical diagnoses and specialist and hospital discharge diagnoses (if registered by GPs)

DDD, defined daily dose; OTC, over the counter; GP, general practitioner.

(e.g. dialysis) at either the international, the national or the regional level. Specific drug-related registries are also available, which are generally aimed at monitoring the effects of risky and costly drugs (e.g. biological drugs used in oncology or rheumatic disease), especially during the initial postmarketing phase. For example, in Italy, there are currently almost 80 drugs, mostly biological drugs, undergoing registry-based monitoring (see Chapter 29). However, these drug-based registries have not yet been systematically explored for scientific purposes, so they mainly represent a strategy by which to keep drug expenditure under control, rather than being useful as a data source for outcomes research studies.

In light of the specific aims of various patient registries, information on drug exposure may have different levels of completeness. Disease registries contain information on the disease itself but not so much on its pharmacological management, while in drug-based registries more detailed information about drug use is available, but there is less on clinical outcomes, especially those occurring after long-term exposure.

Claims databases

Claims databases are widely available (and extensively used) for pharmacoepidemiology and drug utilization research in all developed countries, particularly in Europe and the United States, and increasingly in Asia and Australia.

Claims databases collect data for administrative purposes (i.e. reimbursement of health care services). Through record-linkage techniques, multiple sources of information (drug dispensing, hospital discharge diagnoses, death registry, etc.) can be combined. As for general practice databases, the data are collected longitudinally for large populations, allowing observational studies to be conducted rapidly and cheaply in order to investigate drug–(adverse) event associations.

Depending on the type of clinical outcome under study, different types of data can be considered for outcome ascertainment in claims databases. Some major adverse events can be captured by searching disease codes among primary (and, eventually, secondary) hospital discharge diagnoses, reasons for health care services payment exemption and the death registry, if available. It is essential also to search codes among secondary discharge diagnoses, which may have a tremendous impact in terms of outcome misclassification [23].

In general, for proper assessment of the relationship between a given treatment and its outcome, a limited specificity is more damaging than a limited sensitivity, a 100% specificity of the outcome assessment allowing an unbiased estimate of the measured association irrespective of the sensitivity value [24].

When using claims database, outcome identification is expected to be highly specific when diagnoses are based on hospital records, but lower when they are based on out-of-hospital identification of diseases (e.g. by general practitioners (GPs) or primary care specialists).

With respect to outcome identification via hospital discharge diagnoses, the main limitation is that medical events that do not lead to hospitalization cannot be captured. As an example, more than one-third of pneumonia cases are cared for directly by GPs, without any hospitalization [25]. In the context of drug safety studies, this limitation should be taken into account as a form of outcome misclassification, which may eventually bias risk estimates.

Some claims databases can also be supplemented with outpatient laboratory test results, thus increasing the sensitivity of the coding algorithms for the identification of certain outcomes (in which laboratory tests are part of the diagnostic work-up, e.g. alanine aminotransferase and aspartate aminotransferase for acute liver injury, creatininemia for chronic kidney disease [26]) and allowing for better confounding adjustment in outcomes research studies [27].

In order to extract data concerning outcomes from claim databases, specific coding algorithms must be developed based on terminology used for coding events and the availability of additional information (e.g. clinical notes as free-text unstructured information, laboratory values, etc.). Hence, validation studies through medical chart review should be performed to assess the accuracy of terminology-specific (e.g. ICD9-CM, ICD10) disease codes and additional criteria (e.g. free-text search) for outcome identification [28].

However, national privacy regulations in several countries prevent individual medical records from being thoroughly reviewed. Thus, sensitivity analyses that verify the robustness of findings by applying credible sensitivity and specificity ranges to the source of outcome information are often the only practical option for exploring the possible effects of outcome misclassification.

Same considerations regarding misclassification hold true for the comorbidities that are potential confounders of drug–outcome associations.

Information about drug exposure is derived from dispensing data, which generally capture only information about drugs reimbursed by national health systems. Drugs that are dispensed over the counter, herbal remedies and drugs that are administered in hospital cannot easily be tracked through this source. In an Italian rheumatology specialist centre, a survey of around 1000 patients with rheumatoid arthritis or osteoarthritis found that, in addition to the prescribed nonsteroidal antiinflammatory drug (NSAID), almost 20% used over-the–counter (OTC) NSAIDs for the treatment of conditions other than disease-related pain (e.g. dental pain, headache, etc.) [29]. Therefore, underestimation of exposure in patients with autoimmune disorders must be taken into account when conducting outcomes research studies concerning NSAIDs.

Claims databases contain no information on whether a dispensed medication is filled by the patient themselves. This is strongly influenced by patient adherence to drug treatment and may vary even across different molecules belonging to the same class, raising the potential for risk estimation bias due to nonrandom exposure misclassification in drug safety studies.

General practice databases

A number of general practice databases have been run for several decades, mostly in Europe, where GPs act as gatekeepers of national health care systems and are involved in the provision of most health care services to the public [30].

An increasing number of European countries have nationwide electronic medical record databases, which are created through a network of GPs. Some of the most frequently used GP databases for pharmacoepidemiology studies include The Health Improvement Network (THIN) database, the Clinical Practice Research Datalink (CPRD) and Qresearch in the United Kingdom, the Integrated Primary Care Information (IPCI) database in the Netherlands, Base de datos para la Investigacion Farmacoepedemiologica en Atencion Primaria (BIFAP) in Spain and the Health Search and Arianna databases in Italy.

In contrast to claims databases, hospitalized events are not generally captured by GPs unless specialists' discharge letters are subsequently keyed into the electronic archive. On the other hand, GPs may register signs and symptoms as unstructured free-text information, which can be extremely helpful for both outcome identification and validation by medically trained researchers. The use of free-text information for outcome ascertainment has been investigated in the IPCI, where the low granularity of International Classification of Primary Care (ICPC) terminology for the identification of medical events is compensated by extensive use of free-text search and subsequent manual validation.

In the context of the EU-ADR project, a study has been conducted to explore the possible effects of outcome misclassification of upper gastrointestinal bleed (UGIB) in UGIB-related safety studies using two GP databases (IPCI and Health Search; UGIB was searched for using both disease codes and free-text key words) and two claims databases (Aarhus and the Tuscany regional database, which captured only hospitalized UGIB cases) [28]. This validation study demonstrated that using the most specific coding algorithm for the automatic identification of UGIB cases in both GP and claims databases does not significantly affect the risk estimate of drug-related UGIB, but reduces the precision of such a risk estimate.

As regards information on drug exposure, this is generally captured through GPs' prescriptions and so has the same limitations as claims databases. In addition, several studies have shown that prescriptions of specific classes are more likely not to be ultimately dispensed by a pharmacy (i.e. the patient does not take the prescribed medicines; see Section F).

In a US study, 195 930 e-prescriptions were matched to dispensing data in order to explore whether they were ultimately filled. It was found that more than 20% were not. Nonadherence was common for newly prescribed medications used to treat chronic conditions such as hypertension (28.4%), hyperlipidemia (28.2%) and diabetes (31.4%) [31].

Networks of multiple health care databases

Several international initiatives have shown the great potential of combining multiple health care databases for the postmarketing assessment of drug and vaccine safety in clinical practice. However, integrating databases containing different types of data and using different drug and disease terminologies, and drawn from different underlying populations and health care systems, is extremely challenging and requires local expertise. Previous experience in the United States, Europe and Asia has demonstrated groundbreaking work in multi-database studies, which provide examples of how to extract harmonized data from different databases and how to handle and store data, as well as key lessons on which work models to adopt for analyses and how to interpret results [22].

The combination of multiple databases is particularly promising for the assessment of vaccine safety, which requires quick answers, and for the study of rare diseases and rare drug exposure, which requires a very large study population in order to provide sufficient statistical power. On the other hand, further efforts are needed to optimize and standardize the whole process of data extraction, handling, analysis and interpretation, while adhering to national privacy legislations.

One of the first international initiatives combining multiple databases was the EU-ADR Project (www.euadr-project.org), launched in 2008 under the auspices of the European Commission's Seventh Framework Programme [32]. EU-ADR was a collaboration of 18 public and private institutions, representing academic research, primary care practice, health services administration and the pharmaceutical industry. It ended in 2012. A computerized integrated framework for the detection of drug safety signals was developed from eight population-based databases (both administrative claims and GP records) in four European countries (Denmark, Italy, the Netherlands and the United Kingdom), covering around 25 million citizens.

Projects such as EU-ADR, the US Food and Drug Administration (FDA)-promoted Mini-Sentinel (minisentinel.org) and Observational Medicinal Outcomes Partnership (OMOP) (omop.fnih.org) and the EU-funded Pharmacoepidemiological Research on Outcomes of Therapeutics by a European Consortium (PROTECT) (www.imi-protect.eu) have also demonstrated the great potential of combining multiple health care databases, not only for drug safety studies, but also in the area of signal detection, where this approach may complement traditional spontaneous reporting systems.

The experience of prescription databases among the Nordic countries represents an important reference for pharmacoepidemiological research. Overall, these databases cover a population of 25 million individuals, and they have frequently been linked to other registries (e.g. census, hospital patient, cancer and medical birth registries) as a source of data for outcomes studies [33].

Patient-reported outcomes measures and patient-reported experience measures

Despite claims and general practice databases being widely used in pharmacoepidemiology, they are limited by the fact that they cannot adequately capture patient-centred outcomes. Increasing interest in such outcomes is demonstrated by the fact that large-scale research projects on this topic have been funded by organizations such as the US Patient Centered Outcome Research Institute (PCORI; www.pcori.org).

Patient-reported outcome measures (PROMs) provide information on the effectiveness of care delivered to patients as perceived by the patients themselves. These data add an important perspective on health care services that might not be captured using other sources, such as patient registries and general practice and claims databases, which cannot provide patient-oriented measurement of provided services. This has led to a significant expansion of the development and application of questionnaires, interview schedules and rating scales measuring health and illness states from the patient's perspective. PROMs currently make a real contribution to clinical outcomes feedback in the UK National Health Service (NHS) and in the United States.

While PROMs provide information on the safety and effectiveness of clinical outcomes, patient-reported experience measures (PREMs) provide information on patients' overall health care experience. This can give a broader view of quality of care, including patients' perceptions of waiting times and health care workers' bedside manners. Together, PROMs and PREMs can be used to provide a comprehensive overview of quality of care and to enable its improvement in the future. The association between PROMs and PREMs is a particular focus of research. Beyond giving a broader view of quality of care, measurement of patient-reported outcomes in clinical trials offers a unique patient perspective on the impact of treatment on functioning and well-being (health-related quality of life) [34,35].

Studies in primary care settings have reported a range of findings on the relationship between patient experience and quality of clinical care, ranging from no association [36,37] to low association [38,39]. Studies in secondary care settings suggest somewhat clearer associations [40,41], but there are relatively few of these compared to studies in primary care [42]. Variation between PROM and PREM associations may result from key methodological differences between studies using PREMs and PROMs, including in size of study population, choice of quality indicators and whether associations are derived from individual, health care practice or health insurance data [43].

Conclusion

In the area of outcomes research, it is essential to carefully evaluate the potential of different types of data source (general practice databases, claims databases and patient registries) to capture information on drug exposure, outcomes and potential confounders.

In general, when using either claims or general practice databases, it is important to carry out sensitivity analyses in order to explore the potential effects of exposure and/or outcome misclassification and, more specifically, to evaluate the magnitude of possible biases due to such a misclassification. Residual confounding due to absence of relevant information in health care databases, which are maintained for purposes other than research, must always be considered in the interpretation of results. Nevertheless, claims and general practice databases are to be preferred to registries in case of rare or long-term adverse outcomes that require readily available clinical data from large populations and long-term follow-up.

The combination of multiple health care databases offers even greater opportunity to investigate associations of rare drug exposure and rare outcomes, but it is methodologically challenging and requires time and effort to set up the data infrastructure. Database networks are in development in several countries worldwide and promise to increase the potential of postmarketing vaccine and drug safety assessment.

Finally, increasing efforts should be made by the scientific community to take into account patient-centred outcomes when investigating the effects of health care interventions. One of the most notable improvements in the area of outcomes research has been the development of methodologies for the integration of large health care databases (e.g. administrative claims and health care databases that collect resource utilization data, clinical outcomes data, etc.) with patient-centred outcome information, which may allow for more patient-oriented clinical research.

Acknowledgment

Dr Janet Sultana at the University of Messina contributed to the editing of this chapter.

CHAPTER 42

Drug utilization research and pharmacoeconomics

Cara Usher[1], Kathleen Bennett[1], Lorenzo G. Mantovani[2] & Dyfrig Hughes[3]

[1] *National Centre for Pharmacoeconomics, St James's Hospital, Ireland*

[2] *Department of Statistics, School of Medicine, University of Milano, Italy*

[3] *Centre for Health Economics & Medicines Evaluation, Bangor University, United Kingdom*

KEY POINTS

- Drug utilization studies provide insights into patterns of drug use over time, efficiency of drug use, cost-effectiveness and outcomes of use, particularly the economic consequences of use in the real-world setting.
- Information from drug utilization studies can provide clinical and economic outcome data for use in economic evaluations of pharmaceuticals.
- Drug utilization studies are often used in pharmacoeconomics in relation to choice of comparator drug, information on prevalence/incidence of disease, understanding treatment pathways, comparative safety and effectiveness, adherence and persistence and costs of drugs.
- Drug utilization studies are important in the application of local formularies and guidelines and their impact on pharmacoeconomics.

Introduction

Global expenditure on prescription medicines is expected to exceed USD1 trillion by 2017 [1]. An ageing population, increasing multimorbidity and technological advances all mean that the year-on-year rise in the total costs of medicines is likely to continue. Pharmacoeconomics is the discipline concerned with optimal allocation of resources to maximize population health from the use of medicines.

Economic evaluations in health care are conducted to inform decisions on health care resource allocation; they include estimating costs and consequences (effects). Economic analyses seek to make explicit criteria that may be used in deciding different uses for scarce resources. Economic analyses or evaluations can be defined as 'the comparative analysis of alternative courses of action in terms of both their costs and consequences' [2] and have been widely applied in health policy, including in the assessment of prevention programmes (such as vaccination, screening and health promotion), diagnostics, treatment interventions (such as drugs and surgical procedures), organization of care and rehabilitation.

Pharmacoeconomic analyses are commonly used to determine whether the use of a new drug is likely to represent value for money for the health care system. It should be noted that pharmacoeconomic analyses are comparative in nature, so they require information on the costs and effects of alternative treatments, and costs and effects need to refer to the use of the drug and its comparator in a specific indication. In light of this, the price of a new drug, its level of reimbursement and its overall cost-effectiveness profile are highly dependent on the position of that drug in overall therapy. Again, the natural way to address the position of a new drug in therapy is to use a drug utilization study aimed at reporting the use of currently available therapies with

Drug Utilization Research: Methods and Applications, First Edition. Edited by M. Elseviers et al.
Published 2016 by John Wiley & Sons, Ltd.

the same indication. In this context, drug utilization research is also key to pharmacoeconomic analyses, as it helps select appropriate and relevant comparator treatments and describe current courses of care (and related costs) applicable to potential candidates for the new drug.

Moreover, drug utilization studies are also helpful in addressing the transferability of evidence from the highly selected populations generally enrolled in phase III randomized controlled trials (RCTs) to the unselected ones of everyday clinical practice.

All techniques of economic evaluation involve the same explicit consideration and calculation of the use of resources and overall costs. However, each method of evaluation handles consequences differently. The perspective of an economic evaluation determines which costs are to be valued [3]. This perspective might be narrow (e.g. the payer) or broad (e.g. the health service provider or society). It is not just the cost of the medicine that is considered within economic evaluations, but the total costs related to treatment, including, for example, diagnostic tests, procedures, hospitalizations, outpatient care and primary care clinic attendance.

Challenges in health care decision-making

Health care payers are charged with the responsibility of deciding whether or not to fund particular therapeutic approaches, based on balancing the costs and benefits of the therapy. Commonly, health care payers have to decide whether or not to recommend treatments that either cost less and deliver fewer benefits than alternatives or (more commonly) cost more but deliver potentially greater benefits. Interpreting and analysing the clinical evidence base therefore plays a pivotal role in reaching a decision.

Common difficulties with the evidence from the health care payer's perspective include inappropriate comparisons, use of intermediate outcomes, inadequate duration of follow-up, different study populations and lack of data on resource use and economic impact. These problems were highlighted in a review of industry submissions to the Australian [4] and Canadian [5] insurance agencies.

An additional difficulty facing health care payers and decision-makers is that early technology assessment (i.e. on new innovative technologies) carries the risk of allowing inappropriate decisions to be made (a treatment that is cost-ineffective could be recommended for use in practice; subsequent removal may be difficult once reimbursed) or a treatment that is truly cost-effective not being recommended. Further difficulties in decision-making, in addition to costs and effects, relate to the impact of the new technology on specific subgroups of patients. There is also a need to balance equitable resource use across different disease or therapeutic areas. Underlying all of these difficulties is the need to ensure that decisions are taken in a fair and transparent manner.

Health care payers and decision-makers involved in coverage and payment policies are increasingly seeking information on 'real-world' outcomes on which to base their decisions. This is because early data from clinical trials do not always reflect what happens in practice, which is important in making decisions on policy. Policies are being developed globally that recognize the importance of evidence that goes beyond information collected during RCTs mandated by regulatory authorities as part of marketing approval.

The aim of this chapter is to show how real-world data, in the form of drug utilization studies, can provide clinical and economic outcome data that can be readily incorporated into economic evaluations of pharmaceuticals.

Frameworks of economic evaluation

A growing number of jurisdictions now request economic data to support their decision-making processes in various health technology domains. This approach was first used in Australia [6] and Ontario, Canada [7] in making decisions about funding for new medicines, and it has been used by several managed care groups in the United States. Recently, the UK National Institute for Health and Care Excellence (NICE) has undertaken technology appraisals that include analysis of the cost-effectiveness of interventions such as medicines, medical devices and medical procedures [8]. The burden on manufacturers and researchers has increased as more jurisdictions have started to demand economic data, especially as various national guidelines now require local data or the use of specific methods.

Consensus has been reached on a framework for the conduct and reporting [9] of economic evaluations, and it is generally recognized that a complete economic evaluation considers both effectiveness and cost. Additionally:

1 The perspective of the evaluation must be defined explicitly. This might be the health care payer, a governmental agency, a hospital or society.
2 All relevant health outcomes and costs should be included in the analysis and valued sensibly.
3 Costs and outcomes should be discounted to present values.
4 Analyses must be incremental, in that they compare differences in the costs and outcomes of an intervention (or interventions) with a reference case.
5 Sensitivity analyses should be included to test the robustness of conclusions.
6 The incremental cost-effectiveness ratio (if reported) should be stated in terms of the willingness-to-pay threshold for that jurisdiction, so that the economic attractiveness of the programme can be compared with that of another.

Mathematical modelling is a framework that permits the integration of facts and values linked to outcomes of interest to health care decision-makers. The purpose of modelling is to synthesize evidence on clinical and economic outcomes in a form that can help in decisions about clinical practice and health care resource allocation. Models synthesize evidence on health consequences and costs from many different sources:

1 example clinical trials;
2 databases of routinely collected data (for use of resources, costs, treatment patterns and harms; see Chapter 4);
3 epidemiological data (for incidence, prevalence, and disease progression);
4 expert opinion (for treatment patterns and use of resources);
5 patient surveys (for health utilities and resource use);
6 reference sources (for unit costs and tariffs).

While it is broadly acknowledged that RCTs provide a 'gold standard' of product efficacy, they are often conducted in selected populations under carefully controlled conditions. In addition, they are often expensive, explanatory and not pragmatic in nature, and are underpowered to provide robust evidence on drug safety. Information needs are, therefore, greater than can be provided in clinical trials [10]. It is often appropriate to project the results of clinical trials beyond the time horizon of analysis, to capture predicted lifetime costs and benefits.

Models are also used to test the robustness of underlying assumptions and uncertainties [11]. The range of modelling techniques used for medical and economic decision-making has advanced greatly [12,13] as modellers have become familiar with more sophisticated modelling techniques. Models can range from a simple decision-tree approach (with limited ability to reflect time) to state-transition models, which are often well suited to decision-making as they conceptualize the decision problem in terms of a set of 'states' that individuals can 'transition' between [14]. Another common framework used in health care is the individual-based model or 'microsimulation' model. While these frameworks do not capture interactions (or dynamic modelling) as exhibited though infectious disease, modelling is an approach that has been developed to handle interaction between individuals. The evolution of these mathematical frameworks over the last decade has assisted in the decision-making process globally [15], but concerns exist over their credibility [16–18], which is why the International Society for Pharmacoeconomics and Outcomes Research (ISPOR) has issued guidelines for good practice in modelling [19].

Using the components of an economic evaluation, it is possible to show where drug utilization studies can inform analyses and ultimately benefit the decision-maker. Any study that gathers information on the costs and effects of a therapeutic intervention can inform the pharmacoeconomic process. Drug utilization studies can be utilized to obtain just this type of information. This is the basis of the relationship between pharmacoeconomic studies and drug utilization studies.

Choice of comparator drug

For any evaluation, it is imperative to have a clear and appropriately specified decision problem defined in advance. In the context of decisions about a new technology, this requires a statement about the intended patient population/subpopulations of interest and the comparators to the new technology. Comparator can include therapeutic options that are likely to be displaced by the new intervention, 'doing nothing', 'current practice' and the 'most cost-effective alternative'. This type of information can be readily accessed from claims or administrative databases at low cost in a short period of time. Other information that can be retrieved from drug utilization studies includes information on the delivery of the technology (e.g. the intensity or frequency of treatment, the drug dosage schedule, the route and duration of administration). The role that drug utilization studies can play in pharmacoeconomic studies is further strengthened upon examination of the transferability of economic evaluations between jurisdictions. In the case of pharmaceuticals, licenses may differ between jurisdictions, and this can affect the clinical applications of the new product or the comparator. Differences in clinical practice in individual jurisdictions may influence the specification of treatment strategies. Drug utilization studies allow patterns of use to be examined, but do not always contain information about diagnosis or outcomes, and therefore can be limited in their application.

Identifying the incidence/prevalence of disease (morbidity data)

Information on the prevalence and/or incidence of disease is often required in pharmacoeconomic evaluation (e.g. in decision analytic modelling or cost-of-illness studies). In most countries, this information can be obtained through official statistics (e.g. World Health Organization (WHO) Health for All) or through local registries or databases (e.g. the Clinical Practice Research Datalink (CPRD) in the UK: www.cprd.co.uk). However, it may not be available for all diseases or may represent only a subset of the population (e.g. hospital discharge information). Therefore, drug utilization studies are often considered an alternative source of information on morbidity, based on specific treatment data. Where the indication is not available, treatment data can be used as a proxy for the disease in certain well-defined cases (e.g. antidiabetes medication) where there are no other indications and they are not used in combination with other treatments. These approaches have been used to develop validated comorbidity scores such as the chronic disease score [20] and risk adjustment measure (RxRisk) [21]. Prevalence data from drug utilization studies are derived from all cases having at least one prescription for the drug (sometimes with more than one prescription, when considering chronic use). Incidence data are based on a new prescription dispensed after a period of non-use of the drug (from 6 months to several years). There are limitations to the use of drug utilization studies in estimating prevalence or incidence in this way, as some cases may not be detected because they were not treated (e.g. lifestyle intervention in diabetes) and sometimes treatment may be given for other reasons.

When using drug utilization data for pharmacoeconomic modelling studies, it is often necessary to include the prevalent and/or incident use of alternative treatments; drug utilization studies are useful for this. In cost-of-illness studies, only drug costs for specific conditions are derived from drug utilization studies, and these may not reflect real costs if there are high levels of associated copayments or other costs. In addition, the costs of medical services (including primary and secondary care) associated with any disease cannot be extrapolated from drug costs. These are just some limitations to the use of drug utilization data in measuring morbidity; others include the lack of validation against diagnostic data, poor quality or insufficient detail of information and bias in the selection of study populations.

Describing current treatment pathways or disease management patterns and contributing to cost-of-illness studies

Using colorectal cancer as an example, advances in treatment in recent years have had a notable impact on costs, especially in view of the high acquisition costs of the combined chemotherapy regimens and biological agents [22]. Over the past decade, there has been a marked increase in the complexity of chemotherapy (e.g. from 5-fluorouracil (5-FU) with or without leucovorin to multiagent regimens containing capecitabine, irinotecan or oxaliplatin). Second- and third-line options for treating metastatic disease have been developed [23]. In addition, the biological targeted agents bevacizumab and cetuximab were approved for the treatment of metastatic disease in 2004 [24]. The impact of these new biologicals on the overall cost of care of patients with colorectal cancer is described by Tilson et al. [25], who linked data from a university teaching hospital database with a national cancer registry containing information on the utilization of the newer biological agents and developed separate treatment pathways for each stage of colon and rectal cancer. The results of this study established for the first time the cost of managing colorectal cancer in the Irish health care setting and highlighted how cost estimates were sensitive to the use of chemotherapeutic drugs.

Comparative effectiveness and safety

Information regarding the comparative effectiveness of therapies is now recognized as an important parameter in economic evaluation. Globally, health care payers, prescribers, pharmacists and patients require data on the comparative effectiveness and safety of prescription drugs in routine use. Although explanatory RCTs are the gold standard for determining a drug's efficacy against placebo, it is well recognized that the results of such studies may not accurately reflect the effectiveness of therapies delivered in clinical practice [26–28]. In addition, clinical decisions usually involve choices among therapies, yet the manufacturers or sponsors of trials have limited motivation to test new drugs against existing therapies [29]. Policymakers, payers and providers are therefore continually turning to the analysis of large secondary databases, which can help answer a variety of questions. For example, when there is no head-to-head RCT or prospective observational study data available, drug utilization studies can be conducted using secondary data to examine the differences in benefit of various treatments, including drugs in the same or different drug classes. Even if there are published head-to-head clinical trials, there may be clinically important differences in treatment effectiveness in real-world usage compared with the RCTs, perhaps driven by differences in target population or patient adherence. Also, RCTs are frequently designed to examine intermediate outcomes, so it may be desirable to examine the magnitude of benefit of true outcome measures (e.g. morbidity or disability) over a longer period of time.

Comparative effectiveness studies based on secondary data face similar challenges to other pharmacoepidemiological and health services research studies, however. Concerns over a study's validity will limit the translation of its results into policy and practice. The ISPOR has issued a Good Research Practice guide for conducting comparative effectiveness research studies using secondary data sources [30].

Information on the safety of a particular drug is an essential part of its pharmacoeconomic evaluation, as adverse drug events (ADEs) and other safety concerns need to be evaluated. Drug utilization studies can be used to provide estimates of any ADEs or adverse drug reactions (ADRs), particularly in post-authorization safety studies (PASSs; see Chapter 39). Information on patient characteristics (e.g. age, gender, socioeconomic group), event frequency, effect size and cost can be collected as part of these studies and included in cost-effectiveness studies, economic modelling or cost-of-illness studies.

Medication adherence

Medication adherence can be defined in relation to persistence and adherence [31]. Nonpersistence and suboptimal adherence are associated with worse clinical outcomes and increased health care expenditure [32], and have a significant impact on morbidity and mortality. When medications are not taken as prescribed (nonadherence) or not continued for the intended duration (nonpersistence), this often leads to reduced effectiveness, potentially prolonged illness and wasted medicine. Medication nonadherence and nonpersistence are of particular relevance to pharmacoeconomics, due to the increased costs associated with extra visits to primary and secondary care and the costs of medicines not taken [33]. Therefore, when conducting pharmacoeconomic studies, the level of anticipated adherence and persistence to treatment – which is often derived from drug utilization studies – should be factored in. The methodology and usefulness of adherence assessment are discussed in Section F.

Costs of drugs

Drug costs, for both study and comparator drugs, are an essential element in any economic evaluation. The cost of concomitant drugs used to treat adverse events can also be important. Calculating the cost of a drug regimen involves not only the price of the drug but also the impact of any wholesale discounts, pharmacy costs or wastage (owing to package or vial size) [34]. Depending on the country or region, the drug cost burden is usually shared in varying degrees between government and other third-party payers and patients. Given the complexities existing between supply-side (e.g. wholesalers, retailers etc.) and demand-side (e.g. group purchasing organizations) intermediaries, drug acquisition costs may vary in complex and nontransparent ways. Given this background, drug costing for economic evaluation is complicated and, to some extent, jurisdiction-specific. The complexity is compounded when one considers that each economic evaluation is carried out from a specific perspective (e.g. hospital, government, payer, patient, societal) and that the different perspectives reflect different objectives and so involve different costs. Administrative databases, based on locally reimbursed data, can therefore be a potential source of cost data, which will usually allow incorporation of aspects of adherence and persistence, long-term utilization, local tariffs, etc. The ISPOR Drug Cost Task Force Report is recommended as a useful guideline for good research practice in measuring drug costs for economic evaluation [35].

Budget impact analysis

Budget impact analyses (BIAs) are increasingly required, along with economic evaluations, as part of the reimbursement submission by industry. Where an economic evaluation asks, 'Does the intervention in question provide value for money?', the BIA simply asks, 'Can we afford it?. A BIA will typically address expected changes in the expenditure of a health care system (i.e. the financial consequences) after the new intervention is adopted. Therefore, given the highly local nature of health systems globally and the varying perspectives of decision-makers, a BIA does not provide a single estimate applicable to all decision-makers, but rather a framework that allows decision-makers to view financial estimates applicable to their setting. A typical BIA will incorporate the size and characteristics of the eligible population, the use of the current and new intervention, the costs of the current and new intervention and the use and costs of other condition-related health care services. Populating the BIA with data relevant to the budget holder can be a challenge but, again, local drug utilization studies can prove suitable sources for these elements.

For this purpose, data on expected and observed use are very useful. For instance, in England, the Health and Social Care Information Centre publishes statistics on the use of NICE-appraised medicines in the National Health Service (NHS) [36]. Estimates of anticipated prescription volume are calculated from eligible patient population estimates and reported as defined daily doses (DDDs). Observed use of medicines is obtained from routine data on prescriptions dispensed in the community (supplied by the NHS Business Services Authority) and use of medicines in hospitals (supplied by IMS Health). Drug usage data are converted to physical quantities and, where appropriate, to DDDs in order to allow comparison with the estimates.

In a recent report [36], comparisons between expected and observed use were made for 15 medicines in 9 groups. Actual use by the NHS in England was higher than the predicted use for two groups, lower for three and about equal for four (Table 42.1). There are several caveats to this analysis, including a lack of robust prevalence and incidence data at the national level, difficulty in controlling for the presence of multiple indications for some medicines and the fact that medicines may be recommended as one of a number of treatment options. However, such analyses of medicines use, linked with

Table 42.1 Expected and observed use of NICE-appraised medicines in 2012.

Source: Health and Social Care Information Centre 2014 [36]. Copyright © 2014, Health and Social Care Information Centre. Reproduced by permission under Open Government Licence.

Technology	Ratio of expected to observed use[a]
Alzheimer's disease: donepezil, galantamine, rivastigmine, memantine	1.48
Carmustine implants	0.84
Diabetes (type 2): exenatide and liraglutide	0.97
Diabetes (type 1 and type 2): insulin glargine and insulin detemir	1.03
Ranibizumab	0.95
Renal cell carcinoma: sunitinib and pazopanib	0.68
Riluzole	0.65
Temozolomide	2.09
Trastuzumab	0.97

[a]A ratio less than 1 shows that actual use was lower than expected; a ratio greater than 1 indicates that actual use was higher than expected.

decisions based on clinical effectiveness and cost-effectiveness, serve to highlight the need to account for variances in prescribing, especially as the NHS is required to provide funding and resources for medicines recommended by NICE.

Performance-based risk sharing

There has always been considerable uncertainty at product launch about the ultimate real-world clinical and economic performance of new medicinal products. This uncertainty, and the concomitant financial risk to the payer for a new treatment that does not work as anticipated, has increased with the rising price of new treatments. If payers are reluctant to adopt, manufacturers face the risk of reduced revenue. Performance-based risk sharing involves a plan by which the performance of a product is tracked in a defined patient population over a specified period of time and the level of reimbursement is based on the health and economic outcomes achieved. Such a scheme represents a mechanism for reducing uncertainty through greater investment in evidence collection while a drug is in use within a health care system. A study by Carlson et al. [37] identified 116 cases of this type of arrangement for medicines and other medicinal products since 1997, with numbers growing in more recent years [37,38]. An example of a performance-based risk-sharing scheme from France involved the use of dipeptidyl peptidase-4 (DPP4) inhibitors ('gliptins') in patients with type 2 diabetes. Initially, the manufacturer wanted to set a premium price based on evidence of the durability of effect (involving HbA_{1C} lowering); however, the pricing committee applied a condition that the manufacturer would retrospectively pay back the difference between the agreed-upon price and the initial price for all sales if claims of durability were not met. All new DPP4 inhibitors have been subject to the same agreement.

Developing local formulary/clinical practice guidelines

The need for cost containment upon the introduction of new treatments is now more relevant than ever, with the increasing volume of drugs prescribed and products made available. Decision-makers at all levels are faced with difficult choices about which drugs to use to treat patients. Restricted formularies can provide one approach to containing costs by allowing hospital and community prescribers to decide on the treatments that will be made available or reimbursable. A formulary may include less expensive medicines and provide a basis for negotiation with the pharmaceutical industry where several treatments are available. Use of formularies will often lead to less variability across hospitals and practices and better-quality prescribing in general, which benefits patients and their outcomes. The WHO provides some broad criteria to be considered in making formulary decisions (Box 42.1) [39].

Box 42.1 World Health Organization (WHO) criteria for consideration of new medicines.

- Efficacy.
- Effectiveness and safety.
- Quality (of both the drug and the supply chain).
- Availability of clinical expertise and laboratory services.
- Availability of the drug.
- Cost estimates (including the costs of the drug, of hospitalization and of investigations).
- Comparative efficacy (where the drug does not represent a major advance over existing formularies).

Clinical practice guidelines are used to provide guidance on best practice and are often based on available evidence. Adherence to guidelines can be problematic, because medicines recommended for the standardized care of single diseases often lead to adverse events when used in patients with comorbidities. However, like restricted formularies, they can provide a consistent and cost-effective standard of care.

Communicating to prescribers

Prescribers are often routinely provided with marketing materials by industry representatives. Governmental and medicines agencies responsible for medicine management and prescribing also communicate with prescribers about safe, effective and cost-efficient prescribing. These external factors may have a modest or a large impact on prescribing behaviour, and drug utilization studies can be used to evaluate this impact (see Chapter 38), particularly around costs. There is also communication between prescribers and pharmacists, which is another important element.

Assessing the impact of health policy initiatives

An important strength of most retrospective databases is that they allow researchers to examine medical care utilization as it occurs in routine clinical care. They often provide large study populations and long observation periods, allowing for examination of specific subpopulations. In addition, retrospective databases provide a relatively inexpensive and expedient approach to answering the time-sensitive questions posed by decision-makers. For example, Mamdani et al. [40] used an interrupted time-series design to assess the impact of the restriction of fluoroquinolones in Ontario on rates of antibiotic prescription and infectious disease-related hospitalization among elderly individuals who were dispensed antibiotics. Historical trends were used to establish an expected drug utilization rate in the absence of a policy change, which was compared with observed rates following the implementation of the drug policy. The findings suggested that formulary restrictions on fluoroquinolones aimed at decreasing use among an elderly population could be implemented effectively without adversely impacting on hospital admission rates.

Drug utilization studies can also be used to assess the impact of cost-containment measures on the utilization of and expenditure on drugs. For example, in a study of a series of measures implemented to lower the prices of generic and off-patent medicines in Ireland, a national prescription claims database was used to examine the volume of and expenditure on prescription items over a 6-year period during which various changes were introduced to the pricing mechanism for pharmaceuticals (e.g. pharmacy mark-up, wholesale margin, etc.) [41]. The findings suggested that expenditure had decreased and highlighted the need for a more structured pricing format for generics in Ireland.

CHAPTER 43

Assessment of quality of prescribing using quality indicators

Petra Denig[1], Flora Haaijer-Ruskamp[1] & Lisa Pont[2]

[1]*Clinical Pharmacy and Pharmacology, University of Groningen, University Medical Center Groningen, The Netherlands*

[2]*Australian Institute of Health Innovation, Macquarie University, Australia*

KEY POINTS

- Three domains of the prescribing process are commonly targeted by prescribing indicators: (i) decision to prescribe; (ii) choice of medication; and (iii) monitoring of medication treatment.
- These domains can be connected to different quality aspects, including underprescribing, overprescribing, timely prescribing, first-line medication, inappropriate medication and medication continuation.
- Many prescribing indicators are available, covering a wide range of quality aspects, with good face and content validity.
- Clinical relevance and predictive validity remain uncertain for several indicators – particularly drug-oriented indicators.

Introduction

Quality indicators are tools for measuring quality of care as defined by scientific evidence and/or expert consensus [1]. As described in Chapter 12, they can be classified as structure, process or outcome indicators. Prescribing quality indicators have been defined as 'a measurable element of prescribing performance for which there is evidence or consensus that it can be used to assess quality' [2]. In other words, they focus on the process of prescribing drug treatment. This process includes the decision to prescribe medication, the choice of medication and the monitoring, including adjustment or discontinuation, of prescribed medications. Quality indicators have been developed and implemented across a range of therapeutic areas.

Prescribing quality indicators are commonly defined at an aggregated level. Indicators can be used to provide information on resource use at the government level and to monitor quality and assess policy at the national or regional level. Quality indicators are also used locally to assess the quality of prescribing at the health care professional or organizational level, to stimulate reflection on current practice and to encourage quality improvement. In addition, indicators are used in research evaluation to determine changes in quality over time or after an intervention. More recently, indicators have been used for accreditation and provision of financial incentives for clinicians and organizations. Such use often involves the setting of minimum accepted quality standards, or benchmarks, which form an important element of quality assessment.

In Chapter 12, different types of prescribing quality indicator were introduced, including drug-oriented and disease-oriented indicators. Drug-oriented indicators are based on drug utilization patterns, irrespective of the indication for which the drugs are being prescribed. Disease-oriented indicators describe the quality of

Drug Utilization Research: Methods and Applications, First Edition. Edited by M. Elseviers et al.
Published 2016 by John Wiley & Sons, Ltd.

prescribing in relation to the condition for which a drug is being prescribed. Both types of indicator can become patient-oriented by assessing prescribing in relation to specific patient characteristics, such as age and comorbidity.

The objective of this chapter is to provide a conceptual framework to delineate the quality aspects related to the prescribing process that are commonly assessed using prescribing indicators, and to present and discuss the value of such indicators. This framework can be used to develop or select a comprehensive set of indicators in a given therapeutic area. To illustrate the possibilities and limitations, we present examples from two common therapeutic areas. Furthermore, we discuss several general quality indicator sets applied in practice and explore their use for different purposes.

Conceptual framework

In general, health care should be effective, safe, timely, patient-centred and efficient [3]. When applying these criteria to the prescribing process, the effectiveness of each medication needs to be weighed in relation to its safety, suitability and cost. Different options, including nonpharmacological alternatives, must be compared to one another when deciding whether or what to prescribe. Good prescribing has been defined by the World Health Organization (WHO) as comprising six steps (Box 43.1) [4]. Currently, most prescribing quality indicators focus on the decision to prescribe a medication and the choice of agent (step 3) [5]. Some focus on suitability in specific cases (step 4). For example, suitability can be assessed in terms of effectiveness or safety, considering dose contraindications or interactions. Few indicators for the assessment of adequate monitoring of medication have been proposed, although it has been argued that such quality indicators are much needed [6]. Also, only a few quality measures have been developed for assessment around setting goals and informing or involving patients in the prescribing process (steps 1, 2 and 5). These are mainly questionnaire-based measures assessing patient experience, such as the indicator based on the Global Satisfaction Scale of the Treatment Satisfaction Questionnaire for Medication.

Box 43.1 The six-step treatment plan.

- **Step 1** Define the patient's problem.
- **Step 2** Specify the therapeutic objective:What do you want to achieve with the treatment, based on the problem and the patient's needs?
- **Step 3** Define therapeutic options: Which treatment is indicated (including ***decision to prescribe***)?What is the most effective, safe, suitable and cheap treatment for this objective (***medication choice in general***)?
- **Step 4** Verify the suitability of first-line treatment:Check effectiveness and safety in this specific case (***patient-oriented choice***).
- **Step 5** Start the treatment. Give information, instructions and warnings.
- **Step 6** Monitor treatment (***evaluate, adjust, discontinue treatment***).

Source: Data from [4].

Thus, the general domains targeted with prescribing indicators concern: (i) the decision to prescribe, (ii) choice of medication, and (iii) monitoring of medication treatment. Table 43.1 presents a conceptual framework connecting these general domains to the different quality aspects that are commonly assessed, with examples of drug-oriented and disease-oriented prescribing quality indicators.

The first domain focuses on the decision to prescribe any (or additional) medication treatment, and thus on the clinical need for such treatment. Indicators developed to assess this domain focus on measuring the extent of under- or overprescribing, as well as the timelines of prescribing. Since positive indicators are generally preferred, several of these indicators assess the extent of 'no underprescribing' rather than focussing on the negative 'underprescribing'. Most of these indicators are disease-oriented, since they assess quality within the context of a specific disease and require data that include clinical information, such as condition. However, in some cases, clinical need can be determined using prescription data only, such as when one drug is needed to mitigate harm from another drug (Table 43.1) or when clinical need can be inferred unambiguously from medication use.

The focus of the second domain is on the choice of medication. Quality aspects focus on the prescribing of appropriate or inappropriate drugs. Assessed at an aggregate level, the effectiveness and safety of prescribed medication are considered core dimensions for assessing appropriateness. For many of these indicators, effectiveness and safety are assessed relative

Table 43.1 Conceptual framework connecting domains and quality aspects with indicators.

Source: Most examples from [5,32,41,48].

Domain	Quality aspects	Drug-oriented	Disease-oriented
Decision to prescribe	(No) underprescribing or unmet need	Medication to prevent side effects from another medication is (not) prescribed, e.g. ***percentage of patients on strong opioid medication (not) receiving laxatives***	Indicated medication is (not) prescribed, e.g. ***percentage of patients with asthma receiving chronic short-acting beta agonists who do (not) receive inhaled corticosteroid*** Treatment recommended for indication is prescribed, e.g. ***percentage of patients with diabetes receiving a flu vaccination***
	(No) overprescribing	Volume of drugs with known overprescribing or restricted indication, e.g. ***percentage of patients receiving antibiotics (stratified by age and gender)*** Medication is duplicated, e.g. ***percentage of patients using more than one drug from the same therapeutic class***	Medication prescribed is not indicated or treatment that is not indicated is avoided, e.g. ***percentage of patients with acute bronchitis who are not receiving an antibiotic prescription*** Medication intensification is not indicated, e.g. ***percentage of patients >80 years old with a systolic blood pressure <150 mmHg for whom medication treatment with antihypertensives is intensified***
	Timely prescribing		Medication is initiated in a timely manner after an event, e.g. ***percentage of patients with ischaemic stroke receiving antithrombotic therapy by the end of hospital day 2*** Medication is intensified in a timely manner, e.g. ***percentage of hypertensive patients with blood pressure >140/90 mmHg who have an increase in dose of initial drug, change to a drug from another class or addition of a second drug from another class***
Medication choice	Prescription of first-line medication	Medication is first-line within a therapeutic class, e.g. ***percentage of patients prescribed an antibiotic receiving a guideline recommended antibiotic*** Medication is best value for money or most cost-effective choice, e.g. ***percentage of drugs prescribed by generic name***	Medication is first-line for an indication, e.g. ***percentage of patients with heart failure receiving an angiotensin-converting enzyme (ACE) inhibitor or angiotensin receptor blocker (ARB)***
	Prescription of second-line or inappropriate medication	Medication is not first-line but is prescribed as initial treatment, e.g. ***percentage of elderly patients receiving nonsteroidal antiinflammatory drugs (NSAIDs) without having first received paracetamol*** Medication is second-line and prescribed after first-line treatment, e.g. ***percentage of patients receiving an ARB after having received an ACE inhibitor*** Medication is inappropriate and should not be prescribed, e.g. ***percentage of patients receiving long-acting sulfonylurea derivatives***	Medication is inappropriate and should not be prescribed for a specific indication, e.g. ***percentage of elderly patients with dementia but no psychosis receiving antipsychotics*** Medication is not first-line for a specific indication, e.g. ***percentage of elderly patients with chronic obstructive pulmonary disease (COPD) receiving theophylline without a long-acting beta agonist or antimuscarinic***

(continued)

Table 43.1 *(continued)*

Domain	Quality aspects	Drug-oriented	Disease-oriented
	Contraindications	Medication is high-risk and should not be prescribed in elderly patients, e.g. ***percentage of patients >65 years old receiving NSAIDs for more than 28 days***	Medication is contraindicated in patients with a specific concurrent condition, e.g. ***percentage of asthma patients receiving a beta blocker***
	Interactions	Medication has undesired interaction, e.g. ***percentage of patients receiving verapamil in combination with a beta blocker***	
	Dose	Prescribed dose is too low, e.g. ***percentage of patients initiating on simvastatin 20 mg/day*** Prescribed dose is too high, e.g. ***percentage of patients on verapamil or ciclosporin or a human immunodeficiency virus (HIV) protease inhibitor receiving simvastatin >10 mg/day***	Prescribed dose is too high for a specific indication, e.g. ***percentage of patients with renal impairment receiving digoxin >0.125 mg/day***
	Duration	Prescription duration is too short, e.g. ***percentage of male patients receiving nitrofurantoin <7 days***	Effective duration of treatment, e.g. ***percentage of patients with a new episode of major depression receiving antidepressant medication for at least 180 days***
Treatment monitoring	Timely adjustments	Relevant tests are conducted to monitor the effectiveness or safety of a specific medication, e.g. ***percentage of patients on lithium therapy with a record of lithium levels in the therapeutic range***	Medication is discontinued or decreased following a specific indication or event
	Medication continuation	A minimum proportion of days is covered by a medication, e.g. ***percentage of patients with at least two antiretroviral drug prescriptions on two unique dates who met the proportion-of-days-covered (PDC) threshold of 90% during the measurement period***	Medication is continued for chronic use, e.g. ***percentage of patients discharged with a diagnosis of myocardial infarction who received persistent beta-blocker treatment for 6 months after discharge***
	Medication discontinuation	Medication is prescribed for too long, e.g. ***percentage of patients aged over 50 receiving hormone replacement therapy for ≥5 years***	Treatment is continued too long, e.g. ***percentage of elderly patients with dementia and psychosis receiving risperidone for ≥12 weeks***

to each other, with the risk–benefit balance determining what is considered first-line or second-line therapy or what may be seen as an inappropriate drug at both the population and the individual levels. Resource utilization and costs can be incorporated by including the efficiency of the prescribed treatment, focusing on value for money (Table 43.1). Such efficiency indicators are often relative to the local context and time, and may need modification when used across different locales. Furthermore, the focus can be on suboptimal prescribing (or misprescribing) of appropriate medication (e.g. regarding dosing or duration; Table 43.1). Such indicators may focus on suboptimal effect (e.g. underdosing or too–short duration) or on safety aspects of the prescribed medication (e.g. overdosing or contraindication). Indicators assessing medication choice can be defined in general (drug-oriented) or linked to specific indications (disease-oriented) or subpopulations (patient-oriented).

In the third domain, the focus is on monitoring the effectiveness and safety of the medication after it has been prescribed. This includes subsequent evaluation of whether the treatment needs continuation, adjustment or discontinuation. Some indicators assess whether safety aspects related to specific medication are sufficiently monitored (e.g. related to therapeutic drug levels or relevant biochemistry). Other indicators have been developed to assess adequate continuation or adherence to medication intended for chronic use (Table 43.1).

Diabetes and cardiovascular risk management

As a first example, we present an overview of prescribing indicators developed for type 2 diabetes and related cardiovascular risk management. A systematic review of the international literature identified a large number of such prescribing quality indicators [7]. In general, these indicators are derived from evidence-based guideline recommendations and have adequate content validity.

Decision to prescribe

In this therapeutic area, there are various indicators determining whether treatment is prescribed when indicated. Most of them assess whether patients with a given condition have received prescriptions for specific drugs or drug classes, such as the indicator looking at patients with diabetes and proteinuria who are treated with angiotensin-converting enzyme (ACE) inhibitors. These are relatively simple disease-oriented indicators targeting potential underprescribing (Box 43.2). Usually they incorporate one or more medication classes that are considered indicated for a specified condition.

Box 43.2 Examples of simple indicators targeting the decision to prescribe.

No underprescribing or unmet need in relation to diagnosis (disease-oriented)

- Percentage of patients with diabetes aged ≥40 years who have a current prescription for a statin [8].
- Percentage of patients with a history of myocardial infarction treated with antiplatelet medication, beta-blocker, angiotensin-modifying medication and lipid-modifying medication (or statin) [9,10].
- Percentage of patients with diabetes and a diagnosis of proteinuria or micro-albuminuria (or hypertension) who are treated with angiotensin-converting enzyme (ACE) inhibitors (or angiotensin receptor blocker, ARB) [10,11].

Guidelines for the management of diabetes and related cardiovascular risk factors also provide treatment recommendations when target values (e.g. blood glucose levels, blood pressure) have not been achieved. These recommendations can be used to incorporate individual patient need into quality indicators [12]. One example of this is an indicator that looks at the percentage of patients who are adequately treated (i.e. patients who are either well controlled or receiving multiple drugs when they are insufficiently controlled; see Box 43.3). Similar indicators relating treatment intensity (or level of medication use) to target values in diabetes have been used in Dutch general practice as a quality improvement measure (Figure 43.1) [13]. All such indicators provide a static or cross-sectional image of prescribing at a specific point or period in time. In this way, they can identify a possible need for action, such as low treatment intensity, but they do not assess whether the indicated medication is being prescribed in a timely manner.

Action indicators, also called 'tightly linked indicators' [14], are a specialized subset of indicators that assess timeliness for medication initiation or changes in response to

Box 43.3 Examples of indicators targeting patient-specific need to prescribe (or not).

No underprescribing or unmet need

- Percentage of patients with coronary artery disease who have a blood pressure <140/90 mmHg OR who have a blood pressure ≥140/90 mmHg and were prescribed two or more antihypertensive medications during the most recent office visit [16].

Timely prescribing

- Percentage of uncomplicated hypertensive patients aged 18–60 with blood pressure >140/90 mmHg who are on medication and who have a change in pharmacological therapy (e.g. increase in dose of initial drug, change to a drug from another class or addition of a second drug from another class within a defined period of time) [17].

Overprescribing

- Percentage of patients with systolic blood pressure <130 mmHg who are receiving three or more blood pressure-lowering drugs OR who had an increase in dose within 120 days after the index date OR who started a new blood pressure-lowering drug class within 120 days after the index date) AND who don't have systolic blood pressure ≥130 mmHg within the next 120 days [18].

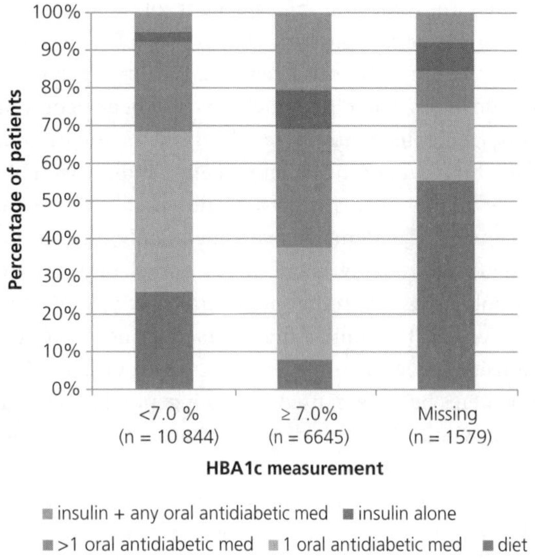

Figure 43.1 Disease-oriented diabetes management indicators, relating diabetes control (HbA1c mmol/l) to antidiabetic drug treatment, provided as feedback to Dutch general practitioners (GPs) as part of the Groningen Initiative to Analyse Type 2 Diabetes Treatment (GIANTT) project. Left bar: number of patients who reached the target and are considered adequately treated. Middle bar: number of patients who did not reach the target. Underprescribing or unmet need is assumed for those who received no medication or only one oral antidiabetic drug (38%). HbA1c, glycated haemoglobin A1c.

Source: Translated and adapted from http://www.giantt.nl [13].

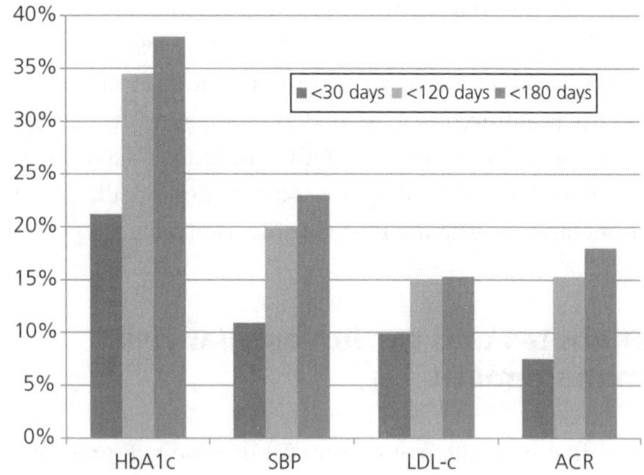

Figure 43.2 Percentage of diabetic patients with treatment intensification within 30, 120 or 180 days following identification of a risk factor. HbA1c, glycated haemoglobin A1c; SBP, systolic blood pressure; LDL-c, low-density lipoprotein cholesterol; ACR, albumin–creatinine ratio.

Source: Sidorenkov et al. 2011 [19]. Copyright: © 2011 Sidorenkov et al.

an identified need. They mainly focus on undertreatment and on increasing doses or adding drugs to regimens when needed [15]. An example of such an indicator is the initiation or intensification of drug treatment within a defined timeframe after an elevated HbA1c or blood pressure reading has been identified (Box 43.3).

Assessment of prescribing decisions using action indicators showed that Dutch general practitioners (GPs) were more likely to intensify diabetes medication following elevated HbA1c levels than to intensify antihypertensive medication following elevated blood pressure levels (Figure 43.2) [19]. A comparison of action and cross-sectional disease-oriented indicators for the management of diabetes found that action indicators gave a more accurate picture of quality when compared to a detailed evaluation of treatment quality; cross-sectional indicators focusing on the percentage of uncontrolled patients receiving medication tended to overestimate prescribing quality [20]. Action indicators were found to be predictive of better short-term outcomes in patients with diabetes [21,22].

Recently, a new type of prescribing indicator has been applied to the assessment of potential overtreatment regarding blood pressure and glucose-lowering treatment in patients with diabetes (Box 43.3) [18,23]. This follows growing concern that patients may be overtreated due to incentives to achieve strict target levels [24,25]. However, this is an area lacking evidence-based guidance on how quality indicators might be defined [26], and further validation is warranted.

Medication choice

There are many prescribing indicators focusing on medication choice in diabetes and related cardiovascular risk management (Box 43.4). Their interpretation with respect to quality can be difficult. It is not always clear to what extent an indicator is clinically relevant and has predictive validity in terms of patient outcomes, especially with drug-oriented indicators that focus on a single preferred medication within a therapeutic class. In many cases, this is primarily cost-driven. A systematic review of studies that examined the predictive validity of diabetes quality indicators found no studies that had assessed the relationship between drug-oriented indicators and patient outcomes [27].

Box 43.4 Examples of indicators focusing on medication choice.

First-line medication

- Percentage of biguanides of all oral antidiabetic drugs [28].

First-line medication based on costs

- Percentage of patients prescribed simvastatin among all patients prescribed a statin [29].

Second-line medication

- Percentage of patients prescribed an angiotensin receptor blocker (ARB) following trial of an angiotensin-converting enzyme (ACE) inhibitor among all patients prescribed ARBs [30].

Dosing

- Percentage of users of low-dose thiazides among all diuretic users [28].

Contraindications

- Percentage of patients with diabetes and heart failure who receive a thiazolidinedione [31].

Other indicators assess whether a choice of medication is appropriate for an individual's clinical situation (e.g. regarding contraindications; Box 43.4). The interpretation of such disease-oriented indicators with respect to quality is usually more straightforward.

Monitor and (dis)continue treatment

Several indicators have been developed that focus on the provision of adequate laboratory monitoring for safe prescribing of specific cardiovascular drugs [32]. One example is an indicator looking at patients on diuretics or ACE inhibitors who have not had their urea and electrolytes checked (Box 43.5). Medication continuation indicators in this field measure whether indicated chronic treatment is continued or consistently provided over a specified period (Box 43.5), which may reflect either patient or prescriber actions. One difficulty with such indicators is that the underlying reason for discontinuation of treatment may be justifiable, (e.g. because of side effects) [33]. Additionally, most indicators do not include a measure of timeliness, which may further complicate interpretation in terms of quality.

Box 43.5 Examples of indicators focusing on medication monitoring and continuation.

Monitoring

- Percentage of patients treated with potassium-sparing diuretic who had no urea and electrolytes check in the last 48 weeks [32].

Medication continuation or persistence

- Percentage of patients discharged with a diagnosis of acute myocardial infarction who received persistent beta-blocker treatment for 6 months after discharge [11].

Medication safety in the elderly

Medication safety, particularly in the elderly, has been identified as a priority throughout the world. It is therefore not surprising that many indicators have been developed to monitor this issue. Different approaches have been taken in the development of medication safety indicators for the elderly, each with their own merits and limitations. Some indicator sets focus mainly on the choice of inappropriate medications, whereas others address several domains of prescribing. Furthermore, several sets of criteria have been developed to assess the quality of treatment at the individual patient level. Such criteria can also be applied at the practice or population level, when adequately detailed data are available about all patients. This results in an indicator which expresses the percentage of patients fulfilling the criteria.

Potentially inappropriate medication lists

Indicators based on avoidance of potentially inappropriate drugs in the elderly have long been used to identify medication safety issues in the population. Among the first used for this purpose were the Beers criteria in the 1990s, which have been updated several times since [34]. The focus is on medication choice. These drug-oriented indicators, based on such lists of 'drugs to avoid, have shown to be associated with hospitalizations, adverse drug reactions (ADRs) and health-related quality of life [35,36]. The Beers criteria are widely used, especially in the United States, and are included in the Healthcare Effectiveness Data and Information Set (HEDIS) standard indicators set (Box 43.6) [37]. Despite this, there is considerable debate around their use [38], including their international relevance [39]. Alternative lists have been developed in Canada, France, Norway and Australia, partly to include inappropriate drug–disease combinations [39], and recently the PRISCUS list was developed for use in Germany [40].

Box 43.6 Examples of drug-oriented safety indicators and criteria for the elderly.

HEDIS inappropriate medication indicator, based on the Beers criteria [37]

- Percentage of patients ≥65 years who received at least one high-risk medication.

Drug-oriented STOPP criteria [41]

- Patients ≥65 years old with aspirin >150 mg/day.
- Patients ≥65 years old on warfarin and nonsteroidal antiinflammatory drugs (NSAIDs).

ACOVE medication indicators applicable to administrative data [47]

- IF a vulnerable elder is taking a monoamine oxidase (MAO) inhibitor THEN they should not receive medications that interact with MAO inhibitors for at least 2 weeks after termination.
- IF a vulnerable elder is prescribed an oral hypoglycemic drug THEN chlorpropamide should not be used.

The Screening Tool of Older Persons' Prescriptions (STOPP) criteria were first published in 2008 [41] and are now widely used [42]. The original list consisted of 65 criteria identifying potentially inappropriate or high-risk medications, drug–drug combinations, dosages and/or medication durations for the elderly. Only 10 of the STOPP criteria are exclusively drug-oriented (see Box 43.6 for examples), with the remainder being disease-oriented. The disease-oriented criteria often concern the use of contraindicated or high-risk drugs. The STOPP criteria have been correlated with preventable adverse events [43].

In conjunction with the STOPP criteria, a Screening Tool to Alert to Right Treatment (START) was developed. The STOPP/START criteria have recently been updated, and various adaptations of the original lists have been made for specific countries or settings [42,44,45]. Together, they cover most domains of prescribing for a variety of therapeutic areas.

Quality-of-care indicators

The Assessing Care of Vulnerable Elderly (ACOVE) indicators were developed in the United States in 2000 to improve and monitor the quality of care of the vulnerable elderly [46,47]. A number of medication-related indicators are included in this list, focusing on the domains of (i) prescribing indicated medications or underprescribing, (ii) avoiding inappropriate medications or misprescribing and (iii) education, continuity, documentation and medication monitoring. These are all defined as IF–THEN statements, but several have been translated into medication indicators that can be assessed at an aggregated level. There is considerable overlap between the ACOVE indicators and both the Beers and STOPP lists.

General sets that include safety indicators for the elderly

There are a number of general sets of prescribing indicators, not specifically for the elderly, that include safety indicators for elderly and older populations (Box 43.7). For example, a set developed in the United Kingdom includes several indicators for patients aged >65 years, focusing on the dose and duration of benzodiazepines and nonsteroidal antiinflammatory drugs (NSAIDs) [48]. A set developed in Scotland includes a number of safety indicators for patients aged ≥65, ≥75 and ≥85 years, focusing on high-risk medication, excess duration, interactions and contraindications [32]. Those indicators concerning high-risk medications and interactions are similar to the Beers and STOPP criteria.

Drug burden scales

Several measures or scales have been developed to assess the exposure of elderly patients to anticholinergic or sedative medications based on drug choice and dosage. Examples are the Drug Burden Index (DBI) and

Box 43.7 Examples of disease-oriented safety indicators and criteria for the elderly.

Duration

- Initiation of benzodiazepine for ≥21 days in a patient aged >65 years with depression [48].

Second-line medication

- Prescription of theophylline without use of long acting beta2-agonist or antimuscarinic in a patient aged ≥65 years with chronic obstructive pulmonary disease (COPD) [32].

Contraindications

- Prescription of tricyclics antidepressants in a patient aged ≥65 years with dementia [32].

the Anticholinergic Drug Scale (ADS). These have been developed primarily for individual medication reviews of older patients with potential medication safety concerns. Higher scores are associated with poorer physical and cognitive functioning in the elderly [49]. These measures are not currently included in quality indicator sets, and further evaluation as an indicator of medication safety in the elderly is needed.

Polypharmacy

Polypharmacy, defined as taking multiple drugs simultaneously, is used as a prescribing indicator in many countries. Although not exclusively intended for the elderly, it is often applied in this population. The association between polypharmacy and medication safety (including drug interactions and drug-related hospital admissions) has been demonstrated [50]. The advantage of polypharmacy as an indicator is that it is usually easy to calculate. There is, however, no standard definition of polypharmacy, with definitions differing from five or more drugs in the Netherlands to ten or more drugs in Sweden. The WHO prescribing indicator set includes 'the average number of drugs per encounter' as a measure of the degree of polypharmacy. Since there appears to be a linear relation between number of drugs taken and drug-related problems, a strict cut-off to identify polypharmacy is of limited clinical value [51]. The major limitation with all polypharmacy measures is that their relevance for complex patients with multimorbidity is questionable, due to the lack of differentiation between 'legitimate' and 'unnecessary' polypharmacy – and yet this is exactly the population where most polypharmacy is found.

Prescribing quality indicators in practice

Prescribing quality indicators may be used for a variety of different purposes. Aggregate indicators are applied for internal use by health care professionals to receive feedback on prescribing and to identify issues for improvement in local, regional and national quality assessment programmes. Using feedback and audit is one of the more effective strategies by which to improve prescribing quality [52], and several countries use general drug-oriented indicator sets to support prescribers or policymakers in reviewing prescribing patterns. Examples of such services can be found in the United Kingdom and the Netherlands. In the United Kingdom, indicators based on Electronic Prescribing Analysis and Cost (ePACT) data are used by the Health & Social Care Information Centre to support national policy [53]. In the Netherlands, the Monitor Prescription Behaviour provides reports on 22 quality-of-prescribing and drug-preference indicators and on 4 prescribing-volume indicators, which are calculated from reimbursement data drawn from a national datacentre for health care insurers [54]. These indicators are included in the Dutch health care performance report to support national policy [55], but are also provided to individual GPs in order to improve their prescribing behaviour.

To promote rational drug use in developing countries, a small set of prescribing indicators is recommended by the WHO [56]. These indicators do not measure all relevant aspects of prescribing but provide a simple tool for quickly assessing a few critical ones. These include: (i) average number of drugs per encounter; (ii) percentage of drugs prescribed by generic name; (iii) percentage of encounters with an antibiotic prescribed; (iv) percentage of encounters with an injection prescribed; and (v) percentage of drugs prescribed from an essential drugs list or formulary. Results with these indicators can point to particular issues in need of more detailed examination.

Indicators are also used for cross-national comparisons of drug use. For example, the European Surveillance of Antimicrobial Consumption Network (ESAC) published a set of 12 drug-specific and 21 disease-specific quality indicators for outpatient antibiotic use in Europe [57,58]. The drug-specific indicators are volume-based, either expressing defined daily doses (DDDs) per 1000 inhabitants per day or using ratios of broad- to narrow-spectrum antibiotics. The disease-specific indicators express percentages of patients with a specific diagnosis receiving (i) antibacterials for systemic use, (ii) recommended antibacterials or (iii) quinolones.

In addition to clinical practice, prescribing indicators are used in intervention studies to monitor and improve prescribing. For example, the Data Driven Quality Improvement in Primary Care Trial (DQIP) applies a fairly comprehensive set of medication quality and safety criteria that can be implemented using routine primary care datasets [32]. These criteria focus on: (i) indicated and preferred drug treatment for common conditions, such as cardiovascular diseases, diabetes, asthma and osteoporosis; (ii) high-risk medications, including antiplatelet agents, NSAIDs, diuretics and corticosteroids; (iii) drug use in high-risk populations, including the elderly and patients with chronic kidney disease; (iv) drug–drug interactions; (v) dosing; and (vi) tests to monitor effects/safety. The DQIP criteria were developed to facilitate the identification of patients at risk of preventable drug-related morbidity in the United Kingdom, but it is anticipated that they could serve a range of other purposes.

In the last decade, there has been increasing external use of indicators in benchmarking, accreditation and pay-for-performance programmes to demonstrate that adequate levels of quality have been achieved. Such programmes have been implemented by policymakers, professional organizations and health insurance companies. Commonly, they include a wider range of quality indicators than simple prescribing. For example, in the United Kingdom, the Quality and Outcomes Framework links part of GPs' income to their performance on quality indicators, including some prescribing indicators [10,59]. In the United States, the Integrated Healthcare Association programme is a large nongovernmental incentive programme that includes indicators on proportions of days covered by medication, generic prescribing, appropriate treatment and high-risk medication [60].

Conclusion

Hundreds of prescribing indicators can be found for a wide range of disease topics, through databases such as the National Quality Forum [11] and the National Quality Measures Clearinghouse [5]. The majority of indicators included in these databases are drawn from the United States, but they do include some sets from other countries. As a collection of indicators, they are far from complete, and one must search literature databases and the websites of professional organizations in order to identify currently used indicators of treatment quality in specific fields.

With the large number of prescribing quality indicators available it is important to select and use valid ones that target relevant problems, and not just pick the ones that are easiest to apply. There are currently no general guidelines or standards for the development and selection of quality indicators [61]. We have presented a framework that can be used for the primary selection of potential indicators covering relevant domains of prescribing quality. The next step is to identify indicators that can be made into valid quality measures. This includes operationalizing them into measures for the available data sources (see also Chapter 12).

Looking at the cases of diabetes and cardiovascular risk management and medication safety in the elderly, many indicators are currently in use, covering a wide range of quality aspects. They are commonly based on guideline recommendations and are generally accepted, ensuring both face and content validity. There is, however, uncertainty about the clinical relevance and predictive value of several of the more simple, mostly drug-oriented indicators. Use of an indicator with poor predictive validity may lead to poorer outcomes in some patients, rather than improving the quality of care as intended. Although such indicators can be helpful for internal use, caution is indicated in using them in health policy, particularly when linking them to financial or performance incentives. With the increased accessibility of clinical patient data, opportunities to develop and use more sophisticated prescribing quality indicators with good predictive validity are increasing.

CHAPTER 44

Quality indicators for patient care in pharmacy practice

Hanne Herborg
Pharmakon, Danish College of Pharmacy Practice, Denmark

KEY POINTS

- Pharmacies can improve the quality of drug utilization in multiple ways, and pharmacy errors can lead to serious adverse events.
- The international Good Pharmacy Practice (GPP) guideline encourages countries to set quality standards in four areas: distribution of medical products; medication therapy management; professional performance; and improvement of the effectiveness of health care systems.
- The main direct mechanisms by which pharmacies can influence drug utilization are: (i) dispensing of prescribed medicines; (ii) self-medication support and sale of over-the-counter (OTC) medicines; and (iii) cognitive activities (e.g. patient information and counselling).
- In relation to dispensing of prescribed medicines, quality improvement has particularly been focused on to dispensing errors, prescription interventions, dose dispensing and patient counselling.
- In relation to self-medication, documented quality issues include inappropriate self-medication, inappropriate product request, inappropriate (too-high) intended duration of use (including abuse) and inappropriate dosage.
- In relation to cognitive activities, a key concept is pharmaceutical care aimed at preventing, identifying and resolving drug-related problems and improving health outcomes.

Introduction

The pharmacy is a supplier of medicines, both over the counter (OTC) and on prescription from prescribers. Therefore, pharmacies can influence drug utilization and medication safety via multiple mechanisms (direct and indirect). The scope of this chapter is pharmacy practice, but limited to roles involving direct patient care.

There are three mechanisms that directly affect patients: (i) dispensing of prescribed medicines; (ii) self-medication support and sale of OTC medicines; and (iii) cognitive activities. Cognitive activities are delivered either in connection with the sale/supply of individual medicines (e.g. patient information and counselling) or as additional separate services (e.g. medication therapy management/pharmaceutical care), which usually cover a patient's drug therapy.

Dimensions of quality in pharmacy practice

Ensuring the quality of the prescribing, dispensing and use of medicines is integrated in the overall role and function of a pharmacy. Dimensions of quality in pharmacy practice have been described in many different frameworks across different countries. In this chapter, we use the international guideline for Good Pharmacy Practice (GPP) as our main framework because it describes the totality of pharmacy practice based on an international consensus. The GPP is a joint World Health Organization (WHO)/International Pharmaceutical Federation (FIP) guideline describing standards of quality for pharmacy activities. It states that 'The mission of pharmacy practice is to contribute to health improvement and to help patients with health problems to make the best use

Drug Utilization Research: Methods and Applications, First Edition. Edited by M. Elseviers et al.
Published 2016 by John Wiley & Sons, Ltd.

of their medicines' [1]. It identifies four main roles for pharmacists in serving individual patients and society as a whole (see Box 44.1). The focus in this chapter is on the roles that involve giving direct care to patients (i.e. Role 1E: 'Dispense medical products' and Role 2: 'Provide effective medication therapy management').

The GPP was supplemented in 1998 with a version aimed specifically at developing countries [2]. This version recommends national standards for premises, dispensing, containers, labelling, self-medication, products, patient instructions, record-keeping, health information, patient counselling and pharmaceutical care. It puts more emphasis on a stepwise implementation process and has more of a focus on basic system elements, such as labelling and containers.

Box 44.1 Pharmacy roles and functions according to the Good Pharmacy Practice (GPP guideline) [1].

Role 1: Prepare, obtain, store, secure, distribute, administer, dispense and dispose of medical products

Function A: Prepare extemporaneous medicine preparations and medical products.
Function B: Obtain, store and secure medicine preparations and medical products.
Function C: Distribute medicine preparations and medical products.
Function D: Administer medicines, vaccines and other injectable medications.
Function E: Dispense medical products (including patient information).
Function F: Dispose of medicine preparations and medical products.

Role 2: Provide effective medication therapy management

Function A: Assess patient health status and needs.
Function B: Manage patient medication therapy.
Function C: Monitor patient progress and outcomes.
Function D: Provide information about medicines and health-related issues.

Role 3: Maintain and improve professional performance

Function A: Plan and implement continuing professional development strategies to improve current and future performance.

Role 4: Contribute to improving effectiveness of the health-care system and public health

Function A: Disseminate evaluated information about medicines and various aspects of self-care.
Function B: Engage in preventive care activities and services.
Function C: Comply with national professional obligations, guidelines and legislations.
Function D: Advocate and support national policies that promote improved health outcomes.

Pharmaceutical care may or may not be linked to dispensing. The basic elements can be an integrated part of the dispensing process (Role 1E), but more advanced pharmaceutical care will often be delivered to individual patients as medication therapy management, medication review or medication use review, or else to institutions as clinical pharmacy (Role 2).

Self-medication support also involves direct patient care in pharmacies. In the 1996 version of the GPP, assessing symptoms, recommending self-care (including nonprescription medicines, NPM) and referral to physicians were given an independent role: 'Self-care'. These functions are now included in Role 4A: 'Disseminate evaluated information about medicines and various aspects of self-care', but may also involve the dispensing process (Role 1E).

Indirect mechanisms, such as influencing the rational use of medicines in other health care settings (aspects of Role 4), are not within the scope of this chapter, but these activities should be mentioned as they may have a considerable effect on the quality of drug utilization. Preventive care activities (Role 4B) will also not be discussed here, as they are focused not on the quality of drug utilization, but on using the pharmacy as a point of care in order to achieve other public health outcomes.

We will first discuss pharmacy interventions in direct patient care (dispensing, self-medication and medication therapy management/pharmaceutical care), illustrating each area with examples of intervention studies, before reviewing some validated indicators and discussing the application of quality indicators in pharmacy practice.

Pharmacy interventions and intervention studies

The interventions included in this section are delivered directly from pharmacists/pharmacies to patients. Clinical pharmacy services delivered in hospitals, general practitioner (GP) surgeries or institutions such as nursing homes or homes for disabled people are not included.

Dispensing

The main steps of the prescription dispensing process can be described as shown in Box 44.2 [3,4]. Hence, dispensing a medicine in a pharmacy is not only a logistic task but has an integrated focus on avoiding prescribing errors, avoiding dispensing errors and avoiding errors in use by the patient.

The dispensing process will vary between countries. However, in most countries, dispensing involves only the actual prescription and does not *per se* include an assessment of the patient's entire medication regimen, as would be the case in medication therapy management (Role 2B).

According to the GPP, the dispensing process in pharmacies requires, as a minimum, standards for:

- providing appropriate facilities, trained personnel, standard dispensing practices and documentation;
- assessing and evaluating all paper and electronic prescriptions received;
- considering the therapeutic, social, economic and legal aspects of the prescribed indication(s) before supply, as well as generic substitution;
- ensuring patient confidentiality at the point of dispensing and providing written and oral information so that patients can derive maximum benefit from treatment.

Box 44.2 The pharmacy dispensing process [3,4].

Accept and check prescription

- Prescription details, patient identification, script validity

Review and process

- Check prescribing safety and appropriateness, dispensing history, patient-specific factors
- Perform calculations
- Resolve problems

Select, prepare and check

- Select and dispense products
- Package, label and assemble dispensed products

Supply and counsel

- Supply prescription to patient/carer; recheck
- Counsel patient/carer on safe and appropriate use and answer patient queries

Ensure stock management and documentation

- Monitor and maintain stock levels routinely
- Implement documentation routinely

The quality of pharmacy dispensing has been widely studied. In particular, researchers have focused on (i) dispensing errors, (ii) pharmacy prescription corrections, (iii) dose dispensing and (iv) the quality of pharmacy counselling and of the information provided to patients. A systematic review of the quality of private pharmacy services in low- and middle-income countries has shown that these countries experience quality problems in relation to dispensing [5]. Virtually all reviewed studies identified deficiencies in the quality of current professional practice. In particular, the authors highlighted a lack of pharmacists or other trained personnel, provision of incorrect advice for common symptoms and inappropriate supply of medicines (e.g. sale of prescription medicines over the counter).

Dispensing errors

The incidences, types and causes of dispensing errors were reviewed by James et al. [6] in the United Kingdom, the United States, Australia, Spain and Brazil. They found that incidences varied by setting, dispensing system, research method and definition. The most common errors in community and hospital pharmacies were dispensing wrong drug strength, form or quantity, or labelling medications with incorrect directions.

Beso et al. [7] studied the frequencies and causes of dispensing errors in a UK hospital pharmacy. They estimated that errors were identified at the final check stage in about 2% of all dispensed items and that about 1 in 100 were missed, resulting in an error rate of 0.02% outside the pharmacy. The majority of the errors involved slips in picking products and assumptions that the correct products were picked.

Knudsen et al. [8] studied prescription corrections and dispensing errors in Danish community pharmacies. They found a frequency of 0.1/1000 prescriptions for dispensing errors and 0.2/1000 for dispensing near-misses. The cases that reached patients were analysed in depth and it was found that most of the errors, and the potentially most serious ones, occurred in what was termed the 'transcription stage' of the dispensing process; that is, in the packaging, labelling and assembly of dispensed products [9].

The factors identified in these studies as contributing to dispensing errors were quite similar: handwritten prescriptions, look-alike/sound-alike drugs, misleading phrasing of names or dosages, lack of effective control of prescription labels and medicines, low staffing, outdated computer software, high workload, interruptions, distractions, inadequate lighting, a culture in which errors were seen as being inevitable and reliance on others to identify and rectify errors.

Prescription interventions

Pharmacies have the responsibility to correct problematic prescriptions issued by physicians. Studies of intervention rates are carried out in many countries, and it has been a trend to evaluate the health economic value of prescription interventions using expert panels to estimate costs and savings [10,11]. Overall intervention rates are low, but the absolute number of interventions is very high as dispensing prescriptions is such a common procedure.

As examples of prescription intervention rates, a New Zealand study found a rate of 64 interventions per 1000 prescription items, of which 52 per 1000 concerned bureaucratic and generic substitution issues. Clinical interventions were recorded at a rate of 13 per 1000 items [12].

A prospective electronic registration aimed at updating the Knudsen et al. [8] study on pharmaceutical interventions in prescription problems in Denmark found a rate of 10.2 interventions per 1000 prescriptions, with 32% being of clinical and 68% of administrative nature [13]. The estimate by Knudsen et al., based on retrospective pharmacy registrations, found a rate of 2.3 per 1000 prescriptions for prescription corrections, illustrating the importance of data collection methods.

Prescription interventions have also been used to evaluate the safety of electronic prescriptions. Warholak & Rupp [14] documented an intervention rate of 3.8% for e-prescriptions in US pharmacies (4.1% for new prescriptions and 2.2% for refills). Most interventions were to supplement omitted information (31.9%), especially missing directions for use. Dosing errors were also quite common (17.7%). Another US study compared electronic versus traditional prescriptions in two pharmacies [15] and found that the difference in intervention rates between e-prescribing (11.7%) and handwritten prescriptions (15.4%) was not statistically significant, whereas faxed and telephone prescriptions required fewer interventions. Such results show that prescriptions corrections in pharmacies are necessary even with the emergence of new technology.

Dose dispensing

Dose dispensing is delivered by pharmacies in both hospital and community settings. In some countries, automated dose dispensing (ADD) technology is widely disseminated (e.g. the Nordic countries and the Netherlands). Like e-prescribing, dose dispensing has the potential to improve packaging errors and patient safety, but again it comes with new error types and requires evaluation [16–18]. A recent systematic review of the literature on dose dispensing in primary care concluded that the evidence for the influence of ADD on the appropriateness and safety of medication use is limited. The findings suggest that patients using ADD have more inappropriate drugs in their regimens but that ADD may improve medication safety in terms of reducing discrepancies in medication records [19].

Patient counselling

The pharmacy dispensing process includes the provision of patient information and counselling. This function is essential to the quality of drug use.

A systematic review reported counselling rates varying from 8 to 100% depending on the research methods used and the type of prescription [20]. Higher rates were found in counselling consumers with new versus regular prescriptions. Information on directions for use, dosages, medicine names and indications was given more frequently than information on side effects, precautions, interactions, contraindications and storage.

As an example, a US study found that some form of oral communication related to a medication was reported in 68% of encounters [21]. At least one risk information item was provided in 22% of encounters. Direct encounters between pharmacists and patients, strict state regulations mandating that pharmacists counsel patients with new prescriptions and private areas for prescription pick-up were significant predictors of patients receiving oral counselling. Svartstad et al. [22] studied the use of written information in eight US states and found that provision of patient leaflets was routine practice, occurring with 87% of prescriptions dispensed.

Many countries are focusing on improving patient information and counselling, and the use of simulated patients/pseudocustomers is common. Extended counselling using structured processes is on the increase, in order to make sure that vulnerable patient groups receive more focused counselling [23,24].

Self-medication

Self-medication is part of the self-care that people engage in so as to maintain their health and prevent and deal with illness [25]. Pharmacists are often the only health professionals consulted in relation to this type of medication use.

Self-medication legislation and practice differ greatly between countries, according to national policies and traditions. Pharmacy guidelines on self-medication typically comprise assessment of needs and symptoms, recommendation of safe and effective NPM products, referral to a physician (if appropriate), counselling on medicines use, follow-up, nonpharmacological self-care and customer satisfaction [26–29].

A nationwide Australian study assessed the rates and clinical significance of pharmacy NPM interventions [30], finding an average rate of 5.66 per 1000 unit sales, which varied with clinical significance. It was estimated that Australian pharmacies perform 485 912 NPM interventions per annum, 101 324 of those avert emergency medical attention or serious harm.

Several studies have demonstrated that pharmacy counselling can improve drug use in self-medication. Drug-related problems related to self-medication are common, and pharmacy interventions can identify and solve them. This has been documented in several countries, and models for evidence-based self-care counselling have been developed and evaluated [31–34].

In a German study, 100 community pharmacists were asked to document 100 consecutive customers presenting symptoms or requesting OTC drugs [35]. Drug-related problems were found in 17.6% of cases. Four types made up almost 75% of all problems identified: inappropriate self-medication (29.7%), inappropriate product request (20.5%), inappropriate (too-high) intended duration of use (including abuse) (17.1%) and inappropriate dosage (6.8%). The most frequent pharmacy interventions were referral to a physician (39.5%) and switching to a more appropriate drug (28.1%). In a Danish study using similar methods, drug-related problems were identified in 21.0% of pharmacy customers [36].

Guideline compliance has been evaluated in many countries, using different methods and producing varying results. A Scottish study found that few NPM consultations were fully guideline-compliant [37]: 6.6% showed sufficient information gathered, 13.2% showed adequate advice/information provision, 46.1% showed personal involvement of a pharmacist, 21.1% showed particular care of specific patient groups and 28.9% showed pharmacist involvement with specific NPMs.

An Australian study of the implementation of standards of practice for NPMs comprised three visits by pharmacy educators [38]. At visit 1, the lowest levels of compliance were to standards relating to the documentation process (44%) and customer care and advice (46%). By visit 2, more than 80% of pharmacies had met most criteria. This had improved further at visit 3.

The previously mentioned systematic review of the quality of private pharmacy services in low- and middle-income countries showed that the quality of self-medication was an area of concern [39]. A multicomponent intervention study to improve dispensing practices in Vietnam and Thailand illustrated the problem, but also demonstrated improvement in the key indicators, showing significant improvement following the intervention in reducing the dispensing of illegal steroids (29 vs 62% in Hanoi and 25 vs 44% in Bangkok), reducing the dispensing of low-dose antibiotics (69 vs 90% in Hanoi) and increasing the supply of counselling and information (11 vs 30% for steroids and 51 vs 81% for antibiotics in Hanoi).

In summary, pharmacies play a key role in ensuring the quality of self-medication. However, in many health care systems there are issues with guideline implementation.

Medication therapy management and pharmaceutical care

With Role 2, the GPP guideline sets pharmacies the responsibility to provide effective medication therapy management. This role focuses on medication safety and relies on the concept of ***pharmaceutical care***.

Hepler & Strand [40] define pharmaceutical care as 'the responsible provision of drug therapy for the purpose of achieving definite outcomes that improve a patient's quality of life'. It usually covers all of a patient's drug therapy. The key components are:

- identifying potential and actual drug-related problems;
- resolving actual drug-related problems;
- preventing drug-related problems.

Pharmaceutical care is a collaborative function in health care systems. From this perspective, it is comparable to the systems approach in the patient safety literature [41], where all parties involved in health care processes – here the medication use system – contribute to avoiding adverse events and patient harm.

At the same time, pharmaceutical care is provided directly to individual patients and is in this context a key function for pharmacies [42]. The Pharmaceutical Care Network Europe (PCNE) decided in 2013 on a definition of pharmaceutical care that emphasizes this aspect: 'Pharmaceutical Care is the pharmacist's contribution to the care of individuals in order to optimize medicines use and improve health outcomes' [43]. The pharmaceutical care process has been described by Strand et al. [44] as a quality cycle with the components shown in Box 44.3.

The focus of pharmaceutical care differs between countries, as does the terminology. Many regard patient counselling in relation to dispensing as a basic level of care. Others emphasize medication therapy management with continuous follow-up. When provided as a service to individual patients as part of a care plan, pharmacies counsel on adherence, lifestyle and other health- and patient-related issues.

The journal *Annals of Pharmacotherapy* published a series of review articles describing pharmaceutical care in community pharmacies in 13 different countries in 2005–07 [45–57]. These articles give a most varied insight into the provision of patient care in this setting.

Systematic reviews of pharmaceutical care interventions

A considerable number of systematic reviews have been published in this area, documenting whether pharmaceutical care processes do in fact achieve intended patient outcomes. The results vary from no clear effect to a valuable contribution to health care outcomes.

Box 44.3 The pharmaceutical care process.

Establish therapeutic relationship

- Ensure patient involvement

Assess

- Ensure that all drug therapy is indicated and safe, and that patient can and will comply with instructions
- Identify drug therapy problems

Enact care plan

- Resolve drug therapy problems
- Achieve goals of therapy
- Prevent drug therapy problems

Evaluate

- Record actual patient outcomes
- Evaluate status as progress in meeting goals of therapy
- Reassess for new problems

Provide continuous follow-up

- Follow up, reassess and document

Table 44.1 presents an overview of 21 systematic reviews. The studies included were produced in the period 2004–13 and review between 4 and 298 articles each, with an average of 24 studies per review (disregarding the largest study). With regard to areas of care, eight reviews concern general pharmaceutical care/clinical pharmacy provided by pharmacists [58–66], while thirteen are disease-specific, focusing on the following disease areas: diabetes (1) [67], cardiovascular disease (CVD)/hypertension (3) [68–70], diabetes and CVD (2) [71,72], heart failure (1) [73], osteoporosis (1) [74], chronic pain (1) [75], dyslipidaemia (1) [76], depression/mental illness (2) [77,78] and antibiotics (1) [79]. Five reviews have a specific focus on interventions in community pharmacy/outpatients and two on hospital pharmacy/inpatients, while fourteen have no specific setting.

Fifteen of the reviews concluded that evidence supported a positive effect of pharmacist-provided patient care. Most of these addressed disease-specific interventions involving dyslipidemia, hypertension, chronic pain, diabetes, CVD, osteoporosis, heart failure, depression/mental illness and antibiotics. Five positive reviews involved general pharmaceutical care or clinical pharmacy. Three specifically concerned hospital pharmacies and four community pharmacies.

Six reviews found limited or no evidence for the value of pharmacist-provided care. The reviews with weak evidence were in the areas of community/general pharmaceutical care, community/adherence in chronically medicated, community/diabetes and CVD, elderly/adherence and Hypertension.

All reviewers found studies that did not show effect. One systematic review registered that for all outcomes measured, between 0 and 57% showed effect.

Several reviewers pointed to methodological quality problems and called for more high-quality studies. Despite these methodological issues, however, the evidence from the systematic reviews shows a positive effect of pharmacist-provided care in a very large number of the outcome measures shown in Table 44.1. The pattern is that documentation for health improvement, medication use measures and satisfaction is good, but documentation for other humanistic and economic outcomes is less so.

Table 44.1 Systematic reviews of pharmaceutical care interventions.

Ref.	Title	Number of studies	Conclusion on evidence	Conclusion on methods	Results (significant effects)	Results (limited or no effect)	Area of care
Chisholm-Burns et al. [58]	US Pharmacists' Effect as Team Members on Patient Care: Systematic Review and Meta-analysis	298	Pharmacist-provided direct patient care has favourable effects across various patient outcomes, health care settings and disease states	None	Hb A1c, LDL cholesterol, blood pressure, ADEs, medication adherence, patient knowledge, quality of life, general health	Humanistic outcomes were variably favourable	General
Blalock et al. [60]	The Effect of Community Pharmacy-Based Interventions on Patient Health Outcomes: A Systematic Review	21	Evidence supporting the effectiveness of pharmacist-provided direct patient care services delivered in the community pharmacy setting is more limited than in other settings	None	Of 134 outcomes registered, 50 (37.3%) demonstrated beneficial intervention effects	The percentage of studies reporting favourable findings ranged from 50% for blood pressure to 0% for lipids, safety outcomes and quality of life	General Community
Kaboli et al. [61]	Clinical Pharmacists and Inpatient Medical Care: A Systematic Review	36	The addition of clinical pharmacist services to the care of inpatients generally resulted in improved care, with no evidence of harm. Interacting with the health care team on patient rounds, interviewing patients, reconciling medications and providing patient discharge counselling and follow-up all resulted in improved outcomes	Future studies should include multiple sites, larger sample sizes, reproducible interventions and identification of patient-specific factors that lead to improved outcomes	ADEs, ADRs and medication errors were reduced in 7 of 12 trials. Medication adherence, knowledge and appropriateness improved in 7 of 11 trials. Shortened hospital stays were seen in 9 of 17 trials	One study reported higher health care use Some did not show improvement	Clinical Pharmacy Inpatient
Van Wijk et al. [62]	Effectiveness of Interventions by Community Pharmacists to Improve Patient Adherence to Chronic Medication: A Systematic Review	18	Currently, it is impossible to identify an overall successful adherence-improving strategy performed by pharmacists	More well-designed and well-conducted studies on the effectiveness of interventions are needed	Eight studies showed significant improvement to adherence. Counselling, monitoring and education during weekly or monthly appointments showed some effect	Eight studies did not show any effect	Chronic medication Adherence Community

(continued)

Table 44.1 *(continued)*

Ref.	Title	Number of studies	Conclusion on evidence	Conclusion on methods	Results (significant effects)	Results (limited or no effect)	Area of care
Nkansah et al. [63]	Effect of Outpatient Pharmacists' Nondispensing Roles on Patient Outcomes and Prescribing Patterns	43	Most included studies supported the role of pharmacists in medication/therapeutic management, patient counselling and provision of health professional education with the goal of improving patient processes of care and clinical outcomes, and of educational outreach visits on physician prescribing patterns	Heterogeneity in study comparison groups, outcomes and measures makes it challenging to make generalized statements	Therapeutic duplication, total number of medications prescribed, prescribing patterns. Quality of life subdomains	Improvement in most clinical outcomes, although not always statistically significant	Nondispensing roles Outpatients
George et al. [64]	A Systematic Review of Interventions to Improve Medication Taking in Elderly Patients Prescribed Multiple Medications	8	Reviewers were unable to draw firm conclusions in favour of any particular intervention	Inconsistent methodology and findings. Until further evidence is obtained from single-intervention strategies, combinations of educational and behavioural strategies should be used	Regularly scheduled patient follow-up plus multicompartment dose administration aid was an effective strategy for maintaining adherence in one study, while group education combined with individualized medication cards was successful in another. Medication review by pharmacists with a focus on regimen simplification was found to be effective in two studies	Only 4 of 8 studies demonstrated a significant improvement in adherence	Adherence in elderly multimedcated patients
Graabaek & Kjeldsen [65]	Medication Reviews by Clinical Pharmacists at Hospitals Lead to Improved Patient Outcomes: A Systematic Review	31	The pharmacist interventions were well implemented, with acceptance rates from 39 to 100%. The 10 controlled studies generally showed a positive effect on medication use and costs, satisfaction with the service and positive but insignificant effects on health service use	Studies using rigorous designs, large sample sizes and comparable outcome measures are required	Medication use, costs, satisfaction	Several outcomes were statistically insignificant	Clinical Pharmacy Hospital
Hanlon et al. [66]	Can Clinical Pharmacy Services Have a Positive Impact on Drug-Related Problems and Health Outcomes in Community-Based Older Adults?	14	Large multicentre studies are required to test the cost-effectiveness of clinical pharmacy services for the community-based elderly and the impact of these services on such health outcomes as use of health services, timed functional-status measures and ADRs	Future large multicenter studies are required	Considerable evidence that clinical pharmacy interventions reduced the occurrence of drug-related problems in the elderly	Limited evidence that such interventions reduced morbidity, mortality or health care	Clinical Pharmacy Elderly Community

Rubio-Valera et al. [77]	Effectiveness of Pharmacist Care in the Improvement of Adherence to Antidepressants: A Systematic Review and Meta-analysis	6	Pharmacist intervention is effective in the improvement of patient adherence to antidepressants	Data limited, particularly outside United States	Adherence: pooled OR 1.64		Antidepressants adherence
Aguiar et al. [68]	Pharmaceutical Care in Hypertensive Patients: A Systematic Literature Review	16	Few studies showed statistically significant improvement in blood pressure	Lack of hardiness and many important limitations were common. Improvements to research design are recommended	Systolic blood pressure was the most positively impacted outcome		Hypertension
Charrois et al. [76]	A Systematic Review of the Evidence for Pharmacist Care of Patients with Dyslipidaemia	21	Enhanced pharmacist care improves lipid parameters – notably LDL levels – in patients with dyslipidaemia	Mean total cholesterol results were highly heterogeneous Adherence data could not be analysed	Mean LDL, mean total cholesterol, target lipid parameters, having lipid panel recommended, having changes in lipid-lowering therapy	Adherence	Dyslipidaemia
Machado et al. [69]	Sensitivity of Patient Outcomes to Pharmacist Interventions. Part II: Systematic Review and Meta-analysis in Hypertension Management	28	Systolic blood pressure is sensitive to pharmacists' interventions	Other outcomes may also be sensitive, but more high-quality studies are needed	Systolic blood pressure 39 outcomes (57%) were sensitive to pharmacists' interventions	Diastolic blood pressure, quality of life, adherence	Hypertension
Bennett et al. [75]	Educational Interventions by Pharmacists to Patients with Chronic Pain: Systematic Review and Meta-analysis	4	Pharmacist-delivered educational interventions seem to reduce adverse events and improve satisfaction, but their clinical benefit in pain intensity is debatable	Deeper understanding and evaluation of the active components of these interventions is needed	Average pain, adverse effects, patient satisfaction	Interference from pain in daily life, self-efficacy	Chronic pain education
Evans et al. [71]	Diabetes and Cardiovascular Disease Interventions by Community Pharmacists: A Systematic Review	40	Unproven clinical significance	Poor study quality, time-intensive interventions and unproven clinical significance warrant the need for further high-quality studies		No specific intervention emerged as superior	Diabetes and CVD community

(continued)

Table 44.1 *(continued)*

Ref.	Title	Number of studies	Conclusion on evidence	Conclusion on methods	Results (significant effects)	Results (limited or no effect)	Area of care
Santschi et al. [72]	Pharmacist Interventions to Improve Cardiovascular Disease Risk Factors in Diabetes: A Systematic Review and Meta-analysis of Randomized Controlled Trials	15	Supports pharmacist interventions (alone or in collaboration with other health care professionals) to improve major CVD risk factors among outpatients with diabetes		Systolic blood pressure, diastolic blood pressure, total cholesterol, LDL cholesterol, BMI	HDL cholesterol	Diabetes and CVD
Altowaijri et al. [70]	A Systematic Review of the Clinical and Economic Effectiveness of Clinical Pharmacist Intervention in Secondary Prevention of Cardiovascular Disease	59	The involvement of a pharmacist demonstrated the ability to improve CVD outcomes through educational intervention, medicine management intervention or a combination of both. These interventions resulted in improved CVD risk factors, improved patient outcomes and reduced numbers of drug-related problems, with a direct effect on CVD control		68% of the outcomes reported showed that clinical pharmacy services were associated with better improvement in patients' outcomes compared with a control group		CVD Economic effectiveness
Elias et al. [74]	The Impact of Pharmacist Interventions on Osteoporosis Management: A Systematic Review		Data support a potential role for pharmacists in helping reduce gaps in osteoporosis management through identification of high-risk patients	More research is needed			Osteoporosis
Wubben & Vivian [67]	Effects of Pharmacist Outpatient Interventions on Adults with Diabetes Mellitus: A Systematic Review	21	Overall improvement in A1C for patients in a diverse group of settings and across multiple study designs. The results suggested that pharmacist interventions can reduce long-term costs	Findings limited by flaws in study designs, including the high potential for selection bias in the study populations	Glycaemic control (A1C), use of resources		Diabetes

von Gunten et al. [79]	Clinical and Economic Outcomes of Pharmaceutical Services Related to Antibiotic Use: A Literature Review	43	The most frequently observed outcomes with a positive impact were appropriateness of prescribing and cost savings. The vast majority of studies used multiple interventions in conjunction with pharmacists' recommendations to physicians. Coupled with the use of practice guidelines or educational strategies, these interventions demonstrated a positive impact on economic and clinical outcomes	Data are still sparse and sometimes contradictory; therefore, further studies with randomized controlled designs are needed	Appropriateness of prescribing, costs, length of hospital stay (mixed results)	Other measure outcomes: drug use, prescriptions, length of treatment, dose intervals, switch to oral route, mortality rate, treatment failure	Antibiotics
Ponniah et al. [73]	Pharmacists' Role in the Post-Discharge Management of Patients with Heart Failure: A Literature Review	7	Demonstrated the effectiveness of pharmacists' interventions in reducing the morbidity and mortality associated with heart failure	Using the Jadad scoring method, none of the studies achieved a score of more than 2 (out of a maximum of 5), indicating the potential for bias	Unplanned hospital readmissions, death rates, compliance medication knowledge	Number of hospitalizations (one study)	Heart failure
Bell et al. [78]	Community Pharmacy Services to Optimize the Use of Medications for Mental Illness: A Systematic Review	22	Some evidence that pharmacists can contribute to optimizing the use of medications for mental illness in the community setting	More well-designed studies are needed	Adherence, potentially inappropriate prescribing		Mental health community

LDL, low-density lipoprotein; ADE, adverse drug event; ADR, adverse drug reaction; OR, odds ratio; CVD, cardiovascular disease; BMI, body mass index; HDL, high-density lipoprotein.

Examples of individual studies in pharmaceutical care

Pharmaceutical care research has been taken up in both Western and – in the last decade – non-Western countries. Studies provide evidence for the frequency of drug-related problems in these health care settings, but also for pharmaceutical care delivered by pharmacies as a means to solve them.

As an example, the value of pharmaceutical care for patients with diabetes has been documented in the US-based Asheville study. This study showed that community pharmacy-delivered pharmaceutical care improved both haemoglobin A1c and patient satisfaction with pharmacy services in diabetes patients, with an 87% increase in direct medical disease-specific costs (USD52 per patient per month) on a short-term basis, but with decreased all-diagnosis costs [80]. The percentage of patients with optimal haemoglobin A1c increased from about 40% at baseline to more than 60% during the first 18 months of follow-up. In a 5-year follow-up, cost outcomes showed a reduction of USD1200 (39%) per patient per year in total mean direct medical costs [81]. The service has been implemented on a routine basis in the city of Asheville [82].

Another example is a long-term Brazilian programme for elderly diabetes patients [83], which showed improvement in adherence (50.5% of adherent patients at baseline versus 83.5% after 36 months) and significant improvements in the number of patients reaching adequate values for blood pressure (26.8% at baseline versus 86.6% after 36 months), fasting glucose (29.9% at baseline versus 70.1% after 36 months), haemoglobin A1c (3.3% at baseline versus 63.3% after 36 months), triglycerides (47.4% at baseline versus 74.2% after 36 months) and total cholesterol (59.8% at baseline versus 80.4% after 36 months). The results were verified in the intervention group but remained unchanged in the control group.

The value of pharmaceutical care for asthma patients has been documented in a series of therapeutic outcome (TOM) studies conducted in seven European countries and coordinated by the PCNE. A Danish study showed that TOM intervention could influence drug utilization (use of beta-agonists and preventive steroids); with time, the regimens changed more toward consensus guidelines among TOM patients. There were on average 2.4 changes in drug therapy per TOM patient. The largest number of changes (49%) involved inhaled corticosteroids [84]. The programme showed significant improvement in inhalation errors, knowledge, asthma symptom status, days of sickness and health- and asthma-related quality of life [85]. Economic analyses showed increases in drug costs but savings on lost working days, resulting in the programme paying for itself after 23 months [86]. German studies showed similar results and documented an effect on peak flow and self-efficacy [87,88].

As an example of non-disease-specific interventions, home medication review (HMR) services have been intensively evaluated. HMR is now delivered to community-dwelling older people on a routine basis by pharmacists in Australian primary care. Retrospective research using the Medication Appropriateness Index (MAI) documented that 99% of patients had at least one inappropriate rating at baseline, and more than 50% had a cumulative MAI score >15. The mean MAI score at baseline was 18.6, which decreased to 9.3 after HMR. The number of patients with a cumulative MAI score ≤15 increased after the HMR service [89].

A Dutch study of HMR intervention patients using five or more different drugs documented 10 potential drug-related problems per patient; 58% of all recommendations involved a drug change. In all, 27% of all drug-related problems were identified during patient interviews and 74% from medication and clinical records; those identified during patient interviews were more often assigned higher clinical relevance [90].

Review of existing and validated quality indicators

Indicators used in pharmaceutical care intervention research

Intervention research in pharmacies has been most widely performed in the field of pharmaceutical care. Pharmaceutical care intervention evaluations generally use the structure–process–outcome framework described by Donabedian [91].

Practically all intervention studies follow a number of process variables. In fact, it is a methodological challenge for this research that many studies only provide information at process level, even when links to outcomes are not firmly established.

Outcomes research is often based on the so-called ECHO model described by Kozma et al. [92], which suggests that in pharmacoeconomic research, interventions should be evaluated with respect to economic, clinical and humanistic outcomes.

Table 44.2 provides an overview of the types of process and outcome measures used in intervention research.

Table 44.2 Evaluation of pharmaceutical care interventions – process and outcome measures.

Type of measure	Typical measurements
Process measures	
Performance measures	Number of services/interventions delivered (e.g. medication reconciliation, medication review, medication use review, etc.)
	Number/proportion of patients in target group receiving intervention/service
Pharmaceutical care/ counselling process	Degree of implementation according to quality manual for intervention (e.g. advice-giving, pharmaceutical care process, service process)
	Degree of expert agreement on identification of drug therapy problems
Problem detection	Drug therapy problems identified (number, type)
	Risk factors predicted
	Patient-perceived problems identified
	Pharmaceutical care issues identified
	ADEs, ADRs and medication errors detected
Intervention registration	Pharmacist recommendations (number, type)
	Pharmacist counselling (number, type)
	Solutions accepted by patient
	Solutions accepted by physician
Implementation	Prescription changes
	Changes in drug utilization indicators
Outcome measures	
Clinical outcomes	
Final	Mortality
	Morbidity (e.g. symptoms, side effects, duration of illness, severity of illness, etc.)
	PDRM
Intermediate	Clinical measurements (e.g. blood pressure, HbA1C, lipid profiles, lung function, weight, BMI, etc.) – value or target
	Medication appropriateness
	Health care contacts (hospital admission, emergency contacts, GP contacts, etc.)
Humanistic outcomes	
Final	Health-related quality of life (general or disease-specific)
	Functionality in daily living
	Work status
	Patient perceived health benefits
	Patient satisfaction
Intermediate	Patient knowledge and beliefs
	Patient self-efficacy
	Patient attitudes
	Patient behaviour (e.g. adherence, lifestyle changes, etc.)
Economic outcomes	
Final	Cost-effectiveness or cost benefit for society or health care
	Cost-effectiveness or cost benefit for payers
	Patient costs
	Pharmacy business viability
Intermediate	Drug expenditures
	Health care resources

ADE, adverse drug event; ADR, adverse drug reaction; PDRM, preventable drug-related morbidity; BMI, body mass index; GP, general practitioner.

The table is based on evidence reports from the Danish Evidence Database for Pharmacy Practice [93] and the systematic review studies in Table 44.1. The table distinguishes between final and intermediate outcomes [94], where final outcomes at, for example, patient level can be categorized according to the 5Ds model suggested by Lohr [95] (death, disease, disability, discomfort and dissatisfaction). Final outcomes can be difficult to access in pharmacy-driven projects or may require more statistical power than is realistic in practice research. Hence, intermediate outcomes (including effects on drug use) are also important evaluation measures.

Indicators for drug-related problems

Most common in pharmaceutical care research is the development of indicators for drug-related problems or drug therapy problems. Nearly all pharmaceutical care intervention studies will have a focus on drug-related problems and document drug-related problem interventions.

The drug-related problem concept has been described by Hepler & Strand [96] as 'an event or circumstance involving drug treatment that actually or potentially interferes with the patient's experiencing an optimum outcome of medical care'. These authors describe eight categories that allow for risk of treatment failure and risk of new medical problems caused by drug therapy to be checked: (i) untreated indications; (ii) improper drug selection; (iii) subtherapeutic dosages; (iv) failure to receive drugs; (v) overdosage; (vi) adverse drug reactions (ADRs); (vii) drug interactions; and (viii) drug use without indication.

Reviews have described different categorization systems used as drug-related problem indicators [97,98]. More than 20 tools have been published, but few have been validated, and there is no common consensus on their use. However, validity and usability have been documented for some categorization systems [99], including the PCNE system, the Swedish Westerlund model [100], the Spanish Revised Granada Consensus [101] and the Scottish classification system for issues identified in pharmaceutical care practice [102].

Indicators for preventable drug-related morbidity

While drug-related problem indicators have a process focus, pharmaceutical care researchers have also been active in developing outcome indicators for preventable drug-related morbidity (PDRM). These indicators are intended to form an important bridge between processes and outcomes of care and could in future be used in conjunction with other performance indicators for drug utilization [103]. The PDRM indicators combine outcomes and processes and aim to capture the essence of the pharmaceutical care approach, which is to prevent drug-related morbidity. Hence, they are used to identify patients who have experienced a potential adverse drug-related outcome and record whether they have also experienced a pattern of care involving inappropriate medication.

Box 44.4 Examples of indicators for preventable drug-related morbidity (PDRM).

Management: Concurrent use of two or more oral/topical nonsteroidal antiinflammatory drugs (NSAIDs) for 2 weeks or more.
Outcome: Dyspepsia or upper gastrointestinal (GI) bleed or GI perforation or GI ulcer or anaemia. The indicators belong in 3 pairs of managment and outcome indicators.
Management: Use of a long-half-life hypnotic-anxiolytic.
Outcome: Fall or broken bone.
Management: Use of an inhaled short-acting bronchodilator more than once daily or at night in an asthmatic patient with no regular inhaled 'preventer' therapy (corticosteroid or cromoglicate or nedocromil).
Outcome: General practitioner (GP) surgery or hospital contact due to asthma symptoms.

The PDRM indicators have been validated in several countries [104–106]. Pharmacy-relevant examples of the indicator format are shown in Box 44.4 [107]. The PDRM indicators have primarily been used in pharmacoepidemiological research, but Portuguese research has demonstrated that they have the potential for use in outcomes research and pharmacy quality improvement as well [108].

Validated indicators for patient care in pharmacy practice

Validated pharmacy indicators are available in the literature. In addition to overall frameworks for assessing pharmacy quality, a number of indicators for specific processes have been published. An overview of examples is given in Table 44.3.

Odedina & Segal [109,110] developed the Behavioral Pharmaceutical Care Scale (BPCS), which addresses the pharmaceutical care process. This scale was validated in the United States [109] and later adapted for use in a large European study conducted in 13 countries [110].

Bissel et al. [111] focused on the general counselling and advice-giving process in the pharmacy and published a validated set of criteria for assessing this process. The eight criteria are: (i) General communication

Table 44.3 Validated Pharmacy Indicators

Category	Reference	Title/aim	Type	Content	Country/region for validation
Specific process indicators					
	Odedina, Segal [109], Hughes CM, Hawwa AF, Scullin [110]	Behavioral Pharmaceutical Care Scale (BPCS)	Process	Instrument for observing pharmacy behaviour. Three main dimensions (direct patient care activities, referral and consultation activities and instrumental activities	USA, Europe
	Bissel, Ward, Noyce [111]	Criteria for Assessing the Appropriateness of Patient Counselling in Community Pharmacies	Process	The instrument assesses 5 criteria: rational content of advice, rational product choice, and referral to another health professional	UK
Total pharmacy frameworks					
	Azzopardi [112,113]	Validation instruments for community pharmacy	Structure	7 tools covering following areas: The setting of the community pharmacy, Dispensing a prescription, Responding to symptoms, Communicating with the patient, Equipment and professional services available in a community pharmacy, Consumer Services, Health Professionals	Malta
	Roberts, Keith [114]	Performance Evaluation System in a Correctional Managed Care Pharmacy	Process/ performance	7 performance indicators in the following 7 areas: clinical interventions, dispensing errors, missing medications, misshipments, pharmacist productivity, support staff productivity, pharmacy unit audits	USA
	Curtiss, Fry, Avey [115]	Framework for pharmacy services quality improvement: Grid and Self-Assessment Tool	Structure	More than 250 tasks in 7 core focus areas: Drug therapy management, Health programmes and services, Patient assessment and drug therapy, Distribution system and health information, Drug therapy monitoring and adjustment, Medical benefits provision, Health system assessment of results of drug therapy management for individuals and populations	USA
	Trap et al. [116]	An indicator-based tool for systematic assessment and reporting of good pharmacy practice (GPP)	Structure	34 indicators in 5 areas: System, Storage, Service, Dispensing, Rational use	Africa
	de Bie et al. [117]	Indicators for community pharmacy care	Structure Process Outcome	42 indicators in 6 areas: Patient counselling, Clinical risk management, Compounding, Dispensing, Monitoring of medication use , Quality management	Netherlands

skills; (ii) What information is gathered?; (iii) How is the information gathered?; (iv) Issues to be considered before giving advice; (v) Rational content of advice; (vi) How is advice given?; (vii) Rational product choice; and (viii) Referral to another health professional.

In the handbook 'Validation Instruments for Community Pharmacy' [112,113], Azzopardi described a set of validated tools by which to score community pharmacy practice. The tools cover the following areas: the setting of the community pharmacy; dispensing a prescription; responding to symptoms; communicating with the patient; equipment and professional services available in a community pharmacy; consumer services tool; health professionals.

Roberts & Keith [114] presented the development of a performance indicator system designed to evaluate the performances of departments within a managed care organization. The indicator system allows departments to be scored on a quarterly and an annual basis on a percentage scale in the following areas: clinical interventions, dispensing errors, missing medications, misshipments, pharmacist productivity, support staff productivity, pharmacy unit audits.

Curtiss et al. [115] presented a Framework for Pharmacy Services Quality Improvement, which comprises a Grid and Self-Assessment Tool allowing pharmacy organizations to score the relevance and importance of more than 250 tasks in seven different functional areas and attach action plans to the instrument.

Trap et al. [116] developed and validated an indicator-based tool for the systematic assessment and reporting of good pharmacy practice, which has been validated for use in Ethiopia, Uganda and Zimbabwe. The instrument comprises 34 structure indicators in the following five areas: system, storage, service, dispensing, rational use.

De Bie et al. [117] developed and validated a set of indicators for community pharmacy care, which have been used to inform pharmacy quality standards in the Netherlands. The set contains 42 structure, process and outcome indicators in the following six areas: patient counselling (6), clinical risk management (10), compounding (7), dispensing (3), monitoring of medication use (11), quality management (5).

Satisfaction with pharmacy services is a key quality dimension and has been widely measured. A review of studies in community pharmacy found 24 articles measuring patient satisfaction [118]. Of these, eleven measured satisfaction with general services, six with intervention services and seven with cognitive services. Most studies measured satisfaction as a multidimensional construct, but few instruments were validated.

Some validated instruments are available, however. As an example, Larson et al. [119] validated and updated an instrument for measuring satisfaction in pharmaceutical care. The instrument has two dimensions: friendly explanation (including items related to friendliness of care, the setting of care and medication counselling) and managing therapy (including items dealing with the concept of pharmaceutical care, managing drug therapy and solving therapy problems). In Slovenia, Horvat & Kos [120] developed and validated a questionnaire (PSPP-Q) that focuses on issues expressed as important by patients, services (and the supporting structure) and items of relevance to the individual pharmacy [120].

The European Directorate for the Quality of Medicines & HealthCare under the Council of Europe (EDQM) has in recent years focused on pharmacies and pharmaceutical care as a key part of the responsible provision of pharmaceutical therapy. It aims to develop European quality indicators for pharmaceutical care and to that end has commissioned an initial report which – based on interviews and literature – suggests the following indicator types should be developed [121]:

- performance/medicines substitution;
- hospital admission, frequency and duration (after pharmacy or nurse-led interventions);
- number of interventions (pharmacy and nurse-led interventions);
- number of drug-related problems/medication errors;
- patient satisfaction;
- regular customers/trust/patient–pharmacist relationship;
- process indicators (on key elements of pharmaceutical care, e.g. counselling, documentation);
- health status indicators (e.g. morbidity rates).

The work on indicator development and validation is currently taking place in working groups [122].

Application of quality indicators in pharmacy practice

Quality indicators are in widespread use in pharmacy practice today, used by individual pharmacies, pharmacy chains, hospital owners, professional organizations, insurance providers, and local/national health authorities.

Measuring quality is not easy in this field, as we have only a few numerical targets compared to prescribing. However, the degree of compliance with structure indicators can be a quantifiable measure, and this is commonly used.

Quality audits of individual pharmacies take place in most countries, carried out by health authorities, quality agencies and owners (e.g. chains or managed care organizations). They use indicators to follow performance.

The GPP guideline encourages countries to set national standards for pharmacy practice, and such standards are indeed issued by professional organizations in many countries [123–126]. National standards comprise sets of indicators, which will often to a large extent be structure indicators, where pharmacies are required to document that they have sufficient quality in their processes, organizations, facilities, documentation systems and so on. Pharmacies may also have to document quality measurements, some of which may be publicly published or benchmarked on a national level or between groups of pharmacies.

Many pharmaceutical care services are delivered as special services, coupled to a fee for service arrangement [127,128]. These services usually have documentation instruments, used to document performance and send claims to payers. Such instruments may or may not rely on research and validated indicators.

Only in a few countries do authorities publish national performance indicators to measure and benchmark the quality of pharmacy-delivered patient care. However, there is a trend in that direction, as the previously mentioned work by EDQM illustrates [121].

In spring 2014, the American Society of Health System Pharmacists (ASHP) announced that it was working together with national authorities to establish a set of national pharmacy indicators, but these are not yet published [129].

The Swedish drug agency, Läkemedelsverket, decided to launch a set of national quality indicators to measure professional quality in Swedish pharmacies following a liberalization of the pharmacy system. The indicators were to cover patient safety, accessibility and quality, and a suggested set of 21 were included in a hearing process [130]. The result was the following five national indicators [131]:

- Is it possible, both through the pharmacy's website and by phone, to preorder prescription drugs and to be notified by the pharmacy when they are ready to pick up?
- Does the pharmacy provide written instructions and counselling on the human and animal use of nonprescription drugs?
- Is there a wheelchair-accessible private space for individual counselling?
- Does the pharmacy provide time-booked counselling?
- Does the pharmacy have a documented approach to handling errors?

In 2009, the Dutch Health Care Inspectorate (IGZ) started asking pharmacies to provide data on 42 indicators of pharmacotherapeutic care. These indicators have also been used by Dutch health care insurers to determine whether pharmacists qualify for higher fees. The original indicators covered the following themes: patient records, contraindications, intolerances, interactions, drug delivery, internal error registration, patient assistance, patient experiences with care delivery, pharmacy compounding and pharmacotherapy policy. The indicators have been criticized and revised several times, and they are still under development by the Royal Dutch Pharmacists Association.

Finally, indicators are used at the individual pharmacy level in daily practice [132]. Examples of indicators followed at this level are given in Box 44.5.

The transparency that can be achieved by working with publically available indicators of pharmacy quality has great potential in documenting the value that pharmacies deliver in health care, medication safety and drug utilization. This is true both at the level of the individual pharmacy and on national and international levels.

Box 44.5 Examples of quality indicators at the individual pharmacy level.

- Percentage of substitution
- Level of service
- Quality of stock
- Number of prescription lines per day
- Number of prescriptions-related actions per day
- Number of documented changes to prescriptions
- Number and type of actions per year
- Number of care conversations per licensed staff member
- Number of care modules and activities per month
- Number of complaints and appraisals
- Patient satisfaction survey
- Personnel satisfaction survey
- Staff competence
- Pharmaceutical care modules and projects
- Pharmacy side effect reports
- Manufacturer drug recalls and pharmacy actions
- Complaints and appraisals

CHAPTER 45

Interventions that influence prescribing decisions and drug utilization

Jens Søndergaard[1], Dorte Gilså Hansen[1] & Debra Rowett[2]

[1]*Research Unit of General Practice, Institute of Public Health, University of Southern Denmark, Denmark*

[2]*Drug and Therapeutics Information Service, Repatriation General Hospital, South Australia, Australia*

KEY POINTS

- Interventions that influence the prescribing, dispensing and use of medicines can be broadly categorized as professional, organizational, financial, structural and regulatory.
- Interventions should be designed and implemented using evidence- and theory-based best practice.
- Drug utilization data can be used to support the needs assessment, design and implementation of interventions, and to measure the effect of such interventions.

Introduction

Medicines have made a profound contribution to the prevention and treatment of human disease, but there is considerable heterogeneity in benefits and harms across diseases, age groups and countries [1]. Parallel to the pharmacotherapeutic advances and commensurate with the increased prevalence of use of medicines, there has been a growing recognition of the significant burden associated with the harm caused by medicines to individual patients and their cost to society [2–9].

Our understanding of the patterns of drug use has evolved substantially across this time: initially, through data collected from paper-based clinical records, wholesalers and national health insurance databases [10–12], and more recently, through secondary analysis of electronic medical records. This has made population-level analysis of drug utilization linked to clinical data a reality. Drug utilization data is now accessible from hospital, residential aged care and community care settings.

These evolutions have brought insight into patterns of drug use and variability in prescribing. Research continually produces new findings that can contribute to improving the quality and safe use of medicines and the cost-effectiveness of health care more generally, through efficient and economic use of medicines.

However, simply identifying the problem or generating new research evidence is rarely sufficient to successfully and consistently change practice [13–15]. A wide range of interventions have emerged to promote the systematic uptake of research findings and other evidence-based practices into routine practice.

Despite significant resources invested in the research and implementation of these interventions, it remains a consistent finding that they have variable success, with obvious implications for the quality of patient care [14,16–20]. Research aimed at improving our understanding of how to design and evaluate interventions and how to use theory in the implementation of complex interventions is increasingly being undertaken in order to identify what factors modify the effectiveness of interventions [21–30].

The aim of this chapter is to provide illustrative examples of interventions that influence prescribing, with a focus on professional (educational) interventions [31]. Interventions to influence the prescribing,

Drug Utilization Research: Methods and Applications, First Edition. Edited by M. Elseviers et al.
Published 2016 by John Wiley & Sons, Ltd.

dispensing or use of medicines are widely employed by a range of stakeholders, including health insurers, health system payers, professional groups, academic researchers and individual clinicians seeking to improve their own practice. The motivation, goals and objectives of each stakeholder can and do vary, and it is an ongoing challenge to balance the many conflicting demands, especially in the face of increasing fiscal restraint in most countries [32–34]. This chapter is not intended to be a systematic review of the range of interventions that have been developed to influence prescribing over the past 30 years. For further reading, see some of the many reviews on this subject [16–18,35–38].

Classification of interventions

The many different strategies for influencing prescribing practices and the performance of prescribers have typically been developed based on different theoretical perspectives and assumptions about changing behaviour and habits [27,39]. Intervention methods are typically characterized as educational, organizational, financial and regulatory – or as the 4Es: education, engineering, economics and enforcement [40]. Although the literature includes a variety of terms by which to describe interventions, with new ones emerging over time [29], the Cochrane Effective Practice and Organisation of Care Group (EPOC) taxonomy [31], the Intervention Taxonomy (ITAX) [25], the 4Es [40] and the Behaviour Change Wheel [27] are the most commonly used. The EPOC taxonomy was originally developed in 2002 by the EPOC editorial team as a framework for characterizing EPOC interventions, and has been modified to incorporate new terms (see Table 45.1). The use of a common taxonomy for the content, structure and delivery of interventions is important in comparing and testing interventions in real-world settings [22,25,27,40]. A searchable database containing research into intervention strategies has been developed. It seeks to identify

Table 45.1 Effective Practice and Organisation of Care Group (EPOC) taxonomy of interventions

EPOC professional intervention	Description
Distribution of educational materials	Published or printed recommendations for clinical care, including clinical practice guidelines, audiovisual materials and electronic publications. May be delivered personally or through mass mailings.
Educational meetings	Participation in conferences, lectures, workshops and traineeships by health care providers.
Local consensus	Inclusion of providers in discussions, to ensure that they agree that the chosen clinical problem is important and the approach to managing it is appropriate.
Educational outreach visits (academic detailing)	Giving providers information in their practice settings, with the intent of changing their practice. Includes feedback on provider performance.
Local opinion leaders	Use of providers nominated by their colleagues as influential. Investigators must state explicitly that their colleagues have identified them.
Patient-mediated interventions	Collecting new clinical information (not previously available) directly from patients and giving it to the provider (e.g. depression scores from an instrument).
Audit and feedback	Summary of the clinical performance of health care over a specified period of time. May include recommendations for clinical action. May be obtained from medical records, computerized databases or direct patient observation.
Reminders	Patient- or encounter-specific information, provided verbally or in writing, designed or intended to prompt a health professional to recall information or avoid wrong actions. Usually encountered through their general education, in the medical records or through interactions with peers. Includes computer-aided decision support and drug dosages.
Marketing	Use of personal interviewing, group discussions, 'focus groups' or surveys of targeted providers to identify barriers to change, followed by design of an intervention that addresses these barriers.
Mass media	Varied use of communication that reaches large numbers of people, including television, radio, websites, newspapers, posters, leaflets and booklets, alone or in conjunction with other interventions. Targeted at the population level.

which interventions work and in what circumstances, and to alter behaviours of health technology prescribing, practice and use [41].

Interventions can occur at the individual clinician/health professional level (micro-level), at a group or team level (meso-level) or at an organization/policy/regulatory level (macro-level) [39,42,43].

Educational/professional interventions

Educational interventions (4Es) and professional interventions (EPOC) are designed to influence prescribing clinicians to modify their practice performance using clinical information strategies [14,40,44,45]. Information or knowledge is provided in the form of face-to-face education and training and/or written materials (e.g. pamphlets, websites). These interventions build on formal basic training, which can vary considerably. A range of strategies may be implemented, with varying effects (Table 45.2). There is not one strategy to suit all circumstances, nor any precise guidance on which combinations are more effective in multifaceted interventions. With respect to influencing prescribing patterns, those systematic reviews that have examined interventions targeting individual professionals show educational outreach (academic detailing), audit and feedback, use of local opinion leaders and reminders (for drug dosing) to be generally effective [16–18,35–38,41,46].

Another way of thinking about professional interventions is that some interventions primarily operate inside the doctor–patient consultation and others primarily operate outside it. Interventions that can be considered to operate outside the consultation include drug legislation and policy that influences licensing of and access to medicines, management support systems, didactic educational meetings at venues at a distance from the practice setting, local consensus processes and passive dissemination of information in medical journals and clinical guidelines. Other interventions have been targeted directly at patient behaviour (e.g. increased prescription charges, copayments and generic substitution programmes). Interventions operating inside the doctor–patient consultation include computerized decision support systems, pop-up reminders and patient-specific reminders at the time of the consultation. Academic detailing is designed to be implemented as close as possible to the real-time decision-making within the consulting room.

Printed educational material

Printed educational material is widely used worldwide to influence prescribing patterns. However, there is evidence of only a marginal impact when it is used as a standalone intervention and compared to no intervention [47,48]. For example, clinical guidelines are often disseminated as printed materials. Despite this being a common approach to influencing prescribing, simply making them available does not improve physicians' practice. The lesson is not, however, that clinical guidelines are of no value, but that implementation of clinical guidelines requires consideration of the context in which they will be used and of the importance of making more active interventions to facilitate their uptake in practice [27].

Audit and feedback

Audit and feedback are widely used either alone or as a key component of multifaceted interventions. This is one of the most studied health care quality improvement interventions [19,22]. The most recent Cochrane systematic review and meta-analysis of audit and feedback included 140 randomized clinical trials [19].

Feedback can be given in a written, electronic or verbal format, and may include recommendations on clinical action. It frequently involves giving physicians information about their practices or patient health outcomes that can be compared with other practices or with external standards (e.g. clinical guidelines). The format may be aggregated where there is no information about individual patients or, in some settings, where the information becomes more detailed with the inclusion of additional patients. Aggregate data are 'far away' from the individual user and more 'translation' has to be done in order to interpret them. There is thus a great risk that different conclusions will be reached about the quality of prescribing.

Actions, decisions, and behaviour are guided by habits, customs, assumptions and beliefs, and by the values of one's peers. Prevailing practices and social norms often define behaviour. Hence, it might be assumed that feedback including peer comparisons is more powerful than feedback without comparisons.

Identifying the key factors that contribute to audit and feedback interventions that are more or less

Table 45.2 Overview of educational (4Es) and professional (EPOC) interventions.

4Es [40]	EPOC category [44]
Education	***Professional interventions***
Range from simple distribution of printed materials to more intensive strategies, such as educational outreach visits by trained facilitators, monitoring of prescribing against agreed guidance (with further interventions, if required) and various consensus processes	Include (i) distribution of educational materials, (ii) educational meetings, (iii)local consensus, (iv) educational outreach visits (academic detailing), (v) local opinion leaders, (vi) patient-mediated interventions, (vii) audit and feedback, (viii)reminders, (ix)marketing and (x) mass media
Economics	***Financial interventions***
Include changes in insurance and reimbursement systems, patient copayment (including tier levels), positive and negative financial incentives for physicians and rebate schemes for overprescribing of agreed drugs Also include devolving drug budgets to physicians, with penalties and incentives	*1. Provider interventions* Include (i) fees-for-service, (ii) prepayments, (iii) capitations, (iv) provider-salaried services, (v) prospective payments, (vi) provider incentives, (vii) institution incentives, (viii) provider grants/allowances, (xi) institution grants/allowances, (x) provider penalties, (xi) institution penalties and (xii) formularies *2. Patient interventions* Include (i) premiums (insurance plans), (ii) copayment, (iii) user fees, (iv) patient incentives, (v) patient grants/ allowances and (vi) patient penalties
Engineering	***Organizational interventions***
Include organizational/managerial interventions, disease management programmes and interventions designed to optimize medication use in nursing homes Include prescribing targets, structured programmes for the introduction of new drugs and changes in task delegation	*1. Provider-oriented interventions* Include (i) revision of professional roles, (ii) clinical multidisciplinary teams, (iii) formal integration of services, (iv) skill mix changes, (v) continuity of care, (vi) satisfaction of providers with the conditions of work and with material and psychological rewards and (vii) communication and case discussion between distant health professionals *2. Patient-oriented interventions* Include (i) mail-order pharmacies (versus traditional pharmacies), (ii) presence and functioning of adequate mechanisms for dealing with patients' suggestions and complaints, and (iii) consumer participation in the governance of health care organization
Enforcement	***Regulatory interventions***
Include regulations by law, prescribing restrictions, prior authorization schemes and compulsory prescribing and dispensing restrictions	Any intervention that aims to change health services delivery or costs by regulation or law (may overlap with organizational and financial interventions) Include (i) changes in medical liability, (ii) management of patient complaints, (iii) peer review and (iv) licensure
	Structural interventions
	Include (i) changes to the setting/site of service delivery, (ii) changes in physical structure, facilities and equipment, (iii) changes in medical records systems, (iv) changes in the scope and nature of benefits and services, (v) the presence and organization of quality monitoring mechanisms, (vi) the ownership, accreditation and affiliation status of hospitals and other facilities and (vii) staff organization

successful is complicated by poor reporting of both intervention components and contextual factors in the literature [22]. However, further study of the Cochrane systematic review reveals that feedback is most effective when delivered by a supervisor or respected colleague, presented frequently, featuring both specific goals and action plans, aiming to decrease a targeted behaviour, targeting lower baseline performance and being delivered to non-physicians [49].

Method of delivery may be important to impact. Unsolicited prescriber feedback can be regarded negatively as intrusive, insulting and a hassle, leading to worse practice [50–52]. Recent advances in technology have allowed prescribers to receive feedback that can be individualized to specific patients [53], and clinical audit software can now generate audit data in real time.

Feedback to physicians on their prescribing patterns has been used in many countries in an attempt to improve practice (Box 45.1) [19].

Box 45.1 Example of audit and feedback.

> In Denmark, in an innovative and successful example, audit and feedback are encouraged by agreement between general practitioners (GPs) and the administrative authorities. An advanced information technology (IT) system has been developed in order to provide on-time feedback to GPs [51]. In some instances, the feedback is based on administrative data, while in others it is based on data from the GPs' own patient filing systems or on other independent data. In 2006, Danish GPs were invited to implement a data capture module. Data from the participating practices are automatically sent to the National Danish General Practice Database (DAMD) [94]. In return, the DAMD provides feedback to the GPs on each patient's treatment and quality of care. Data collected automatically include all drug prescriptions, all diagnoses of patient contacts, all disbursement codes and all laboratory data recorded in the patient file. Once a year, a pop-up appears on participating GPs' computers (Figure 45.1), which records data not otherwise available in the electronic journal system (i.e. the GPs can fill in further nonstructured information regarding diabetes care (e.g. information on diet, exercise and smoking habits) and whether or not the patient had been to the ophthalmologist and chiropodist).

Reminders, alerts and computerized decision support systems

Reminder systems are often implemented in health care settings. They have been used for many years. Manual paper reminders (involving no computers) range from simple notes attached to the front of every chart to more sophisticated reminders given under specific conditions for specific types of patient. Computer-generated reminders using physicans' patient record systems are generally delivered to health professionals when they are making decisions regarding treatment. Early systematic reviews showed that reminders to health care professionals could be effective in promoting change in practice across a variety of clinical areas and settings [54–59], including test ordering, vaccination, drug selection, dosing, prescribing and general disease management.

The effect of a reminder is influenced by how easily it fits within normal workflow. It is also important to understand and recognize 'reminder fatigue' and the impact that overriding reminders have on effectiveness. A recent systematic review assessed the effectiveness of computerized decision support systems featuring rule- or algorithm-based software integrated with electronic health records and evidence-based knowledge [60]. The authors found large between-study heterogeneity in interventions, settings, diseases and study designs. The results complement other analyses showing that computerized decision support systems are best oriented to directly affecting process outcomes (recommendation adherence), with decreasing impact on morbidity and mortality [60].

Academic detailing

Academic detailing is a proven intervention for influencing prescribing and has consistently been shown to influence prescribing behaviour [16–18,37,61]. It is also referred to as 'educational outreach' and 'educational visiting' – the term 'academic detailing' became widely adopted following a 1983 study by Avorn and Soumerai [61]. It involves one-to-one visits by trained academic detailers [62] to doctors, as close to where they deliver care and undertake prescribing as possible (e.g. GPs' consulting rooms, hospital wards). Academic detailers are trained to provide evidence-based information to clinicians in an interactive, educational encounter.

One of the key features of successful academic detailing is a sound understanding of the clinical content of the programme to be implemented. It is important that the academic detailer has excellent knowledge and can present both sides of an issue and is aware of any gaps

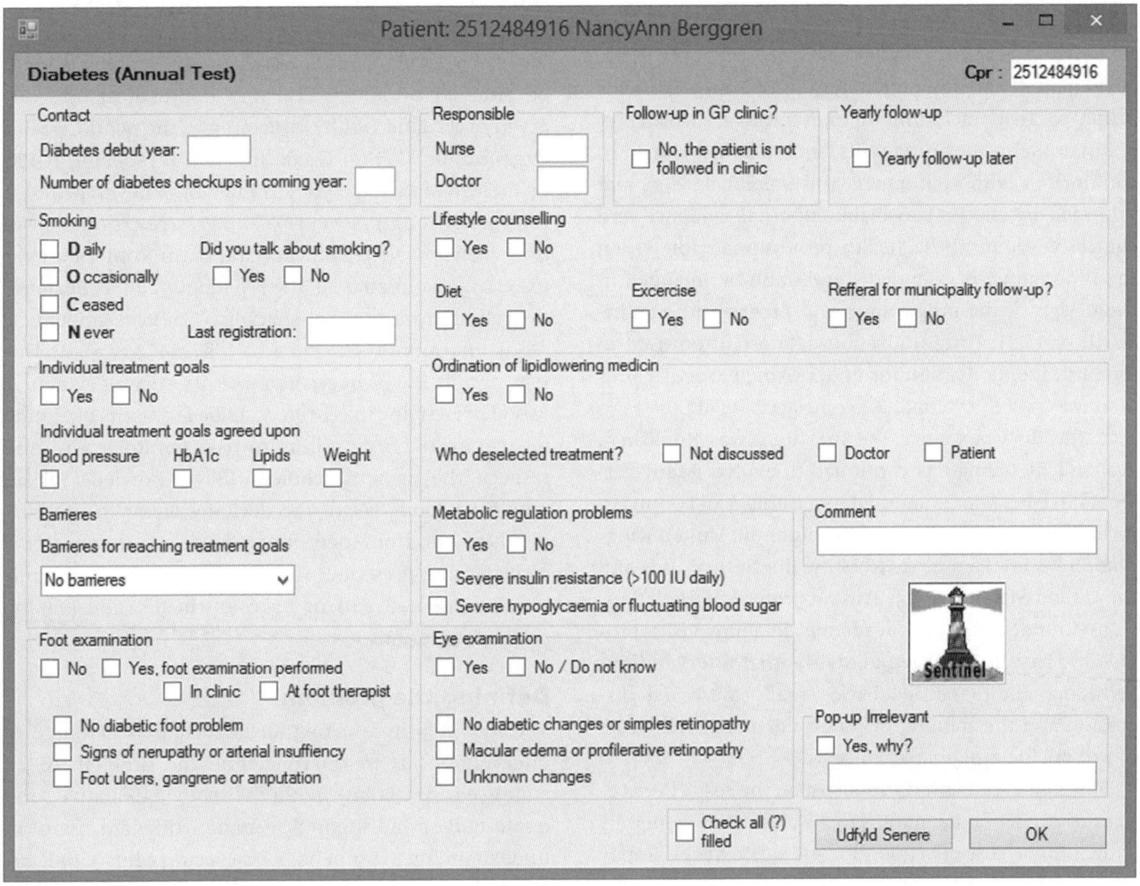

Figure 45.1 Danish data capture form.

in the evidence. Academic detailers must be critical thinkers and able to engage in deep conversations about the area of practice they are discussing. Training of academic detailers should include capability and competency assessment. A key principle of academic detailing is that its message is concise and of clear relevance to patient care. As with other interventions, the term 'academic detailing' is often used to refer to a variety of interventions, some bearing little or no relationship to the principles outlined here, and it is important to review the methodologies of studies that claim to be using this technique in order to confirm the nature of the intervention being implemented.

During a visit, key messages that are developed *a priori* and informed by the best available current evidence are discussed flexibly, responding to the doctor or other health professional's particular circumstances, needs and questions as they arise. The focus of the visit is on engaging with the doctor to move the educational interaction beyond simple communication of information or facts to an understanding of existing behaviour and identification of the key motivations for current behaviours and barriers to behaviour change. This technique is based on encouragement to achieve 'voluntary action' rather than coercion or enforcement. It recognizes the importance of building a trusted collaborative professional relationship between the academic detailer and the doctor receiving the educational intervention. Some authors have noted the potential for academic detailing to be a cognitive de-biasing strategy, which has important implications for future prescribing decision-making and the sustainability of change [63,64].

Academic detailing interventions should be based on academic detailing principles, using a social marketing framework as the theoretical basis for their planning, development and implementation [62,65–69]. The education package, including the 'key messages' for delivery in academic detailing visits, should be developed in conjunction with key experts and opinion leaders and informed by the best available external evidence and clinical wisdom. Those health professionals for whom the programme is intended should also be included in the design of the programme and programme materials (Box 45.2). Drug utilization data are often used to establish the motivation for undertaking particular programmes and to evaluate outcomes [18,70,71].

In the 30 years since the first RCT was published, academic detailing has continued to evolve. Many services have been implemented in a number of countries, including Australia, Canada, Belgium, the United Kingdom, Sweden, Denmark, Norway, the Netherlands and the United States [18,72]. Trusted professional relationships founded through academic detailing visits provide the basis for engagement with other interventions, including audit and feedback, small case-based discussion and the training of junior doctors in the basics of prescribing and pharmacology.

Only a few studies have reported on the cost-effectiveness of academic detailing [16,73], but they generally show it to be cost-effective [70,74,75]. However, it may not be so in all settings or for all prescribing, dispensing and medicine use issues [74,76]. Its general cost-effectiveness has seen academic detailing translated into national and regional funded programmes by governments and health insurance providers.

Box 45.2 Questions to consider when developing an academic detailing intervention.

- Is there a public health issue?
- Is there a drug utilization issue?
- Is there good evidence in the published literature?
- Is it controversial?
- Will the programme capture the attention of an individual doctor?
- Is it about new treatment?
- Is it about comparative effectiveness?
- Is it new knowledge about old treatment?
- Is there evidence of harm to patients?
- What are the barriers and facilitators?

Developing an intervention strategy

Ideally, a level of competency in prescribing should be attained by all medical and nonmedical prescribers in accordance with, for example, the World Health Organization (WHO) Guide to Good Prescribing (GPP) or prescribing competency frameworks developed at a regional or country level [77–79]. Prescribers often form their view of a drug's efficacy and harm from their own experience and that of their patients and colleagues, as well as from medical specialists, clinical guidelines, regulatory authorities and advertising [78,80–84]. This may or may not be in accordance with current evidence. 'Good prescribing' has been described in terms of aiming to 'maximize effect; minimize risk; minimize cost and respect [the] patient's choices' [85]. Knowledge about medicines alone is not the deciding factor in optimizing outcomes from medicine use; nor is it simply a case of increasing prescriber training [86]. Good communication skills and patient inclusion in decision-making are also important.

Defining the problem

The first step in selecting an intervention or range of interventions is to clearly define the problem to be addressed. Different methods (both qualitative and quantitative) and theoretical frameworks are useful in understanding why behaviours occur, who is the target audience and what is the nature and scope of the problem. Drug utilization research can contribute significantly at this stage by defining medicine use problems, including prescribing, dispensing and patient use (see Chapter 46).

Understanding motivating factors for current behaviour

It is important to understand the beliefs and motivations that might contribute to observed prescriber behaviours and to the context in which they take place. Prescribing decisions are commonly made in the face of uncertainty about the diagnosis, the effectiveness of a given medicine in an individual patient, past history of effectiveness, allergies, adverse effects, how the patient will use and adhere to the medicine, interactions with other drugs, the complex interplay of disease progression and the emergence of new conditions.

In addition to prescribing decisions about individual medicines, prescribing in the context of multimorbidity has its own set of problems. Multimorbidity is increasingly becoming the norm for many older people, but there is limited evidence and a dearth of guidelines in this area [87–89]. Most guidelines focus on a single disease or condition, although this is changing.

Time pressures and other resource limitations impact prescribing decision-making, as do meeting patients' expectations and balancing the burden of prescribing decisions (cost, complexity of medication regimens, investigation and monitoring, follow-up) [90,91]. The complex health care environments in which clinicians work also have a powerful influence on prescribing choices, because of issues related to access and affordability of medicines.

A combination of interventions is often used, and there is much to be learned about in which settings and for which problems this is likely to be most cost-effective [22,92]. Also, combined interventions targeted at both prescribers and patients have been widely used (e.g. to reduce antibiotic use and antibiotic resistance) [93].

Conclusion

Quality development programmes should be based on deep insight into the components that contribute to the success of an intervention. Interventions will need to evolve to embrace the complexity of an ageing population (with increasing multimorbidity) and an increasingly integrated team-based practice (with multiple people involved in decision-making related to prescribing). This is an important area of development for drug utilization research. Sound methods will be required to inform the design and evaluation of interventions into the future.

CHAPTER 46

Development, delivery and evaluation of implementation programmes

Elizabeth Roughead & Andrew Gilbert

School of Pharmacy and Medical Sciences, University of South Australia, Australia

KEY POINTS

- Successful implementation of drug utilization research relies on the measurement of utilization of medicines.
- The development of implementation programmes to improve medicine use is equally critical to achieving successful outcomes.
- The lack of application of theoretical behavioural frameworks to the development and delivery of health implementation programmes has led to poor results.
- Greater application of theoretical frameworks of behavioural and organizational change to implementation research is considered likely to promote the uptake of research findings into practice and to solve problems identified in current practice.
- Theoretical models of behavioural and organizational change drawn from the fields of health promotion and health psychology demonstrate the central place of drug utilization research in implementation programmes aimed at improving medication use.

Introduction

Drug utilization research is undertaken to identify potential problems with medicine use, with the ultimate aim of improving medicine use and thus health outcomes. Critical to the successful implementation of drug utilization research is the measurement of utilization of medicines. Equally critical to achieving successful outcomes where suboptimal care or gaps in practice have been identified is the development of implementation programmes aimed at improving medicine use. Rigorously evaluated interventions to improve medicine use in health care have had mixed results [1–7]. The lack of application of theoretical behavioural frameworks to the planning and delivery of health implementation programmes is considered to have contributed to this [8]. Greater application of theoretical frameworks of behavioural and organizational change to implementation research is likely to promote the uptake of research findings into practice and to solve problems identified in current practice [8]. In this chapter, we will use theoretical models of behavioural and organizational change [9], particularly those from the fields of health promotion and health psychology, to demonstrate the central place of drug utilization research in implementation programmes aimed at improving medication use.

There are three stages in the development of implementation programmes aimed at changing or improving medication or health service activities: development, delivery and evaluation [10]. Each stage relies on information from drug utilization research and stakeholder engagement. Further, each stage calls on a consistent mixture of aspects of theoretical models of learning and behavioural change drawn from the areas of psychology and health promotion.

Many theories drawn from behavioural science [11–15], communication science [16,17], social marketing [18,19] and community development and organizational change [10,20–24] can be used to inform the development, implementation and evaluation of health promotion programmes. Some of these models were developed for models of behavioural change in patients

Drug Utilization Research: Methods and Applications, First Edition. Edited by M. Elseviers et al.
Published 2016 by John Wiley & Sons, Ltd.

(e.g. Bandura's social cognitive theory), but many were designed for use by organizations (e.g. Green and Kreuter's health programme planning).

The integrative approach to health promotion planning [24] argues that health-related problems should be analysed within each individual theoretical model in order to enable robust programmes to be developed. Each theory offers a different perspective on factors contributing to the problem. Analysis in this manner enables many contributing factors to be identified and, as a result, comprehensive interventions which address all the identified factors to be developed. This can increase the likelihood that a programme will be successful. This type of analysis can also broaden the scope and depth of evaluations, because a greater variety of outcomes can be articulated and subsequently evaluated.

Theoretical models of behavioural and organizational change

We will describe the application of the PRECEDE-PROCEED health programme planning model [10] to the planning, delivery and evaluation stage of successful implementation programmes and discuss the underlying behavioural theories, including social cognitive theory [11,12] and the transtheoretical model of behaviour change [13–15]. We will also discuss the role of underlying behavioural theories in providing a range of perspectives that can help guide change. The success of programmes aimed at controlling tobacco use in Australia illustrates the value of this approach [25].

In the ***planning stage***, the PRECEDE-PROCEED model [10] identifies that there should be a needs assessment, which should include stakeholder consultation and an epidemiological analysis. From a drug utilization research perspective, the epidemiological analysis involves medication-related problem identification. The choice of intervention is also made in the planning stage; this will be underpinned by an evidence base, available resources and stakeholder engagement. Later in the chapter, we will explore how stakeholder consultation assists in framing the programme and its delivery and how both stakeholder consultation and epidemiological analysis contribute to planning an evaluation that is based on measurable and agreed outcomes.

In the ***delivery stage***, individual behaviours are often the target of drug utilization research interventions. We will examine how behavioural theories support the place of drug utilization research in changing behaviour through raising awareness, improving knowledge and promoting skill development among clinicians and patients, as well as providing motivation for action.

For the ***evaluation stage***, we will highlight how the evaluation must connect with the medication-related problem analysis undertaken at the beginning of the intervention. In any evaluation, all stakeholders must have the opportunity to interpret outcome data from their own perspective.

The next section examines in more detail the theoretical models that support each stage in a successful intervention.

Theoretical models supporting successful implementation programmes

PRECEDE-PROCEED

PRECEDE-PROCEED [10] incorporates individual behavioural change, organizational change and public health principles. PRECEDE is an acronym for Predisposing, Reinforcing and Enabling Constructs in Educational Diagnosis and Evaluation. This aspect of the model highlights the need to identify factors that predispose individuals towards given health-related behaviours, alongside those that enable and reinforce health-related behaviours. The PROCEED component of the model recognizes the influence of the wider environment on health. PROCEED is an acronym for Policy, Regulatory, and Organizational Constructs in Educational and Environmental Development. This aspect of the model draws attention to the need for organizational support or change and for interventions that develop a supportive environment within which educational strategies can be conducted. Within this aspect of the model, interventions also need to address the regulatory, political and organizational factors that may impact on the success of any education programme targeted towards individuals.

The model uses a diagnostic approach to determine the focus of the health promotion programme and recommends three diagnostic steps be undertaken prior to programme planning: a social diagnosis, which involves consultation with stakeholders to identify health and social issues of concern to the stakeholders; an epidemiological diagnosis, which involves consultation with health professionals and examination of epidemiological data to determine health concerns and priorities; and a behavioural diagnosis, to determine the behaviours that contribute to the cause or resolution of the health problems, including predisposing, enabling and reinforcing factors. Drug utilization research is central to the epidemiological analysis and supports the social diagnosis. Providing epidemiological data to stakeholders and consulting with stakeholders to understand what data mean can provide further insight into problems and potential solutions.

Individual behavioural change theories, arising from social psychological theories, are embedded within the PRECEDE-PROCEED model. When considering individual behavioural change, an individual's awareness, attitudes, knowledge, skills, perceived ability and motivation all impact on the likelihood of enacting any given behaviour. The role and impact of awareness, attitudes, knowledge, skills, perceived ability and motivation on behaviour are described in individual behavioural change theories.

Theory of reasoned action and planned behaviour

The theory of reasoned action and planned behaviour [26,27] highlights the importance of attitudinal awareness and social norms in influencing behavioural change. It was developed to help understand and predict behavioural intentions. The theory has three components: behavioural intention, attitude and subjective norm. It hypothesizes that behaviour is based on rational decisions and that an individual – or an organization – considers the consequences of a behaviour before performing or implementing it. A person's intention to undertake a particular behaviour depends on their attitude – positive or negative – towards the behaviour and how they think others want them to act. This is known as 'perceived social pressure' or 'subjective norm'. Thus, a person's attitude plus subjective norm forms behavioural intention. In keeping with this theory, interventions to change behaviour may need to target social norms and attitudes. This alone is insufficient to effect behavioural change. The theory does not take into account the control an individual has over their behaviour (volitional control), nor that an individual may not have full volitional control due to external factors (e.g. organizational rules within the institution where an individual is employed) .

The theory of planned behaviour [27] was developed as an extension of the theory of reasoned action [26] and includes the understanding that behaviour is also influenced by environmental, nonvolitional factors. A lack of supportive environmental or organizational factors is considered a barrier to behavioural change. The theory also includes perceived behavioural control as a predictor of behaviour. Behavioural control refers to a person's perceived ease or difficulty in performing a behaviour, as well as barriers or facilitators that influence that behaviour. Behavioural control is considered to be determined by both internal (skills, abilities, knowledge) and external (resources, opportunities) factors. The theory suggests that there will be a higher intention to perform a behaviour if an individual has a positive attitude towards the behaviour, a favourable subjective norm and greater perceived behavioural control. This is similar to the ideas expressed in Rotter's locus of control model, which suggests that internal rather than external control of reinforcements drives behaviour [28,29].

The theory of planned behaviour [27] explains that a person is less likely to perform a given behaviour if they perceive that opportunities for performance do not exist. Based on this theory, interventions targeting attitudes, knowledge, skills, social norms and opportunities for performing behaviours in a supportive environment are key to changing behaviour.

Bandura's social cognitive theory

Social cognitive theory [11] provides further insight into individual behavioural change. It recognizes that people learn not only through personal knowledge, practice and experience but also by observing the behaviours and actions of others (vicarious learning). The ability to learn from the behaviours and actions of others is called 'modelling'. This theory provides insight into why opinion leaders and peer educators, acting as models, can be powerful in interventions supporting behavioural change. In this theory, human behaviour is viewed as a three-way relationship, where cognitive, behavioural and environmental factors all influence one another. This relationship is known as 'reciprocal determinism'. Bandura speculates that although the environment can influence a behaviour and a person, through reciprocal determinism the behaviour and person also influence the environment.

Four conditions must be fulfilled for learning:

1 Paying attention to the new material or modelled behaviour.
2 Retaining the information. Retention is aided through symbolic representation, rehearsal and repetition. Retention of information allows for subsequent planning and anticipation of the consequences of modelling or implementing the new behaviour.
3 Reproducing the behaviour. Reproduction occurs when an individual has gained the necessary abilities and knowledge through trial and error.
4 Providing motivations or incentives. This determine whether the new behaviour will be enacted. Motivations and incentives include the benefits or inhibitions associated with the behaviour. These may be direct, observed or self-produced.

Bandura's social cognitive theory [11] expands on Rotter's locus of control [29] and argues that expectations of outcomes are influenced by whether a person thinks they will succeed or not. The term 'self-efficacy' is used to indicate an observer's confidence in their ability to act and implement an observed behaviour successfully. High self-efficacy means that a person is more likely to engage in novel behaviours. Such an able individual is active and tends to succeed in the new behaviour. Those with low self-efficacy are less likely to engage in a new behaviour and less likely to persist with the change.

Application of these theoretical models to the three stages of implementation programmes: development, implementation and evaluation

Stage 1: developing an implementation programme

Drug utilization research has been highly successful in developing methods by which to review medicines use, collect relevant data and identify and classify medication-related problems [30]. This information is critical to the development stage of any intervention; however, it is not sufficient. Interventions initiated with only drug utilization research data often have little impact, and some have unexpected outcomes [31].

Box 46.1 Example of a multifaceted programme.

> A multifaceted programme to improve benzodiazepine use in a regional setting in Australia was effective in reducing use by 19% [33]. Part of the reason for the success was the initial planning phase: the intervention was chosen only after stakeholder consultation with the medical practitioners and pharmacists in the region. The decision was supported by an epidemiological analysis. Data from the Australian National Health Survey and the Australian Longitudinal Study of the Ageing both showed high and prolonged use of benzodiazepines.

Successful programmes use an assessment process (e.g. Box 46.1). These assessments identify and engage key stakeholders, consider necessary resources and their availability and plan the outcome evaluation, all of which is supported by the drug utilization research. Stakeholders participate in the framing and planning of the intervention and in developing outcome measures. These processes are consistent with the PRECEDE-PROCEED model [10].

When considered collectively, the previously detailed behavioural theories highlight the need within the planning phase to understand current levels of awareness of the target problem (smoking, obesity), to understand current attitudes to the problem and attitudes to potential solutions, to identify current knowledge and knowledge deficits and to identify current levels of skill and motivation within targeted individuals and organizations (Figure 46.1). Additionally, the identification of social norms, role models and motivators is also required. This highlights the importance of social diagnoses (e.g. smoking while pregnant because family and friends all smoke) and behavioural diagnoses (e.g. reading in bed, alcohol use at bedtime, etc.), in addition to drug utilization research, before any programme is implemented. By showing the results of drug utilization research to participants at the planning stage, awareness, attitudes and knowledge can be assessed by tests. Evaluation planning is also required, and will be informed by the epidemiological, social, behavioural and environmental diagnoses, with measureable evaluation indicators needing to be planned for each of the elements to be targeted [32].

Stage 2: programme delivery

Ultimately, programmes to improve prescribing, use of medicines and health care require changes in behaviour among individuals and organizations. In the previous

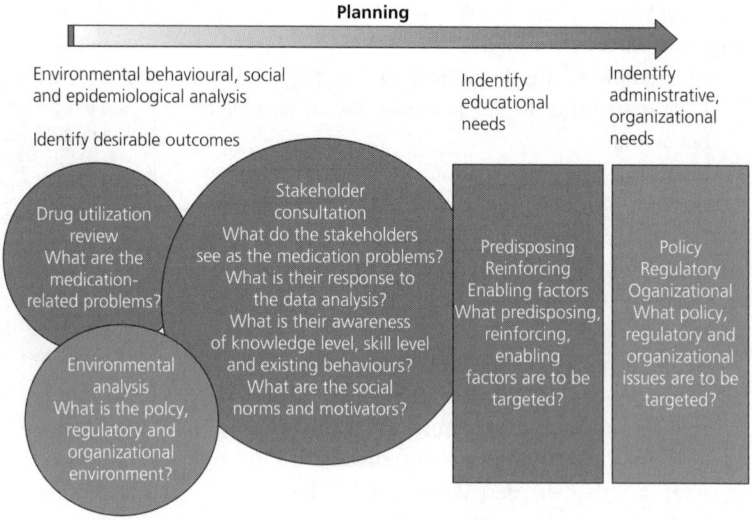

Figure 46.1 Health development stage.

section, we described a range of theories that highlight the importance of awareness, knowledge, skill planning and motivation for action in facilitating behavioural change. One further model, the ***transtheoretical model*** [14], also known as the stages of behaviour change model, is particularly relevant to intervention delivery. This model posits that change occurs in a continuous, cyclic process. Behaviour usually does not change suddenly, but occurs as a participants move around the ***stages of change cycle***, from:

1 precontemplation, where they are not aware of any problems; to
2 contemplation, where awareness is raised of potential problems; to
3 preparation, where they seek out information to respond to problems; to
4 action, where they trial new behaviours; and to
5 maintenance, where if the behaviours have been successful and motivation continues, they maintain the new behaviour.

The model also describes the processes of change that people use in order to progress through the stages [15], discussed in more detail later in the chapter. The model acknowledges that relapse is common and identifies strategies to encourage those who relapse to move back into the five stages of change at a level that meets their needs.

At the precontemplation stage, an individual has no current or future intentions to change. In the contemplation stage, they start to think about change and are aware that an issue exists. The process of consciousness-raising helps a person find information and develop awareness in order to move from precontemplation to contemplation. Thus, interventions raising awareness are used when people are at this stage. Promotion and advertising – or social marketing to raise awareness of brands or issues – is an intervention that targets people at this stage of change. Many interventions that use printed materials have been found to have small or negligible effects on outcomes [34,35]. From a theoretical point of view, this may be expected, but evaluation of the impact on awareness may be more appropriate when considering the stage of change to be targeted. Warning messages concerning product safety also target this stage of change; however, as there are five stages of change, warning messages alone will not be sufficient to move a person to the action stage, as messages about alternative behaviours will not have been provided. From a theoretical perspective, this is why studies assessing the impact of warning messages alone often find they fail to influence prescribing [36,37]; however, they have been demonstrated to improve reporting of adverse reactions, suggesting they are effective in raising awareness [38,39].

As described in social cognitive theory [11], individuals also learn through feedback as a direct result of their own experience; this is described as 'dramatic relief' within the transtheoretical model [15]. Negative experiences increase the reluctance to adopt a desired behaviour. This has been observed when the experience of a serious adverse event reduces prescribing of appropriate therapies in individuals or across a population.

For example, warfarin initiation for patients with atrial fibrillation fell by 21% in the 3 months after one physician's patient experienced a major bleeding event [40]. This highlights the importance of developing interventions where behaviours are realistic and achievable, so that negative experiences are not created.

Individuals also learn through observation of models and respond to social norms and environmental events; this is known as 'environmental reevaluation' in the transtheoretical model [15]. Interventions involving change champions, opinion leader education or peer education are all based on the knowledge that observation of models supports behavioural change. These interventions are generally successful [41], although results are mixed. The theories suggest that the success of these interventions is dependent upon the opinion leader being identified as a role model by the target audience. Where the target audience does not identify the person as a role model or believes that the modelled behaviour is not within its capacity to achieve, the strategy is unlikely to succeed.

Social cognitive theory [11] highlights the importance of providing opportunity for reflection in learning. The transtheoretical model [15] identifies this process of change as self-reevaluation, where an individual evaluates the new behaviour and comes to an understanding of whether a change in behaviour would be of benefit to them. Audit and feedback and academic detailing interventions both enable practitioner reflection on performance and thus facilitate behavioural change at this stage. However, they may fail without participant engagement of a sort that ensures cognitive processing and thus reflection on performance. Use of theory to underpin these interventions and so increase success is increasingly recognized [42,43]. However, an insufficient number of programmes have utilized theory to date to allow us to test whether its application improves effect [44].

Analysis of peer education programmes for consumers has demonstrated that one of the mechanisms by which they facilitate learning is through provision of the opportunity for self-reflection [45] (Box 46.2). Where the outcome of this reflection is positive, this process facilitates the progress of an individual into the third stage of behavioural change: preparation. In the preparation stage, the person has the intention to change and makes appropriate plans for how to undertake the necessary change processes. Interventions targeting this stage of change need to provide resources supporting change, such as information on the appropriate medicines to prescribe, guidelines, protocols and information on skill planning. Social cognitive theory describes the need for individuals to believe they can undertake the new behaviour, which is also called self-efficacy [12]. Within the transtheoretical model [15], it is described as 'self-liberation', and is the process required to move a person from the preparation stage to the action stage (fourth stage). Self-liberation is about people believing that they are able to change and making a firm commitment to change. Decisional balance [15] is also considered important in the transtheoretical model, and reflects an individual's relative weighing of the positives and negatives of change. The balance of positives and negatives informs decision-making and is another core construct in the transtheoretical model [15]. Within pharmaceutical marketing, sample supply and product familiarization programmes target this stage of change, allowing people to trial the new product. Role models, peer educators and use of opinion leaders, where they are accepted by the targeted audience as models, also target this stage of change, promoting the idea that the behaviour is achievable.

Box 46.2 Example of a theory-based educational programme.

> The use of theory-based educational programmes, including social cognitive theory, the theory of planned behaviour and operant learning theory, were assessed in examining the impact of an educational programme on management of upper respiratory tract infections among medical practitioners [46]. The study found that medical practitioners' confidence in their ability to manage upper respiratory infections without antibiotics (their self-efficacy) and the anticipated consequences of their actions (their decisional balance) were important predictors of their intended behaviour. Educational interventions based on different theories could impact on beliefs differently.

The fourth stage is where, by enacting the new behaviour successfully, a person's direct experience may change their attitude so that they can continue to meet their goals.

The final stage is the maintenance stage, where new attitudes and behaviours are supported to prevent relapse [14]. The process of change involved in moving individuals into this final stage is termed 'reinforcement management' [15]. For an individual to maintain a new behaviour, they must seek and use supports for maintenance. The behaviour needs continual reinforcement, and stimuli that encouraged old behaviours must be avoided in order to prevent relapse. This stage of change highlights the need for interventions to include reinforcement of messages over time and to provide feedback over time in order to maintain motivation to perform the new behaviours.

The stages of change model [14] is particularly relevant to the implementation of interventions aimed at improving medicine and health service use. The model acknowledges that within a population, individuals will be at different stages of change. Some individuals will be unaware problems exist, while others will already be enacting the new behaviours. This is why, when tested, single-strategy interventions are often found to give poor results; they are only relevant to those who are at the correct stage of change. In order to successfully address problems with medicine use, the theories suggests that a multistrategic approach is required (Figure 46.2). The intervention will need to include strategies to raise awareness of potential problems (e.g. warning messages concerning safety issues, 'advertisements' on the extent of problem medicine use) and resources to develop knowledge about what to do in response to these problems (e.g. guidelines, printed information, lectures). Interactive activities are required to promote reflection and self-evaluation, which is why case studies, audit and feedback and academic detailing can support behavioural change. Opportunities for the planning of self-efficacy and motivation can be provided through the use of feedback, opinion leaders and peer educators, as well as other incentives such as continuing professional planning points and financial incentives. Finally, as the model suggests people move through stages over time and there is potential for relapse, successful interventions will need to include repetition and reinforcement of messages and activities over time.

Drug utilization research can be embedded throughout the intervention [47]. The initial medication-related problem analysis may form the evidence base for – and be included in – the awareness-raising activities. Audit and feedback are particularly valuable for skill development and motivation, with the audit activities providing opportunity for reflection and rehearsal and subsequent feedback in response to actions providing motivation to improve or maintain performance. Academic detailing, due to is interactive nature, also provides opportunity for attention, rehearsal and reinforcement, all critical elements to successful behavioural change. It can be applied across all the stages of change. Role models, peer educators and opinion leaders can also be used to assist transition across all the stages of change, including awareness raising, knowledge building, skill planning, motivation and reinforcement, offering different messages to people at different stages in the change cycle.

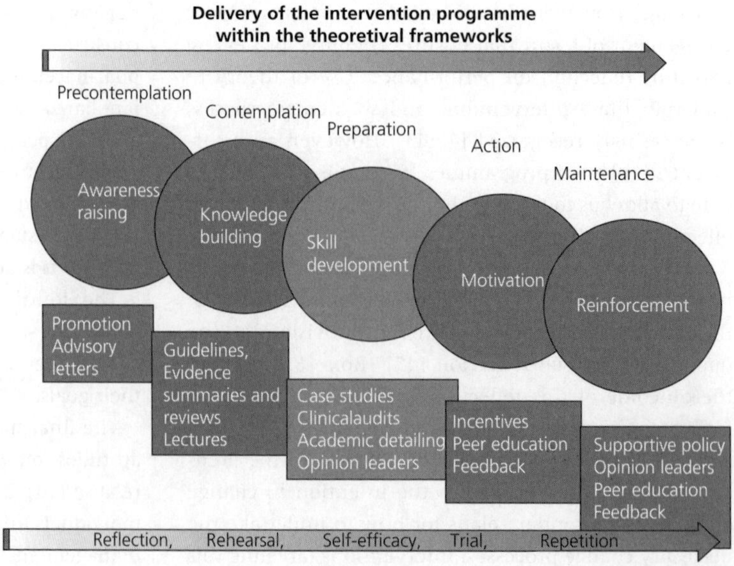

Figure 46.2 Intervention programme delivery stage.

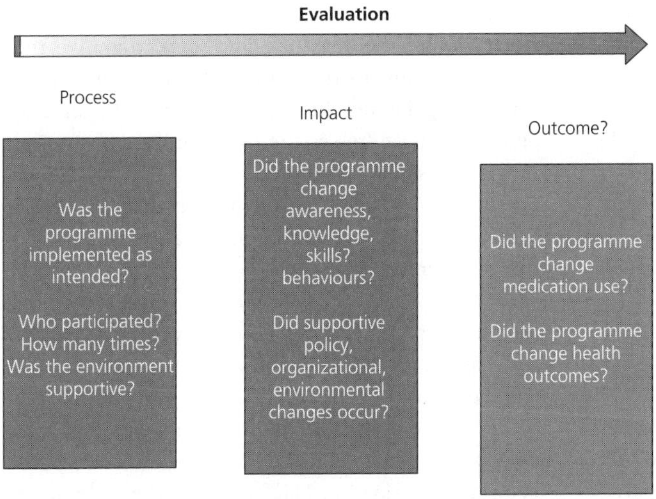

Figure 46.3 Evaluation stage.

Stage 3: evaluation stage

Successful programmes will have developed evaluation plans during the planning stage of health programme planning. Importantly, the evaluation plan will be consistent with the implementation plan and based on drug utilization research. All stakeholder groups should be included in discussions about the measurement of key indicators and the interpretation of results, as the results of an evaluation are more likely to be considered and responded to by stakeholders if they can see that their input has been valued.

Conclusions about the success or failure of an intervention must be based on knowledge that the programme was implemented as intended. Implementation programmes may fail not because the programme itself is flawed, but because it was not implemented as intended. For this reason, the evaluation plan requires measurement of the process, the impact and the outcome of the intervention. Thus, process, impact and outcome indicators are required within an evaluation plan (Figure 46.3; Box 46.3) [10].

Process measures are designed to monitor whether the programme is implemented as intended and include measures of participation. Impact measures are designed to measure changes in awareness, knowledge, skills or behaviours and are a measure of the programme's immediate effects. Impact measures may include measures of the targeted population's responses to intervention materials or events. Outcome measures may relate to intermediary markers of change, including changes in medication use, and may relate to the long-term outcomes of the intervention and related changes in health outcomes. Outcome indicators include measures of changes in the use of health services and mortality or morbidity (e.g. hospitalizations for specified conditions).

Drug utilization research again plays a central role in the evaluation, remeasuring the extent of medication-related problems in order to provide evidence of the intervention effect. However, evaluations limited to drug utilization research data alone may not provide the full story concerning why an intervention was successful or not. Process measures of programme implementation and reach must underpin any interpretation of the drug utilization research results before interventions can be considered a success or a failure. Additionally,

Box 46.3 Example of the use of evaluation measures.

Process, impact and outcome measures were a feature of the evaluation of a national campaign to reduce inappropriate antibiotic use in Australia [48]. Evaluation measures included campaign awareness and message recall, health professional opinions on the value of the campaign, changes in consumer knowledge, changes in consumer-reported use of antibiotics for coughs and colds and changes in antibiotic utilization. Evaluation methods and data sources for these indicators included national annual surveys of consumers, national surveys of health professionals and drug utilization data. The programme found positive changes in consumer awareness, attitudes and beliefs, demonstrating that it achieved its behavioural objectives and reduced antibiotic use nationally.

the evaluation must be relevant to the epidemiological and social diagnosis identified in programme planning. If the goal of the programme was awareness raising only because the majority of the targeted population was unaware of the problem, then the evaluation should be limited to assessing programme reach and changes in awareness only. Subsequent programmes aimed at moving participants to the next stages of change would then need to be developed, implemented and evaluated.

Conclusion

In this chapter, we have described theoretical frameworks of behavioural and organizational change and implementation research that have application to drug utilization research. We have highlighted the importance of the social, behavioural and environmental diagnosis in addition to the epidemiological (drug utilization research) diagnosis at the programme planning stage. Critical to this element is the involvement of stakeholders in all aspects of programme planning, intervention and evaluation, as is the need to address wider environmental and organizational issues in order to encourage behavioural change. We have described the application of behavioural theories including social cognitive theory and the transtheoretical model to intervention planning and highlighted the importance of a multistrategic approach that addresses the target group's awareness, knowledge, skill planning and motivation to change, and the need for the intervention to include opportunities for rehearsal, repetition, reevaluation, trial and error and reinforcement.

We have also described the role of drug utilization research in intervention delivery, particularly with regards to its position as the evidence base for awareness-raising activities and its role in motivation and reinforcement strategies to support continued behavioural change. Further, we have explained the need for an evaluation plan that is intrinsically linked to the epidemiological, social and behavioural diagnosis undertaken at the beginning of the process.

Finally, we have highlighted the need for an evaluation of the processes, impacts and outcomes of the intervention, in order to ensure that the programme was implemented as intended, impacted on the intermediary stages of the targeted behavioural change and had the desired effect on health outcomes [31].

CHAPTER 47

Towards a better understanding of prescribing-enhancement interventions

Frank May

Drug and Therapeutics Information Service, Repatriation General Hospital, Daw Park, South Australia

School of Pharmacy, Faculty of Health and Behavioural Sciences, University of Queensland, Australia

KEY POINTS

- Prescribing is an art practised in the context of multilayered uncertainties.
- Prescribing constitutes a relatively small part of the therapeutic relationship between patients and health professionals.
- Definitional difficulties around processes, mechanisms, outcomes and contexts confound many contemporary evaluations of the effectiveness of interventions designed to influence prescribing.
- Prescribing enhancement tactics in standard health care settings are complex interventions. As such, evaluative techniques are needed which can explore the interplay of theorized mechanisms with the varied contexts in which such interventions are applied.
- Future research exploring the effectiveness of prescribing enhancement interventions needs to extend beyond conventional randomized controlled trials (RCTs).

Introduction

Despite appearing to be a relatively trivial matter, the act of prescribing therapy in order to achieve better health outcomes has many complex dimensions underlying it. Since ancient times, prescribing has been believed primarily to be an art form. Deep knowledge of the nature and likely progression of disease and of the probable outcomes of different therapeutic regimes has always been the basis for the mystique attributed to it [1].

Today, scientific evidence and clinical experience are considered to be core components of wise prescribing. Patient preferences have recently been added to this mix, to make up the now familiar triad of elements of 'evidence-based medicine' (Figure 47.1) [2]. Before considering interventions which might enhance prescribing, it is necessary to examine the way in which these three components interact with one another in the contemporary context.

The context of prescribing

In most medical education settings, prescribing is not taught as a specific discipline, but rather is left to be learned in practice in the final experiential years of training. However, as a means to prepare medical undergraduates for an expected lifelong career of ongoing professional learning, medical educators generally pay a greater degree of attention to clinical aspects of pharmacology and therapeutics during later years of the academic programme [3].

As a result, there is asymmetry between clinical experience, which is steadily enriched during a lifetime of practice, and knowledge and understanding of the rapidly evolving sciences underpinning medical practice, which are generally gained early in a medical career. Individual propensity to share with patients and to engage them in decisions about prescribed therapeutic regimes is also particularly influenced one way or the other by subspecialty teachers and professional mentors in the early years of practice [4].

Drug Utilization Research: Methods and Applications, First Edition. Edited by M. Elseviers et al. © 2016 John Wiley & Sons, Ltd.
Published 2016 by John Wiley & Sons, Ltd.

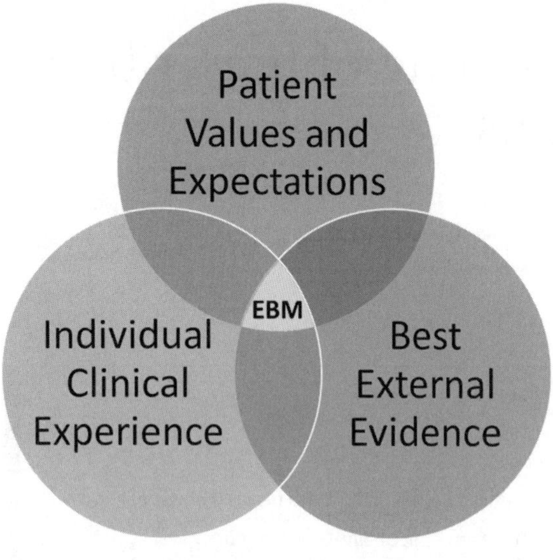

Figure 47.1 'Evidence-based medicine', as formulated in the Cochrane Library and illustrated by the EBM Triad.

Source: Reproduced with permission of Nancy Clark, The EBM Triad. © Florida State University College of Medicine.

There is a profound and irreducible uncertainty surrounding both diagnostics and therapeutics in the practice of medicine [5], and prescribing is a prime example of this. In primary practice, a key general practice educational text states that 'No disease-specific diagnosis is possible in 25–50% of patient visits to family physicians' [6]. Reflecting this uncertainty, major diagnostic error discovered at autopsy is relatively common. A 23.5% median rate of 'major error' has been noted in a systematic review of 26 autopsy series [7]. In one such series, false-negative diagnoses constituted two-thirds of such errors, and false positives the other third [8].

Apart from such prevalent uncertainty at many levels, there are myriad other contextual factors influencing prescribing decisions. Among others, these include social, attitudinal, demographic, financial, health system, education, knowledge and experience factors [9].

The indeterminate nature of pharmacotherapeutics

While keeping in mind the levels of uncertainty about underlying diagnostic issues and the frequently inadequate accounting for patient values in prescribing decisions [10], there is a fundamental underlying indeterminacy about prescribing choices in therapeutics. As discussed by Dowie [11], there can be no guaranteed correct decision when it comes to prescribing a particular therapy for a particular patient's circumstances. In therapeutics, there is no 'gold standard' or absolute definitional certitude as is customarily available in diagnostics. One may be uncertain as to whether a patient has a particular diagnosis, but inevitably diagnoses are definable by either criteria or exclusion and explicitly codified in textbooks of medicine. In the case of therapeutics, however, there can be no such categorical definitions of an invariably 'correct' therapy.

This reality about the nature of therapeutics has important ramifications when it comes to evaluating the quality of prescribing. Without careful study of individual clinical circumstances, it is usually difficult (with the exception of the use of frankly toxic substances/doses) to be categorical about the quality of prescribing [12].

In a number of countries, notably the United Kingdom, the availability of aggregated third-party payer data has led to an extensive industry built around examining prescribing trends over time at different levels of prescriber specificity [13]. This type of data has been successfully used for both short-term economic and direct cost-reduction purposes [14]. There is a hope that this type of data might also be used to encourage better-quality prescribing, with prescribing quality indicators being regularly published in the United Kingdom [15]. However, even with increasingly sophisticated use of such information, including linkage to practice data about individual patients, without mediation by academic detailers there is scant evidence that this form of intervention has been particularly beneficial in clinical care (as opposed to reducing direct costs).

The essential indeterminacy of therapeutics militates against the usefulness of this type of cost-focused data in enhancing prescribing. There is also a risk of perverse outcomes resulting from misreadings of the meaning of such data. Finding oneself in the lowest decile of prescribers for compound analgesics, for example, can lead to a belief that more should be prescribed; even more hazardously, being at the 50th percentile potentially leads to a sense of complacency about the judiciousness of one's ongoing prescribing. It has long been known that prescribing patterns more closely relate to practice demography than to standards of prescribing rectitude [16,17].

This problem of perverse outcomes from tactics which successfully change prescribing practices constitutes a significantly underinvestigated issue. Those tactics which involve use of control and financial or institutional power over prescribers to achieve change are particularly prone to such unintended consequences [18,19].

Classification of interventions which influence prescribing

There is a large body of literature describing the results of efforts to influence prescribing both at the individual level and at a more macro, community or nationwide level. A considerable amount of this research has been performed out of academic interest, but another prevalent reason for such investigations has been the wish of third-party payers to obtain better value from (or to reduce the cost of) medicines. A framework for classifying interventions supporting such objectives has recently been proposed [20] and used extensively in Europe [21]. This framework, termed the '4Es' approach, is based on long-standing mass-communication theory [22], adding the term 'economics' to the three customary 'E's of education, engineering and enforcement.

Unfortunately, investigations by manufacturers of medicines and other therapeutic devices into the results of their proprietary efforts to influence prescribing in favour of particular products are largely missing from the literature.

Extensive work has been done to classify and analyse different types of intervention which, to a greater or lesser degree, influence prescribing and other activities in the organization of health care. This work has been led by the Cochrane Effective Practice and Organization of Care Group (EPOC) [23], which began its work in July 1994 as the Behaviour Change Group, 2 years after the first Cochrane centre was established in Oxford in 1992. In March 1998, EPOC assumed its current name, and today it has its centre in Ottawa, Canada, with active staffed satellites in England, Norway, France and Australia. Figure 47.2 outlines a taxonomy of interventions for influencing the structure of health care as defined by this group. Full details of its elements are available from the EPOC website [24].

In parallel with and supported by EPOC, the Canadian Agency for Drugs and Technologies in Health (CADTH) maintains a publicly accessible database for health care professionals, which provides access to current evidence on the effectiveness of strategies specifically designed to improve drug prescribing and use [25]. This database uses roughly the same structure for interventions as those defined by the EPOC taxonomy, and provides high-level summaries of multiple systematic reviews of primary literature. For example, a total of 74 separate systematic reviews are currently tabulated in the case of the 'educational meeting' tactic within the 'professional interventions' strategy group. Summaries of these 74 individual reviews are available directly from the website, as are listings of the primary studies included in each systematic review.

Definitions, boundary delineations and outcome and context problems

Systematic reviews developed through the Cochrane EPOC group are of value in providing considered overviews of tactics for enhancing prescribing in high-quality primary research studies, mostly of experimental design. However, despite the deep and carefully delineated structures of EPOC's analytical work, the usefulness of these materials in evaluating the relative strengths of the effects of these different interventions is limited.

There are considerable difficulties associated with definitions of individual interventions and of the overlap and boundaries between them. These difficulties result from the complex, mutually entangled nature of interventions and the wide variety of contexts in which their effects have been observed.

The educational outreach visit tactic from the professional interventions strategy acts as a useful model for exploring these difficulties. EPOC defines educational outreach visits as 'Use of a trained person who met with providers in their practice settings to give information with the intent of changing the provider's practice. The information given may have included feedback on the performance of the provider(s)' [24]. Notable among EPOC's professional intervention strategies, educational outreach visiting (or academic detailing) frequently spearheads many of the other tactics. For example:

- Educational materials are likely to be delivered as well as, or instead of, an educational outreach one.
- As there is no restriction on whether a 'trained person' should meet one-to-one with a provider or with a group of providers, an educational outreach visit can be classed as an 'educational meeting' as well as, or instead of, an educational outreach one.
- The skilful trained person may well use 'local consensus processes' in their encounter with a provider.

Professional interventions

- **Distribution of educational materials**
- **Educational meetings**
- **Local consensus processes**
- **Educational outreach visits**
- **Local opinion leaders**
- **Patient-mediated interventions**
- **Audit and feedback**
- **Reminders**
- **Marketing**
- **Mass media**

Financial interventions

- **Provider interventions**
  - Fee for service
  - Prepaid
  - Capitation
  - Provider salaried service
  - Prospective payment
  - Provider incentives
  - Institution incentives
  - Provider grant/allowance
  - Provider penalty
  - Institution penalty
  - Formulary
- **Patient interventions**
  - Premium
  - Copayment
  - User fees
  - Patient incentives
  - Patient grant/allowance
  - Patient penalty

Organizational interventions

- **Provider-orientated interventions**
  - Revision of professional roles
  - Clinical multidisciplinary teams
  - Formal integration of services
  - Skill mix changes
  - Continuity of care
  - Interventions to boost morale
  - Communication and case discussion with distant health professionals
- **Patient-orientated interventions**
  - Mail-order pharmacies
  - Presence and function of patient suggestions and complaints
  - Consumer participation in governance of organization
- **Structural interventions**
  - Changes in site of service delivery
  - Changes in the physical Structure of facilities and equipment
  - Changes in medical record systems
  - Change in the scope and nature of benefits
  - Presence of quality-monitoring systems
  - Ownership, accreditation and affiliation of facility
  - Staff organization

Regulatory interventions

- **Changes in medical liability**
- **Management of patient complaints**
- **Peer review**
- **Licensure**

Figure 47.2 Cochrane EPOC group taxonomy of interventions for improvement of care.

Source: http://epoc.cochrane.org/epoc-resources. Reproduced with permission of Norwegian Knowledge Centre for the Health Services.

- The trained person may also fulfil the requirements for classification as a 'local opinion leader'.
- Feedback and perhaps even audit may be part of an educational outreach visit.
- Physical objects, print materials and computer application reminder skills are not infrequently left with the provider after an educational outreach visit.
- Marketing concepts may be incorporated in the approach used during a structured encounter.

Apart from problems of heterogeneity among EPOC's various professional intervention tactics, further sources of context, mechanism and outcome heterogeneity in the educational outreach tactic specifically include:

- The definition of precisely what an educational outreach visit consists of, among different studies of apparently the same tactic (e.g. the location of the visit, the location from which 'outreach' emanated).
- Whether or not third parties are in the room at the time of the visit.
- The conceptual structure of prescribing-enhancement messages.
- The background, training, imprimatur, knowledge and communication skills of 'visitors'.
- The nature of 'reminder' materials left with the prescriber.
- The extent to which an *a priori* trusting relationship has been established between the visitor and the prescriber at the time of the study.
- At baseline, and as defined in each individual study, how far 'actual' naturally occurring practice is located

relative to 'ideal' practice. This gap will influence the observable strength of a tactic, because it is almost certainly harder to measure change in aggregated outcomes when 'actual' practice is nearly the same as 'ideal' practice.

In EPOC's systematic review investigating the effects of the educational outreach visit tactic [26], efforts were made to take account of some of these covariates within the 69 randomized controlled trials (RCTs) that were of sufficient rigour to meet the Cochrane Collaboration's inclusion criteria. These efforts included an analysis of rankings of some of the covariates using metaregression techniques, the primary rankings being notionally assigned by EPOC reviewers. Insufficient numbers of studies were available to demonstrate anything but tendencies within the framework of the metaregression techniques' own, not inconsiderable, conceptual and statistical assumptions.

The authors of this particular review stated that 'Differences in intervention design may explain differences in the results but it is difficult to know if differences are related to the interventions or to the study contexts. Secondly in this review, the contribution of the educational outreach visit to the overall intervention varied from study to study making it difficult to disentangle the relative importance of the educational outreach visit component in those studies in which educational outreach visits were only part of the interventions' [26].

These issues for educational outreach visits are, to a greater or lesser degree, reflected in problems with other tactics listed among EPOC's defined professional interventions.

It is therefore difficult to be confident of estimates of the comparative strengths of the effects of these different tactics, given this level of heterogeneity. However, members of the EPOC group have recently noted when summarizing their gauging of the effectiveness of tactics from professional interventions that 'Generally, similar median absolute effect sizes are reported across the interventions' [27].

In this particular summary, the median absolute 'improvement' size for seven of the professional intervention tactics drawn from EPOC systematic reviews ranged between 4.2 and 12.0%. More significantly, perhaps, the interquartile ranges for included studies ranged between 3.5 and 18.0%, indicating (relatively speaking) very large differences in the outcomes of the high-quality studies included in these separate systematic reviews. It is worth noting that these studies covered professional behaviour change outcomes generally, and not just prescribing. However, enhancement of prescribing specifically made a considerable contribution to these results.

A further disconcerting aspect of EPOC's work is its failure to demonstrate additive effects from sequential addition of multiple different tactics and strategies. This failure was first described in a systematic review of guideline dissemination and implementation strategies [28]. These findings have been underscored in another important summary publication from the EPOC group [27] (see Figure 47.3).

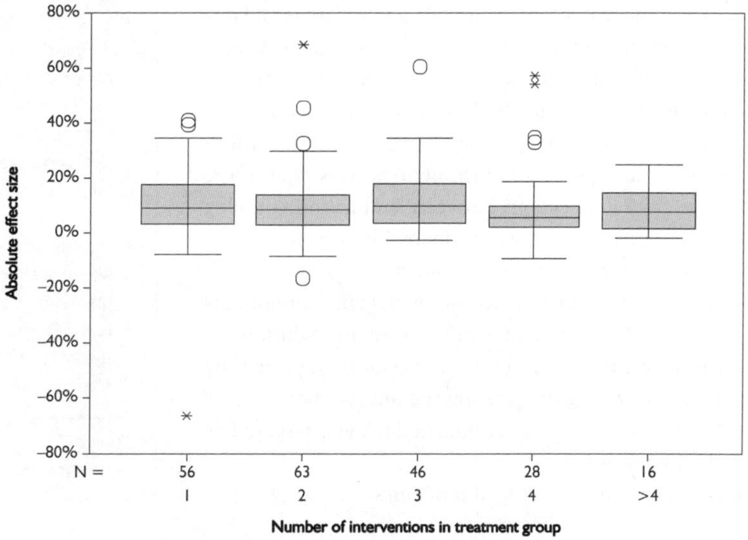

Figure 47.3 Box plots of the effect sizes of multifaceted interventions by number of interventions (strategies included both professional and organizational interventions).

Source: Grimshaw et al. 2004 [28]. Reproduced with kind permission from the UK National Institutes for Health Research.

The authors advance no convincing reason for this counterintuitive finding, apart from postulating that researchers may have lacked a theoretical basis for the inclusion of particular tactics among their multitactic interventions. As a result, it is important to examine possible reasons for these EPOC observations of similar median absolute effect sizes among tactics used to improve health care activities, such as prescribing. It is also important to gain a better understanding of the failure of these analytic methods to observe any additive effects from the simultaneous application of different strategies and tactics.

Complex interventions

In 2000, the British Medical Research Council (BMRC) published guidance on evaluating 'complex interventions' – interventions they suggested were 'built up from a number of components, which may act both independently and interdependently. The components usually include behaviours, parameters of behaviours (e.g. frequency, timing), and methods of organizing and delivering those behaviours (e.g. type(s) of practitioner, setting and location)' [29]. This original guidance document was updated in 2008 to highlight the 'difficulty of standardizing the design and delivery of the interventions, their sensitivity to features of the local context, and the organizational and logistical difficulty of applying experimental methods to service or policy change, and the length and complexity of the causal chains linking intervention with outcome' [30]. The newer guidance was explicitly framed to avoid the assumption that conventional clinical trials provide a template for all different approaches to evaluation, as well as the previous lack of attention to the social, political and geographical contexts in which interventions take place.

In terms of defining what makes an intervention complex, this guidance document affirms that there are no clear delineations between simple and complex interventions. It suggests the following as some of the dimensions which denote complexity:

- Number of, and interactions between, components within the experimental and control interventions.
- Number and difficulty of behaviours required by those delivering or receiving the intervention.
- Number of groups or organizational levels targeted by the intervention.
- Number and variability of outcomes.
- Permitted degree of flexibility or tailoring of the intervention.

From consideration of these dimensions, it is clear that interventions associated with enhancing prescribing must almost invariably be seen as 'complex interventions'. Box 47.1 summarizes some implications for the development and evaluation of complex interventions, quoted directly from the 2008 guidance document.

For the evaluation of interventions that enhance prescribing, this document provides an excellent primer, giving concrete suggestions for both experimental and non-experimental study designs. Through its associated case studies, it elaborates a practical stepwise approach to evaluation design. It uses a major prescribing-enhancement study [31,32] as a means of demonstrating the importance of understanding the underlying processes that cause a complex intervention (subjected to rigorous experimental study) to apparently either succeed or fail.

Overall, this particular study revealed contradictory results after the use of an identical academic detailing intervention for a range of prescribing topics (Specifically, adherence to an aspirin-use guideline relative to adherence to an NSAID use guideline): a 7% improvement in aspirin guideline adherence but a 3% reduction in the case of NSAID guidelines. A subsequent

Box 47.1 Complex interventions: implications for development and evaluation.

- A good theoretical understanding is needed of how the intervention causes change, so that weak links in the causal chain can be identified and strengthened.
- Lack of impact may reflect implementation failure (or teething problems) rather than genuine ineffectiveness; a thorough process evaluation is needed to identify implementation problems.
- Variability in individual-level outcomes may reflect higher-level processes; sample sizes may need to be larger to take account of the extra variability, and cluster- rather than individually-randomized designs considered.
- Identifying a single primary outcome may not make best use of the data; a range of measures will be needed, and unintended consequences picked up where possible.
- Ensuring strict fidelity to a protocol may be inappropriate; the intervention may work better if adaptation to local setting is allowed.

Source: Craig et al. 2008 [29]. Reproduced with kind permission from the UK Medical Research Council.

qualitative study [33] revealed unsuspected, internally consistent underlying barriers among prescribers to the use of the NSAID guideline, which were not present in the case of the aspirin use guideline.

Similarly, when prescribers received the intervention with three or more persons present, the overall outcome from four prescribing-enhancement topics was a statistically nonsignificant 1.4% improvement. However, a highly significant 13.5% improvement was observed when prescribers were seen alone or in the presence of just one additional person. The underlying dynamics and processes contributing to this outcome in the one-to-one/one-to-two settings were found to be different from those applying in larger group contexts, independent of higher proportions of prescriber-attendees at academic detailing sessions in smaller, as compared to larger, practices [32].

In a further UK cluster RCT exploring the usefulness of computerized guidelines for management of asthma and angina in primary care [34], apparent complete failure ensued. Both prescribing and outcome-of-care parameters appeared unchanged by the intervention. However, when a subsequent qualitative review of the attitudes and opinions of primary care participants was performed, a different picture emerged [35]. Barriers to the use of the system were found in the perceived helpfulness of the computerized content, use of the computer system itself and the timing of guideline triggers in the study protocol. Using experimental designs, such computerized systems for prescribing enhancement have been found to be apparently effective in different primary care contexts [36,37].

Randomized studies of complex interventions (such as those designed to enhance prescribing) in which the authors conclude either positive or negative definitive outcomes warrant close examination. Companion studies exploring elements of process, context and mechanism will almost always shed further light on what has been working positively (or negatively) in relation to the desired outcomes. It is clear that without insight into, and knowledge of the processes of prescribing enhancement strategies, randomized trials can produce profoundly misleading conclusions.

However, when such insights and knowledge are indeed available, the following approaches to the evaluation of complex interventions are suggested by the BMRC guidance (according to circumstances and not in any particular order):

- individually randomized trials;
- cluster randomized trials;
- randomized stepped wedge designs;
- preference trials and randomized consent designs;
- N-of-1 designs.

Examples of suitable observational studies, including quasiexperimental designs, cohort studies, case–control designs and process evaluations have been suggested to be appropriate, depending on the circumstances.

A further invaluable source of detailed methodological guidance for observational studies relevant to the enhancement of prescribing practices comes from recent work in North America associated with comparative effectiveness research [38]. Comparative effectiveness research has been defined by the US Institute of Medicine as including not just the relative effectiveness of medicines and devices, but also methods of improving the delivery of care [39]. While this work currently focuses substantially on observational studies within existing (large) computerized databases, its basic premises concerning the interpretation of observational data need to be studied and applied in the evaluation of any complex intervention.

Evolution of methods of evaluating complex interventions

The methods by which an evaluation of a complex intervention takes place – and the exact nature of those methods – have become the subject of much spirited debate.

Within the social sciences literature, there has long been scepticism about the ability to fairly evaluate complex social programmes and interventions [40]. In 1996, two social scientists, Pawson & Tilley [41], put forward the concept of 'real' evaluation of complex systems, a process which relies on the idea that the context of an intervention plus mechanism(s) produces what can be observed as an outcome. A central contention of their work was that investigators need to develop theories about how, for whom and under what conditions complex interventions might work, and then use observational data to examine how context and intervention mechanisms interact to generate outcomes [42].

In 1997, the same authors contrasted this focus on mechanisms and contexts with the classical experimentalist's model of observing a system, then introducing an intervention to some but not all participants in the system and then observing again. They asserted that the experimentalist's model misses the basic point about how an intervention works and the critical role that context plays in its outcomes.

Arguments about such a paradigmatic shift remained largely within the social science sphere until Berwick [43] published a commentary in the *Journal of the American Medical Association* in 2008, discussing some inadequacies of an exclusively experimentalist approach to evaluation of complex social interventions. This commentary developed the case for more careful consideration of Pawson & Tilley's approach: 'Health care researchers who believe that their main role is to ride the brakes on change – to weigh evidence with impoverished tools, ill-fit for use – are not being as helpful as they need to be. "Where is the randomized trial?" is, for many purposes the right question, but for many others it is the wrong question, a myopic one. A better one is broader: "What is everyone learning?"' [43]. Vigorous debate then ensued, at least in the circles of medical science methodologists. In parallel, debate and development of 'real' evaluation concepts also progressed within the social sciences. A recent important review [44] and subsequent discussion of the state of thinking, particularly on the helpfulness of experimental methods going hand in hand with 'realist' approaches [45,46], has led to some significant implications for the evaluation of interventions which enhance prescribing.

In putting forward the view that while the RCT may be the best means by which to examine intervention causality, Bonell et al. [44] affirm 'that RCTs designed primarily to identify whether or not a specific intervention is effective have focused too much on the internal validity of the trial, addressing the question of efficacy rather than broader questions of reach, effectiveness, adoption, implementation and maintenance. This has led to an evidence base that is dominated by high quality RCTs of poorly theorized interventions, with effects that are poorly understood and unlikely to be universally replicated in translation studies or real world implementation. This model of evidence generation is oriented towards "accrediting" as effective specific intervention "products".'

The realist position advocates the formulation of 'middle-range' theories about particular mechanisms that might operate in different contexts to generate specified outcomes – in the current discussion, enhanced prescribing [47]. Through empirical work which tests, refines and better evolves these various hypotheses, a more detailed understanding can be gained of the way in which the contexts themselves influence how mechanisms achieve the goal of enhanced prescribing.

EPOC has provided high-level classifications of different mechanisms by which enhanced prescribing outcomes might be achieved. However, for the future, it is going to be necessary for researchers to dig much deeper into these individual mechanism classifications in order to more closely understand 'how' enhanced prescribing is achieved in different contexts and how these contexts influence the effectiveness of the intervention's approach.

It seems that 'realist' critics of exclusively experimentalist approaches to complex interventions have quite correctly forecast the results of EPOC tabulations and aggregated analysis work, with all high-level tactics (mechanisms) being shown to work (or not work) to a greater or lesser degree in different contexts. As predicted by realist theorists, the addition of multiple high-level tactics (mechanisms) for enhancing outcomes of rigorous experimentalist studies appears to provide no additional power, likely as a result of the widely different contexts and the disparate natures of the measured outcomes in such studies.

The approach suggested by Bonell et al. [44] offers a productive way forward for further research into interventions that enhance prescribing: having first theorized a range of 'middle-range' mechanisms for the enhancement of prescribing through elements of the intervention tactic, before/after observations of comparison (or, where sensible, randomized control) groups not receiving the intervention versus those receiving it should be undertaken. Whether or not the study appears to 'work' overall, a key finding needs to be the reason why positive or negative results are observed in individuals exposed to the theorized elements (mechanisms) of the intervention.

Still-evolving publication standards for such 'realist' studies of prescribing enhancements are now available [47], and preliminary concepts and standards are also available for the publication of reviews extending across all methods of study of a topic (termed 'metanarrative'), including experimentally derived data and materials from other learning approaches [48].

Conclusion

Knowledge of how to reliably enhance prescribing practice remains elusive. A definition of exactly what constitutes 'better prescribing', while seemingly clear in the macrosense, is far less clear when applied to the indeterminacy of a therapeutic relationship between individual prescribers and their patients. Prescribing quality indicators, while perhaps useful in a comparative macrosense, appear to be of marginal utility in the individual therapeutic relationship, and may even prove counterproductive [49]. The use of power and control over prescribers and their prescribing risks perverse outcomes and limits individual learning and growth of clinical experience.

However, the imperative remains to bring the value of hard-won scientific evidence to bear in the decision-making of individual prescribers and their patients.

In past investigations of methods to enhance prescribing, failure to appreciate the extent of confounding of experimentally derived conclusions (as a consequence of underlying complexity) has resulted in delays in understanding which intervention mechanisms work for which prescribers, and in which contexts.

The act of prescribing constitutes only a small part of the therapeutic relationship between a health care professional and a patient. Arguably more than making a well-judged selection of pharmacotherapy with the active involvement of the patient, the relationship experience of patient and prescriber powerfully predicates ongoing therapeutic success or failure [50,51]. When looking for enhancements in prescribing, it must be appreciated that these relationships represent the keys to resultant health outcomes.

A better understanding of the natural history of individual prescribing, such as was commenced by Denig & Haaijer-Ruskamp [52,53] in the early 1990s, seems important. Development of 'realist' studies testing theorized mechanisms of bringing about prescribing enhancement in different contexts for defensible outcomes is a further exciting area for development. The uptake of new tools and standards in observational research [38,54] will assist in this process. Better understanding of the place of experimental studies, systematic reviews and aggregation of learnings from all research literature (together with associated limitations) will also be important for the future.

It is probably now time to again acknowledge the indeterminacy and 'art' of therapeutics, confident that our understanding of its underpinnings is continuing to advance as a result of the gift of our sciences to health care.

PART 4
Epilogue

CHAPTER 48

The many futures of drug utilization research

Hubert G.M. Leufkens[1], Frank May[2,3] & Nicky Britten[4]

[1]*Division of Pharmacoepidemiology and Clinical Pharmacology, Utrecht Institute for Pharmaceutical Sciences, Utrecht University, The Netherlands*

[2]*Drug and Therapeutics Information Service, Repatriation General Hospital, Daw Park, South Australia*

[3]*School of Pharmacy, Faculty of Health and Behavioural Sciences, University of Queensland, Australia*

[4] *University of Exeter Medical School, United Kingdom*

Introduction

Drug utilization research has a wide range of historical antecedents, from political outrage over unexplained differences in drug prescribing behaviour to technical support for policymakers in charge of drug budgets. It is an eclectic discipline, focusing on all aspects of medicine use, utilizing a wide array of qualitative and quantitative methods and bringing together many scientific spheres. Over the last couple of decades, it has become a mature and valued part of the health care sector. It allows comparisons of countries, regions, populations, GP practices and hospitals in terms of how they prescribe, dispense and use medicines. Such comparisons have many policy and regulatory dimensions: drug utilization research may fuel new policies or regulatory measures, or it may be used to assess the efficiency or risk–benefit ratio of existing ones. Many analysts have argued that any policy or regulatory measure concerning medicines that does not have a well designed drug utilization research chapter is a waste of energy.

Drivers of the future

What the precise future of drug utilization research will be remains uncertain. However, (i) the nature of the output of future pharma research and development, (ii) the validity and quality of methods for the quantification of disease exposures and outcomes and (iii) how society handles and values new therapeutic options will be critical drivers of that future. The first will determine the ***contents*** of the field, the second the ***methods*** and the third the ***soul***. The future of drug utilization research will be shaped by all three drivers, independently and together. Contents will be mainly an external factor; methods and soul are intrinsic to the field.

Promises for the future

There are many challenges in emerging clinical and public health fields, including cancer, multiple sclerosis (MS) and hepatitis C, which need to be tackled based on sound and valid drug utilization research data. These include regulatory challenges, such as which patients might benefit most from new products, how to manage apparent safety concerns and policy issues and how insurance coverage can be sustainable, given high prices. From the perspectives of both policymakers and regulators, we should anticipate a strong future of 'integrative' drug utilization research. This must combine methods, involve a mix of both quantitative and qualitative approaches, capture data on drug exposure and outcomes and be open to lateral 'learning'. Such learning will be key to 'integrative' drug utilization research, ensuring synergy with 'confirming'. Increasingly sophisticated and more widely generalized use of secondary data is likely to become the norm, resulting from intensified recording of clinical data in electronic health records (EHRs). This, too, should contribute to ongoing learning.

The challenge for the drug utilization research community is to reach global integration, bringing

Drug Utilization Research: Methods and Applications, First Edition. Edited by M. Elseviers et al.
Published 2016 by John Wiley & Sons, Ltd.

together Europe and Australasia (mostly universal-coverage health care systems), Canada (private and public systems), the United States (private health insurers and health maintenance organizations) and Africa, Asia and Latin America (health care systems for low/middle-income countries and up and coming economic powers).

Caveats for the future

While it has advantages for the drug utilization researcher, the advent of larger databases containing administrative or clinical data also brings new responsibilities. It is tempting to think that studies using such data will be effective in influencing health policy and will result in actual changes in health care. However, drug utilization researchers must be aware of the danger of oversimplifying secondary data to 'yes' or 'no' statements (expressed digitally as '1' and '0'), particularly when assessing exposure, covariates and outcomes. We must avoid both overinterpretation of drug utilization data and blindness to the subtleties underlying them.

Digitized data generated through regular health care delivery may not always have the required levels of precision. For frontline health care workers, the care of patients is of paramount importance – not the creation of perfect datasets. They need to be supported and encouraged to create better medical documentation, based on highly structured clinical records and sophisticated end-user terminologies, enabling the wider health workforce to participate in valid secondary use of data.

Drug utilization research, particularly that using digitized third-party payer data, also needs to be accompanied by judicious sensitivity analyses and systematic sample-checking. Recommendations for policy action will produce more consistent health care outcomes if these forms of validation are routinely applied in our work.

Moreover, sloppy data, poor analysis and ill-conceived medicines policies can lead to unintended outcomes. Drug utilization research must strive to avoid becoming part of this problem, and instead contribute to its solution. This can be achieved by effective engagement between drug utilization researchers, clinicians and policymakers.

The role of patients

Drug utilization researchers need to consider who will be impacted by their work. Patients are the end users of all medicines. This brings us back to the soul of the discipline. How will society and, ultimately, patients handle and appreciate new therapeutic options? How much attention do we pay to the patients' own perspectives when we interpret data on nonadherence? Are we aware of the epistemological and social contexts in which medicines are used by patients?

Two options are available to us. First, researchers could make patients the focus of their research. Or, second, patients could become research partners.

In the first case, taking patients' perspectives seriously may lead to the investigation of new topics and real-life problems. We need to understand how patients manage complex medicines regimens in real life, how we can harness their expertise in self-management of chronic disease and how we can best support them. We need to conduct pragmatic clinical trials that include comorbid patients taking multiple medicines. New research topics could include the determination of minimum effective doses, the effectiveness and safety of drug and nondrug treatments in situations of variable implementation and how forgiving particular drugs are when not taken as prescribed.

In the second case, it has been argued that if the users of research, including patients, are involved in setting research agendas, then the results are more likely to be useful and less likely to be wasted. There is no reason why patients should not be involved in all stages of the research cycle, as is already done in other settings. Patient involvement could contribute to shaping the research agenda. The European Medicines Agency (EMA) has recognized the value of patient voices in the evaluation of medicines and has included them in the licensing and development of new pharmacotherapeutic interventions. More accurate tools for recording treatment burden and gathering patient-reported outcomes are needed. These should be developed together with patients in order to find the most effective and least disruptive schemas for drug treatment while ensuring affordability and equitable access.

The field of drug utilization will gain content and soul if this focus and cooperation with patients can be established. A prerequisite is that this systematic cooperation and alliance between patients and researchers should develop independently, ideally supported by publicly funded organizations.

Conclusion

There are many futures possible for drug utilization research. There will always be much to learn and many new methodologies to develop. Collaboration between researchers, policymakers, payers and patients will ultimately result in drug utilization research becoming a robust source of valuable intelligence in the life cycle of medicines.

Acknowledgements

This document is based on a compilation of three presentations (given by each of the authors) at the Final Session of the EuroDURG Conference in Groningen (29 August 2014), entitled 'Future Perspectives of Drug Utilisation Research'. These presentations were inspired by a 20-year-old article: Leufkens H, Haaijer-Ruskamp F, Bakker A, Dukes G. Scenario analysis of the future of medicines. *BMJ* 1994;**309**(6962):1137–40. The compilation of this epilogue was endorsed by the authors and by the members of the editorial board.

Glossary

Chapter 7 Individual-level drug utilization analyses

Incidence rate Used in epidemiology to express the rate of newly diseased in a population. For example, 'the incidence rate of insulin use is 12 new users per 1000 person-years'.

Kaplan–Meier technique Used in drug survival analysis to chart the rate at which drug users discontinue their current drug treatment, while accounting for censoring.

Lorenz curve In drug utilization, a graph of the proportion of drug use that is accounted for by a given proportion of the most intensive drug users. For example, '1% of insulin users account for 4.5% of insulin use'.

Prevalence proportion The epidemiological term for the proportion of a population with a given characteristic at a given point in time. For example, 'the prevalence proportion of insulin use is 89 per 1000 inhabitants'.

Waiting-time distribution In drug utilization, the distribution of individuals' times from the beginning of a time window until their first observed redemption of a prescription within it. It may be used both visually and formally to estimate key features of drug use: duration of prescriptions, incidence, prevalence and chronicity of treatment.

Chapter 8 Measurement of drug expenditure

Clawback A funding element in a reimbursement system allowing third-party payers to recoup (part of the) discounts/rebates granted by various stakeholders, e.g. wholesalers and pharmacists.

Copayment The insured patient's contribution towards the cost of a medical service covered by the insurer. Can be expressed as a percentage of the total cost of the service or as a fixed amount. Copayment is a form of out-of pocket payment.

Copayments may be designed in different formats. With regard to copayment applied to medicines, commonly applied variants in European countries are prescription fees, percentage reimbursement /copayment rates and, to a lesser extent, deductibles.

Discount A price reduction granted to specified purchasers under specific conditions prior to purchase.

Dispensing fee A type of remuneration to reward pharmacies for their service of filling prescriptions. Normally it is a fixed fee that pharmacies are allowed to charge per prescribed item, independent from the price of the medicine.

Drug utilization 90% (DU90%) The number of drugs accounting for 90% of drug use. This is the 90% of the total volume of defined daily doses (DDDs). There are three quality prescribing indicators that this method can be used for:

1 The range of prescribing: how many individual medicines account for the DU90% segment; a relatively limited number of pharmaceutical products within a drug group is indicative of higher-quality prescribing.
2 Adherence to guidelines: the proportion of DDDs of guideline recommended drugs can be related to the whole number of DDDs in the DU90% segment, with a higher index expected for those prescribers who practice evidence-based medicine.
3 Cost-effectiveness of prescribing: the difference in the cost per DDD of those drugs in the DU90% segment compared to the remaining 10% is expected to be higher for those prescribers who are consistently cost-effective in their choices.

See Bergman et al. European Journal of Clinical Pharmacology. *1998;**54**(2):113–18; Teichert et al.* European Journal of Clinical Pharmacology. *2007;**63**(12):1171–7.*

Ex-factory price, manufacturer price, ex-manufacturer price The manufacturer's posted price. Discounts or other incentives offered by manufacturers result in an actual price that is lower than the ex-factory price.

External price referencing, international price comparison The practice of using the price(s) of a medicine in one or several countries in order to derive a benchmark or reference price for the purposes of setting or negotiating the price of the product in a given country.

List price The prices that purchasers display as those at which they are prepared to sell their products and/or the prices regulated by legislation. The prices of products as quoted in the purchaser's price list, catalogue, Web site or advertisements, or in a national price list/formulary etc. They are not necessarily actual transaction prices. Depending on the country and/or the product, they may or may not include delivery and installation costs, VAT and other indirect taxes on products, discounts, surcharges and rebates, invoiced service charges and voluntary gratuities. Certain pharmaceutical transactions, such as setting payment rates to pharmacies, may be based on list prices.

Managed-entry agreements An arrangement between a manufacturer and payer/provider that enables access to (cover-

Drug Utilization Research: Methods and Applications, First Edition. Edited by M. Elseviers et al.
Published 2016 by John Wiley & Sons, Ltd.

age/reimbursement of) a health technology, subject to specified conditions. These arrangements can use a variety of mechanisms to address uncertainty about the performance of technologies or to manage the adoption of technologies in order to maximize their effective use or limit their budget impact.

Types of managed entry agreements include Access with Evidence Development (AED), Conditional Coverage, Conditional Treatment Continuation (CTC), Coverage with Evidence Development (CED), Only in Research (OIR), Only with Research, Outcome Guarantees, Patient Access Schemes (PASs), Pattern or Process Care, Performance-Based Agreements, Performance-Based Health Outcome Reimbursement Schemes, Performance-Linked Reimbursement, Price Volume Agreements and Risk Sharing Schemes (RSSs).

Margin The percentage of the selling price that is profit.

In the case of pharmaceutical distribution, a wholesale or pharmacy margin is one type of remuneration awarded to distribution actors such as wholesalers and pharmacies for their services.

The wholesale margin is the gross profit of wholesalers, expressed as a percentage of the wholesale price (pharmacy purchasing price).The pharmacy margin is the gross profit of pharmacies, expressed as a percentage of the pharmacy retail price.

Mark-up A defined (linear or percentage) amount is added on to the cost of a good to create a profit (either linear or regressive at the wholesale and/or retail levels). In the case of the pharmaceutical distribution, it is one type of remuneration awarded to distribution actors such as wholesalers and pharmacies for their services.

The wholesale mark-up is the gross profit of wholesalers, expressed as a fixed or percentage add-on to the ex-factory price.

The pharmacy mark-up is the gross profit of pharmacies, expressed as a fixed or percentage add-on to the wholesale price (or pharmacy purchasing price).

Medical device A medical device is any instrument, apparatus, appliance, software, material or other article, whether used alone or in combination, including the software intended by its manufacturer to be used specifically for diagnostic and/or therapeutic purposes and necessary for its proper application, intended by the manufacturer to be used with human beings for the purpose of:

- diagnosis, prevention, monitoring, treatment or alleviation of disease
- diagnosis, monitoring, treatment, alleviation of or compensation for an injury or handicap;
- investigation, replacement or modification of the anatomy or of a physiological process;
- control of conception;

and which does not achieve its principal intended action in or on the human body by pharmacological, immunological or metabolic means, but which may be assisted in its function by such means.

Medicine price Price related to one or more medicines.

It may relate to different market segments (e.g. outpatient vs. inpatent market, reimbursement segment) and may be defined at different price types.

Nonprescription medicines, over-the-counter (OTC) medicines Medicines which may be dispensed without a prescription. In some countries, they are available via self-service in pharmacies and/or other retail outlets (e.g. drugstores). Selected OTC medicines may be reimbursed for certain indications in some countries.

Nonreimbursable medicines Medicines which are not eligible for reimbursement (i.e. coverage by public payers). Their costs are not covered by third-party payers, and have to be fully paid out of pocket by the patient.

Out-of-pocket payments The amount a person has to pay for all covered health care services for a defined period (often a year). It includes fixed copayments (e.g. a prescription fee), percentage copayments and deductibles.

Pharmacy purchasing price, wholesale price The price charged by wholesalers to the retailers (usually community pharmacies). It includes any wholesale remuneration (e.g. mark-up).

Pharmacy retail price The price charged by community pharmacies to the general public. It includes any pharmacy remuneration, such as a pharmacy mark-up or dispensing fee. It can be a gross pharmacy retail price (including value-added tax/VAT) or a net pharmacy retail price (excluding VAT).

Prescription-only medicines (POMs) Medicines that can be dispensed only on a health professional prescription.

Price Price is the value component of expenditure. The value of one unit of a product, for which the quantities are perfectly homogeneous not only in a physical sense, but also in respect of a number of other characteristics.

Price type The level (e.g. ex-factory price, pharmacy purchasing price, pharmacy retail price) at which a medicine price is set.

The price type reflects the perspective of the targeted stakeholders (e.g. industry, pharmacy, patient).

Price-volume agreements Agreements that focus on controlling financial expenditure, with pharmaceutical companies refunding over-budget situations.

Rebate A payment made to the purchaser after the transaction has occurred. Purchasers (either hospitals or pharmacies) receive a bulk refund from a wholesaler, based on sales of a particular product or total purchases from that wholesaler or manufacturer over a particular period of time.

Reference price system The third-party payer determines a maximum amount (= reference price) to be reimbursed for medicines with a given active ingredient or in a given therapeutic class. If the price of the medicine exceeds the reference price, the insured party must pay the difference between the reimbursed fixed amount (reference price) and the actual pharmacy retail price of the medicine, in addition to any copayments (e.g. prescription fees) or percentage copayment rates.

Reimbursable medicines Medicines that are eligible for reimbursement. Costs of reimbursable medicines may be fully or only partially (a specific percentage) covered by third-party payers. The opposite of nonreimbursable medicines.

Reimbursement price The basis for reimbursement of medicines in a health care system, i.e. the maximum amount that will be paid for by a third-party payer. The reimbursed amount can be either the full reimbursement price (e.g.in Austria) or a percentage share of the reimbursement price (e.g. in Denmark).

Remuneration, distribution remuneration The payment made to a health care provider (individual or organization) for services provided. The services may be paid directly by the patient or by a third-party payer. A typical pharmaceutical wholesale remuneration is a wholesale mark-up or margin scheme, and common pharmacy remuneration models are a pharmacy mark-up, pharmacy margin scheme or fee-for-service remuneration.

Risk-sharing agreements A contract between two parties (typically public payers and pharmaceutical companies), who agree to engage in a transaction in which there are uncertainties concerning its final value. Nevertheless, one party, the company, has sufficient confidence in its claims of either effectiveness or efficiency that it is ready to accept a reward or a penalty depending on the observed performance of its product.

Self-medication The treatment of common health problems with medicines especially designed and labelled for use without medical supervision and approved as safe and effective for such use.

Medicines for self-medication are often called 'non-prescription' or 'over-the-counter' (OTC) and are available without a doctor's prescription through pharmacies. In some countries, OTC products are also available in supermarkets and other outlets.

Statutory pricing A pricing system in which medicine prices are set on a regulatory basis (e.g. by law, enactment, decree).

Tax A compulsory transfer of money from private individuals, institutions or groups to the government.

It may be levied upon wealth or income (direct taxation) or in the form of surcharges on prices (indirect taxation). It may be paid to the central government (central taxation) or to the local government (local taxation). Taxation is one of the principal means by which a government finances its expenditure, including health care systems.

Value-added tax (VAT) A sales tax on products collected in stages by enterprises. It is a wide-ranging tax usually designed to cover most or all goods and services, including medicines. The VAT rate of medicines in European Union member states is often lower than the standard VAT rate.

Chapter 11 Multilevel analyses in drug utilization research

AU-ROC Area under the receiver operating characteristics curve.

HCU Primary health care center.

ICC Intra-class correlation.

MLRA Multilevel regression analysis. A statistical technique suitable for the study of outcomes correlated by the existence of multilevel structures. Examples of simple multilevel structures are patients within physicians and physicians within health care centers. Multilevel structures can also be complex (e.g. a patient attending several physicians). To be considered a 'higher level', the candidate category must always condition the information at the lower level. For instance, patients from the same doctor are more likely to receive the same treatment compared to patients from other doctors. MLRA provides an improved estimation of standard errors and a better measurement of medical practice variation and institutional ranking (what is sometimes denominated as 'league tables'). In MLRA, variance is a source of substantive information for understanding the influence of e.g. geographical, institutional or physician levels on individual medication use or other outcomes.

MOR Median odds ratio.

PCV Proportional change in variance.

PWOR Pairwise odds ratio.

VPC Variance partition coefficient.

Chapter 23 Drug utilization in pregnant women

BDS Slone Epidemiology Center Birth Defect Study.

CGDUP study Collaborative Group on Drug Use in Pregnancy study.

EFEMERIS database French prescription database.

EURAP European and International Registry of Antiepileptic Drugs in Pregnancy.

EUROmediCAT Network under the EUROCAT (European Surveillance of Congenital Anomalies) that evaluates the safety of drugs used in pregnancy.

FASS Swedish Physician's Desk Reference.

FDA US Food and Drug Administration.

GPRD UK General Practice Research Database.

OTC drugs Over-the-counter drugs.

Teratogen An agent that causes birth defects or can disturb the development of an embryo or foetus.

Chapter 25 Drug utilization in older people

ACB Anticholinergic cognitive burden, developed by Boustani et al. (2008) and Campbell et al. (2009).

ADR Adverse drug reaction.

ADS Anticholinergic drug scale, developed by Carnahan et al (2006).

ARS Anticholinergic risk scale, developed by Rudolph et al (2008).

Beers criteria One of the first sets of explicit potentially inappropriate prescribing (PIP) criteria. Original publication 1991, newest update by the American Geriatric Society in 2012.

DBI Drug burden index. Measure to determine the anticholinergic and sedative load, developed by Hilmer et al (2007).

PIM Potentially inappropriate medication.

PIP Potentially inappropriate prescribing.

Polypharmacy Concomitant use of medicines. Often defined as concurrent use of ≥5 medicines, but also used as unnecessary prescribing of medications that is clinically not indicated.

PPO Potential prescribing omission.

START Screening Tool to Alert to Right Treatment.

STOPP Screening Tool of Older People's Prescriptions.

Chapter 42 Drug utilization research and pharmacoeconomics

BIA Budget Impact analysis.

CHEERS Consolidated Health Economic Evaluation Reporting Standards.

Clinical effectiveness How well a specific test or treatment works when used in the 'real world', rather than in a carefully controlled clinical trial. Trials that assess clinical effectiveness are sometimes called 'pragmatic trials'.

Cost The economic definition of cost (also known as opportunity cost) is the value of opportunity forgone in the choice of one expenditure over others. Economists' notion of cost extends beyond the cost falling on the health service alone and e.g. includes costs falling on other services and on patients themselves. In considering the production process, costs may be differentiated as follows:

- Average costs: equivalent to the average cost per unit, i.e. the total costs divided by the total number of units of production.
- Fixed costs: those costs which, within a short time span, do not vary with the quantity of production, e.g. heating and lighting.
- Incremental costs: the extra costs associated with an expansion in activity of a given service.
- Marginal costs: the cost of producing one extra unit of a service.
- Total costs: all costs incurred in the production of a set quantity of service.
- Variable costs: those costs which vary with the level of production and are proportional to quantities produced.

Cost–benefit analysis (CBA) Used to value both incremental costs and outcomes in monetary terms and therefore allow a direct calculation of the net monetary cost of achieving a health outcome. The methods used to value gains in quality of life include techniques such as *willingness-to-pay,* where the amount that individuals would be willing to pay for a quality-of-life benefit is assessed.

Cost-effectiveness analysis (CEA) Measures the incremental cost of achieving an incremental health benefit. While cost is measured in monetary terms, effectiveness is determined independently and may be measured in terms of a clinical outcome such as number of lives saved or complications prevented.

Cost-minimization analysis (CMA) A method of calculating drug costs in order to project the least costly drug or therapeutic modality. This method of cost evaluation is the one used most often in evaluating the cost of a specific drug. Cost minimization can only be used to compare two products that have been shown to be equivalent in dose and therapeutic effect.

Cost-of-illness study Aims to identify and measure the total costs attributable to a particular disease. This is not a type of economic evaluation, as it is not used to assess the costs and benefits of alternative interventions or programmes. However, it may provide information that can be used in the context of an economic evaluation of interventions or in estimating the budgetary impact of introducing new health technologies.

Cost-utility analysis (CUA) Used to determine cost in terms of utilities, especially quantity and quality of life. Compares two different drugs or procedures whose benefits may be different and expresses the value for money in terms of a single type of health outcome: quality-adjusted life year (QALY). This allows for easy comparison across different types of health outcome, but still requires value judgements to be made concerning increases in the quality of life (utility) associated with different health outcomes.

CPRD Clinical Practice Research Datalink (formerly GPRD).

Discounting A technique that allows the calculation of present values of inputs and benefits which accrue in the future. Discounting is based on a time preference, which assumes that individuals prefer to forego a part of the benefits if they accrue it now, rather than fully in the uncertain future. By the same reasoning, individuals prefer to delay costs rather than incur them in the present. The strength of this preference is expressed by the discount rate, which is used to calculate present value in economic evaluations.

DMs Decision makers.

Economic evaluation Used to assess the value of health care interventions (i.e. to compare the costs and benefits of a health care intervention in order to assess whether it is worth doing). The aim of an economic evaluation is to maximize the level of health benefits relative to the resources available. It should be used to inform and support the decision-making process.

HCP Health care provider.

Health economics Includes the study of how scarce resources are allocated among alternative uses for the care of sickness and the promotion, maintenance and improvement of health, including the study of how health care and health-related services, their costs and benefits, and health itself are distributed among individuals and groups in society.

Health technology appraisal The process of determining the clinical and cost-effectiveness of a health technology.

Health technology assessment Includes the multidisciplinary activities that systematically examine the safety, clinical efficacy and effectiveness, cost, cost-effectiveness, organizational implications, social consequences and legal and ethical considerations of the application of a health technology – usually a drug, medical device or clinical/surgical procedure.

ISPOR International Society for Pharmacoeconomics and Outcomes Research.

RCT Randomized controlled trial.

Quality-adjusted life year (QALY) A measure of the state of health of a person or group in which the benefits, in terms of length of life, are adjusted to reflect the quality of life.

Utility A term used by economists to signify the satisfaction accruing to a person from the consumption of a good or service. This concept is applied in health care to mean the individual's valuation of their state of well-being deriving from the use of health care interventions.

Index

Drug Utilization Research: Methods and Applications, First Edition. Edited by M. Elseviers et al.
Published 2016 by John Wiley & Sons, Ltd.